BIOMECHANICS
OF THE
UPPER LIMBS

MECHANICS, MODELING
AND MUSCULOSKELETAL INJURIES

SECOND EDITION

BIOMECHANICS
OF THE
UPPER LIMBS

MECHANICS, MODELING
AND MUSCULOSKELETAL INJURIES

SECOND EDITION

ANDRIS FREIVALDS

CRC Press
Taylor & Francis Group
Boca Raton London New York

CRC Press is an imprint of the
Taylor & Francis Group, an **informa** business

CRC Press
Taylor & Francis Group
6000 Broken Sound Parkway NW, Suite 300
Boca Raton, FL 33487-2742

First issued in paperback 2018

© 2011 by Taylor & Francis Group, LLC
CRC Press is an imprint of Taylor & Francis Group, an Informa business

No claim to original U.S. Government works

ISBN-13: 978-1-4200-9119-9 (hbk)
ISBN-13: 978-1-138-07323-4 (pbk)

Visit the Taylor & Francis Web site at
http://www.taylorandfrancis.com

and the CRC Press Web site at
http://www.crcpress.com

Contents

List of Figures

List of Tables

Preface

What Is Biomechanics and Why Study It?

Biomechanics is the science that deals with the internal and external forces acting on the human body and the effects produced by these forces. This book, though, will focus exclusively on the injuries to the upper limbs of the human body. Over the last 20 years or so, there has been a tremendous increase in the number of work-related musculoskeletal disorders (WRMSDs) of the upper limbs. Not only do these preventable injuries cause pain and suffering, they also place an undue financial burden on the individual and on industry in these times of financial crises. By analyzing the forces and their effects on the human body, the ergonomist may have a better insight into the role that various job stressors play in the development of these disorders. This may help in controlling these job stressors more effectively and may require certain modifications to the workplace environment, which could arrest the current epidemic of WRMSDs thereby benefiting both the workers and the companies. Although much effort has already been expended by National Institute for Occupational Safety and Health (NIOSH) and the medical community in understanding WRMSDs and educating the practitioners, further work is still needed, and this book may help in the process.

Why Was This Book Written?

The objectives of this book are to provide practical, up-to-date, engineering-oriented information for graduate students on the biomechanics of the upper limbs. A number of books provide general introductions to cumulative trauma disorders and medical management to the layperson, while several other books provide in-depth information on the biomechanics of manual material handling and lower back problems. However, none of these books focus exclusively on WRMSDs of the upper limbs. This second edition emphasizes the musculoskeletal components involved, the engineering models of these components, and the measurement and prediction of injury potential based on these models. The second edition also covers the current state of research and includes more problems.

For Whom Is This Book Written?

This book is primarily intended as a university textbook for graduate-level engineering or kinesiology students, the future researchers in the area of WRMSDs. A large number of material and technical reports were collected from various sources. I hope that I have been able to distill this material into an effective medium of medical and engineering expertise with the appropriate technical data. The book may also be useful for researchers, industrial ergonomists, industrial hygienists, and medical professionals as a reference text to supplement their professional material.

How Is the Book Organized?

The book is organized into 10 chapters. Chapters 1 through 3 provide an introduction to biomechanics, describe the structure of the human musculoskeletal system, and cover the neuromuscular physiology of the motor control system, respectively. Chapters 4 and 5 present the mechanics and models of the various components of the neuromuscular systems as well as models of the larger systems of the upper limbs. Chapter 6 discusses the various WRMSDs and their associated risk factors. Chapters 7 and 8 present the types of instruments and risk assessment tools than can be used to identify WRMSDs in the industrial workplace. Finally, Chapters 9 and 10 provide specific applications related to hand tools and describe WRMSDs of the upper limbs associated with sitting at computer workstations. Thus, one chapter can be covered roughly every one and a half weeks in a typical semester-long course.

This textbook also attempts to assist the educator by providing numerous examples and problems within each chapter. Moreover, a Web site (http://www2.ie.psu.edu/Freivalds/courses/ie552/index.htm) is available for online notes, background material, solutions, and sample exams. Comments and suggestions for improvement by users of this textbook, especially if any outright errors are detected, are greatly appreciated. This can be done by simply responding to the *OOPS!* button on the Web site or by contacting the author directly via e-mail at axf@psu.edu. As with any Web site, this one will also continually evolve.

Acknowledgments

I would like to acknowledge Professor Don B. Chaffin for providing the training and tools, as well as a model, to proceed with this endeavor. I would also like to thank my graduate students, Neil Davidoff, Lynn Donges, Gerald Fellows, Carol Heffernan, Jesun Hwang, Hyunkook Jang, Dongjoon Kong, Yongku Kong, Kentaro Kotani, Cheol Lee, Brian Lowe, Glenn Miller, Seikwon Park, Shihyun Park, Vishal Seth, Roberta Weston, Heecheon You, and Myunghwan Yun, for working long hours in collecting the research data on which much of this book is based and Professor Neil A. Sharkey for use of his cadaver specimens and laboratory. Last but not least, I would like to express my sincere gratitude to my wife, Dace Freivalds, for her patience, support, and valued assistance on the production of this textbook.

Author

Dr. Andris Freivalds is professor of industrial engineering and the director of the Center for Cumulative Trauma Disorders at The Pennsylvania State University. He received his PhD in bioengineering in 1979 from the University of Michigan while assisting on the development of its 3D Static Strength Prediction Model. He later held a Faculty Summer Research Fellowship at the Bioengineering and Biodynamics Division of Aerospace Medical Research Laboratory at Wright-Patterson Air Force Base in Ohio, during which time he became proficient with and developed a neuromusculature for the Articulated Total Body Model. Since then, Dr. Freivalds has focused his attention on the reduction of cumulative trauma disorders (CTDs) in U.S. industries through ergonomic tool and workplace design. This effort led to the founding of the Center for Cumulative Trauma Disorders with the cooperation of the Ben Franklin Partnership of the Commonwealth of Pennsylvania. This center has served over 90 small companies in Pennsylvania in controlling their workplace hazards for the last 20 years. As part of the services to better quantify and predict the stresses of workers employed on hazardous jobs, the Penn State CTD Risk Index and the "touch" glove were developed, and with the cooperation of the Hershey Medical Center, several retrospective epidemiological studies were conducted to better understand both work factors and individual attributes on an individual's likelihood for developing carpal tunnel syndrome. More recently, he has been working with Dr. Neil Sharkey to measure tendon forces during gripping in cadaver forearms. Much of the above industrial experience has been incorporated into the current textbook as well as an introductory industrial engineering textbook, *Methods, Standards and Work Design* (McGraw-Hill, 2009). He is a fellow of the Ergonomics Society and a member of the Human Factors and Ergonomics Society and the American Society of Biomechanics. In addition, he has mentored 19 PhD students, most of whom are now faculty members at various universities around the world.

1

Introduction to Biomechanics

1.1 What Is Biomechanics?

Biomechanics is mechanics, the science that deals with forces and their effects, applied to biological systems. Traditionally, this has meant the human body at a relatively macro level. However, there need not be any such limitations, since any life form can be studied at any level. More recently, perhaps because of the interest in the development of new drugs and measuring their effects on the body, biomechanical studies have progressed down to the level of a single cell. This book, though, will focus exclusively on the human body and the upper limbs.

Although biomechanics is based solidly on the principles of physics and mathematics developed in the 1600s and 1700s by Galileo, Newton, Descartes, Euler, and others, the first biomechanical observations as related to the function of the muscle and bones of the human body were made already in the early 1500s by Leonardo da Vinci. Borelli, a student of Galileo, published the first treatise on biomechanics, *De Motu Animalium*, in 1680. Later in the 1700s, Ramazzini, whom many consider the first occupational physician, described in detail the forceful and extreme motions in butchering and other jobs leading to the development of musculoskeletal disorders and other diseases.

More recent advances that laid much of the groundwork for later human modeling include Braune and Fischer (1889), Fischer (1906), and A.V. Hill's 50 years of detailed studies on muscle mechanics, ultimately culminating in a Nobel prize in 1922. The cross-over of biomechanics into ergonomics, the science that deals with fitting work to the human operator, probably started with E.R. Tichauer using biomechanical principles to redesign tools for the workplace in the early 1970s. In the 1980s, the National Institute for Occupational Safety and Health (NIOSH) began specifically focusing on workplace-related musculoskeletal disorders (WRMSDs) as part of its Year 2000 Objectives to reduce workplace injuries.

1.2 Basic Concepts

Biomechanical principles can be applied to a system of bodies at rest, termed *statics*, or to a system of bodies in motion, termed *dynamics*. In such systems, bodies may be pushed or pulled by actions termed *forces*. Such forces always act in unison; i.e., if one body is pushing on another body, the second one is pushing back on the first body equally hard.

This is Newton's third law, the *law of reaction*: For every action there is an equal and opposite reaction. Thus, if an operator is pinching or applying a force to a tool or a part, that tool or part is pushing back equally hard, as evidenced by the compression of the skin and underlying tissues.

Newton's first law is the *law of inertia*: A body remains at rest or in constant-velocity motion until acted upon by an external unbalanced force. Newton's second law is the *law of acceleration*: the acceleration of a body is proportional to the unbalanced force acting upon it and inversely proportional to the mass of the body. Mathematically this law is expressed as

$$F = ma \qquad (1.1)$$

where
  F is the force
  m is the mass
  a is the acceleration

A force can be characterized by three factors: magnitude, direction, and point of application. The *magnitude* is a scalar quantity that indicates the size of the push or pull action, e.g., a force of 10 N is twice as large as a force of 5 N. The *direction* of the force indicates the line of action of the force; i.e., a force applied perpendicular or normal to surface of a body will have a different effect than a force applied parallel to the surface, or in a shear direction. Note the direction can range a full 360° in two dimensions, so that a normal force could be either pushing or pulling the body, depending on the angle defined. Typically, for simplicity in modeling and calculations, the magnitude and direction are combined into one quantity termed a *vector*. Finally, the *point of application* of a force on a body is self evident; i.e., the effect on an arm will be quite different if a force (such as a weight) is applied to the hand as opposed as to the elbow.

In this example, the weight acts as an *external force* to the arm, since it acts outside the body, while the muscular forces in the arm are *internal forces*, since they act inside the body. Note also that weight is not the same as mass, the weight being determined by the effect of gravity on the mass of the object and is measured in Newtons (N, named after the English physicist and mathematician Sir Isaac Newton, 1642–1728) while the mass is measured in kilograms (kg). In some situations, a force will be distributed over an area rather than a single point of application. In that case, it is termed *pressure* and defined as

$$P = \frac{F}{A} \qquad (1.2)$$

where
  P is the pressure
  F is the force
  A is the area

If the force is Newtons and area in meters squared, then the units of pressure are measured in Pascals (Pa, named after French mathematician Blaise Pascal, 1623–1662).

Another important concept is the *moment* of a force or *torque*. A moment is the tendency of a force to cause rotation about a point or axis (depending on if one is considering a two-dimensional [2D] or three-dimensional [3D] system). It is defined as the application of a force at a perpendicular distance from the point of rotation or the perpendicular component of a force to a lever arm. Mathematically, the moment equals force times distance or

$$M = r \times F \tag{1.3}$$

where
  M is the moment
  r is the distance

1.3 Coordinate Systems

To define a vector or the direction of a force, a reference coordinate system needs to be defined. In a 2D system, this can be done by dividing the plane into four quadrants using two perpendicular lines are axes (see Figure 1.1a). The horizontal one is defined as the x-axis or *abscissa* while the vertical one is defined as the y-axis or the *ordinate*. The point of intersection of the two axes is known as the *origin* of the system from which all point of applications are defined. Measurements are made in common units along the axes; positive values to the right of the origin on the x-axis and above the origin for the y-axis. Any point of application then can be defined using these coordinates, with (0,0) being the origin and point A in Figure 1.1a being (3,4). Such a coordinate system is termed the *rectangular* or *Cartesian coordinate system* (named after the French mathematician René Descartes, 1596–1650). A third dimension can be easily added by placing the z-axis perpendicular to both the x-and y-axes (see Figure 1.1b).

An alternate coordinate system is the *polar coordinate system* shown in Figure 1.2a. In this system, all coordinates are measured with an angle θ, starting with 0° at the Cartesian x-axis, moving full circle or 360° counter clockwise, and ending back at the same axis, and a distance r defined from the origin of the Cartesian coordinate system. The same point can be converted between the two coordinate systems with the following equations. From the polar to Cartesian system, use the equations:

$$x = r \cos \theta \tag{1.4}$$

$$y = r \sin \theta \tag{1.5}$$

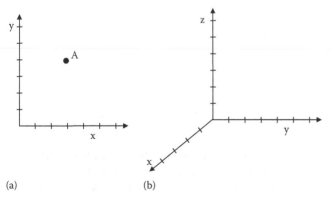

(a)   (b)

FIGURE 1.1
Rectangular or Cartesian coordinate system: (a) two dimensional and (b) three dimensional.

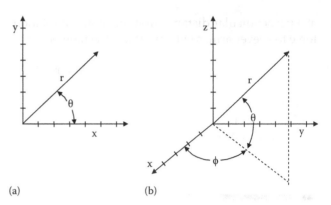

FIGURE 1.2
(a) Polar coordinate system (2D).
(b) Spherical coordinate system (3D).

From the Cartesian to the polar system, use the following equations:

$$r = (x^2 + y^2)^{1/2} \tag{1.6}$$

$$\theta = \tan^{-1}\frac{y}{x} \tag{1.7}$$

For three dimensions, the *spherical coordinate system* with a distance r and two angles θ and φ can be used (see Figure 1.2b). The same point can again be converted between the two coordinate systems. From the spherical to Cartesian system, use the following equations:

$$x = r \sin \theta \cos \varphi \tag{1.8}$$

$$y = r \sin \theta \sin \varphi \tag{1.9}$$

$$z = r \cos \theta \tag{1.10}$$

From the Cartesian to the spherical system, use the following equations:

$$r = (x^2 + y^2 + z^2)^{1/2} \tag{1.11}$$

$$\varphi = \tan^{-1}\frac{y}{x} \tag{1.12}$$

$$\theta = \cos^{-1}\frac{z}{r} \tag{1.13}$$

1.4 Force Vector Algebra

The force vector shown in Figure 1.3 on a 2D Cartesian coordinate system has a direction defined by the line originating at the origin (0,0) and ending at the point of application of (3,4). In vector notation, the direction can be also defined as 3i + 4j, where i and j are termed

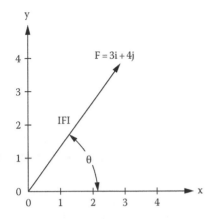

FIGURE 1.3
Cartesian coordinate system with vector 3i + 4j.

the unit coordinate vectors for the x-and y-axes, respectively (k is used for the z-axes). This vector is thus broken down into its x, y components, with a value of 3 for the x component and a value of 4 for its y component. The magnitude of a vector, based on Equation 1.6, is defined as

$$|F| = \left[F_x^2 + F_y^2 \right]^{1/2} \tag{1.14}$$

where
  F_x is the x component of the force vector F
  F_y is the y component of the force vector F

For the above case, the magnitude has a specific value of

$$|F| = [3^2 + 4^2]^{1/2} = 5 \tag{1.15}$$

The directional angle θ (sometimes termed phase angle) can also be found from the components of the force vector from Equation 1.7 or

$$\theta = \tan^{-1}\left(\frac{F_y}{F_x} \right) \tag{1.16}$$

For the above case, the directional angle has a specific value of

$$\theta = \tan^{-1}\left(\frac{4}{3} \right) = 53.13° \tag{1.17}$$

These two values now define the force vector F in polar coordinates as (5, 53.13°) and demonstrates the interchangeability of the notation between the two coordinate systems.

In the generic form, the force vector would be defined in the polar coordinate system as

$$F = (r, \theta) \tag{1.18}$$

where
  r is the magnitude |F|
  θ is the angle

The components along the x- and y-axes are defined as

$$F_x = F\cos\theta \qquad\qquad (1.19)$$

$$F_y = F\sin\theta \qquad\qquad (1.20)$$

For the specific force vector shown in Figure 1.3, the x, y components become

$$F_x = F\cos\theta = 5\cos(53.13°) = 5(0.6) = 3 \qquad\qquad (1.21)$$

$$F_y = F\sin\theta = 5\sin(53.13°) = 5(0.8) = 4 \qquad\qquad (1.22)$$

Two force vectors A and B can be added together to create a resultant force vector C by adding the x and y components (see Figure 1.4). Since A is 5i + j and B is 3i + 4j, then C is simply:

$$C = 5i + j + 3i + 4j = 8i + 5j \qquad\qquad (1.23)$$

This same resultant force vector can also be found graphically by placing the tail of force vector B to the tip of force vector A with the line between the tail of A and the tip of B creating the new resultant force vector C (see Figure 1.4). The same result can also be obtained by adding the tail of A to the tip of B.

One important manipulation of vectors is the vector *cross product* which is used to calculate the moment of the force (from Equation 1.3) which is also a vector, but perpendicular to both the force and distance vectors. The sense of this resultant vector is determined by the *right-hand rule*, in which the fingers of the right hand pointing in the direction of the first vector are curled toward the second vector so as to cover the included angle between the two vectors. The extended thumb will then point in the resultant cross-product vector direction, which will be perpendicular to both of the original vectors. Mathematically, this can be expressed as

$$i \times j = k \quad (j \times i = -k)$$

$$j \times k = i \quad (k \times j = -i) \qquad\qquad (1.24)$$

$$k \times i = j \quad (i \times k = -j)$$

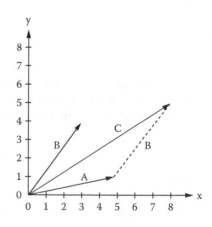

FIGURE 1.4
Addition of vectors A (5i + j) and B (3i + 4j) to create vector C (8i + 5j).

Note, that this cross product also applies to the definition of a 3D Cartesian coordinate system (see Figure 1.2b). Also, any vector crossed on itself (e.g., i × i) is equal to zero, i.e., there is no unique perpendicular vector. There is also the *dot product* of vectors with both requiring the same direction (i.e., i·i) and resulting in a purely scalar value.

1.5 Static Equilibrium

One result of Newton's first law is that bodies are typically studied in *static equilibrium*, which allows for several useful conditions. First, for the body to be in static equilibrium, it must be in *translational equilibrium*. Mathematically, this means that the net forces on the body must be zero or

$$\sum F = 0 \tag{1.25}$$

More practically, the forces are broken down into components by axes and result in

$$\sum F_x = 0 \quad \sum F_y = 0 \quad \sum F_z = 0 \tag{1.26}$$

Secondly, the body must also be in *rotational equilibrium*, which means that the net moments about any point in the body due to the external forces must also be zero. This can be expressed as

$$\sum M = 0 \tag{1.27}$$

To study these conditions in detail, the body or the part of the body of interest is isolated and drawn as a *free-body diagram*. All the known forces are drawn accurately with respect to the magnitude, direction, and point of application. If a force is unknown, a representative arrow is included with an arbitrary direction. If a part of a body is isolated from another or more complete body, arbitrary reactive forces are included at that point of separation. Also, all moments are included.

Example 1.1: Static Equilibrium of the Upper Limb Holding a Weight

Consider the musculature of the upper limb as shown in Figure 1.5. There are three primary muscles involved in elbow flexion: the biceps brachii, the brachioradialis, and the brachialis, and one for elbow extension: the triceps brachii (see Section 2.1 for definitions of these terms). The hand holds a weight at the center of gravity of the hand. It would be of interest to find the muscle forces needed to hold this load at an elbow flexion of 90°. If the weight is merely being held, then this is a simpler case of statics, with no need to consider the dynamic effects from accelerations or initial velocities. Since the triceps is active only during elbow extension, it can be disregarded for elbow flexion. Also, including all three elbow flexors would result in a statically indeterminate situation, i.e., there are too many variables for the given amount of data or no one unique muscle force can be attributed to each muscle. The two smaller muscles are disregarded leaving only the biceps brachii and the simpler case shown in Figure 1.6a.

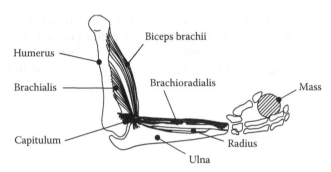

FIGURE 1.5
Musculature of the left upper limb while holding a weight.

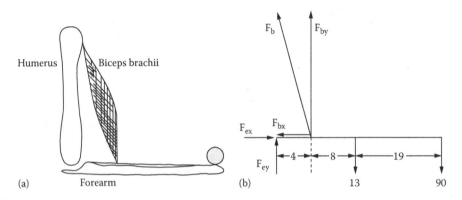

FIGURE 1.6
(a) Simplified upper limb while holding a weight. (b) Free-body diagram of upper limb holding a weight.

Next, the forearm is isolated with all relevant reactive forces as shown in Figure 1.6b. The elbow joint is represented with two unknown reactive force F_{ex} and F_{ey}. The weight of the forearm is represented by a weight or force of 13 N acting downward through the forearm center of gravity, 12 cm distal of the elbow joint. The weight itself and the weight of the hand are represented by a force of 90 N acting downward at a distance of 31 cm from the elbow joint. The biceps brachii is represented by an unknown force F_b acting upward (i.e., lifting the forearm and weight up) at a point 4 cm distally of the elbow joint center of rotation. Since it is acting at an angle, the force is best represented in the vector form with x and y components of the form of Equations 1.19 and 1.20. The angle θ is found from Equation 1.16, where the distance of the origin of the biceps muscle is 30 cm from the elbow:

$$\theta = \tan^{-1}\left(\frac{30}{4}\right) = 82.4° \qquad (1.28)$$

From Equations 1.19 and 1.20, the unknown x and y components of F_b are

$$F_{bx} = F_b \cos\theta = F_b \cos(82.4°) = 0.132\, F_b \qquad (1.29)$$

$$F_{by} = F_b \sin\theta = F_b \sin(82.4°) = 0.991\, F_b \qquad (1.30)$$

Then the unknown biceps muscle force can be represented by

$$F_b = 0.132\, F_b i + 0.991\, F_b j \qquad (1.31)$$

The translational equilibrium of Equation 1.26 yields

$$\sum F_x = 0 = F_{ex} - F_{bx} = 0 \tag{1.32}$$

$$\sum F_y = 0 = F_{ey} + 0.991\, F_b - 13 - 90 = 0 \tag{1.33}$$

Simplification of Equations 1.32 and 1.33 yields

$$F_{ex} = 0.132\, F_b \tag{1.34}$$

$$F_{ey} = 103 - 0.991\, F_b \tag{1.35}$$

The rotational equilibrium of Equation 1.27 can be established at any point, but is most convenient around the elbow joint center of rotation, since this eliminates both reactive components of the elbow joint, neither of which creates a moment around the point through which it passes. Using distances in meters, yields

$$\sum M_e = 0 = (0.04i) \times (0.132\, F_b i + 0.991\, F_b j) + (0.12i) \times (-13j) + (0.31i) \times (-90j) \tag{1.36}$$

The accepted practice is to follow the right-hand rule as the force vector pushes down on its respective lever arm, with clockwise torques considered negative and counter-clockwise torques considered positive. (However, as long as one is consistent, the opposite implementation can be used just as well.) Thus, in the above case, the weight or gravity induced torques are negative, while the muscle force induced torque is positive. Of course, using the vector notation and cross products of Equation 1.24 automatically creates the proper moment, with $i \times i$ terms dropping out, $i \times j$ becoming k and $i \times -j$ becoming $-k$. Simplifying Equation 1.36 yields

$$0.03964\, F_b k = 29.46 k \tag{1.37}$$

$$F_b = 743.2\ N \tag{1.38}$$

Substituting Equation 1.38 back into Equations 1.34 and 1.35 yields

$$F_{ex} = 0.132\,(743.2) = 98.1\ N \tag{1.39}$$

$$F_{ey} = 103 - 0.991 F_b = 103 - 0.991\,(743.2) = -633.5\ N \tag{1.40}$$

In summary, the biceps brachii muscle (in reality, a combination of all three elbow flexor muscles) must exert an internal force of over eight times ($743.2/90 = 8.3$) the external force to maintain equilibrium. To find the individual contributions of each of the three elbow flexor muscles, is an indeterminate situation and requires assumptions about the relative forces, typically determined from relatively muscle cross-sectional areas. Also, there are considerable internal forces sustained in the elbow, especially since it acts as the pivot point for joint rotation.

The combination of forces acting around a pivot point or *fulcrum* (as in Example 1.1) is termed a *lever system*. The external weights or resistive forces are counterbalanced by an effort force, in this case the biceps brachii muscle force. Each acts through a respective moment or lever arm. The ratio of these forces, or of these moment arms, forms a quantity termed the *mechanical advantage* (ma):

$$ma = \frac{r_e}{r_r} = \frac{F_r}{F_e} \qquad (1.41)$$

where
  r_e is the lever arm for the effort force
  r_r is the lever arm for the resistive force
  F_r is the resistive force
  F_e is the effort force

There are three different types of lever systems with different values for the mechanical advantage. In a *first-class lever*, the fulcrum is located between the effort and resistance as in a playground teeter-totter or the erector spinae (F_{es}) muscles acting on the L_5/S_1 vertebra as a fulcrum to maintain an erect trunk position or while lifting a load ($F_{resistance}$ in Figure 1.7a). Note, that in an approximate calculation using the free-body diagram of Figure 1.7b, disregarding alignment angles, and assuming an effort moment arm of 5 cm and a resistance moment arm of 70 cm, the mechanical advantage is

$$ma = \frac{r_e}{r_r} = \frac{5}{70} = 0.0714 \qquad (1.42)$$

This, in reality, is a mechanical disadvantage and may be one of the factors in the high incidence of low-back problems.

The versatility of the first-class lever system is demonstrated by changing the length of the moment arms to have a mechanical advantage that can be either greater or less than one. Thus, unequally heavy children can still use the teeter-totter by repositioning the fulcrum such that they are in relative equilibrium. Most extensor muscles act as first-class levers.

In a *second-class lever*, the resistance is located between the effort and fulcrum and always results in a mechanical advantage greater than one, i.e., the effort is always less than the resistance. Examples include the wheelbarrow, a nut cracker, or a pry bar. However, in the human body, it is difficult to find a true second-class lever. One possibility is the action of the sternocleidomastoid muscle during forceful inspiration (see Figure 1.8a). The sternocleidomastoid muscle originates on the mastoid process of the skull and inserts on both the sternum and clavicle. The clavicle and sternum are tied into the rib cage through the attachments of the various intercostal muscles. Although, the sternocleidomastoid has a relatively direct insertion to the clavicle, which can be represented as a simple effort force F_{stern}, the resistance force is distributed over the length of the clavicle (see Figure 1.8b). Therefore, for some part of

FIGURE 1.7
(a) The lower back modeled as a first-class lever. (b) Free-body diagram of the lower back.

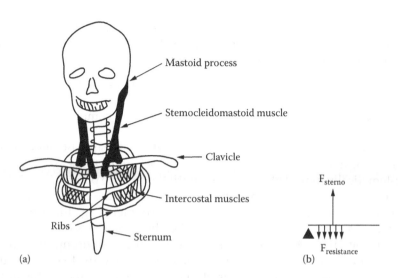

Mastoid process

Stemocleidomastoid muscle

Clavicle

Intercostal muscles

Ribs

Sternum

F_{sterno}

$F_{resistance}$

(a)
(b)

FIGURE 1.8
(a) The sternocleidomastoid muscle and clavicle modeled as a second-class lever. (b) Free-body diagram of the sternocleidomastoid muscle and clavicle.

the clavicle, the resultant pry bar action through the fulcrum at the sternum is a second-class level. (The point of application for a uniform distributed force is simply the midpoint of the distribution. For nonuniform distributions, the center of mass approach of Section 1.4 must be used.)

In a *third-class lever*, the effort is located between the fulcrum and the resistance and always results in a mechanical advantage less than one, or a mechanical disadvantage. The elbow flexion of Figure 1.6 and most other flexor muscles are good example of third-class levels. The mechanical advantage of the biceps brachii from Example 1.1 is

$$ma = \frac{F_r}{F_e} = \frac{90}{743.2} = 0.12 \tag{1.43}$$

It would seem odd that there is again a mechanical disadvantage in the human body. This is typically the case for the upper and lower limbs, with the effort being greater than the resistance. However, there is a tradeoff. With the very short effort moment arms, small changes in muscle length will be amplified into large movements of the ends of the limbs. Thus, the human musculature is designed for speed and movement as opposed to strength.

1.6 Anthropometry and Center of Mass Determination

For the above static equilibrium analyses (see Figure 1.5) and later biomechanical models, several key properties need to be known. Since, typically, the upper limb will be divided into its component segments, the segment link lengths, segment weights, and the location of the *center of mass* (cm, but often termed *center of gravity*, cg, both terms will be used interchangeably here) are needed. For specific cases, the segment link lengths can be measured directly using specialized calipers termed *anthropometers* or indirectly through stereo photography or laser or other optical surface scanning techniques while the segment weights can be determined directly by water displacement techniques (Miller and Nelson, 1976). Note, however, that the volume must be multiplied by a density factor, which is not always specifically known and can vary between individuals:

$$\text{Mass (g)} = \text{volume (cm}^3) \times \text{density (g/cm}^3) \tag{1.44}$$

Specific density factors and segment properties have been compiled for the upper limbs in Table 1.1.

The center of mass values in Table 1.1 have typically been found by the suspension technique of balancing a frozen cadaver segment along each of the three axes (Dempster, 1955). A pin is systematically moved along one axis until the balance point is found. The intersection of the three axial lines through each point determined the center of mass.

For a live person, the center of mass for a given segment, e.g., the arm, can be found through a technique reported by LeVeau (1977). The person lies on a board, supported by a knife edge at one end and a force scale at the other, assuming two different positions relative to that segment, in this case the arm (see Figure 1.9). As the upper limb is allowed to hang naturally, the center of mass for the body moves toward the head, decreasing the reading on the scale. With a few calculations based on simple mechanical principles, the weight of the upper limb can be determined. The full analysis is given in Example 1.2.

Example 1.2: Determining the Weight of the Arm

In the fully prone posture, the body mass W is acting at a distance R from the left support. When the arm is hanging down, the whole body cg will have moved toward the head, with a shorter moment arm of R′, and the scale will show a lower value of S′, than in the first posture with S. Taking moments about the left support for each posture yields

$$SL - WR = 0 \tag{1.45}$$

$$S'L - WR' = 0 \tag{1.46}$$

where L is the distance between the scale and the left support. The corresponding moment arms are then

$$R = \frac{SL}{W} \tag{1.47}$$

$$R' = \frac{S'L}{W} \tag{1.48}$$

Note that in the second case, the whole body center of mass has moved anteriorly due to the movement of the arm.

A useful property for finding the center of mass of individual body segments is the *principle of moments*: the moments of the components must be equal to the moment of the whole. For each posture, this yields

$$WR = R_a W_a + R_b W_b \tag{1.49}$$

TABLE 1.1

Gross Anthropometric Data for the Upper Limbs

	Upper Arm	Forearm	Hand
Link definition[a]	Line between glenohumeral and elbow joint centers	Line between the elbow and wrist joint centers	Line between the wrist joint center and hand center of gravity
Proximal joint[a]	Glenohumeral	Elbow	Wrist
Joint center location[a]	Midregion of the palpable bone mass of the head and tuberostities of the humerus; with the arm abducted 45°, a line dropped perpendicular to the long axis from the acromion bisects the joint	Midpoint on a line between the lowest palpable point on the medial epicondyle of the humerus and a point above the radiale	Midpoint of a line between the radial styloid and the center of the pisiform, in the line with the metacarpal III bone
Segment definition[a]	Acromion to radiale	Tip of elbow to styloid process	Base of hand to end middle finger
Link to segment ratio[b]	0.89	1.07	0.506
Segment dentsity (g/cm³)	1.075	1.125	1.15
Segment length to stature ratio	0.186	0.146	0.108
Segment mass to body mass ratio	0.029	0.018	0.008
Segment cg to segment length ratio (from proximal end)	0.452	0.424	0.397
Moment of inertia (k_{cm}) (10^{-4} kg m²)[b]	141	55	5
Moment of inertia			
(I_a) from proximal end (10^{-4} kg m²)[b]	407	182	19
Radius of gyration to segment length ratio (from proximal end)[d]	0.542	0.526	0.587

(continued)

TABLE 1.1 (continued)

Gross Anthropometric Data for the Upper Limbs

| | Upper Arm | | | | | | Forearm | | | | | | Hand | | | | | |
| | Male | | | Female | | | Male | | | Female | | | Male | | | Female | | |
	5th	50th	95th	5th	50th	95th	5th	50th	95th	5th	50th	95th	5th	50th	95th	5th	50th	95th
Segment link length (cm)[a]	28.6	30.4	32.3	26.1	27.8	29.5	25.6	27.1	28.7	22.7	24.1	25.5	—	—	—	—	—	—
Segment length (cm)[a]	30.3	33.0	35.6	28.3	31.0	33.6	24.6	26.9	29.3	21.2	23.4	25.7	17.8	19.1	20.5	16.9	18.3	20.1
Segment mas (kg)[b]	1.6	2.1	2.8	1.3	1.7	2.5	0.9	1.2	1.6	0.7	1.0	1.4	0.4	0.4	0.6	0.3	0.4	0.5
Distance to cg from proximal end (cm)[b]	12.5	13.2	14.0	11.6	12.1	12.5	11.0	11.7	12.3	9.9	10.4	11.0	6.7	7.0	7.4	6.1	6.4	6.7

Note: See Figure 1.9 for landmarks; detailed data for the fingers are found in Tables 5.5 and 5.6.

[a] Webb Associates (1978).
[b] Dempster (1955).
[c] Roebuck et al. (1975).
[d] Plagenhoef (1966).
[e] Chaffin et al. (1999).

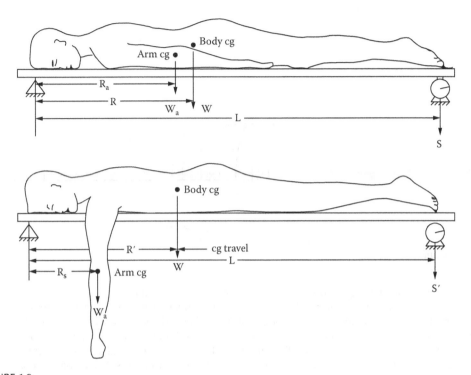

FIGURE 1.9
Method for determining the weight of the arm. (Adapted from LeVeau, B., *Williams and Lissner Biomechanics of Human Motion*, W.B. Saunders Co., Philadelphia, PA, 1977.)

$$WR' = R_sW_a + R_bW_b \qquad (1.50)$$

where
   R_a is the distance to the arm cg
   W_a is the weight of the arm
   R_b is the distance to the body minus the arm cg
   W_b is the body weight minus the arm weight
   R_s is the distance to the arm cg when hanging down, roughly the distance to the shoulder joint

By subtracting Equation 1.50 from Equation 1.49, the unknown value of R_b can be eliminated:

$$R_a - R_s = \frac{W(R - R')}{W_a} \qquad (1.51)$$

Substituting Equations 1.47 and 1.48 into Equation 1.51 yields the final expression for the location of the arm cg from the shoulder joint:

$$R_a - R_s = \frac{L(S - S')}{W_a} \qquad (1.52)$$

Alternatively, Equation 1.52 can be rearranged to yield the weight of the arm:

$$W_a = \frac{L(S - S')}{(R_a - R_s)} \qquad (1.53)$$

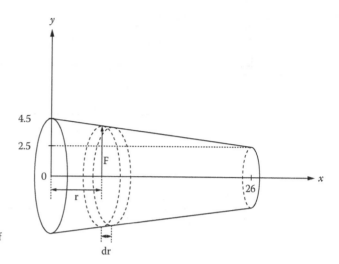

FIGURE 1.10
Method for determining the center of mass of the upper arm.

The center of mass for a given body segment can also be calculated mathematically by extending the principle of moments. Assume that the truncated cylinder shown in Figure 1.10 represents a forearm. This shape can be cut into thin segments of thickness dr, each with a small force vector F representing the segment's weight and each acting a given distance r from the left-hand origin to create many small moments. Adding all the moments together should equal the total weight acting through a lever arm corresponding to the distance to the center of mass. Extending this concept to thinner and thinner segments and using integration to sum these moments, the center of mass can be found mathematically from

$$cm = \frac{\int rF dr}{\int F dr} \tag{1.54}$$

The full details of the analysis are shown in Example 1.3.

Example 1.3: Determining the Center of Mass of the Upper Arm

For the stylized upper arm of Figure 1.10, the weight of each segment is the volume times a density factor. The volume is simply a disk of area $2\pi F$ with thickness of dr. Assume a constant density factor of 1. (In reality, the density factor may vary with segment length, and then an actual value may need to be used.) The relationship of F with respect to r can be expressed as a line with the equation:

$$F = \frac{-r}{13} + 4.5 \tag{1.55}$$

Then, substituting Equation 1.55 into Equation 1.54 and integrating from 0 to 26 yields

$$cg = \frac{\int rF dr}{\int F dr} = \frac{\int (-r^2/13 + 4.5r) dr}{\int (-r/13 + 4.5) dr} = \frac{(-r^3/39 + 2.25r^2)}{(-r^2/26 + 4.5r)} \Bigg|_0^{26} = 11.26 \tag{1.56}$$

Note that a distance of 11.26 cm from the left-hand origin or elbow is roughly 43.3% of the segment length of 26 cm, which corresponds closely to the relative cm locations given in Table 1.1.

1.7 Friction

Friction is the interaction between two surfaces when coming into contact as one slides over the other (see Figure 1.11). The resulting force in the lateral direction is termed the frictional force and depends on how tightly the surfaces are in contact and the material properties of the two surfaces, such as the roughness, which can be defined as the *coefficient of friction*. Mathematically, the frictional force can be expressed as

$$f = \mu N \tag{1.57}$$

where
  f is the frictional force
  N is the normal force
  μ is the coefficient of friction

Theoretically, the coefficient of friction should range from a lower limit of 0 to an upper limit of 1, i.e., the frictional force cannot exceed the normal force applied. However, under certain conditions, such as grasping with the grooved ridges found in the fingertips, frictional coefficients may exceed 1 and perhaps even reach values of 2 (Bobjer et al., 1993). Practically, it ranges from values as high as 0.75 for rubber on rough wood (LeVeau, 1977) to values as low as 0.08 for oiled steel on steel and 0.04 for high molecular weight polyethylene on steel (Weast, 1969). The latter properties are used in the designs used in low-friction artificial joints with coefficients of friction approaching 0.02 (Kitano et al., 2001). However, these still do not approach the coefficient of friction values of 0.003–0.005 found in real synovial joints (Unsworth et al., 1975), which most likely are attributable to the special hydrodynamic properties of synovial fluid described in Section 2.5.2.

The coefficient of friction also depends on movement. It is normally measured at the point where one surface begins to slide with respect to the other, at which point it achieves the maximum value. It then decreases in value as the surfaces begin sliding more quickly. This leads to the classic physics example of static equilibrium: determining the steepest angle at which the block remains stationary without sliding down an inclined plane (see Example 1.4).

Example 1.4: Determination of the Coefficient of Friction on an Inclined Plane

The block of weight W (see Figure 1.12) exerts a normal force N on a surface inclined at an angle of θ. This is also the component of the weight perpendicular to the inclined plane:

FIGURE 1.11
Frictional forces.

$$N = W \cos\theta \tag{1.58}$$

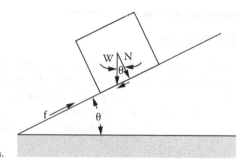

FIGURE 1.12
Determination of the coefficient of friction on an inclined plan.

The frictional force is the component of the weight parallel to the incline:

$$f = W \sin\theta \tag{1.59}$$

Substituting Equations 1.58 and 1.59 into the definition of friction in Equation 1.57 and rearranging yields the coefficient of friction as a function of critical angle of the inclined plane:

$$\mu = \frac{f}{N} = \frac{\sin\theta}{\cos\theta} = \tan\theta \tag{1.60}$$

This is one practical method for finding the maximum coefficient of friction between two surfaces.

Friction can also occur in pulley systems. A fixed pulley changes the direction of a force but not the magnitude of the force (see Figure 1.13a). This principle allows for the reduction of forces in a free pulley, with each strand supporting one half of the weight (see Figure 1.13b).

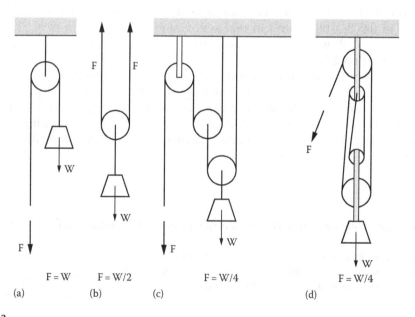

FIGURE 1.13
Pulley systems: (a) one fixed pulley, (b) one free pulley, (c) two free pulleys and one fixed pulley, and (d) block and tackle.

A larger combination of n free pulleys with one fixed pulley (see Figure 1.13c) reduces the force needed to lift the weight to

$$F = \frac{W}{2^n} \qquad (1.61)$$

FIGURE 1.14
Crude pulley with friction.

Such a pulley system is more typically set up as a block and tackle with n free pulleys and n fixed pulleys (see Figure 1.13d).

Although pulleys are assumed to be frictionless, this does not need to be the case. This is especially true for a crude pulley such as simply passing a rope around a pole (see Figure 1.14), where the friction can assist in controlling the lowering of a heavy weight. The relationship between the two forces can be expressed as

$$F_{max} = F_{min} e^{\mu\theta} \qquad (1.62)$$

where
F_{max} is the larger of the two forces determined by movement in that direction
F_{min} is the smaller of the two forces
θ is the angle of contact between the rope and pole (radians)

Example 1.5: Friction on a Crude Pulley

Assuming that the coefficient of friction for a rough rope on a rough pole is approximately 0.5 and the angle of contact is 180° or π radians, then the force needed to lower a weight of 100 kg (equivalent to 980.7 N) is

$$F_{min} = \frac{980.7}{e^{0.5\pi}} = \frac{980.7}{4.81} = 203.9 \text{ N} \qquad (1.63)$$

This force is only one-fifth of that created by the weight itself. On the other hand, this set up would be very disadvantageous to lifting the weight as it would require

$$F_{max} = 980.7 e^{0.5\pi} = 980.7(4.81) = 4717.2 \text{ N} \qquad (1.64)$$

or almost five times as much force as created by the weight itself.

1.8 Dynamics

Dynamics can be subdivided into *kinematics*, which is the study of pure motion, displacement, velocities, and acceleration, and into *kinetics*, which, in addition, studies the forces that produce that motion. Pure motion can either be rectilinear or circular. In the rectilinear case, the displacement vector of a body can be defined along the three axes of the Cartesian coordinate system as

$$s = xi + yj + zk \qquad (1.65)$$

The velocity of that body is the change in displacement with respect to change in time and can be defined as an instantaneous velocity:

$$v = \frac{ds}{dt} \tag{1.66}$$

or as an average velocity:

$$\bar{v} = \frac{\Delta s}{\Delta t} \tag{1.67}$$

and is measured in meters per second. Similarly, the acceleration of that body can be defined as the change in velocity with respect to change in time in an instantaneous sense:

$$a = \frac{dv}{dt} \tag{1.68}$$

or in an average sense:

$$\bar{a} = \frac{\Delta v}{\Delta t} \tag{1.69}$$

and is measured in meters per second squared. The velocity and displacement vectors can be calculated for a given acceleration by integrating once for velocity:

$$v = at + v_0 \tag{1.70}$$

where v_0 is the initial velocity, and integrating twice for displacement:

$$s = \frac{1}{2}at^2 + vt + s_0 \tag{1.71}$$

where s_0 is the initial displacement.

For circular motion, it is easier to use polar coordinates, in which case, the angular displacement is defined as

$$s = r\theta \tag{1.72}$$

The angular velocity and angular acceleration are defined as

$$\omega = \frac{d\theta}{dt} \tag{1.73}$$

$$\alpha = \frac{d\omega}{dt} \tag{1.74}$$

and measured in radians per second and radians per second squared, respectively. For a constant radius r, linear and angular quantities are related as follows:

$$v = r\omega \tag{1.75}$$

$$a = r\alpha \tag{1.76}$$

For studying kinetics, force effects on the body are also included. These forces follow Newton's second law defined previously in Equation 1.1. For circular motion, substituting Equation 1.76 into Equation 1.1, yields

$$F_t = mr\alpha \tag{1.77}$$

where
F_t is the *tangential force* acting at the center of mass of the body
α is the instantaneous angular acceleration of the body
r is the distance of the body center of mass from the point of rotation

A second force acting on the body is the *centrifugal force* F_c acting along the radius of the rotation:

$$F_c = mr\omega^2 \tag{1.78}$$

In terms of calculations moments and the rotational equilibrium analysis of Section 1.4, there is the moment created by the weight of the body acting a distance r, there is the tangential force acting a distance r and a force component due to the mass of the body resisting change in angular velocity known as the *moment of inertia*:

$$M = I_{cm}\alpha \tag{1.79}$$

where I_{cm}, the moment of inertia at the center of mass, is defined as the integral over the volume of the body:

$$I_{cm} = \int r^2 dm \tag{1.80}$$

For a point mass, Equation 1.78 results in

$$I_{cm} = r^2 m \tag{1.81}$$

Experimentally, moments of inertia for body segments are found by suspending frozen cadaver parts and swinging them as a pendulum (Lephart, 1984). The resulting period of oscillation yields an estimate of the moment of inertia:

$$I_0 = \frac{WL}{4\pi^2 f^2}$$

(1.82)

where
I_0 is the moment of inertia at the axis of suspension
W is the weight of segment or mg
L is the distance of center of mass to axis of suspension
f is the period of oscillation

The moment of inertia at the center of mass located a distance L from the axis of suspension is found, by the parallel-axis theorem, to be

$$I_{cm} = I_0 - mL^2$$

(1.83)

More practically, mean values for key body segments determined experimentally are given in Table 1.1.

Another useful parameter relating to moments of inertia is the *radius of gyration*, K. It is the effective distance from the axis of rotation, K, for which a point mass of Equation 1.82 yields an equivalent moment of inertia to the body segment:

$$K = \sqrt{\frac{I_{cm}}{m}}$$

(1.84)

The final rotational equilibrium equation for angular motion of a body can now be defined as the sum of three components:

$$\sum M = r \times mg + r \times F_t + I\alpha$$

(1.85)

Note, that since the centrifugal force acts through the point of rotation, it does not create a moment around the point of rotation.

For certain situations when the forces are not constant, it may be useful to apply concepts of work and energy to solving equations of motion. *Work* is the result of force acting on a body to produce motion and is measured as the product of the magnitude of the force vector times the amount of displacement of the body:

$$W = F \cdot s$$

(1.86)

Note that both vectors need to have the same direction and the dot product results in a purely scalar value. If the force is in Newtons and the displacement in meters, the resulting unit is Joules (J, named after the English physicist James Prescott Joule, 1818–1889).

Energy is the capacity of a system to do work and thus has the same units as work. It can be *potential energy* associated with position in the gravitational field or *kinetic energy* associated with linear displacement of a body. In the first case, it is defined as

$$E_p = mgh \tag{1.87}$$

where
  E_p is the potential energy
  h is the change in height with respect to gravity

In the second case, it is defined as

$$E_p = \frac{1}{2}ks^2 \tag{1.88}$$

where
  k is the spring constant of an elastic body
  s is the linear displacement

Kinetic energy is associated with the energy released during motion of a body and is defined as

$$E_k = \frac{1}{2}mv^2 \tag{1.89}$$

where
  E_k is the kinetic energy
  m is the mass of the body
  v is the rectilinear velocity of the body

The key principle in using work and energy for motion analyses is that work done on a body by a conservative force can be converted to kinetic and potential energies, the sum of which will always be constant for any position of the system, i.e., energy cannot be created or destroyed, but can only be transformed. This is known as the *law of the conservation of mechanical energy*.

Example 1.6: Potential Energy of a Falling Object

The average energy required for skull fracture is approximately 70 Nm. Consider a construction site or steel mill with an overhead crane carrying scrap metal. It would be of interest to determine the minimum height a 2 kg piece of metal would need to fall to cause skull fracture. Equation 1.87, with g being 9.807 m/s², yields

$$70 = 2 \times 9.807 \times h \tag{1.90}$$

Solving for h yields

$$h = \frac{70/2}{9.807} = 3.57 \text{ m} \tag{1.91}$$

This is not a very high height and demonstrates the need for wearing hard hats on industrial sites.

A similar analysis could be applied to the wrist, for an individual trying to break a fall with an outstretched arm after tripping. Considering a large body weight of 70 kg, the height would be very minimal. However, the analysis is quite a bit more complicated since the weight is distributed along the length of the body and other parts of the body may come in contact with the ground first, absorbing some of the impact. Still it is not an uncommon occurrence for an individual in a fall to fracture some of the bones in the wrist or the forearm.

Example 1.7: Kinetic Energy from a Flying Object

Again assume that the average energy required for skull fracture is approximately 70 Nm. Consider a powered lawn mower that picks up a stone weighing 0.01 kg and, through the action of the revolving blades, ejects it from the discharge chute of the mower. It would be of interest to determine the minimum velocity that would cause skull fracture. Equation 1.89 yields

$$70 = \frac{1}{2} \times 0.01 v^2 \qquad (1.92)$$

Solving for velocity yields

$$v = \left(\frac{2 \times 70}{0.01} \right)^{1/2} = 118.3 \text{ m/s} \qquad (1.93)$$

Considering that the peripheral velocity of the blades for some mowers can achieve speeds of up to 100 m/s, it would not be unusual for a sufficiently large stone to cause major injury.

For further background material on biomechanics principles, useful examples, and practical applications to the human body, the reader is referred to LeVeau (1977) and Özkaya and Nordin (1991).

Questions

1. What is biomechanics?
2. Who are some of the historical figures that helped develop biomechanics as a science?
3. What factors characterize a force?
4. What characteristics are found in static equilibrium?
5. Compare and contrast the three different classes of levers. Give an example from the human body for each class.
6. What is the principle of moments? Why is it useful in biomechanics?
7. Define the coefficient of friction. How is it possible for it to exceed the value of 1?
8. What is the difference between kinematics and kinetics?
9. Describe a method for determining the center of mass for a body segment.

10. Describe a method for determining the moment of inertia for a body segment.

11. What is the law of the conservation of mechanical energy? Give an example of where this may be applied.

12. How is the moment of inertia related to the radius of gyration for a body segment?

Problems

1. Consider Example 1.1, except that the included angle is now 135° instead of 90°. How would that change the force required of the biceps brachii and the mechanical advantage? Repeat for 45°. Relate these results to the development of certain types of strength-training equipment.

2. Consider the upper limb bent at 90°. The weight of the upper arm, forearm, and hand are represented by forces of 21, 13, and 4 N, acting through the respective center of gravities as shown below. Find the center of gravity for the combined upper limb system.

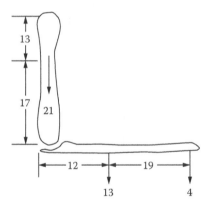

3. Consider the sternocleidomastoid muscle shown Figure 1.8. Discuss the two different lever systems involved and the relative mechanical advantages for the respective ranges on the clavicle for which each type of lever system is applicable.

4. Consider a pilot using night vision goggles (force of 9 N) that are attached to the front of the helmet (force of 18 N). To counteract the resulting large downward torque of the head and consequent fatigue of the neck muscles, the pilot attaches a lead weight to the back of the helmet. Helmet cg is 2 cm in front of neck pivot point; goggle cg is 20 cm anterior of neck pivot point; lead weight cg is 10 cm behind neck pivot point; the head is of uniform density and exerts a force of 40 N. Find the appropriate lead weight that would best balance the head and eliminate neck fatigue. What critical assumption must be made before this problem can be started? Why is this assumption valid? What class of lever system is involved?

5. Traction is applied in line to the arm with a 15 kg weight suspended via three pulleys as shown below. Assuming frictionless pulleys, how much traction is applied to the arm?

6. A patient is being lowered in a frictionless wheelchair down a 30° ramp. The total weight of the patient and wheelchair is 100 kg. A rope tied to a wheelchair takes a half turn around a pipe at the top of the ramp with μ = 0.2. What force must be applied to the rope to control the motion of the chair and patient?

7. A Russell traction (shown below) is used for immobilizing femoral fractures. Assuming μ = 0.05 and neglecting the weight of the leg, what weight is needed to produce a 30 kg traction force on the femur? What important features have been forgotten and usually must be done to the patient in these cases? Measure the angles needed directly from the drawing.

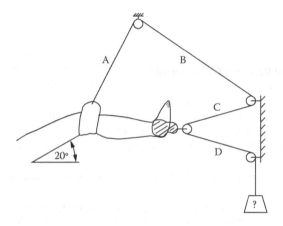

8. Assume that the energy level needed for shoulder fracture is approximately 70 J. What is the minimum weight needed for an object falling from a 10 m height to cause fracture? What is its velocity at impact?

9. The Achilles tendon is located on the posterior aspect of the calcaneus bone as far as possible from the ankle joint (roughly 6 cm) giving the calf muscles (gastrocnemius and soleus) the maximum possible advantage in lifting the body. In addition, this distance changes very little during foot movements. Consider a 98 kg basketball player jumping from the right foot.

   a. Given a foot length of 28.7 cm and a center of gravity location at 12.3 cm from the heel, how much muscle force (i.e., G for gastrocnemius/soleus) is supported by the Achilles tendon at the instant the heel is lifted from the floor?

   b. How much force is (i.e., F) is exerted by the foot on the floor?

   c. What kind of a lever system is this? What is the mechanical advantage of the muscle G? What are the implications of this result?

References

Bobjer, O., Johansson, S.E., and Piguet, S. (1993). Friction between hand and handle. Effects of oil and lard on textured and non-textured surfaces; perception of discomfort. *Applied Ergonomics* 24:190–202.

Braune, W. and Fischer, O. (1889). *The Center of Gravity of the Human Body*, Leipzig, S. Herzel, Verlag.

Chaffin, D.B., Andersson, G.B.J., and Martin, B.J. (1999). *Occupational Biomechanics*, 3rd edn, New York: John Wiley & Sons.

Dempster, W.T. (1955). *Space Requirements of the Seated Operator*, WADC-TR–55-159. Dayton, OH: Aerospace Medical Research Laboratories.

Fischer, O. (1906). *Theoretical Fundamentals for a Mechanics of Living Bodies*, Leipzig, B.G. Teubner.

Kitano, T., Ateshian, G.A., Mow, V.C., Kadoya, Y., and Yamano, Y. (2001). Constituents and pH changes in protein rich hyaluronan solution affect the biotribological properties of artificial articular joints. *Journal of Biomechanics*, 34:1031–1037.

Lephart, S.A. (1984). Measuring the inertial properties of cadaver segments. *Journal of Biomechanics*, 17:537–543.

LeVeau, B. (1977). *Williams and Lissner Biomechanics of Human Motion*, 2nd edn, Philadelphia, PA: W.B. Saunders Co.

Miller, D.I. and Nelson, R.C. (1976). *Biomechanics of Sport*. Philadelphia, PA: Lea and Febiger.

Özkaya, N. and Nordin, M. (1991). *Fundamentals of Biomechanics*. New York: Van Nostrand Reinhold.

Plagenhoef, J.A. (1966). Methods for obtaining kinetic data to analyze human motions. *The Research Quarterly of the American Association for Health, Physical Education, and Recreation* 37:103–112.

Roebuck, J.A., Kroemer, K.H.E., and Thomson, W.G. (1975). *Engineering Anthropometry Methods*. New York: Wiley-Interscience.

Unsworth, A., Dowson, D., and Wright, V. (1975). The frictional behavior of human synovial joints— Art I. Natural joints. *Transactions of the American Society of Mechanical Engineers, Series F, Journal of Lubrication Technology,* 97:369–376.

Weast, R.C., eds. (1969). *Handbook of Chemistry and Physics*. Cleveland, OH: The Chemical Rubber Co., p. F15.

Webb Associates, eds. (1978). *Anthropometric Source Book, NASA 1024*. Washington, DC: National Aeronautics and Space Administration.

2

Structure of the Musculoskeletal System

2.1 Gross Overview of Movements

The musculoskeletal system is a complex system of muscles, bones, and soft connective tissue to produce movement in the human body. The movements are three dimensional, centered around joints but are typically defined in two dimensions along the three major planes (see Figure 2.1): *sagittal*, observing the body from the side, *transverse*, observing the body from directly above the head, and *frontal*, observing the body from the front, i.e., face to face. These movements are defined with the human body in a *standard anatomical position*, as shown in Figure 2.1, with palms facing forward.

Movements of the trunk and neck in the sagittal plane include *flexion*, bending the trunk or neck forward, and *extension*, bending the trunk or neck backward. In the frontal plane, bending the trunk sideways results in lateral flexion, with the *lateral* direction being further away from the midline of the body, as opposed to the *medial* direction, which is closer to the midline. In the transverse plane, rotation of the trunk along the vertical long axis of the body (roughly the spinal column) results in *axial rotation*.

Movements of the shoulder girdle (as opposed to the *glenohumeral joint* or strictly the shoulder joint) in the sagittal or frontal plane include shoulder elevation, the raising the shoulders, and shoulder depression, the lowering of the shoulders. In the sagittal plane, drawing the shoulder forward results in *protraction*, while drawing the shoulders backward results in *retraction*.

Movements of the glenohumeral joint and hip joint in the sagittal plane include flexion, raising of the arm or moving the thigh forward, extension, pushing the arm or thigh backward of the midline. In the frontal plane, *abduction* is the raising of the arm or thigh to the side, while *adduction* is lowering the arm or bringing the thigh closer to the midline. In the transverse plane, rotation of the arm or leg along its long axis outward results in lateral or outward rotation, while rotation of the arm or leg along its long axis inward results in medial or inward rotation.

Note that both the glenohumeral and hip joints are ball-and-socket type of joints, allowing for 3° of rotational freedom.

Movements of the elbow and knee joints in the sagittal plane include flexion, the bending from a fully straightened position or a decrease in the internal angle and extension, an increase of the internal angle back toward the fully straightened position. Note that the elbow and knee joints are basically hinge or pin joints allowing only 1° of rotational freedom.

Movement of the wrist joint including the eight *carpal* bones in the wrist can be defined as follows. In the sagittal plane, flexion is bending the palm upward or closer to the forearm,

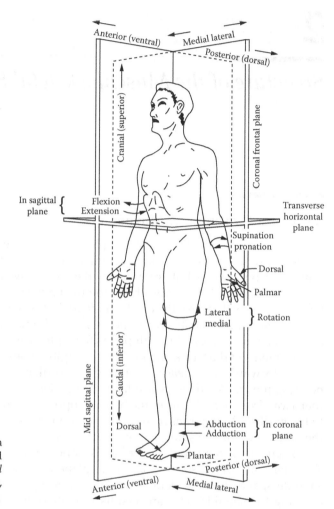

FIGURE 2.1
Standard anatomical posture with major movements shown. (Reproduced from Chaffin, D.B. et al., *Occupational Biomechanics*, 3rd edn., John Wiley & Sons, New York, 1999. With permission.)

while extension is bending the palm back or away from the forearm. In the frontal plane, *radial deviation* is moving the hand away from the trunk and closer to radius bone in the forearm, while *ulnar deviation* is moving the hand closer to the trunk and closer to the ulna in the forearm.

Movement of the ankle in the sagittal plane include flexion or, more specifically, *dorsi-flexion*, the raising of the dorsum or the top part of the foot and extension or *plantar flexion*, moving the sole or the plantar part of the foot downward. If the *tarsal* bones of the foot are also involved, then *inversion* is bringing the sole of the foot inward and *eversion* is moving the sole of the foot outward.

Because of the large number of bones in the hand (see Figure 2.2 or 5.1), there a correspondingly large number of joints and type of movements possible of the hand. The fingers are termed the *phalanges* and the palm is formed by the *metacarpals*. This is one reason why the hand is such a good manipulative device that is difficult to replicate even with the finest robotic controls currently available. The thumb is the first digit, the index finger is the second, the middle finger is the third, the ring finger is the fourth, and the small finger is the fifth. MP refers to the metacarpophalangeal joint and IP refers to interphalangeal joints. MP and IP flexion is movement of the fingers closer to the palm,

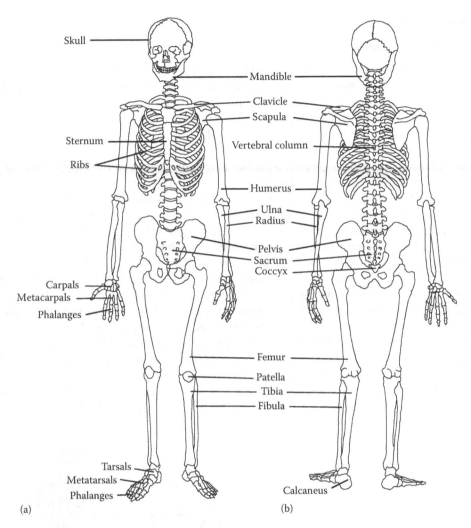

FIGURE 2.2
Major bones of the human skeleton. (a) Anterior and (b) posterior.

i.e., curling the fingers, while MP and IP extension is movement of the fingers away from the palm. Movement of the thumb perpendicularly away from the palm is abduction, with adduction being closer to the palm. Movement of the thumb to oppose other digits pulpy surface to pulpy surface is *opposition*. The hand is considered to have a long axis defined by digit 3. Therefore, movement of digits 2, 4, and 5 away from this axis in the plane of the palm is abduction, with adduction being the return of the digits to their normal position.

Movement of the forearm can also be considered a joint action, because the two forearm bones, the *radius* and the *ulna*, rotate with respect to one another along the long axis. Rotation of the forearm to the palm up position is *supination*, while to the palm down position is *pronation*. Note that in all of these gross movements, there typically will be two opposing motions for each joint, each of which is controlled by a separate set of muscles.

2.2 Skeletal System

The purpose of the skeletal system (see Figure 2.2) is both (1) to provide a rigid system of links, the bones, for the attachment of muscles and the basis of movement and (2) to protect the internal organs. There are a bit over 200 bones in the human body of various sizes, shapes, and mechanical properties. Interestingly, these characteristics can change dramatically in response to external stressors and, thus, living bones can be very dynamic systems.

Bones can be roughly categorized as either *long bones*, found in the extremities, i.e., the femur, the humerus, etc., or as *axial bones*, such as the skull, vertebrae, pelvis, etc. The long bones are characterized by a tubular shaft termed the *diaphysis* and two enlarged rounded ends termed the *epiphysis* (Figure 2.3). The outer edge of the diaphysis is composed of higher mineral content and, thus, denser bone material, *cortical or compact bone*, while the center and epiphysii contains spongier and less dense bone material termed *cancellous or spongy bone*. To better distribute stress in this less dense region, a three-dimensional lattice-like structure of fibers, the *trabeculae*, has evolved. Interestingly, this is one of the very dynamic aspects of bone, with the trabeculae structure adapting to external stress in very visible patterns. This was first characterized by Wolff (1892) as "form follows function," now known as *Wolff's Law*. The center of the diaphysis also contains bone marrow that produces red blood cells and blood vessels carrying away cells and bringing nutrients to the bone. This red blood cell production decreases dramatically by late adolescence with a concurrent increase in fatty deposits in the marrow.

Bone material is composed of cells and an extracellular matrix of fibers and a ground substance. The cells produce the extracellular matrix which determines the

FIGURE 2.3
Diagram of a long bone, shown in longitudinal cross. (Reproduced from Chaffin, D.B. et al., *Occupational Biomechanics*, 3rd edn., John Wiley & Sons, New York, 1999. With permission.)

mechanical properties of bone. The combined effect of the fibers and ground substance provides an additive effect for strength. An apt analogy is reinforced concrete with the concrete producing compressive strength and the rebars providing structural support. These cells are initially called *osteoblasts*, but gradually transform themselves into *osteocytes*, which become mineralized and isolated in the matrix. A third type of cells, the *osteoclasts*, perform a reverse process of gradually reabsorbing the bone structure. This again shows the very dynamic processes occurring in bone, with bone formation and resorption occurring simultaneously, especially in adaptive responses to external stressors and forces. This, however, is very different from the soft connective tissue, which once formed, can only deteriorate, and is a partial explanation for the seriousness of repetitive motion injuries which are slow to heal in connective tissue. On the other hand, bone, when injured, can actually heal to a stronger state than it was initially.

The ground substance is *hydroxy apatite*, a crystalline structure of calcium while the fibers are primarily collagen fibers. During bone formation or *ossification*, the first bone called *woven bone* is laid down at outer edges of the *Haversian canal system* (Figure 2.4), or points of injury or fracture. Gradually, through the parallel arrangement of the collagen fibers and hydroxy apatite crystals, the woven bone becomes a more sheet like *lamellar bone*. With repeated deposits of circumferential lamellae, cortical bone is formed and the overall bone gains strength. Note, this could be considered similar to production of plywood, which increases the overall strength of wood, or the laying down of steel strands in belted tires. Note also that this process follows mechanics principles of obtaining optimum strength. Bending strength is increased with increased moments of inertial,

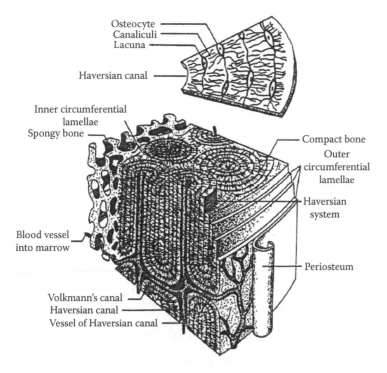

FIGURE 2.4
Diagram of the Haversian system within compact bone. (Reproduced from Chaffin, D.B. et al., *Occupational Biomechanics*, 3rd edn., John Wiley & Sons, New York, 1999. With permission.)

i.e., increasing cross-sectional areas and increasing the area further from the point of rotation, i.e., for the same amount or mass of material, a hollow tube is stronger than a solid tube (see Example 2.1).

Example 2.1: Bending Moments of Hollow Tubes

The elastic deflection of a support beam can be defined as the radius of curvature resulting from a bending moment applied to the beam:

$$\rho = \frac{EI}{M} \tag{2.1}$$

where
  ρ is the radius of curvature
  E is the modulus of elasticity for the given material
  I is the moment of inertia of the cross section of the beam with reference to its axis
  M is the bending moment on the beam

When there is a small bending moment or a very large moment of inertia, the radius of curvature approaches infinity, yielding a straight beam.
  The moment of inertia of a solid beam with a circular cross section is

$$I = \frac{\pi r^4}{4} \tag{2.2}$$

where r is the radius of the circular cross section.
  The moment of inertia of a tube is

$$I = \frac{\pi \left(r_1^4 - r_2^4 \right)}{4} \tag{2.3}$$

where
  r_1 is the outer radius
  r_2 is the inner radius

For a solid tube, r_1 is zero and Equation 2.3 becomes equivalent to Equation 2.2.
  The objective is to maximize the moment of inertia for a given amount of material defined as the area, which for the solid beam is

$$A = \pi r^2 \tag{2.4}$$

and for the tube as

$$A = \pi \left(r_1^2 - r_2^2 \right) \tag{2.5}$$

For example, comparing a solid beam with a 1 cm radius and a tube with an outer radius of 3 cm and an inner radius of 2.828 (i.e., wall thickness of 0.172 cm), yields the same amount of material:

$$\pi(1)^2 = \pi(3^2 - 2.828^2) = \pi \tag{2.6}$$

However, the moment of inertia for the solid beam is

$$I = \frac{\pi}{4} \tag{2.7}$$

while the moment of inertia for the tube is

$$I = \frac{\pi(3^4 - 2.828^4)}{4} = \frac{17\pi}{4} \qquad (2.8)$$

Thus, the moment of inertia for the hollow tube is 17 times larger than for a solid beam of the same amount of material resulting in a 17 times greater resistance to deflection for a given bending moment. This principle is used in the construction of pylons and products where weight is important, such as bicycles. Of course, carrying the principle to extremes would result in walls so thin, that they would be easily damaged from direct pressure or impacts. Similarly, bones have evolved with a greater amount of solid material being deposited on the outer edge for greater strength.

2.3 Mechanical Properties of Bone

Stiffness and strength are important mechanical properties of bone. These are typically established through a *stress–strain curve* (see Figure 2.5) obtained from a bone specimen placed in a testing jig. The load applied per unit area of the specimen is termed *stress*, while the deformation normalized to the initial length is termed *strain*. Initially, in a region termed the *elastic region*, the relationship between stress and strain is linear and repeatable during release of the loading. The slope of this region is the modulus of elasticity and represents the stiffness of the material:

$$\sigma = E\varepsilon \qquad (2.9)$$

where
σ is the stress (in Pa)
E is the Young's modulus of elasticity (in Pa)
ε is the strain (unitless)

Once loading exceeds the *yield point*, the material enters the *plastic deformation region* and will not return to its original shape when unloaded. At a certain point after considerable plastic flow, the material will eventually fail at the *failure point*. The relative material strengths at these points are termed the *minimum yield strength* and *ultimate tensile strength*.

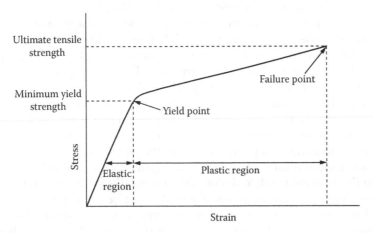

FIGURE 2.5
A typical stress–strain curve for a material in tension.

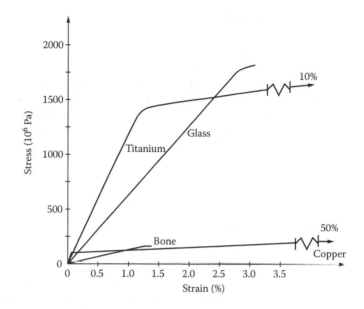

FIGURE 2.6
Stress–strain curves for bone and other materials in tension. Bone—compact bone from human femur. (Modified from Reilly, D.T. and Burstein, A.H., *J. Biomech.*, 8, 393, 1975.) Copper—99.9% pure copper. (Modified from Weast, R.C., *Handbook of Chemistry and Physics*, The Chemical Rubber Co., Cleveland, OH, 1969.) Glass—6 mm strand, SiO_2 with 20% Na_2O. (Modified from Weast, R.C., *Handbook of Chemistry and Physics*, The Chemical Rubber Co., Cleveland, OH, 1969.) Titanium—6Al-4V alloy. (Modified from Weast, R.C., *Handbook of Chemistry and Physics*, The Chemical Rubber Co., Cleveland, OH, 1969.)

Overall bone strength and properties are compared to those of other materials in Figure 2.6. Metals vary in ductility and show a definite plastic region while glass is very brittle and has no plastic region, failing at the end of the elastic region. A stiff metal, such as titanium, has an elongation range of less than 10% before failure, while a ductile metal, such as copper, may elongate up to 50% before failure. Bone has a less definite elastic region, perhaps up to 1% strain, and flows another 2% before failure.

When loaded in *tension* (see Figure 2.7), the ultimate strength of bone is relatively comparable to copper. Not surprisingly due to daily loading, bone is stronger in *compression* but relatively weak in shear loading (see Figure 2.8). Also, because bone is *anisotropic*, its properties are very different depending on the direction of the applied forces as compared to the directional qualities of bone (see Figure 2.9). This would seem quite logical considering the overlapping layers of lamellar patterns. Note also that the above properties apply to cortical bone having quite a dense structure (70%–95%) as compared to cancellous bone, which with a 10%–70% dense structure, is much weaker.

Typical daily loading of bone is compressive by nature and relatively low, around 4 MPa and rarely exceeding 12 MPa, measured during jogging (Carter, 1978). More extreme compressive loadings, as in impacts from falls, can result in fractures, typically found in vertebrae. *Shear* loading is applied parallel to the surface of the structure resulting in deformation of the internal cancellous bone (see Figure 2.4). A relatively typical shear fracture occurs to the femoral condyle during falls especially for older females with weaker bones. Bending fractures can occur when a load is applied at one end of the limb, with the other end relatively fixed, creating bending moment, and causing the limb to bend about the longitudinal axis. One outer surface of the bone is being lengthened through tensile loading, while the opposite outer surface is being compressed. Failure will tend

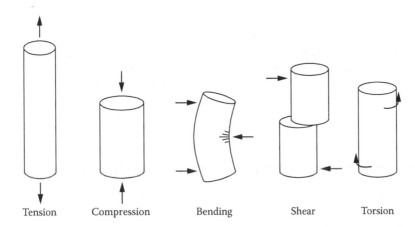

FIGURE 2.7
Schematic representation of various loading modes.

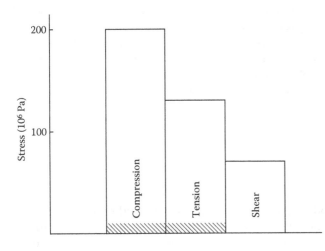

FIGURE 2.8
Ultimate strength at failure for human cortical bone specimens test in compression, tension, and shear. Shaded area indicates stresses experienced during running (Carter, D.R., *J. Biomech.*, 11, 199, 1978). (Adapted from Frankel, V.H. and Nordin, M., *Basic Biomechanics of the Skeletal System*, Lea & Febiger, Philadelphia, PA, 1980.)

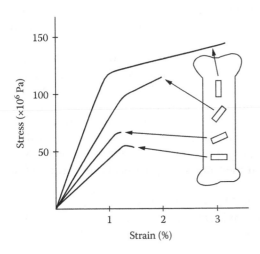

FIGURE 2.9
Stress–strain curves for cortical bone tested in tension in four different orientations. (Adapted from Reilly, D.T. and Burstein, A.H., *J. Biomech*, 8, 393, 1975.)

to occur on the surface subjected to tension, because ultimate tensile strength is lower than ultimate compressive strength in cortical bone. For example, such bending moments may occur during skiing accidents, as the upper body falls forward over the top of a relatively immobile ski and ski boot, resulting in boot-top tibial fractures from falls (Frankel and Nordin, 1980). Torsional fractures may also occur in the same skiing accident, if the long ski tends to twist the tibia and fibula about the long axis.

Bone is very dynamic, changing size, shape, and structure as a result of the mechanical stresses placed upon it. As mentioned earlier, this was first observed by Wolff (1892) who characterized it in his "form follows function" law. Correspondingly, bone mass is deposited or reabsorbed as necessary at the critical locations. The latter is a more critical situation, especially for those immobilized after injuries or in elderly individuals, especially women. Sixty-day immobilization of Rhesus monkeys resulted in more than a 50% loss in compressive strength (Kazarian and Von Gierke, 1969). Full skeletal bone maturity is reached roughly at the age of 30. After age 30, bone loss, exemplified by a decrease in calcium, a decrease in cortical bone thickness and diameter, and a decrease in trabeculae in cancellous bone, occurs steadily, accelerating with increasing age.

Interestingly, a similar bone loss is found in astronauts returning from extended periods in space. The hypothesis is that the lack of mechanical strain in the bone from the lack of gravity leads to bone reabsorption. To prevent such a bone loss, researchers have recommended exercise that maintains stress on bone for astronauts, specifically impact types of exercises that increase the strain rate in bone (Cavanagh et al., 1992). This has resulted in the development and deployment of specialized treadmills in which the astronaut is tethered to the treadmill with an elastic cord so as to maintain contact in the zero-g environment (McCrory et al., 1999).

2.4 Soft Connective Tissue

The soft connective tissue of the body: ligaments, tendons, fascia, and cartilage, provide support and structural integrity to the musculoskeletal system, as well as transmit forces between components. All connective tissue, similar to bone, is composed of cells and an extracellular matrix of fibers and a ground substance. The cells produce the extracellular matrix which determines the mechanical properties of the connective tissue. The ground substance is typically a *proteoglycan*, a polysaccharide with a protein core, some lipids and the ubiquitous water.

There are three main types of fibers: *collagen*, *elastin*, and *reticulin*. Collagen fibers provide strength and stiffness to tissue, elastin fibers provide elasticity, while reticulin merely provides bulk. A stress–strain diagram for collagen (Figure 2.10), indicates a small toe region (up to 1% strain) in which the kinky strands are straightened, a relatively linear elastic region up to roughly 7% strain, and a plastic deformation region until ultimate failure at roughly 10% strain. The stress–strain diagram (Figure 2.11) for elastin is very different with almost pure elasticity (under minimal stress) up to roughly 200%, at which point the fibers have lost their elasticity, become stiff under increasing stress and eventually fail without plastic deformation.

Ligaments connect bone to bone and provide stability at joints. They are typically 90% collagen with relatively straight arrangement of fibers with minimal elasticity (see Figure 2.12). *Fascia* are connective tissue covering organs and muscles. It is very elastic (high percentage

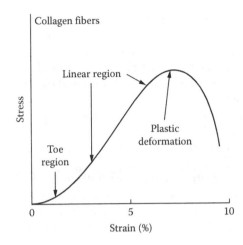

FIGURE 2.10
Stress–strain curve for collagen fibers in tension. (Reproduced from Chaffin, D.B. et al., *Occupational Biomechanics*, 3rd edn., John Wiley & Sons, New York, 1999. With permission.)

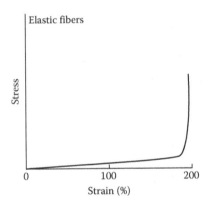

FIGURE 2.11
Stress–strain curve for elastin fibers in tension. (Reproduced from Chaffin, D.B. et al., *Occupational Biomechanics*, 3rd edn., John Wiley & Sons, New York, 1999. With permission.)

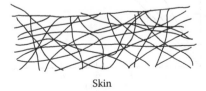

FIGURE 2.12
Schematic diagram of the structural orientation of tendon, ligament, and skin fibers. (Reproduced from Chaffin, D.B. et al., *Occupational Biomechanics*, 3rd edn., John Wiley & Sons, New York, 1999. With permission.)

of elastin) with a very irregular arrangement of fibers, allowing elasticity in all direction. *Cartilage* covers articular bony surfaces and is found also in the ear, nose, and interverte-bral discs. Of the three main types of cartilage, *hyaline cartilage* is found on the epiphysial areas of bone (see Section 2.5), and is a relatively homogenous matrix of collagen fibers. *Fibrocartilage* is present in the intervertebral discs and is composed of collagen and elastin. *Elastic cartilage* if is found in the ear and epiglottis of the throat.

Tendons connect muscle to bone, transmitting the muscle force, in the form of paral-lel bundles of collagen fibers with minimal elasticity. They have a hierarchical structure starting from molecular level with the collagen molecules tightly bound by collagen cross-links to form microfibrils, fibrils, and fibers (Figure 2.13). The fibrils have a slightly kinky structure which leads to the toe region effect in stress–strain curves for both individual collagen fibers (Figure 2.10) and complete tendons (Figure 2.14). The fibrils are embedded in an extracellular matrix of proteoglycans composed primarily of water, around 70% (Ker, 2007; Gupta et al., 2010). This property leads to a high level of viscoelastic properties for

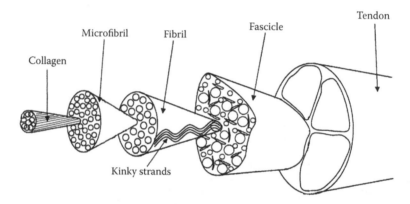

FIGURE 2.13
The hierarchical structure of tendon. (Adapted from Gupta, H.S. et al., *J. Struct. Biol.*, 169, 183, 2010. With permission.)

FIGURE 2.14
Stress–strain curve for three types of human tendons from cadavers. (From Harris, E.H. et al., *Med. Biol. Eng.*, 4, 253, 1966. With permission.)

tendon (Kubo et al., 2002). Tendons are often surrounded by a *synovial* lining sheath, which produces a very low friction synovial fluid to facilitate the gliding of tendons.

Collagen belongs to a special group of polymers whose molecular chains arrange themselves into regions of crystalline order. This structure results in a material that is flexible and relatively inextensible in the fiber direction, ideal for the axial transmission of force (Lanir, 1978). Young's modulus of a crystalline polymer is two or three orders of magnitude greater than that of its noncrystalline counterpart (Wainwright, 1976). Therefore, it could be inferred that forces normal or transverse to the fiber direction could more easily disrupt the structure. This is evidenced by the ratio of axial to normal moduli of 7 in cellophane film (Mark, 1932). However, there is little data is available for the transverse properties of collagen, especially in humans. Lynch et al. (2003) found that transverse modulus for sheep flexor tendons is approximately 200 times less than the axial modulus while Quapp and Weiss (1998) found a ratio of only 23 in human medial collateral ligament. Interestingly in a very recent study, Lake et al. (2010) found no statistical differences for human supraspinatus tendon. However, this is a very complicated multidirectional muscle with many insertion points that is not comparable to the previous tendons. In any case, the structure of tendons needs to be examined more closely because these directional properties probably to affect the likelihood of work-related tendon disorders (see Chapter 6).

2.5 Joints

A joint is the interaction point between two or more bones. There can be three types of joints, the most common of which is the articulating or freely moving joint. A layer of synovial fluid (the same as found in tendon sheaths) is found between the two articulating surfaces of the bones. Thus, these joints are sometimes also called synovial joints. If there is tissue connecting the two bones and it is fibrous such as in the skull, then these are termed fibrous joints. If the tissue is cartilage such as in the intervertebral discs, then these are termed cartilaginous joints.

2.5.1 Articular Joints

In an articular joint (Figure 2.15), the articulating ends of the bones are coved with a 1–5 mm thick layer of connective tissue, the articular cartilage and is surrounded by a synovial membrane (to contain the synovial fluid) and a joint capsule of ligaments. Many

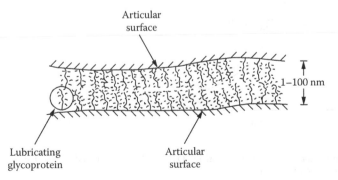

Articular surface

1–100 nm

Lubricating glycoprotein

Articular surface

FIGURE 2.15
Schematic diagram of articular cartilage surface with a monolayer of lubricating proteoglycan. (Reproduced from Mow, V.C. and Ratcliffe, A. In: V.C. Mow and W.C. Hayes (eds.), *Basic Orthopaedic Biomechanics*, 2nd edn., Lippincott-Raven, Philadelphia, PA, 1997. With permission.)

joints (such as the knee) have a disc of fibrocartilage (cartilage with higher collagen content) called a *meniscus* to better distribute forces and protect the bones. In fact, the main purpose of articular cartilage is to spread loads over a larger area and to allow relative movements of the opposing surface with minimum friction and wear. Physiologically, articular cartilage is virtually devoid of both blood and lymph vessels as well as nerves. This has important implications in terms of wear and potential regenerative capabilities.

Hyaline cartilage is primarily composed of the extracellular matrix with relatively few cells. The extracellular matrix is quite high in water content (60%–80%), leaving only 20%–40% solid material widely distributed. Of the solid part, 60% is collagen fibers and 40% is the proteoglycan gel, the ground substance composed of hyaluronic acid protein. The *chondrocyte* cells comprise less than 2% of the material and are arranged in layered zones within the proteoglycan gel (see Figure 2.15). In the superficial tangential zone, the chondrocytes are oblong with their long axes aligned parallel to the articular surface. In the middle zone, the chondrocytes are round and randomly distributed, while in the deep zone the chondrocytes are columnar in arrangement and are perpendicular to the *tide mark*, which acts as a boundary to calcified cartilage and the bone. The collagen fibers are similarly distributed in the cartilage layer: densely packed parallel to the surface in the superficial tangential zone, randomly oriented in the middle zone, and perpendicular to the surface in the deep zone (see Figure 2.16). This latter arrangement and zone is instrumental in anchoring the cartilage to the underlying bone (Mow and Ratcliffe, 1997).

The proteoglycan gel is composed of water and a brush-like appearing polymeric macromolecule based on a hyaluronic acid core with many side units (see Figures 2.15 and 2.16). These molecules are strongly hydrophilic (because of regular fixed negative charges and a high concentration that attempts to dilute itself through osmosis) but are prevented from fully absorbing water and swelling by the collagen network. This constraint on swelling causes an increase in osmotic pressure and tensile stress on the collagen fibers when there is no external stress. When an external stress is applied to the cartilage surface, the internal pressure in the cartilage matrix increases, exceeding the osmotic pressure and causing water to be squeezed out of the cartilage, producing a natural lubricating system (see Section 2.5.2).

Mechanically, articular cartilage can be considered to be a biphasic material, a solid in terms of collagen and a liquid in term of freely moving interstitial water, perhaps, similar to a wet sponge. Correspondingly, it exhibits both elastic and viscoelastic properties under compression, with an initial elastic deformation, followed by a slow creep (see Figure 2.16).

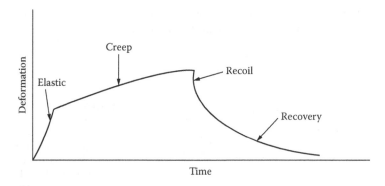

FIGURE 2.16
Stress–strain curve for articular cartilage. (Reproduced from Chaffin, D.B. et al., *Occupational Biomechanics*, 3rd edn., John Wiley & Sons, New York, 1999. With permission.)

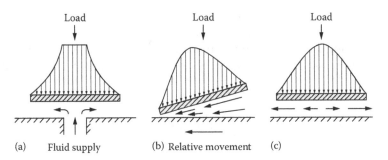

FIGURE 2.17
Diagrams illustrating three modes of joint lubrication: (a) hydrostatic; (b) hydrodynamic; (c) squeeze-film. (Adapted from Frankel, V.H. and Nordin, M., *Basic Biomechanics of the Skeletal System*, Lea & Febiger, Philadelphia, PA, 1980.)

Upon release of the load, initial elastic recoil is followed by a slow recovery (Mow and Ratcliffe, 1997).

2.5.2 Joint Lubrication

As mentioned in Chapter 1, the articular surface has an extremely low coefficient of friction ($\mu = 0.003$–0.005, Linn, 1968; Unsworth et al., 1975), much lower than can be achieved with man-made materials and lubricants. It is thought, that is due to the simultaneous application of three different lubrication mechanisms: hydrostatic, hydrodynamic, and squeeze film lubrication. In *hydrostatic lubrication*, loading of the joint forces the synovial fluid out of the pores of the cartilage, into the space between the articular surfaces (see Figure 2.17a). As the joint is unloaded, the fluid is reabsorbed into the cartilage, similar to a sponge. In this case, the cartilage acts both as the pump and the reservoir for the lubricant.

In *hydrodynamic lubrication*, translational joint motion creates a wedge effect, further forcing synovial fluid between the articular surfaces (see Figure 2.17b). In *squeeze-film lubrication*, even relatively normal pressures, the fluid is squeezed out from the areas of high pressure to areas of lower pressure (see Figure 2.17c). As the pressure in the first area decreases, fluid returns. Thus, there is continual movement of the synovial fluid between the articular surfaces just from the pressures due to normal walking or other activities (Mow and Ateshian, 1997).

2.5.3 Wear and Osteoarthritis

Wear is the removal of material from articulating surfaces, either through abrasion or adhesion of the interfacial surfaces or by fatigue through repetitive stressing and deformation of the contacting surfaces and repetitive exchange of the synovial fluid. Repetitive stressing of the extracellular matrix could cause (1) damage to the collagen fibers, (2) disruption of the proteoglycan gel network, or (3) impairment of the fiber/interfibrillar matrix interface. Repetitive exuding and imbibing of the interstitial fluid may cause a washing out of the proteoglycan molecules from the matrix or a reduction of the cartilage's self-lubricating ability.

Articular cartilage has been found to have a limited capacity for repair and regeneration and if the stresses applied are large and sudden (excessive stress concentration), total

failure can occur. People in certain occupations, such as football players' knees, ballet danc-
ers' ankles, and miners' knees, are especially susceptible to high forces, fractures, damage
to the load-spreading function of the meniscii and ligament ruptures allowing excessive
movement of bone ends. It has been hypothesized that this progression of failure is related
to (1) the magnitude of forces involved, (2) the total number of force peaks experienced,
and (3) the rate of recovery, which is especially critical in some of the current repetitive
motion disorders. Osteoarthritis occurs secondarily to the primary trauma in cartilage in
the form of hemorrhages in the joint space, disorders of the collagen metabolism, degradation of the proteolytic enzymes (Frankel and Nordin, 1980).

2.5.4 Cartilaginous Joints

Cartilaginous joints are primarily found in the intervertebral discs that separate the vertebral bones of the back. The disc consists of the *annulus fibrosus*, the outer onion like fiber
casings, and the *nucleus pulposus*, the gel-like center (see Figure 2.18). As the disc is loaded,
the nucleus pulposus distributes the force uniformly to the outer annulus fibrosus, whose
fibers can withstand the axial tensile stresses. A good analogy would be high pressure
tanks, whose fluid pressure is uniformly distributed to the walls, which are wrapped with
glass fibers having very high tensile strength.

Both surfaces of the disc are covered by cartilage endplates, which are sufficiently porous
to allow the diffusion of fluid across the endplate. Since the disc has no internal blood
supply, this diffusion is its only means for receiving nutrients and eliminating wastes.
This diffusion is accentuated by pressures created by loading of the vertebral column.
Under high loading, fluid is forced out, while under decreased loading, fluid returns to
the disc. As a result, this can lead to a rather large shrinkage of the spine over the course
of a day, 15–20 mm or roughly 1% of overall stature (DePukys, 1935). Anecdotally, astronauts returning from the zero-g space environment and minimal spinal loading have

FIGURE 2.18
Structure of intervertebral disc: A, annulus fibrosus; N,
nucleus pulposus. (Reproduced from Chaffin, D.B. et al.,
Occupational Biomechanics, 3rd edn., John Wiley & Sons, New
York, 1999. With permission.)

experienced spinal expansion two or three times that level. This phenomenon has only been the basis for the development of *stadiometry*, measurement of spinal shrinkage as an indirect assessment of extended spinal loading (Eklund and Corlett, 1984).

Under repeated high loading, there is a tendency for the cartilage endplates to develop to develop microfractures. These can lead to a greater net loss of fluid and an eventual drying up of the nucleus pulposus and permanent shrinkage of the spine. More extreme fractures of the endplates or weakening of annulus fibrosus can lead to *disc herniation*, the bulging of the discs or even more catastrophic extrusion of the gel material. Further complications can result if the extruded material compresses nerve roots with consequent pain (sciatica) or even paralysis. Such events have typically been associated with high compressive forces combined lateral bending or twisting actions on the spine and have led to extensive study and modeling of manual handling of loads.

Questions

1. Compare and contrast cortical and cancellous bone.

2. Describe the structural composition of bone. Give an example of a similar synthetic material.

3. Describe the stress–strain characteristics of bone. How do they compare to those of synthetic materials?

4. What is Wolff's Law? Give several examples of where it may apply to bone.

5. Describe the basic structure of connective tissue.

6. What are the differences between ligaments, tendons, fascia, and cartilage?

7. Compare and contrast the three types of joints.

8. Describe the structure of an articular joint.

9. Describe the structure of hyaline cartilage. How does it compare to the basic structure of bone?

10. Explain why synovial joints have such low coefficients of friction, with respect to joint lubrication.

11. Describe the structure of intervertebral discs.

Problems

1. In addition to being hollow tubes, the long bones typically have larger diameters and thicker walls at the ends. Show the effect these characteristics have on bone strength (i.e., deflection). Note the comparable characteristic used in bicycle frame tubes is termed "double butted."

2. Most support structures (bones, trees, etc.) seem to have a circular cross section. This would imply that a circular cross section is more resistant to bending than other shapes for a given amount of material. Compare the resistance to bending for a hollow square

tube to a hollow circular tube of the same weight. The moment of inertia for a hollow square tube is given by

$$I = \frac{\left(r_1^4 - r_2^4\right)}{12} \tag{2.10}$$

where
    r_1 is the outer radius
    r_2 is the inner radius

3. The stress–strain curve for a material obeying Hooke's law is a line with a positive slope. Draw the experimentally determined stress–strain curve for a tendon. Explain the physiological basis for the differences this curves shows from that of the Hookean material.

References

Carter, D.R. (1978). Anisotropic analysis of strain rosette information from cortical bone. *Journal of Biomechanics* 11:199–202.

Cavanagh, P.R., Davis, B.L., and Miller, T.A. (1992). A biomechanical perspective on exercise countermeasures for long term spaceflight. *Aviation, Space and Environmental Medicine* 63:482–485.

Chaffin, D.B., Andersson, G.B.J., and Martin, B.J. (1999). *Occupational Biomechanics*, 3rd edn, New York: John Wiley & Sons.

DePukys, P. (1935). The physiological oscillation of the length of the body. *Acta Orthopaedica Scandinavica* 6:338–347.

Eklund, J.A.E. and Corlett, E.N. (1984). Shrinkage as a measure of the effect of load on the spine. *Spine* 9:189–194.

Frankel, V.H. and Nordin, M. (1980). *Basic Biomechanics of the Skeletal System*. Philadelphia, PA: Lea & Febiger.

Gupta, H.S., Seto, J., Krauss, S., Boesecke, P., and Screen, H.R.C. (2010). *In situ* multi-level analysis of viscoelastic deformation mechanisms in tendon collagen. *Journal of Structural Biology* 169:183–191.

Harris, E.H., Walker, L.B. Jr., and Bass, B.R. (1966). Stress-strain studies in cadaveric human tendon and an anomaly in the Young's modulus thereof. *Medical and Biological Engineering* 4:253–259.

Kazarian, L.E. and Von Gierke, H.E. (1969). Bone loss as a result of immobilization and chelation: Preliminary results in Macaca Mulatta. *Clinical Orthopaedics* 65:67–75.

Ker, R.F. (2007). Mechanics of tendon, from an engineering perspective. *International Journal of Fatigue* 29:1001–1009.

Kubo, K., Kawakami, Y., Kanehisa, H., and Fukunga, T. (2002). Measurement of viscoelastic properties of tendon structures *in vivo*. *Scandinavian Journal of Medicine and Science in Sports* 12:3–8.

Lake, S.P., Miller, K.S., Elliott, D.M., and Soslowsky, L.J. (2010). Tensile properties and fiber alignment of human supraspinatus tendon in the transverse direction demonstrates inhomogeneity, nonlinearity, and regional isotropy. *Journal of Biomechanics* 43:727–732.

Lanir, Y. (1978). Structure-strength relations in mammalian tendon. *Biophysical Journal* 24:541–554.

Linn, F.C. (1968). Lubrication of animal joints: II. The mechanism. *Journal of Biomechanics* 1:193–205.

Lynch, H.A., Johannessen, W., Wu, J.P., Jawa, A., and Elliott, D.M. (2003). Effect of fiber orientation and strain rate on the nonlinear uniaxial tensile material properties of tendon. *Journal of Biomechanical Engineering* 125:726–731.

Mark, H. (1932). *Physik und Chemie der Cellulos*. Berlin: Springer Verlag.

McCrory, J.L., Lemmon, D.R., Sommer, H.J., Prout, B., Smith, D., Korth, D.W., Lucero, J., Greenisen, M., Moore, J., Kozlovskaya, I., Pestov, I., Stepansov, V., Miyakinchenko, Y., and Cavanagh, P.R. (1999). Evaluation of a treadmill with vibration isolation and stabilization (TVIS) for use on the international space station. *Journal of Applied Biomechanics* 15:292–302.

Mow, V.C. and Ateshian, G.A. (1997). Lubrication and wear of diarthrodial joints. In: V.C. Mow and W.C. Hayes (eds), *Basic Orthopaedic Biomechanics*, 2nd edn, Philadelphia, PA: Lippincott-Raven, pp. 275–316.

Mow, V.C. and Ratcliffe, A. (1997). Structure and function of articular cartilage and meniscus. In: V.C. Mow and W.C. Hayes (eds), *Basic Orthopaedic Biomechanics*, 2nd edn, Philadelphia, PA: Lippincott-Raven, pp. 113–178.

Quapp, K.M. and Weiss, J.A. (1998). Material characterization of human medial collateral ligament. *Journal of Biomechanical Engineering* 120:757–763.

Reilly, D.T. and Burstein, A.H. (1975). The elastic and ultimate properties of compact bone tissue. *Journal of Biomechanics* 8:393–405.

Unsworth, A., Dowson, D., and Wright, V. (1975). The frictional behavior of human synovial joints—Part I. Natural joints. *Transactions of the American Society of Mechanical Engineers, Series F, Journal of Lubrication Technology* 97:369–376.

Wainwright, S.A., Biggs, W.D., Currey, J.D., and Gasline, J.M. (1976). *Mechanical Design in Organisms*. London: Edward Arnold.

Weast, R.C. ed. (1969). *Handbook of Chemistry and Physics*. Cleveland, OH: The Chemical Rubber Co., p. F15.

Wolff, J. (1892). *Das Gesetz der Transformation der Knochen (The Law of Bone Transformation)*. Berlin: Hirschwald.

3

Neuromuscular Physiology and Motor Control

3.1 Introduction to Musculature

There are well over 500 muscles in the body constituting close to 50% of the weight and 50% of the metabolic activity in the body. They are found as three different types: *skeletal muscles* attached to the bones, *cardiac muscle* found in the heart, and *smooth muscle* found in the internal organs and the walls of the blood vessels. Only skeletal muscles will be discussed in detail here because of their relevance to motion. Skeletal muscles are attached to the bones on either side of a joint (see Figure 3.1) by the tendons discussed previously and have the property of actively contracting and shortening, and in doing so, moving the bones. However, because muscle is soft tissue, the reverse action of active lengthening is not possible and a second set of muscles is required to bring the limb back to its original position. Thus, one or several muscles, termed *agonists* or prime movers, act as the primary activators of motion. An opposing set of muscles (typically on the opposite side of the joint) are termed *antagonists*, counteract the agonists and oppose the motion. Typically, one set of muscles is active, while the opposite set is relaxed. For example, during elbow flexion, the biceps or brachioradialis is the agonist (and also a flexor) while the triceps is the antagonist and also an extensor. However, during elbow extension, the triceps becomes the agonist (but is still an extensor), while the biceps becomes the antagonist. The muscle attachments to bones are also given specific names. The *origin* is the most *proximal* attachment, or the one nearest the trunk, while the *insertion* is the most *distal* or distant attachment from the trunk.

In terms of function, skeletal muscles can also be classified as spurt or shunt muscles. *Spurt* muscles originate far from the joint of rotation but are inserted close to the joint. Thus, they have short moment arms and can move the limb very rapidly but are relatively limited in the magnitude of effective strength. *Shunt* muscles are the opposite, with the origin close to the joint and the insertion point far from the joint. This creates a large moment arm and relative stabilizing effect on the joint. For example, in Figure 3.1, the biceps is the spurt muscle and the brachioradialis is the shunt muscle.

Visually, skeletal muscles may have a variety of patterns with muscle fibers arranged either in parallel or obliquely to the long axis of the muscle (Figure 3.2). In *fusiform* muscles, the fibers lie parallel to the long axis, pull longitudinally, and allow for maximum velocity and range of motion, because of the relative length of the fibers. The biceps brachii is a good example of a fusiform muscle. In *pennate* or *unipennate* muscles, the fibers are arranged obliquely to the long axis, similar to the fibers in a bird's feather cut in half. The extensor digitorum profundus in the forearm is an example of a unipennate muscle. In *bipennate* muscles, the fibers are arranged obliquely on both sides of the long axis, as in a

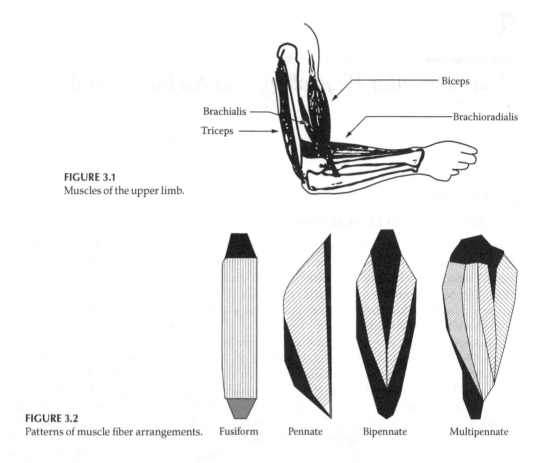

FIGURE 3.1
Muscles of the upper limb.

FIGURE 3.2
Patterns of muscle fiber arrangements.   Fusiform   Pennate   Bipennate   Multipennate

complete bird feather. Examples of bipennate muscles include the interosseous and typically the lumbricals in the hand. At the opposite extreme of parallel muscles are *multipennate* muscles, in which the fibers are relatively short and lie in several different oblique directions. Thus, they have a short range of motion, lower velocities, but can produce more power because of a larger cross-sectional area. The deltoid in the back of the shoulder is a good example of a multipennate muscle.

3.2 Structure of Muscle

The muscle consists of connective tissue in the form of fascia, muscle cells in the form of muscle fibers and nerves. An outer layer of fascia, the *epimysium*, covers the muscle, intermediate layers of fascia, the *perimysium*, subdivide bundles of muscle fibers into *fasciculi*, and inner layers of fascia, the *endomysium*, covers individual muscle fibers (see Figure 3.3). The fascia that binds fibers or groups of fibers extends to the end of the muscle and assists in firmly attaching the muscle and muscle fibers to the bone in the form of tendons. This gradual distribution of fascia throughout muscle tissue is very important in the uniform transmission of force from the active contractile units to the tendon and bone. In addition, muscle tissue is penetrated by tiny blood vessels carrying oxygen and

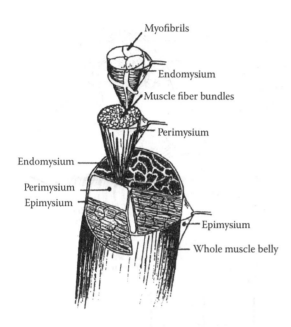

Myofibrils

Endomysium

Muscle fiber bundles

Perimysium

Endomysium

Perimysium

Epimysium

Epimysium

Whole muscle belly

FIGURE 3.3

Transverse section of a muscle showing the various layers of fascia. (Reproduced from Chaffin, D.B. et al., *Occupational Biomechanics*, 3rd edn., John Wiley & Sons, New York, 1999.)

nutrients to the muscle fibers and small nerve endings carrying electrical impulses from the spinal cord and brain.

The muscle fibers or muscle cells are the smallest units in the muscle with independent action and may contain several nuclei. They are approximately 10–60 μm in diameter and range in length from 5 to 140 mm, depending on the size of the muscle. Each muscle fiber is further subdivided into smaller *myofibrils*, 1 μm in diameter, with roughly 1000–8000 of these per fiber. The myofibril contains the ultimate contractile mechanism in the form of protein filaments. There are two types of *myofilaments*: thick filaments comprised of long proteins with molecular heads, called *myosin*, and thin filaments comprised with globular proteins called *actin* (see Figure 3.4).

The two types of filaments are interlaced with various amounts of overlap giving rise to a striated appearance and the alternate name of *striated muscle*. These different bands are shown in Figure 3.4 with a gross division between A-bands (from anisotropic or different characteristics) of both thick and thin filaments and I-bands (from *isotropic* or same characteristic) of just thin filaments. The thin filaments are held together by Z-discs (from the German zwischenscheibe or inter disc), which also define one repeating unit within the myofibril, termed a *sarcomere*. The lighter band of nonoverlapped thick filaments within the A-band is called the H-band (from the German hell for light or not as dark) and is bisected by the M-line (from the German Mittelmembran or middle membrane), a membrane that tends to hold the thick filaments together. The *sliding filament theory* of Huxley (1974) explains muscle contraction as a mechanism by which these filaments slide over one another rather than the filaments themselves being shortened. This theory is supported by the observations that the I-bands and H-bands become narrower until they almost completely disappear. On the other hand, the A-band stays the same width throughout muscle contraction.

The thick filament is roughly 12 nm in diameter and composed of the long myosin molecules. Each myosin molecule (see Figure 3.5) is roughly 150 nm long and consists of a tail composed of *light meromyosin* (LMM) which serves to bind the approximately 180 molecules together into a tight filament. The end of the myosin molecule has a head consisting

FIGURE 3.4
Organization of skeletal muscle from the muscle fibers to the protein filaments. (Adapted from McMahon, T.A., *Muscles, Reflexes, and Locomotion*, Princeton University Press, Princeton, NJ, 1984.)

FIGURE 3.5
Schematic representation of the myosin molecule. (Reproduced from Aidley, D.J., *The Physiology of Excitable Cells*, 2nd edn., Cambridge University Press, Cambridge, U.K., 1985.)

of two subunits of *heavy meromyosin* (HMM), the S_1 and S_2 units. The S_1 unit provides the enzyme activity to cause the formation and breakage of cross bridges with the thin filament while the S_2 unit serves as the actual rotational bridge between the two types of filaments (Aidley, 1985).

The thin filament is a double helix of globular actin (G-actin) molecules 5 nm in diameter. Another protein, *tropomyosin*, serves to bring the globular actins together in a chain, which is then sometimes termed fibrous actin (F-actin). At every seventh actin, there is a third protein, *troponin*, which acts as an inhibitor of the cross bridging to produce muscular contraction (see Figure 3.6).

FIGURE 3.6
Schematic representation of the thin filament. (Reproduced from Ebashi, S. et al., *Q. Rev. Biophys.*, 2, 351, 1969.)

3.3 Basic Cell Physiology

A cell, including the muscle fiber, is composed primarily of *cytoplasm*, which is roughly 80% water but contains *mitochondria* used in the production of energy through metabolism and of a *nucleus* containing genetic material. The cell is surrounded by a *cell membrane*, which is a selective barrier for the passage of nutrients and wastes in and out of the cell. It also serves as the site for the action of hormones and the generation and transmission of electrical impulses. According to the *unit membrane theory* (Figure 3.7), the cell membrane is a bilayer structure roughly 100 Å thick covered with mucopolysaccharide surface. Below the surface is a protein layer followed by a phospholipid layer, which is then reversed for the inner layer. The polysaccharide and protein layers are *hydrophilic*, allowing water molecules to adhere to the surface, while the lipid layers prevent lipid insoluble material to pass through. The thin mucopolysaccharide surface makes the outside different from the inside of the cell allowing a differential charge buildup and a resulting cell potential. Materials can pass through this membrane in one of three different ways. Small charged molecules such as water pass through micropores. Larger molecules such as glucose pass through with the assistance of carrier molecules, while large lipids pass through easily because of their solubility in the lipid structure of the membrane.

The resting cell potential is created by an unequal concentration of ions; a high concentration of sodium (Na^+) and chloride (Cl^-) ions outside the cell and a high concentration of potassium (K^+) ions and negative proteins inside the cell. A relatively large potential of $-70\,mV$ is created by a very small (0.003%) excess amount of total ions. Also K^+ ions are

Mucopolysaccharide

Protein Lipids Protein

Pores
8 Å

FIGURE 3.7
(a) Molecular organization of the cell membrane. (b) Pores in the cell membrane. (Reproduced from Guyton, A.C., *Textbook of Medical Physiology*, W.B. Saunders Co., Philadelphia, PA, 1971.)

(a)   (b)

much more permeable than Na⁺ (about a 30/1 ratio) but, because of the negative intracellular potential, cannot easily diffuse out of the cell. Thus, in steady state, there is continuous balance of concentration gradients versus electrical gradients or potentials. However, there is still a continual leakage of K⁺ ions out of the cell and Na⁺ ions into the cell which is rectified by an active sodium pump bring the K⁺ ions back in and the Na⁺ ions back out.

An active disturbance of the membrane potential for the excitable cells (nerve and muscle cells), termed an *action potential*, creates the means for transmission of information for the activation of muscles and resulting movement. This disturbance can be in the form of hormones, electrical stimulation, chemical neurotransmitters or even spontaneous changes such is in the smooth muscle of the gastrointestinal tract. In an action potential (see Figure 3.8), there is an initial *depolarization* (a positive change in the membrane potential), which changes the permeability of the membrane allowing Na⁺ ions to leak across the membrane down its concentration gradient. The sodium pump cannot keep up and the inside of the cell becomes more positive. At a certain threshold point, around −40 mV, the membrane practically opens up and the Na⁺ ions (P_{Na} in Figure 3.8) flood across the membrane dramatically changing the cell potential to positive values, reaching +30 to +40 mV. However, at the same time, due to the porosity of the membrane, K⁺ ions (P_K in Figure 3.8) are also moving down their concentration gradient out of the cell, with the consequent reversal of cell polarity. Simultaneously, there is a sodium inactivation, shutting down Na⁺ ion permeability with a reversal in the ratio of Na⁺/K⁺ permeability to a value of 1/20. The flow of K⁺ ions out of cell brings the cell potential back to −70 mV, sometimes with a brief hyperpolarization (more negative potential). The dramatic depolarization resulting in the action potential lasts for a brief time period, 1–2 ms. The return to normal steady state takes longer, anywhere from 1 to 15 ms. During this *refractory period*, the membrane cannot be easily stimulated again and the sodium pumps are working to return ionic balance to the cell. Note that once the initial disturbance reaches the threshold level, the process cannot be stopped. This is known as an *all-or-nothing response*. On the other hand, the depolarization

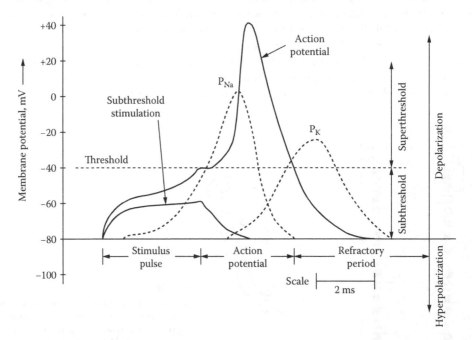

FIGURE 3.8
Formation of an action potential based on changes in Na⁺ and K⁺ ion flow.

process can reverse itself below threshold levels and will later be found to be one of the forms of control mechanisms within the neuromuscular reflex systems.

Note that, strictly speaking, no energy is required to produce an action potential. On the other hand, the sodium pump does require energy (in the form of ATP, discussed in Example 3.1). Also, the actual ion transfer is quite small, and, in fact, should the sodium pumps be poisoned, up to 100,000 action potentials could still be generated before the ion concentrations would be sufficiently equilibrated to prevent further such depolarizations.

Nerve cells, termed *neurons*, are carriers of electrical impulses that initiate muscle contraction (see Figure 3.9). It also has a cell body with mitochondria for energy production and a nucleus with genetic material. More important is the *axon*, the long part of the neuron, which carries the action potential. Many axons are covered by *myelin*, a specialized fatty sheath that forces the action potential to jump between gaps in the myelin, resulting in very high nerve conduction speeds. The *dendrites* are long, extensive branches off the cell body that serve to collect nerve impulses from other neurons. As with the invaginations in the brain, the dendrites greatly increase the surface area of the neuron with a much greater possibility for interconnections between neurons. The interconnection between a neuron and muscle cell is termed a *neuromuscular junction* and consists of a synaptic knob at the end of the neuron, a true gap termed the *synapse*, and the motor end plate, a specialized receptor, on the muscle fiber (see Figure 3.10).

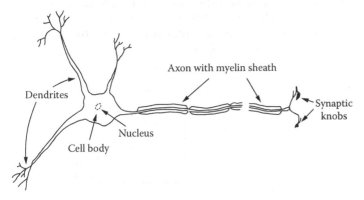

FIGURE 3.9
Schematic diagram of a neuron.

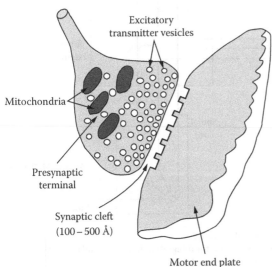

FIGURE 3.10
Anatomy of a synapse showing the synaptic knob and motor end plate. (Reproduced from Guyton, A.C., *Textbook of Medical Physiology*, W.B. Saunders Co., Philadelphia, PA, 1971. With permission from Elsevier Science.)

3.4 Nervous System

Motor control of the muscles initiates in the central nervous system (CNS), which includes the brain, within and protected by the skull, and the spinal cord, passing through and protected by the vertebral column. The brain (see Figure 3.11) can be subdivided into various areas, each of which contains a mass of nerve cells performing certain functions. To increase the motor control and other neural processing capability, the brain has developed deep invaginations, greatly increasing the surface area and thus space for more potential nerve cells, specifically their cell bodies. Among these areas, the *cerebral* or *sensorimotor* cortex covers the top surface of the brain and consists of both a motor part, from which the signals controlling muscle action originate and a sensory part, which receive feedback signals back from the muscles and other parts of the body. The occipital lobe and the *cerebellum*, in the posterior part, process visual information and feedback control for muscles, respectively. The frontal lobe is connected with emotion, the *basal ganglia* with motor processing, and the *brain stem* with sensory processing.

The spinal cord carries various nerve pathways to the periphery of the body, the main ones being the *pyramidal tract*, involved in direct motor control and the *extra pyramidal tract*, also involved in motor control but through a more circuitous pathway (see also Section 3.10). Once the nerves exit the spinal cord, they become part of the peripheral nervous system. The peripheral nervous system is subdivided into an *efferent* part, which carries information from the CNS to either muscles, through the motor system, or to the heart and other organs, through the autonomic system, and an *afferent* or sensory part, which carries information back to the CNS, either from the muscles, through the somatic system or from

FIGURE 3.11
Schematic diagram of the CNS showing pyramidal and extrapyramidal tracts. (Adapted from McMahon, T.A., *Muscles, Reflexes, and Locomotion*, Princeton University Press, Princeton, NJ, 1984.)

TABLE 3.1

Types of Neurons

Size	Group	Subgroup	Myelination	Size (μm)	Speed (m/s)	Function
Large	A	α (Ia)	Yes	12–20	72–100	Annulospiral
		α (Ib)	Yes	12–20	72–100	Golgi tendon organs
		β (II)	Yes	4–12	24–72	Flower spray
		γ (II)	Yes	1–4	6–24	Touch, somatic efferent
		δ (III)	No?	<1	0.6–2	Pain
Small	B		Yes	1–4	3–15	Visceral afferent/efferent
Very small	C	(IV)	No	<1	0.6–2	Pain, temperature, visceral efferent

Source: Adapted from Matthews, P.B.C., *Mammalian Muscle Receptors and their Central Actions*, Edward Arnold, Ltd., London, U.K., 1972.

organs, through the visceral system. Each of the tracts or pathways in the CNS or nerves in the peripheral nervous system are composed of thousands of smaller neurons, which vary considerably both size and function as summarized in Table 3.1. These will become more important in Section 3.10 regarding reflex pathways and motor control.

3.5 Excitation–Contraction Sequence

The generalized excitation–contraction sequence of a nerve impulse traveling from the brain and causing a muscle contraction is as follows. An action potential originates in the motor cortex of the brain and travels down the pyramidal tract to the neuromuscular junction. There, a chemical neurotransmitter, acetylcholine (ACh), is released from vesicles in the synaptic knob. The ACh molecules diffuse across the synapse, to the motor end plate on the muscle fiber (see Figure 3.10).

The ACh attaches to a receptor, causing a small potential at the motor end plate, termed a miniature end-plate potential (MEPP). All of the MEPPs, from many ACh molecules, summate to create a motor end-plate potential, which creates an action potential in the muscle fiber, in a one-to-one response. Eventually, an enzyme, cholinesterase, breaks down ACh into choline and acetic acid which separately diffuse back to vesicles to be reformed into ACh.

Note that the neuromuscular junction is a very critical point in the neuromuscular system and a variety of poisons and drugs can have some very powerful effects here. Curare blocks the receptor sites, preventing muscle contraction (e.g., respiratory muscles) and eventually causing the individual to asphyxiate. Cocaine blocks the reuptake of choline and acetic acid, allowing continual stimulation, until the ACh is used up. Botulism blocks the release of ACh and thus prevents the excitation of muscle. The disease myasthemia gravis causes a decrease in ACh receptor sites, reducing the motor end-plate potential, and eventually reducing the strength of muscle contraction.

The muscle action potential changes the membrane permeability of a series of tubules and sacs surrounding the myofibrils, termed the *sarcoplasmic reticulum,* so as to release stored calcium ions (Ca^{2+}) into the filaments (see Figure 3.12). The calcium ions cause a change in the troponin–tropomyosin–action complex on the thin filament removing an inhibition and allowing the further interaction between actin (A) and myosin (M) to occur. Troponin is a complex molecule with three subunits: troponin-T, which binds to tropomyosin; troponin-C,

Myofibrils

← T system tubule
← Terminal cisternae
← Intermediate cisternae
← Fenestrated collar

Sarcoplasmic reticulum

Triad

FIGURE 3.12
Schematic diagram of the sarcoplasmic reticulum surrounding myofibrils. (Reproduced from Peachey, L.D., *J. Cell Biol.*, 25, 209, 1965.)

which binds with the calcium ions; and troponin-I, which is the actual inhibitory unit. Specifically, calcium ions cause the troponin complex to pull the tropomyosin out of the receptor site, which is occupied by the S_1 unit of myosin to form a bond.

At this point, some energy is required and is provided by the most basic energy molecule, adenosine triphosphate (ATP). With the addition of some magnesium ions (Mg^{2+}), the ATP begins to be split (*hydrolized*) by the S_1 unit of HMM:

$$ATP \cdot M \Rightarrow ADP \cdot P_i \cdot M \tag{3.1}$$

A contortional change occurs in the S_1 head, allowing bonding to occur between the action (A) and myosin (M):

$$ADP \cdot P_i \cdot M + A \Rightarrow A - M \cdot ADP \cdot P_i \tag{3.2}$$

The ATP is completely hydrolyzed, leaving a true bond in the form of a cross bridge between the thick and thin filaments:

$$A - M \cdot ADP \cdot P_i \Rightarrow A - M + ADP + P_i \tag{3.3}$$

To break the actin–myosin bond, a fresh ATP molecule is needed:

$$A - M + ATP \Rightarrow A + M \cdot ATP \tag{3.4}$$

Then, the myosin molecule is free to advance to the next G-actin molecule and repeat the previous steps in forming another cross bridge. For relaxation of the muscle, the Ca^{2+} ions are released from troponin and are taken back up into sarcoplasmic reticulum. This last step again requires energy in the form of ATP.

Example 3.1: Metabolism, Energy, and ATP

ATP is created by the metabolism of the basic foods we eat: carbohydrates, fats, and proteins. This metabolism can occur in two different modes: *aerobic*, requiring oxygen, and *anaerobic*, not using oxygen. Aerobic metabolism uses a slow biochemical pathway, the citric acid or Krebs cycle, to generate 38 ATPs for each glucose molecule, the basic unit of carbohydrates.

$$C_6H_{12}O_6 + 6O_2 \Rightarrow 6CO_2 + 6H_2O + 38\ ATP \qquad (3.5)$$

On the other hand, anaerobic metabolism utilizes a fast glycolytic enzyme to break down the glucose molecule into two lactate molecules and produce two ATPs.

$$C_6H_{12}O_6 \Rightarrow 2C_3H_6O_3 + 2\ ATP \qquad (3.6)$$

The lactate molecule in the extracellular fluid of the body forms *lactic acid*, which is a direct correlate of fatigue. Thus, there is tradeoff—aerobic metabolism is slow but very efficient, while anaerobic metabolism, is very fast but inefficient and gives rise to fatigue.

Overall, there are several key steps in the excitation–contraction sequence. The calcium ions are critical in inhibiting the troponin inhibitor. Energy, in the form of ATP, is needed for contraction, relaxation, and also Ca^{2+} ion uptake. If somehow ATP production is completely stopped, the muscle cannot relax. This is the reason for rigor mortis in dead animals. The myosin molecule serves two functions. The S_2 unit bonds with actin to form the cross bridge while the S_1 unit acts as an enzyme to split ATP.

3.6 Motor Units

The *motor unit* is the functional unit of muscle, defined as one motor neuron (sometimes termed a *motoneuron*) and all of the muscle fibers innervated by the branches of the motor neuron axon. Motor units can vary in size considerably, from as low as 10 muscle fibers in the external rectus of the eye muscles, to as high as 2000 in the gastrocnemius in the calf. These muscle fibers are not clumped together but are distributed throughout the muscle, leading to a more distributed force production. Also, once an action potential is produced in the motor neuron, it travels down all of the branches of the motor neuron and activates all of the muscle fibers that it innervates in another type of all-or-nothing response. The ratio of muscle fibers to motor neuron is termed the *innervation ratio* and is important in determining muscle properties as discussed further in the next section.

3.6.1 Types of Motor Units

There are three types of motor units based on the functional characteristics of the component muscle fibers such as electrophysiological and biochemical properties. Typically, the slow-twitch fibers (Type I or SO) are small with relatively low force but use aerobic metabolism and thus are good for sustained long-term effort without undue fatigue. On the opposite extreme, fast-twitch fibers (Type IIB or FG) are large and respond quickly with high amounts of force, but fatigue quickly because of anaerobic metabolism. In between are fast but fatigue-resistant fibers (Type IIA or FOG) with moderate levels of force and moderate levels of fatigue due a reliance on both types of metabolism. The slow-twitch fibers are

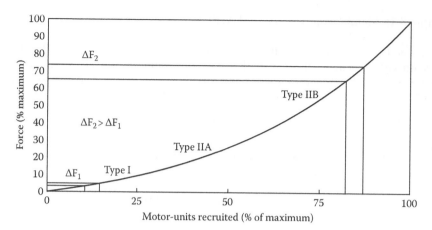

FIGURE 3.13
Motor-unit recruitment demonstrating the size principle and precision in motor control.

typically small and found in smaller motor units, i.e., they have small innervation ratios. This leads to very precise control of force development and movement because each additional motor-unit provides a small increase in force, i.e., ΔF_1 in Figure 3.13 (also a shallower slope). The fast-twitch fibers are typically found in large motor units with large innervation ratios leading to larger jumps in force with each additional motor-unit recruited and thus less precise control, i.e., compare ΔF_2 to ΔF_1 in Figure 3.13 (also a steeper slope).

The above process is a very specific, orderly recruitment of motor units by the size of the neuron, with the smallest slow twitch, Type I fibers recruited first, followed by the intermediate fast, fatigue-resistant, Type IIA fibers, and, finally, by the largest fast twitch, Type IIB fibers. This *size principle*, first postulated by Henneman et al. (1965), exists because the threshold for creating an action potential and firing the motor neuron is overcome more easily in the smallest neurons. For a given number of impulses from other neurons, the excitatory potentials summate most easily across the soma and the dendrites. In larger neurons, the same numbers of excitatory potentials are dispersed over a much larger surface area. Note that in terms of work design, it is inadvisable to perform precise activities immediately after heavy work. Some of the smaller motor units may have fatigued and larger ones will have been recruited with less precise control.

Typically, a muscle will have all three types of fibers, but in varying quantities. Some muscles, such as the soleus in the calf will have a preponderance of slow-twitch fibers, while others such as the brachioradialis will have a preponderance of fast-twitch fibers. To some degree, the characteristics of the fibers can be modified through specific training as in high-level sporting activities. However, to a large degree, the distribution of fibers is genetically determined. Thus, some individuals with a large proportion of slow-twitch fibers will naturally be distance runners, while other individuals, with a large proportion of fast-twitch fibers will naturally be sprinters or power lifters. A general summary of motor-unit characteristics is provided in Table 3.2.

3.6.2 Motor-Unit Twitch

When the motor end plate of a muscle fiber is stimulated via the transfer of ACh molecules, the MEPP causes an action potential to travel down the muscle fiber releasing calcium ions from the sarcoplasmic reticulum and initiating the excitation–contraction sequence.

TABLE 3.2

Motor-Unit Characteristics

Characteristic	Type of Motor-Unit		
	I/SO	**IIA/FOG**	**IIB/FG**
General label	Slow oxidative	Fast oxidative, glycolytic	Fast glycolytic
Contraction velocity	Slow	Fast	Fast
Tetanic frequency (Hz)	~30	~50–60	~100
Metabolism	Oxidative, aerobic	Fast oxidative + glycolytic, aerobic + anaerobic	Glycolytic, anaerobic
Fatigability	Fatigue resistant	Intermediate	Fast fatigable
Twitch force	Low	Medium	High
Twitch time (ms)	~120	~60–80	~20
Size of fibers/motoneurons	Small	Intermediate	Large
Color	Red	Red	Pale
Proportion			
Brachioradialis	35%	—	65%
Biceps	40%	—	60%
Triceps	32%	—	68%
Soleus	80%	—	20%

The resulting contraction is called a twitch response and varies in size and duration depending on the type of muscle and muscle fibers involved, but not on the size of the stimulus since for a motor-unit, the responses is an all-or-nothing response. There is always an initial *latency period* or a delay before a rise in tension is seen. This is due to the conduction time of the action potential down the muscle fiber and into the sarcoplasmic reticulum as well as the time for the calcium ions to be released from the sarcoplasmic reticulum.

Should the muscle fiber be stimulated again before the first twitch has died away, the second twitch reaches a higher force level. This is a potentiating effect since during the relaxation period (an especially during the contraction period), there are still some calcium ions found in the myofibrils (termed the *active state*). Therefore, the protein filaments have not been completely inhibited and are easier to stimulate, resulting in a larger contraction. If the stimulation is repeated at higher frequency bursts (shorter interstimulation interval times), the resulting force output becomes even higher resulting in a steady force level termed unfused *tetanus*. Eventually, with even higher frequencies, the ripples between successive twitches disappear resulting in a fused tetanus with an even larger force output (see Figure 3.14). However, this is

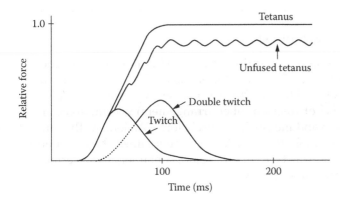

FIGURE 3.14
Twitch and tetanus. Sufficiently high frequency stimuli cause twitch forces to summate to yield a steady force termed tetanus.

the maximum force that can be produced by this motor-unit at this given frequency termed *tetanic frequency*. Higher frequencies will not yield any more increases in force. This tetanic frequency varies from a low of roughly 30 Hz in the soleus to over 300 Hz in the eye muscles. However, for the muscles in the upper limbs, the upper frequency is closer to 100 Hz.

The magnitude of muscle contraction, thus, depends to a large extent on the frequency of stimulation, but also on the magnitude of stimulation, in which case, a greater number of motor units will be recruited. Note that two mechanisms for increasing muscular contraction are not completely independent. Based on the size principle and orderly recruitment of motor units, the smaller motor units have lower tetanic frequencies, while the larger motor units have higher tetanic frequencies.

Muscle contractions at a gross external level can be characterized in the following ways.

Static or *isometric* contractions refer to force production without changes in muscle length. Dynamic contractions refer to conditions under which muscle length changes. If the muscle is shortening, then it is *concentric*. If the muscle is lengthening, then it is *eccentric*. Eccentric contractions are relatively uncommon is everyday life; walking or running downhill or trying to maintain control of a load to heavy to lift up are a couple of examples. Dynamic contractions can be *isotonic*, in which the muscle force remains constant, or *isokinetic*, in which the muscle contracts at a constant velocity, or *isoinertial*, in which the muscle contracts at a constant acceleration. These constraints are imposed so as to have a controlled set of conditions in measuring or comparing dynamic muscle contractions.

Maximum muscle tension is determined by the number of muscle fibers involved. This, obviously, cannot be counted and is typically approximated by the cross-sectional area of the muscle, taken perpendicular to the fibers at the largest point of the muscle, called the belly. This tension or force factor ranges from 40 to 80 N/cm^2 depending on the researcher and the methods used to determine cross-sectional area. This is a relatively simple procedure for fusiform muscle in which the fibers are relatively parallel. However, for multipennate muscles the fiber arrangement varies considerably and no perpendicular cut can be easily achieved. Therefore, most researchers use the volume of the muscle (as determined by the weight of the muscle divided by the density) divided by length to obtain an average cross-sectional area. Note that, muscle cross section increases during muscle contraction due to the overlapping of filaments. However, muscle fibers also shorten during contraction causing the overall volume of the active muscle to remain constant.

3.7 Basic Muscle Properties (Mechanics)

Most of the basic muscle properties were determined by A.V. Hill and his colleagues at the University College, London, between 1910 and 1950 on isolated muscle preparations. These studies are summarized nicely in Hill's (1970) last treatise. Typically a frog's sartorius muscle (having the ideal parallel or fusiform fiber arrangement) was mounted in an apparatus for stimulating the muscle and measuring muscle force. As long as the muscle was kept in an oxygenated saline solution, the muscle fibers maintained their properties for several days. Since the preparation was typically in a glass container, it was termed in vitro as opposed to in vivo, or within a living body.

3.7.1 Active Length–Tension Relationship

The tension developed during muscle contraction is a nonlinear function that depends very specifically on muscle length. Maximum tension is found near the length that the muscle occupies in a relaxed state in the body, or *resting length*, and then drops off as either the muscle shortens or lengthens (see Figure 3.15). At the resting length (position 3), there is maximum overlap between the thin filaments and the entire cross-bridging zone of the thick filament, i.e., all myosin heads have a corresponding G-actin molecule for attachment. The plateau area between positions 2 and 3 results because of the lack of myosin heads in the H-band, and as result, even though the muscle fiber lengthens, no cross bridges are lost. However, at longer lengths, the tension drops off linearly because with each added increase in length the fewer cross bridges are available. This drop off continues until roughly 170%–180% of resting length (position 4), at which point, no overlap between the myosin heads and G-actin molecules is possible and no tension is produced.

When the muscle fiber shortens, on the other hand, the opposite thin filaments overlap and interfere with the bonding to myosin to actin reducing tension. At position 1, or roughly 60% of resting length, there is complete interference of the thin filaments and no cross bridging is possible. Consequently, no force is produced. Also then thick filaments collide with the Z-disks, further complicating any possible cross bridging. This has been supported by electron micrographs, the complete disappearance of the I-bands and the narrowing of the A-bands.

This nonlinear length–tension relationship has been utilized in the development of various strength training devices (such as the Nautilus) to provide the appropriate level of external resistance as the limb and muscles move through its range of motion.

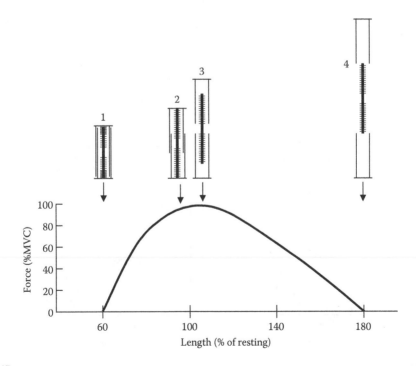

FIGURE 3.15
Active length–tension relationship in a muscle with corresponding sliding filament relationships. (Adapted from Gordon, A.M., et al., *J. Physiol.*, 184, 170, 1966.)

3.7.2 Passive Length–Tension Relationship

The above property was a characteristic of stimulated muscle fibers, thus an active muscle property. However, muscle does not consist solely of the protein filaments, but also contains an extensive soft connective tissue network, primarily fascia composed of elastin. The passive properties of such tissue can be easily observed by recording the force as the passive (no electrical stimulation) muscle is stretched (see Figure 3.16). The rate of tension increase is linear per applied stress:

$$\frac{d\sigma}{d\ell} = \alpha\sigma \tag{3.7}$$

Integrating both sides yields:

$$\sigma = k\ell^{\alpha\ell} \tag{3.8}$$

When the muscle is stimulated, the tension changes dramatically because of the added effect of active contraction. The total muscle tension then becomes the combined effect of the active and passive force components (see Figure 3.17) with a pronounced dip at 120%–150% of resting length. This dip becomes more pronounced as the amount of fascia decreases in the muscle preparation. Thus, multipennate fibers, such as the deltoid, with short fibers and relatively large amount of connective tissue will show almost a

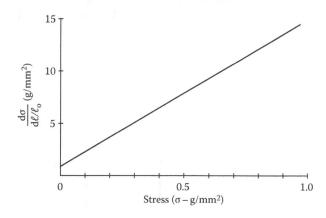

FIGURE 3.16
Passive length–tension relationship in a muscle. The stress-to-strain rate is a linearly increasing function of stress. (Adapted from Pinto, J.G. and Fung, Y.C., *J. Biomech.*, 6, 597, 1973.)

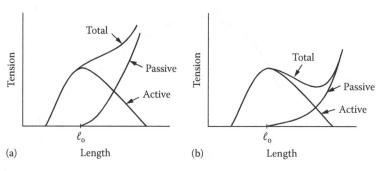

FIGURE 3.17
Combined active and passive length–tension relationships in (a) bipennate and (b) fusiform muscles. (Adapted from McMahon, T.A., *Muscles, Reflexes, and Locomotion*, Princeton University Press, Princeton, NJ, 1984.)

continual increase in muscle tension, while purely parallel-fibered muscle with relatively little connective tissue, such as the biceps, shows considerable dip. Note that a typical range of motion experienced by an in vivo muscle would be on the order of 80%–120% resting length.

3.7.3 Velocity–Tension Relationship

It can be easily observed that during concentric motion, as the velocity of the movement increases, the amount of force developed by muscle decreases (see Figure 3.18). Two factors contribute to this effect: (1) less efficient bonding in the cross bridges with more rapid sliding of the filaments past each other and (2) a damping effect of the fluid-filled muscle tissue. This relationship, also known as the force–velocity relationship, was first observed by Fenn and Marsh (1935) and later used by Hill (1938) to develop the first model of muscle. Interestingly, for eccentric motions, the tension developed by the muscle can increase to a higher value than observed in an isometric state (Katz, 1939). This is probably due to the fact that breaking the protein cross bridges requires more force than to hold them at their isometric limit. Also, the external force must overcome latent viscous friction still present from the shortening stage (Winter, 1991). Eccentric contractions result in greater stress on and consequent micro trauma to the soft connective tissues within the muscle as evidenced by the greater soreness in eccentric exercise such as downhill running.

For the concentric part of the curve, Hill (1938) proposed an empirical quantitative formulation of the hyperbolic shape:

$$(T+a)(v+b) = (T_0 + a)b \qquad (3.9)$$

where
  T is the tension
  T_0 is the isometric tension
  v is the velocity

FIGURE 3.18
Hill's velocity–tension relationship. Note increase in force for eccentric and peak power at $0.3v_{max}$. (Adapted from McMahon, T.A., *Muscles, Reflexes, and Locomotion*, Princeton University Press, Princeton, NJ, 1984.)

Note, that the asymptotes of the hyperbola are not zero, but instead T = −a and v = −b. A normalized form allows one to compare different muscles with one equation:

$$v' = \frac{(1-T')}{(1+T'/k)} \tag{3.10}$$

where $v' = v/v_{max}$, $T' = T/T_0$, $k = a/T_0 = b/v_{max}$.
For most muscles, k ranges between 0.15 and 0.25.
The total mechanical power available from a muscle can be expressed as:

$$\text{Power} = Tv = \frac{v\,(bT_0 - av)}{(v+b)} \tag{3.11}$$

and maximum power (depending on the value of k) occurs at roughly $0.3\,v_{max}$ and $0.3\,T_0$ and almost reaches a value of $0.1\,T_0 v_{max}$. The advantage of maintaining an optimum velocity is demonstrated in bicycling, in which the rider will gear up or down depending on the external conditions of slope, wind, etc., to maintain in optimum pedaling speed.

3.7.4 Active State Properties

The active state was originally meant to refer to the condition a contracting muscle is in as opposed to a resting state. More specifically, it refers to the residual tension in a muscle related to the amount of calcium remaining in the muscle filaments, at which time a greater force can be produced with a second stimulation. This was first demonstrated by Ritchie (1954) in a set of *quick release* experiments. The quick release of a stop mechanism (see Figure 3.19) exposes the muscle to a constant load with a stimulation occurring at increasing times after the release. The muscle shortens against the load until the connection to the force transducer is taught registering additional force on the transducer. After a sufficiently long period of time, the muscle has completed its contraction phase exhibiting

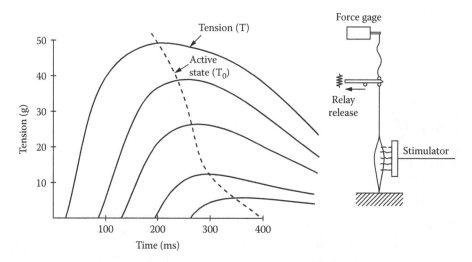

FIGURE 3.19
Quick release experiments defining the active state function. (Reproduced from Ritchie, J.M., *J. Physiol.*, 125, 155, 1954. With permission.)

minimal or no force on the transducer. The maximum point of the resulting set of curves defines the active state tension T_0 as function of time (and corresponds to the relaxation time for a twitch).

3.7.5 Developments Leading to Hill's Muscle Model

In a second set of quick release experiments, a load was attached to the muscle. The mechanism maintains the muscle in isometric tetanus appropriate for its length. After the release of the catch, the muscle is allowed to shorten (not held at constant length) but is regulated by the constant force of the load. The amount of shortening depends on the difference in force generated before and after the release. Hill suggested that there is some sort of a spring or *series elastic element* in the muscle (see Figure 3.20), which has a unique length for every tension level and is not dependent of velocity. This element probably corresponds to the tendon structure and has a slope value of maximum tension over a 2% change in muscle resting length.

The passive tension curves suggest that there must also be a *parallel elastic element* which resists passive stretching. This may represent the different types of fascia and membranes that are parallel to the filaments. The velocity–tension relationship (i.e., muscle force is greatest when velocity is zero) suggests that there is a dynamic resistance to movement or that force is dissipated while overcoming an inherent viscous resistance. Therefore, Hill proposed that the contractile element is pure force generator with a parallel nonlinear *damping element* or dashpot. All of the proposed elements can be combined into a four-element muscle model frequently termed Hill's model (see Figure 3.21). The model can also be expressed mathematically as a series of differential equations, which when solved will explain many of the basic mechanical properties of muscle. However, solution of these equations will left until Chapter 4 when the introduction of Laplace transforms will allow for an easier solution of these equations.

3.7.6 Fatigue and Endurance

It can be easily shown that a maximum force (tetanic frequency, full motor-unit recruitment) can only be maintained for short period of time, 6 s, whereas a relatively low value of

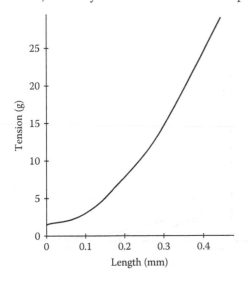

FIGURE 3.20
Length–tension relationship for the series elastic component. (Adapted from Jewell, B.R. and Wilkie, D.R., *J. Physiol.*, 143, 515, 1958.)

FIGURE 3.21
Hill's four-element model with a contractile component generating tension, T_{CE}.

15% of maximum can be maintained for extended periods of time, perhaps several hours. This corresponds exactly with the point at which the mechanical action of a contracting muscle becomes large enough to start compressing the weak (in compression) walls of arteries and occluding blood flow. As the muscle force increases, less blood reaches the working muscle with a corresponding decrease in oxygen availability. This means that the muscle must rely on smaller amount of aerobic metabolism and a greater amount of glycolytic metabolism with concurrent fatigue. At roughly 70% max the blood flow is completely occluded and fatigue (as defined by the ability to maintain the given contraction level) occurs very quickly. This phenomenon (see Figure 3.22) was first observed by Rohmert (1960) in the muscles of the upper limbs and can be quantified as a simple hyperbolic relationship with an asymptote at roughly 15% of maximum strength:

$$T_{end}(s) = \frac{1236.5}{(\%max - 15)^{0.618}} - 72.5 \tag{3.12}$$

In addition to the depletion of nutrients in the muscle fibers, muscle fatigue may also occur in the neuromuscular junction due to a depletion of ACh, in the nervous system with a depletion of ions to produce the action potentials, or perhaps in the protein filaments themselves with decrease in contractility of the cross bridges. Note, that full recovery from a maximum contraction of a 5 s duration may require a minimum of at least 2 min if not more, and has led to standardized procedures to be used in properly

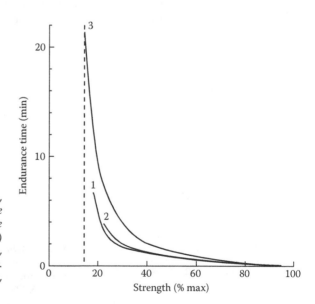

FIGURE 3.22
Endurance curves for various muscles. 1, Arm, leg, trunk. (From Rohmert, W., *Internationale Zeitschrift für Angewandte Physiologie Einschliesslich Arbeitsphysiologie*, 18, 123, 1960.) 2, Upper limbs pulling. (From Caldwell, L.S., *J. Eng. Psychol.*, 2, 155, 1963.) 3, Biceps, triceps. (From Monod, H. and Scherrer, J., *Ergonomics*, 8, 329, 1965.)

assessing human strength (Chaffin, 1975). However, in terms of overall work efficiency, it is best to use short work–rest cycles. This does not allow the muscle to go into anaerobic metabolism and also utilizes the quick recovery of myoglobin stores as so aptly demonstrated by Åstrand et al. (1960b).

3.8 Energy, Metabolism, and Heat Production

Heat production in muscle was measured as early as 1848 by Helmholtz, but the real work was done by A.V. Hill and his colleagues from 1910 to 1950. To measure very small changes of heat production occurring in isolated muscle tissue samples, a very sensitive instrument such as the *thermocouple* was needed. A thermocouple works on the principle of two dissimilar metals (typically copper and nickel), which when connected, create an electrical potential and current proportional to the surrounding temperature. Thus, when properly calibrated, the thermocouple becomes a very sensitive thermometer. Because the temperature changes for a single twitch in a muscle fiber are very small, on the order of 0.003°C, the sensitivity of the thermocouple needed to be improved. By connecting many thermocouples in series to yield a thermopile and using a sensitive galvanometer to measure very small currents, Hill was able to detect temperature changes as small as 0.000001°C.

Resting heat (H_{rest}) is a basic steady state heat of muscle tissue, the simple consequence of the tissue being alive. This is a very small number, amounting to 0.0002 cal/g/min., and will be very much exceeded by the heat production occurring during active contraction. In both isometric and isotonic contractions, an *activation heat* (H_{act}) appears 10–15 ms after the stimulus, begins to increase rapidly and reaches a maximum long before tension is fully developed (see Figure 3.23). It coincides with the active state and, thus, is prolonged during tetanus. It also varies as a function of fiber length.

In an isotonic contraction, there is also additional heat termed the *heat of shortening* (H_{shor}). It was demonstrated by Fenn (1923) that a muscle which shortens produces more heat that when it contracts isometrically. Thus, it is sometimes called the *Fenn effect*, but the true relationship was refined by Hill (1938). In his experiments, a muscle was isometrically tetanized. It was then released and allowed to shorten against a load. With increasing loads, additional heat was produced with the extra heat (the difference between

FIGURE 3.23
The activation heat rises quickly even before tension is developed. (Adapted from Hill, A.V., *Proc. Royal Soc.*, 141, 314, 1953.)

shortening and no shortening) being due to true physical work being done. This physical work is the product of the force exerted and the distance the muscle moved.

The activation heat and heat of shortening are sometimes termed *initial heat* because they occur during muscle contraction as opposed to after the contraction, which is termed relaxation or recovery heat (H_{relax}). This relaxation heat can be liberated over a period of several minutes after contraction and corresponds to the muscle recovering oxygen and regenerating lactate to glucose and is up to 50% greater than the initial heat.

There may be two other types of heats involved in muscle contraction. During eccentric contractions, the lengthening muscle also produces heat (H_{leng}) but it is much less than is produced in isotonic concentric type work. This evidenced by hikers sweating profusely while going uphill and putting on extra clothing while going downhill. Part of this difference may be explained by the larger tension created during eccentric contractions and part due to energy being absorbed by bones and other connective tissues of the musculoskeletal system. This may explain the surprising soreness experienced after such downhill walking. Muscle may also show thermoelastic heat (H_{therm}). Most materials exhibit normal thermoelasticity, expanding when heated and cooling slightly when forcibly stretched. Rubber-like materials exhibit the opposite effect, heating when forcibly stretched. A muscle actually shows both effects; a resting muscle rubber thermoelasticity, while an active muscle normal thermoelasticity.

In summary, the various heats can be combined into the following total heat (H_{tot}) for an isotonic contraction:

$$H_{tot} = H_{rest} + H_{act} + H_{shor} + H_{relax} + H_{therm} \qquad (3.13)$$

with H_{shor} being replaced by H_{leng} for eccentric contractions and H_{shor} eliminated for isometric contractions.

These heats correspond to chemical activity in the muscle primarily the hydrolysis of ATP. ATP is regenerated from creatine phosphate (CP) an intermediary chemical compound:

$$ADP + CP \Rightarrow ATP + Cr \qquad (3.14)$$

where Cr is the basic creatine molecule.

During work or exercise, the initial energy will come from ATP, which is regenerated by CP. While the ATP stores in muscle fiber are used up almost instantly, CP can provide energy for 10 s or more (see Figure 3.24). However, the ATP and CP have to be continually

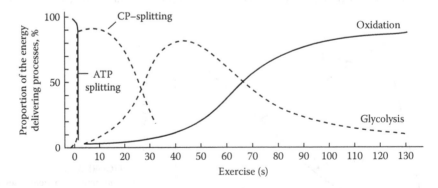

FIGURE 3.24
Schematic representation of energy sources during intense work. (Reproduced from Chaffin, D.B. et al., *Occupational Biomechanics*, 3rd edn., John Wiley & Sons, New York, 1999.)

TABLE 3.3

Percent Metabolic Energy Sources for Different Activities

| | Anaerobic | | Aerobic |
Activity	ATP + CP	Glycogen	(Oxidative)
Weightlifting	98	2	0
Tennis	70	20	10
100 m run	95	5	0
1500 m run	20	60	20
Marathon run	0	5	95
Century bike ride	0	5	95

regenerated through the Krebs cycle. For high workloads, energy will be provided quickly through glycolysis but this leads to higher concentrations of lactate and fairly quick fatigue. For lower workloads, the aerobic contribution increases (see Table 3.3) and keeps pace with the work load for extended periods of time. This was demonstrated very nicely by Åstrand et al. (1960) in an experiment in which subjects exercised at a constant workload of 412 W (see Figure 3.25). Those subjects that exercised for 10 s and took 20 s rest were able to complete the full 30 min, at low blood lactate levels, while those that exercised for 60 s and took 120 s breaks had extremely elevated blood lactate and could not even complete a 30 min, bout of exercise.

FIGURE 3.25

Blood lactate concentration in high intensity work performed in various work–rest cycles. (Reproduced from Åstrand, P.O. and Rodahl, K., *Textbook of Work Physiology*, McGraw-Hill Book Co., New York, 1986. With permission.)

During the shorter bouts of work, only ATP, CP, and some of the oxygen stored in muscle (*myoglobin*) was utilized. During the rest breaks, these sources were replenished with minimal penalty. For longer bouts of work, the muscle utilized the glycolytic process to produce energy quickly at the penalty of elevating blood lactate and incurring fatigue. Thus, the optimum arrangement of work is to have short, frequent work–rest cycles.

Note also the role of glycogen in the energy production process. By increasing the amount of carbohydrates in the diet (*carbohydrate loading*) 2 or 3 days prior to an intense physical activity, the concentration of glycogen in the muscle can be increased from 1.5 g per 100 g of muscle to 2.5 g (or even higher levels with more extreme dietary changes) with an associated increase in endurance for that sustained activity.

For more details on muscle physiology and mechanics please refer to McMahon (1984), Aidley (1985), Jones et al. (1986), and Winter (1991).

3.9 Receptors

Receptors are specialized nerve cells that provide the CNS about external stimuli. Typically, they respond only to the specific stimuli they have evolved for, with increasing output in the form of higher frequency action potentials with increasing magnitudes of stimulation. Thus, the photoreceptors in the retina respond only to light and the hair cells in the inner ear to sound pressure waves. They can be classified as *exteroreceptors*, those that respond to a conscious sensation such as above two examples, or as *proprioreceptors*, those that respond to unconscious sensations, such as those related to motor control discussed below. Most receptors also have the basic property of *accommodation*, in which they adapt to a constant level stimulus by decreasing the rate of firing (see Figure 3.26).

3.9.1 Muscle Spindles

Muscle spindles are modified muscle fibers that are thinner and shorter and have specialized neural receptor endings. They typically are located in parallel to the regular muscle fibers and respond to changes in fiber length and velocity changes. The muscle spindles have a connective tissue capsule giving rise to the name spindle or *fusiform* (see Figure 3.27). The muscle fibers within the spindle are termed *intrafusal* fibers while

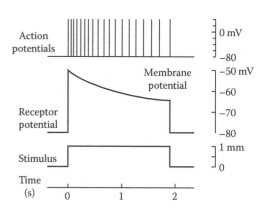

FIGURE 3.26
Receptor properties showing generation of action potentials and accommodation.

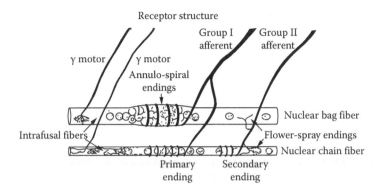

FIGURE 3.27
Schematic representation of nuclear bag and nuclear chain fibers and primary and secondary endings in a muscle spindle. (From Matthews, P.B.C., *Mammalian Muscle Receptors and Their Central Actions*, Edward Arnold, Ltd., London, U.K., 1972.)

the regular muscle fibers outside the spindle are termed *extrafusal* fibers. Note that the extrafusal fibers are greater in numbers, larger in size (100 μ versus 20 μ in diameter and 10–20 cm versus 5 mm in length) and produce much more force. Also, the distribution of muscle spindles varies considerably according to the muscle; whereas the small muscles such as the interosseus of the fingers may have up to 120 spindles per gram of muscle, large muscle such as the gastrocnemius may have only 5 or fewer spindles per gram of muscle. This again has considerable implications for control, with the former allowing for very fine control and the latter with less fine control.

Muscle spindles have two types of receptors: *primary* and *secondary* endings. The primary endings, also known as the *annulospiral* are found in the equatorial region of the spindle where there are few fibers (see Figure 3.27). They generally are sensitive to both the displacement of the muscle as well as the rate of displacement or velocity changes, and usually show a phasic response, with a 5 s transient peak and then a slower decay of about 1 min back to the baseline of no firing (see Figure 3.28). They are innervated by Ia or α afferents and have a fairly low threshold.

The secondary endings, also known as *flower spray* endings, are found in the polar regions of the spindle, where there are many fibers (see Figure 3.27). They are sensitive only to displacements, showing a tonic response, with a 5 s transient peak and then a fairly uniform firing rate proportional to the stretch (see Figure 3.28). They are innervated by II or β nerve afferents and have a fairly high threshold. Both endings together are typically referred to as *stretch receptors*. A comparison of the two muscle receptors (as well as other receptors) is provided in Table 3.4.

The intrafusal muscle fibers are of two distinct types: *nuclear-bag* and *nuclear-chain* fibers (see Figure 3.27). The nuclear bag fibers are about 8 mm long and have swollen equatorial regions, while the nuclear chain fibers are half as long with no central swelling. All nuclear

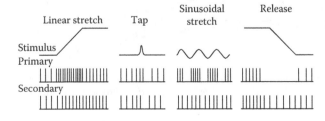

FIGURE 3.28
Typical response of primary and secondary endings to different types of stretch. (Reproduced from Matthews, P.B.C., *Mammalian Muscle Receptors and Their Central Actions*, Edward Arnold, Ltd., London, U.K., 1972. With permission.)

TABLE 3.4

Summary of Receptor Characteristics

Characteristic	Muscle Spindles		Golgi Tendon Organs	Proprioreceptors	Pacinian Corpuscles
	Primary Ending	Secondary Ending			
Afferent fiber	α (Ia)	β (II)	α (Ib)	γ?	γ?
Velocity (m/s)	80–125	50–80	80–125	6–20	6–20
Sensitivity	High	Low	High	—	—
Gain (AP/s/unit)	100/mm	10/mm	20–180/kg	2/degree	—
Threshold, static	Low (~50 μm)	High (~500 μm)	20–200 g	Low	Medium
Threshold, dynamic	Low (~5 μm)	—	—	High (5°/ms)	Low (20 μm/2 ms)
Adaptation	1 min.	4–5 h	3 s	Hours	6 ms

Source: Adapted from Matthews, P.B.C., *Mammalian Muscle Receptors and Their Central Actions*, Edward Arnold, Ltd., London, U.K., 1972.

bag and most nuclear chain fibers have primary endings, while all nuclear chain and some nuclear bag fibers have secondary endings. A typical muscle spindle will have two nuclear bag fibers and four to five nuclear chain fibers.

3.9.2 Golgi Tendon Organs

Golgi tendon organs are specialized encapsulated fascicles of dense collagen which are offshoots from the primary tendon at the tendon–muscle junction. The fascicles, typically five, project into the muscle mass on the way to becoming attached to a bundle of extrafusal muscle fibers (see Figure 3.29). Branches of Ib or α sensory (afferent) nerves intertwine among the five bundles of collagen fibers, which in a relaxed Golgi tendon organ are spread open to reduce pressure upon the nerve endings lying between them. During tension, these bundles straighten and crowd together, compressing the nerve endings and creating electrochemical changes in the nerve (Bridgman, 1968). Thus, the Golgi tendon organs respond to forces imposed upon them by postural and locomotor activity, which could in the form of passive forces developed by the muscle stretch and active forces resulting from muscle contraction. They have a surprisingly low threshold (see Table 3.4) with the contraction of a single motor unit sometimes being sufficient to excite the tendon organ. The response is a slowly adapting one (time constant = 3 s) with a threshold to active tension being lower than passive tension. As opposed to muscle spindles, which are in parallel to extrafusal fibers and measure muscle length, Golgi tendon organs are in series with the extrafusal fibers and measure muscle tension.

FIGURE 3.29
Schematic representation of a Golgi tendon organ: (a) tendon, (b) α afferent neuron, and (c) muscle fibers. (Reproduced from Matthews, P.B.C., *Mammalian Muscle Receptors and Their Central Actions*, Edward Arnold, Ltd., London, U.K., 1972. With permission.)

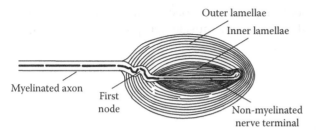

FIGURE 3.30
Schematic representation of a Pacinian corpuscle. (Reproduced from Quilliam, T.A. and Sato, M., *J. Physiol.*, 129, 167, 1955. With permission.)

3.9.3 Other Receptors

Other receptors involved with motor control include Pacinian corpuscles and joint proprioreceptors, proprioreceptor referring to motor function. Pacinian corpuscles are pressure sensitive receptors found on the fascia between muscles in the loose connective tissues near joints. Deformations of the outside covering are transmitted through its lamellae to the central nerve ending (see Figure 3.30). The responses are very phasic, adapting in 6 ms or less.

Joint proprioreceptors are of two basic types: Ruffini type (see Figure 3.31) and free nerve endings. The Ruffini type are of a tonic nature showing a 10 s transient and then maintaining a constant rate of firing proportional to the joint angle last for hours. Furthermore, they show a long-term adaptation, such that it takes more than 10 min, of baseline rest the same angular excursion will produce the same response. The response is bell shaped (see Figure 3.32) with maximum sensitivity for a small range of specific angles. In addition, there are also sensitive to the angular velocity of movement,

100 μm

FIGURE 3.31
Schematic representation of a Ruffini type ending found in joint capsules. (Reproduced from Matthews, P.B.C., *Mammalian Muscle Receptors and Their Central Actions*, Edward Arnold, Ltd., London, U.K., 1972. With permission.)

FIGURE 3.32
Bell-shaped response of joint propriorectors. Note the narrow range of angles to which the receptors respond. (Reproduced from Matthews, P.B.C., *Mammalian Muscle Receptors and Their Central Actions*, Edward Arnold, Ltd., London, U.K., 1972. With permission.)

the discharge increasing for movements toward the specific angle and decreasing for movements away. For further information on muscle receptors, please refer to Matthews (1972).

3.10 Reflexes and Motor Control

Axonal conduction of action potentials is a fundamental process in neural activity. Interconnections through synapses with other neurons or muscle fibers, as at the neuromuscular junction, are another component in this activity. For the motoneuron, at the neuromuscular junction, this was an excitation of the muscle fiber. At other locations, this process could be inhibitory. Furthermore, the motoneuron serves as an efferent pathway, away from the CNS, while other neurons serve as an afferent pathway, sending sensory information from receptors back to the CNS in the form of feedback. Thus, a set of neurons sending stimulus information to the CNS and receiving information back from the CNS, resulting in an appropriate response, can be considered as a system with a feedback loop. If this response is involuntary, i.e., does not require a conscious decision, then it is termed a *reflex*. A variety of such reflex pathways forms the basis for motor control and will be discussed in greater detail.

3.10.1 Stretch Reflex

The *stretch reflex* is the simplest reflex (see Figure 3.33) consisting of five components. The first is the muscle spindle, the receptor that receives and process the stimulus, in this case, a stretch on the spindle. The second is an afferent neuron serving as the input pathway to the CNS. For the stretch reflex the afferent neuron is typically the largest neuron, the α or Ia type. The afferent neuron enters the spinal cord through the dorsal horn of the spinal cord and synapses on a motoneuron. Note that the synapse occurs in the central H-shaped

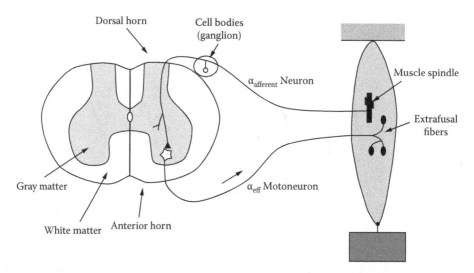

FIGURE 3.33
Schematic representation of a stretch reflex.

darker region of the spinal cord termed *gray matter* as opposed to the *white matter* or lighter region are surrounding it. The gray matter receives its color from the motoneuron cell bodies while the white matter receives its color from the myelin sheaths of the descending pyramidal and extrapyramidal tracts. Note that the cell body for afferent sensory neuron is located outside of the spinal cord in a complex of numerous other such cell bodies, termed a *ganglion*.

The third component is the motoneuron cell body, which serves as an integrating center of information. In the simplest stretch reflex, only one afferent input is required. However, in reality, the cell body is innervated with numerous other afferent inputs, some of which could also be inhibitory. The excitatory inputs depolarize that section of the motoneuron cell body in the form of excitatory post synaptic potentials (EPSPs), similar to the MEPPs at the neuromuscular junction, except that it does not necessarily produce a one-to-one response. Other innervating neurons, with a different neurotransmitter, may hyperpolarize the motoneuron cell body, creating inhibitory post synaptic potentials (IPSPs), which then make it more difficult for the neuron to be depolarize and fire an action potential. All of the EPSPs and IPSPs travel down the cell body membrane to the base of the axon, where all of the potentials summate and finally determine whether there is sufficient depolarization to create an action potential. Thus, the motoneuron cell body acts as a true integrating center or central processing unit.

The fourth component is the efferent path of the motoneuron. Again this neuron is typically the largest α or Ia type so as to provide the fastest conduction velocity. The fifth component is the effector or the extrafusal fibers of the muscle, which contract upon stimulation. A typical stretch reflex is the *patellar reflex* tested by a physician tapping just below the knee of a free-hanging leg with a mallet. A vigorous tap stretches the tendon of the quadriceps muscle, which, after a brief delay, contracts the muscle, raising the leg slightly and relieving the stretch on the tendon. Failure to react indicates some problem in one of the components of the reflex arc, requiring further testing. This type of reflex is also sometimes termed a monosynaptic reflex because only one synapse is required.

Example 3.2: Timing Sequence of a Stretch Reflex

The timing sequence of a patellar tap reflex can be calculated as follows. The annulospiral, synapse, neuromuscular junction, and end plate all have approximately 1 ms delays. The large α neurons conduct action potentials at a minimum of 100 m/s. Assuming a knee tap and the neuron stretching 0.5 m to the L_5/S_1 level of the spinal cord, nerve conduction in either direction requires 5 ms (=0.5/100). In addition, the extrafusal fibers need a minimum of 20+ ms to generate enough force to contract and move the muscle. As a result there is a minimum of a 34 ms delay before any muscle contraction would be apparent.

Element	Time (ms)
Annulospiral	1.0
α_{aff}	5.0
Synapse	1.0
α_{eff}	5.0
Neuromuscular junction	1.0
End-plate potential	1.0
Force buildup	20.0
Total	34.0

FIGURE 3.34
Activation of the annulospiral endings of a muscle spindle by (b) stretching the entire muscle or by (c) intrafusal contraction. (a) Resting length. (Adapted from Schmidt, R.F., *Fundamentals of Neurophysiology*, Springer Verlag, Heidelberg, Germany, 1975.)

3.10.2 γ-Loop Control

Muscle spindles consist of both stretch receptors and intrafusal contractile fibers. The latter serve as a means for controlling the gain of the stretch receptors. Contraction of the intrafusal fibers produces a stretch and excitation of the annulospiral comparable to that caused by an external mechanical stretch (see Figure 3.34). A combination of both events would produce an even larger stimulation of the stretch receptors with a consequently more forceful contraction of the extrafusal fibers.

The intrafusal fibers are innervated by smaller neurons of γ size (see Table 3.1), which emanate from the anterior horn of the spinal cord. Within the gray matter area, collaterals of the α afferent neurons make synaptic connections with γ neuron cell bodies in addition to α efferent motoneurons (see Figure 3.35). Should the initial stretch stimulus to the muscle spindle be weak, the resulting stimulus through the stretch reflex of Figure 3.34 may not be sufficient to fully contract the muscle and relieve the initial stretch. However, in the meantime, the α afferent neurons have sent a signal through the γ efferent neurons to the intrafusal fibers. Those fibers being much smaller in size would, according to size principle of Henneman et al. (1965), have a much greater likelihood of being fired. The resulting contraction on the annulospiral would increase the stretch stimulus sufficiently to eventually, after going around the stretch reflex again, fire the extrafusal fibers. However, the resulting timing sequence of 82 ms (see Example 3.3) would be considerably longer than timing sequence of 34 ms (see Example 3.2) for a pure stretch reflex. Note, also, that since several synapses, are involved the γ-loop is one type of a polysynaptic reflex.

Such γ control is a vital part of a length control system that the body uses to maintain an upright position while under the influence of gravity. As a result, many of the muscles, especially those in the neck, back, and lower limbs, are continually in a state of lower or higher tension, which is referred to as muscle tone. γ Control also plays a part in *tremor*, the physiological oscillation seen during sustained muscle contractions. For example, observe the tremor at the end of a finger tip while holding the arm extended (this amplifies the tremor seen at the fingertip!). Eventually some of the motor units will fatigue requiring

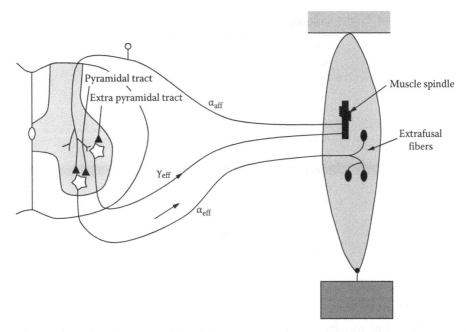

FIGURE 3.35
Schematic representation of a stretch reflex with the γ-loop.

the recruitment of additional motor units, typically larger ones. Much of this recruitment process proceeds through the γ-loop. With larger and larger motor units being recruited, the increases in force will become more discrete and noticeable as tremor. The γ-loop time lag of 82 ms (see Example 3.3) would yield physiological oscillations of approximately 12 Hz (=1000/82). This compares very favorably to the values measured experimentally by Lippold (1970).

γ Control is a factor in whiplash injuries from auto collisions. An unsupported head for a seat-belted occupant would have the tendency to swing forward violently, stretching the neck muscle spindles very quickly. This would result in a maximal stimulation of both the α efferent motoneurons and the γ efferents with a consequently maximal contraction of the neck muscles. The resultant sudden change in head acceleration from a positive to a negative value gives rise to the whiplash effect. The use of head restraints lessens the range motion of the head, thus reducing the magnitude of the acceleration change and the consequent injury.

Example 3.3: Timing Sequence of γ-Loop Control

The timing sequence of a stretch reflex with added γ-loop control can be calculated as follows. The annulospiral, synapse, neuromuscular junction, and end plate all have approximately 1 ms delays. The large α neurons conduct action potentials at a minimum of 100 m/s. Assuming a knee tap and the neuron stretching 0.5 m to the L_5/S_1 level of the spinal cord, nerve conduction in either direction requires 5 ms (=0.5/100 s). The γ neuron for the same length of 0.5 m but a slower speed of 25 m/s requires 20 ms (=0.5/25 s). The fastest muscle fibers need a minimum of 20+ ms to generate sufficient. As a result there is a minimum of a 82 ms delay before any major muscle contraction would be apparent.

Element	Time (ms)
Annulospiral	1.0
α_{aff}	5.0
Synapse	1.0
γ_{eff}	20.0
Neuromuscular junction	1.0
Intrafusal force buildup	20.0
Annulospiral	1.0
α_{aff}	5.0
Synapse	1.0
α_{eff}	5.0
Neuromuscular junction	1.0
End-plate potential	1.0
Extrafusal force buildup	20.0
Total	82.0

3.10.3 α–γ Coactivation

Voluntary control of movement originates in the sensorimotor cortex with an action potential generated in the pyramidal neuron that stretches (in the case of leg movements) along the full length of the spinal cord through the pyramidal tract (see Figure 3.11). The pyramidal tract neurons then directly innervate the large α efferent motoneurons. Since these are large neurons with only one synapse involved, the result is a very quick time to initiate a movement. However, the tradeoff is that there is a massive contraction of the extrafusal fibers resulting in a fairly ballistic type of movement with rather low precision.

Other neurons from the sensorimotor cortex will make various connections in the cerebellum and the basal ganglia, passing through the loosely defined extra pyramidal tract, and eventually reach the same level of the spinal cord as pyramidal neuron. There the extra pyramidal neurons innervate γ efferents resulting in more controlled movements. Note, that without the latter γ control, movements would be limited in magnitude because, with only α stimulation, the extrafusal fibers would contract, with corresponding contraction of the muscle spindles and removal of any further γ-loop activity. With simultaneous extra pyramidal tract activity, both α_{eff} and γ_{eff} are stimulated simultaneously, giving rise to a maximum extrafusal muscle contraction and maximum movement. This is known as α–γ coactivation (McMahon, 1984).

3.10.4 Reciprocal Inhibition

The stretch receptors also form an inhibitory reflex pathway, through an interneuron, to the antagonistic muscle (solid lines in Figure 3.36). Activity in the α afferent neuron results in both the excitation of the same side agonist extrafusal muscle fibers and the inhibition of the antagonistic extrafusal fibers. Termed *reciprocal inhibition*, this prevents the simultaneous activity of both sets of muscles, unless there is a conscious voluntary decision to override it. Should the muscular exertion be reversed (i.e., agonist becomes antagonist and vice versa), then identical reciprocal inhibition pathways exist to again prevent simultaneous activation of the muscles (dotted lines in Figure 3.36).

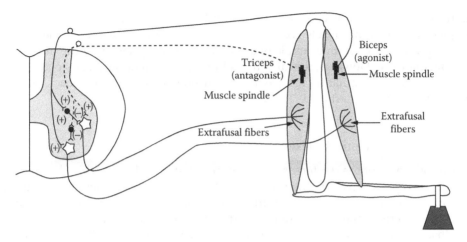

FIGURE 3.36
Schematic representation of a stretch reflex with reciprocal inhibition.

3.10.5 Clasp-Knife Reflex

The Golgi tendon organs also provide feedback in regulating motion and thus form another reflex pathway as well (see Figure 3.37). The tendon organs are innervated by the largest α fibers, which also enter the dorsal horn of the spinal cord. However, instead of innervating directly on the α motor neuron, the action potentials are sent through an intermediary inter neuron which causes an inhibition on the α motor neuron. Upon a sudden force, such as jumping from a height with relatively stiff legs (with completely locked legs, bone and joint mechanics take over, resulting in potentially severe injuries), the Golgi tendon organs send a strong signal (high frequency firing of action potentials) to the spinal cord, which

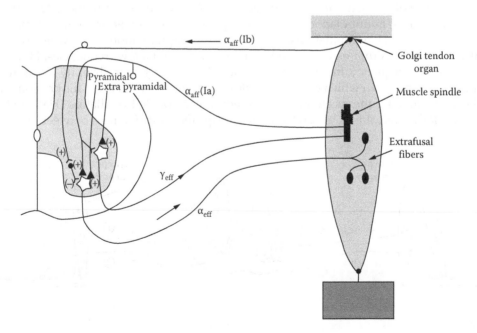

FIGURE 3.37
Schematic representation of the clasp-knife reflex with Golgi tendon organs.

through the inter neuron becomes a strong inhibitory signal on the α_{eff} motor neuron. Consequently, extrafusal muscle contraction declines dramatically and the legs collapse as in a clasp knife. This is an example of a protective reflex, preventing the muscles from overproducing force. However, it is also thought that Golgi tendon organs play a broader more complex role in regulating muscle tension through continuous feedback rather than a purely reactive role (Stuart et al., 1971).

3.10.6 Other Polysynaptic Reflexes

There are collaterals of the α efferent motor neuron that branch off within the gray matter of the spinal cord, synapse via interneurons called *Renshaw cells*, back to the parent cell body. With the signal passing through the interneuron, an inhibitory signal is provided, which acts to decrease the activity of the α efferent motor neuron. This is a form of negative feedback, guaranteeing that weak motoneuron activity is transmitted undisturbed to the extrafusal muscle fibers, while excessive activity is dampened to prevent hyperactivity of the muscles.

In addition to reciprocal inhibition, which occurs to the antagonistic muscle, various other reflexes, known as *crossed* or *contralateral* reflexes, will occur to the other side of the body. For example, in Figure 3.38, a quick push on the underside of the right forearm, will cause the extensors (triceps) to be stimulated causing elbow extension. This is a stretch reflex of the extensors (agonists) and reflex 1. Simultaneously, through reciprocal inhibition, the lateral antagonistic flexors (biceps brachii) are inhibited through reflex 2. In addition, the contralateral muscles of the left arm are also affected. The contralateral flexors (biceps brachii) are stimulated allowing the elbow to flex in reflex 3. Simultaneously, through a more complex form of reciprocal inhibition, the crossed extensors (triceps) are inhibited, allowing full elbow flexion in reflex 4.

The existence of crossed reflexes, as discussed above, would seem to indicate a superiority of alternating manipulations (180° out-of-phase) of the finger or hand over parallel (completely in-phase) manipulations. In fact, such out-of-phase motions, in which one finger flexes while the other extends, can be easily maintained a low frequencies. However, as soon as the frequency increases to a critical level, one finger abruptly shifts to an in-phase relationship, in which both fingers flex in parallel (Kelso, 1981). This phenomenon has been explained quite nicely in terms of nonlinear, coupled oscillators (Haken et al., 1985). Similarly, Freivalds et al. (2000) found no significant differences between in-phase

FIGURE 3.38
Schematic representation of polysynaptic and crossed reflexes: 1, stretch reflex (monosynaptic); 2, reciprocal inhibition; 3, crossed flexor reflex; and 4, crossed extensor reflex.

and out-of-phase hand movements while performing various Purdue Pegboard tasks. Apparently, training, practice, and voluntary factors determined at higher CNS levels can override the basic reflexes.

The full complexity of the reflex system can be difficult to ascertain. Matthews (1961) attempted a census on the cat soleus muscle to find the relative number and distribution of various neuromuscular components. Within roughly 25,000 extrafusal muscle fibers, he found 150 α motor neurons, 45 Golgi tendon organs, and 50 spindles within which were 50 primary (annulospiral) endings, 70 secondary (flower spray) endings and 300 intrafusal fibers with 100 γ neurons. Undoubtedly, all of the interconnections, directly and indirectly through interneurons, at the spinal level, between all of these components cannot be easily mapped. For further information on reflexes and motor control please refer to Schmidt (1975), McMahon (1984).

Questions

1. Discuss the tradeoffs in the arrangement of muscle fibers.
2. Discuss the structure of muscle both at the gross and at the microscopic levels.
3. What is the sliding filament theory?
4. How is an action potential produced?
5. Compare and contrast pyramidal and extrapyramidal tracts in terms of motor control.
6. How is muscle contraction produced?
7. How is energy produced and utilized in the contractile process?
8. What is a motor unit?
9. What are the different types of motor units?
10. How is motor control affected by the size principle and orderly recruitment?
11. What is tetanus and how does it relate to the active state function?
12. What is an isometric muscle contraction? How can an isometric contraction lead to muscle force, i.e., if the muscle does not move, can cross bridging not occur? Explain.
13. What is an isotonic muscle contraction? Is it truly isotonic? Explain.
14. Explain the basis for an active length–tension relationship.
15. Explain the basis for the velocity–tension relationship.
16. What is the active state function? How was it first determined?
17. What is muscle fatigue and where does it occur? That is, what components of the musculoskeletal system may contribute to overall muscle fatigue?
18. What are the different components of heat production in muscle?
19. Describe the structure of a muscle spindle and relate to the reception of sensory input.
20. What is a Golgi tendon organ?
21. What other proprioreceptors may be important in motor control?
22. Describe the pathway and components of a stretch reflex.
23. What effect does γ-control have on motor control?
24. What is α–γ coactivation?

25. What is reciprocal inhibition?

26. What role does the Golgi tendon organ have in motor control?

27. What role does a Renshaw cell have in motor control?

28. What is a contralateral reflex?

29. Consider some of the various types of strength-training programs or equipment that have been promoted over the years. What are the physiological bases for these? (For example, consider the Charles Atlas program of pressing on the opposite sides of a doorway!)

Problems

1. Quantitatively support Henneman's size principle. (Hint: Consider the surface area of a sphere.)

2. Using Hill's force–velocity and power curves shown in Figure 3.18:
   a. Derive the normalized form of Hill's force–velocity equation (Equation 3.10).
   b. Derive the power equation in its standard form (Equation 3.11).
   c. Show that the power curve peaks at approximately $0.3\,v_{max}$ and has an approximate value of $0.1\,T_0 v_{max}$. (Hint consider $0.15 < k < 0.25$, where $k = a/T_0 = b/v_{max}$.)

3. How does muscle endurance time change as the force level in a muscle contraction doubles from 20% to 40% of maximum force? What may explain this result?

4. What is the time advantage of α–γ coactivation over simple γ-loop control?

References

Aidley, D.J. (1985). *The Physiology of Excitable Cells*, 2nd edn, Cambridge, U.K.: Cambridge University Press.

Åstrand, I., Åstrand, P.O., Christensen, E.H., and Hedman, R. (1960b). Myohemoglobin as an oxygen store in man. *Acta Physiologica Scandinavia* 48:454–460.

Åstrand, P.O. and Rodahl, K. (1986). *Textbook of Work Physiology*. New York: McGraw-Hill Book Co.

Bridgman, C.F. (1968). The structure of tendon organs in the cat: A proposed mechanism for responding to muscle tensions. *Anatomical Record* 162:209–220.

Caldwell, L.S. (1963). Relative muscle loading and endurance. *Journal of Engineering Psychology* 2:155–161.

Chaffin, D.B. (1975). Ergonomics guide for the assessment of human static strength. *Journal of the American Industrial Hygiene Association* 35:201–206.

Chaffin, D.B., Andersson, G.B.J., and Martin, B.J. (1999). *Occupational Biomechanics*, 3rd edn, New York: John Wiley & Sons.

Ebashi, S., Endo, M., and Ohtsuki, I. (1969). Control of muscle contraction. *Quarterly Reviews of Biophysics* 2:351–384.

Fenn, W.O. (1923). The relation between the work performed and the energy liberated in muscular contraction. *Journal of Physiology* 58:373–395.

Fenn, W.O. and Marsh, B.S. (1935). Muscle force at different speeds of shortening. *Journal of Physiology* 85:277–297.

Freivalds, A., Kong, D.J., and Murthy, S. (2000). Clarification of the 'Symmetrical use of both hands' principle of motion economy. *International Journal of Industrial Ergonomics* 7:52–56.

Gordon, A.M., Huxley, A.F., and Julian, F.J. (1966). The variation in isometric tension with sarcomere length in vertebrate muscle fibres. *Journal of Physiology* 184:170–192.

Guyton, A.C. (1971). *Textbook of Medical Physiology*. Philadelphia, PA: W.B. Saunders Co.

Haken, H., Kelso, J.A.S., and Brinz, H. (1985). A theoretical model of phase transitions in human hand movements. *Biological Cybernetics* 51:347–356.

Henneman, E., Somjen, G., and Carpenter, D. (1965). Excitability and inhibitability of motoneurons of different sizes. *Journal of Neurophysiology* 28:599–620.

Hill, A.V. (1938). The heat of shortening and the dynamic constants of muscle. *Proceedings of the Royal Society* 126B:136–195.

Hill, A.V. (1953). Chemical change and mechanical response in stimulated muscle. *Proceedings of the Royal Society* 141:314–320.

Hill, A.V. (1970). *First and Last Experiments in Muscle Mechanics*. Cambridge, U.K.: University Press.

Huxley, A.F. (1974). Muscular contraction. *Journal of Physiology* 243:1–43.

Jewell, B.R. and Wilkie, D.R. (1958). An analysis of the mechanical components in frog's striated muscle. *Journal of Physiology* 143:515–540.

Jones, N.L., McCartney, N., and McComas, A.J., eds. (1986). *Human Muscle Power*. Champaign, IL: Human Kinetics Publishers, Inc.

Katz, B. (1939). The relation between force and speed in muscular contraction. *Journal of Physiology* 96:45–64.

Kelso, J.A.S. (1981). On the oscillatory basis of movement. *Bulletin of the Psychonomics Society* 18:63–65.

Lippold, O.C.J. (1970). Oscillation in the stretch reflex arc and the origin of the rhythmical, 8–12 c/s component of physiological tremor. *Journal of Physiology* 206:359–382.

Matthews, P.B.C. (1961). Muscle spindles and their motor control. *Physiological Reviews* 44:219–288.

Matthews, P.B.C. (1972). *Mammalian Muscle Receptors and their Central Actions*. London, U.K.: Edward Arnold, Ltd.

McMahon, T.A. (1984). *Muscles, Reflexes, and Locomotion*. Princeton, NJ: Princeton University Press.

Monod, H. and Scherrer, J. (1965). The work capacity of a synergic muscular group. *Ergonomics* 8:329–338.

Peachey, L.D. (1965). The sarcoplasmic reticulum and transverse tubules of the frog's sartorius. *Journal of Cell Biology* 25(Pt. 2):209–232.

Pinto, J.G. and Fung, Y.C. (1973). Mechanical properties of the heart muscle in the passive state. *Journal of Biomechanics* 6:597–616.

Quilliam, T.A. and Sato, M. (1955). The distribution of myelin on nerve fibres from Pacinian corpuscles. *Journal of Physiology* 129:167–176.

Ritchie, J.M. (1954). The effect of nitrate on the active state of muscle. *Journal of Physiology* 125:155–168.

Rohmert, W. (1960). Ermittlung von erholungspausen für Statische Arbeit des Menschen (Determination of recovery times for human static work). *Internationale Zeitschrift für Angewandte Physiologie Einschliesslich Arbeitsphysiologie* 18:123–164.

Schmidt, R.F. (1975). *Fundamentals of Neurophysiology*. Heidelberg, Germany: Springer Verlag.

Stuart, D.G., Mosher, C.G., and Gerlach, R.L. (1971). Properties and central connections of Golgi tendon organs with special reference to locomotion. In: B.Q. Banker, R.J. Przybylski, J.P. van der Meulen, and M. Victor (eds), *Research in Muscle Development and the Muscle Spindle*. Amsterdam, the Netherlands: Excerpta Medica, pp. 437–464.

Winter, D.A. (1991). *Biomechanics and Motor Control of Human Movement*, 2nd edn, New York: John Wiley & Sons.

4

Modeling of Muscle Mechanics

4.1 Laplace Transforms and Transfer Functions

A transform is a means of converting a number or an expression into another form that can be more easily manipulated and then inversely converted back to the original form of number or expression. Consider that before the advent of computers, logarithms were commonly used to simplify multiplication and long division (see Figure 4.1).

The Laplace transform (named after the French mathematician, Pierre Simon Laplace, 1749–1827) is a specific transformation for a function f(t) defined as

$$\mathcal{L}[f(t)] = F(s) = \int_0^\infty f(t)e^{-st}dt \tag{4.1}$$

where $s = \sigma + j\omega$, a complex number.

For f(t) to be transformable it must meet the requirement that $\int_0^\infty |f(t)|\, e^{-\sigma t}dt < \infty$ for all real and positive σ. This is typically not a problem for most engineering functions, since $e^{-\sigma t}$ is a powerful reducing agent acting on the function f(t).

As an example, perhaps the simplest Laplace transform is for a constant of value one. However, all functions being transformed using the Laplace operator should have a value of 0 for t < 0. Thus, the value of one should, technically, be defined as a *unit-step function*, u(t), which is equal to 0 for t < 0 and equal to 1 for t ≥ 0. The resulting Laplace transformation yields

$$\mathcal{L}[u(t)] = \int_0^\infty e^{-st}dt = \left.\frac{-e^{-st}}{s}\right|_0^\infty = \frac{1}{s} \tag{4.2}$$

As a second example consider the exponential function f(t) = e^{at}. Note that this function is also only defined for values of t ≥ 0; otherwise its value is zero.

$$\mathcal{L}[e^{at}] = \int_0^\infty e^{at}e^{-st}dt = \int_0^\infty e^{-(s-a)t}dt = \left.\frac{-e^{-(s-a)t}}{(s-a)}\right|_0^\infty = \frac{1}{(s-a)} \tag{4.3}$$

With these two equations, a set of transform pairs has been established for two functions. This means that one does not need to perform the cumbersome integration repeatedly, but needs only to look up the appropriate transform. Thus, a table with similar transforms

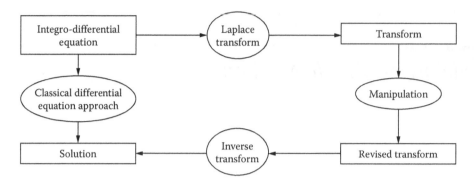

FIGURE 4.1
Algorithmic comparison of Laplace transforms with classical differential equation approach.

for other functions has already been established (see Table 4.1). However, not all functions will have the same exact form as in Table 4.1. In that case, several basic theorems listed in Table 4.2 will assist the user in the process of manipulating and calculating the transforms.

The inverse Laplace transform is defined as

$$f(t) = \frac{1}{2\pi j} \int_{\sigma - j\infty}^{\sigma + j\infty} F(s)e^{st}ds \qquad (4.4)$$

but is generally not used, because of the uniqueness property, which states that there cannot be two different functions having the same Laplace transform F(s). Therefore, typically the Laplace transform table (Table 4.1) is used in reverse to determine the original function f(t):

$$\mathcal{L}^{-1}\{\mathcal{L}[f(t)]\} = \mathcal{L}^{-1}[F(s)] = f(t) \qquad (4.5)$$

4.1.1 Partial Fraction Expansion

Practically, to find the inverse Laplace transform, a *partial fraction expansion* of the polynomial function is performed through either the *algebraic approach* or the *residue approach* using differentiation. The first is conceptually very simple but may lead to computational difficulties for large functions. The second works well until repeated roots lead to complex differentiation. For most of our examples, the algebraic approach should suffice.

For the algebraic approach perform the following steps:

1. Express the transform as a ratio of polynomials (numerator over denominator) as $P(s)/Q(s)$.
2. Should the power of $P(s)$ be greater than the power of $Q(s)$, use long division to reduce the power of the numerator to less than the power of the denominator.
3. Manipulate the polynomial in the denominator $Q(s)$ as a product of factored polynomials in the form of

$$Q(s) = s(s + s_1)(s + s_2)^2(s^2 + as + b) \cdots \qquad (4.6)$$

where s_1, s_2 are termed roots and will yield the exponents for the inverse transform of Equation 4.3 (or Transform 4 in Table 4.1) Note that, through manipulation, the factor $s^2 + as + b$ can be expressed as $(s + \alpha)^2 + \beta^2$, where α and β represent

TABLE 4.1

Table of Transforms

	f(t)a	F(s)
1.	1 or u(t)	$\dfrac{1}{s}$
2.	t	$\dfrac{1}{s^2}$
3.	$\dfrac{t^{n-1}}{(n-1)!}$	$\dfrac{1}{s^n}$
4.	e^{at}	$\dfrac{1}{s-a}$
5.	te^{at}	$\dfrac{1}{(s-a)^2}$
6.	$\dfrac{1}{(n-1)!}t^{n-1}e^{at}$	$\dfrac{1}{(s-a)^n}$
7.	$\dfrac{1}{a-b}(e^{at}-e^{bt})$	$\dfrac{1}{(s-a)(s-b)}$
8.	$1-e^{at}$	$\dfrac{-a}{s(s-a)}$
9.	$\dfrac{1}{\omega}\sin \omega t$	$\dfrac{1}{s^2+\omega^2}$
10.	$\cos \omega t$	$\dfrac{s}{s^2+\omega^2}$
11.	$1-\cos \omega t$	$\dfrac{\omega^2}{s(s^2+\omega^2)}$
12.	$\sin(\omega t+\theta)$	$\dfrac{s\sin\theta+\omega\cos\theta}{s^2+\omega^2}$
13.	$\cos(\omega t+\theta)$	$\dfrac{s\cos\theta-\omega\sin\theta}{s^2+\omega^2}$
14.	$e^{-\alpha t}\sin \omega t$	$\dfrac{\omega}{(s+\alpha)^2+\omega^2}$
15.	$e^{-\alpha t}\cos \omega t$	$\dfrac{s+\omega}{(s+a)^2+\omega^2}$
16.	$\sinh \alpha t$	$\dfrac{\alpha}{s^2-\alpha^2}$
17.	$\cosh \alpha t$	$\dfrac{s}{s^2-\alpha^2}$

Source: Van Valkenburg, M.E., *Network Analysis*, Prentice-Hall, Englewood Cliffs, NJ, 1964. With permission.

real numbers in place of complex conjugate roots that may occur with a complete expansion of that factor.

4. Expand the factors as separate expressions with a polynomial in the numerator of a power lower than the denominator, with unknown constants. For factors that have a power, known as repeated roots, multiple fractions will have to be used, one for each power. Note that the numerator should include s terms up to one power less than found in the denominator.

TABLE 4.2

Basic Theorems for Laplace Transforms

1. Transform of linear combinations	$£[af_1(t) + bf_2(t)] = aF_1(s) + bF_2(s)$
2. Transform of derivatives	$£[d/dt(f(t))] = sF(s) - f(0^+)$
3. Transform of integrals	$£[\int f(t)dt] = F(s)/s$
4. Transform for time shift	$£[f(t - c)] = e^{-cs} £[f(t)]$
5. Transform for s-shift	$£[e^{bt} f(t)] = F(s - b)$
6. Transform for t-factor	$£[t^n f(t)] = (-1)^n d^n/ds^n F(s)$

5. The resulting expression will be of the following form:

$$\frac{P(s)}{Q(s)} = \frac{a_1}{s} + \frac{a_2}{(s + s_1)} + \cdots + \frac{a_3}{(s + s_2)} + \frac{a_4}{(s + s_2)^2} + \frac{a_2 s + a_6}{(s + a)^2 + \beta^2} \tag{4.7}$$

6. Obtain a common denominator for the right-hand side of Equation 4.7, equate the numerators, and solve for the unknown coefficients a_i. Obviously, this will involve several equations in several unknowns. The more equations there are, the more difficult the process becomes.

   For the residue approach, perform the following steps:

7. Multiply both sides of Equation 4.7 by the root term, i.e., $(s + s_1)$:

$$\frac{P(s)(s + s_1)}{Q(s)} = \frac{a_1(s + s_1)}{s} + a_2 + \frac{a_3(s + s_1)}{(s + s_2)} + \frac{a_4(s + s_1)}{(s + s_2)^2} + \frac{(a_5 s + a_6)(s + s_1)}{(s + \alpha)^2 + \beta^2} \tag{4.8}$$

8. Evaluate at $s = -s_1$. All right-hand terms, except for a_2, will become zero and

$$a_2 = \frac{P(s)(s+s_1)}{Q(s)} \bigg|_{s=-s_1} \tag{4.9}$$

9. For repeated roots, multiply Equation 4.7 by the highest power of the root term, i.e., $(s + s_2)^2$:

$$\frac{P(s)(s + s_2)^2}{Q(s)} = \frac{a_1(s + s_2)^2}{s} + \frac{a_2(s + s_2)^2}{(s + s_1)} + a_3(s + s_2) + a + \frac{(a_5 s + a_6)(s + s_2)^2}{(s + \alpha)^2 + \beta^2} \tag{4.10}$$

10. Evaluate at $s = -s_2$. All terms, except for a_4, become zero.

11. Then differentiate both sides with respect to s and evaluate at $s = -s_2$ yielding the value for a_3. Obviously, there may be some difficulty in the differentiation. For higher powers, second and third derivatives are required. Note that sometimes, a combination of the two methods can be used more effectively in combination, than each method separately.

Example 4.1: Complex Conjugate Roots by the Algebraic Method

The initial Laplace function is

$$\frac{P(s)}{Q(s)} = \frac{s+5}{(s+3)(s^2+4s+5)} \tag{4.11}$$

Using Step 4, expand Equation 4.11 as partial fractions, reaching Step 5:

$$\frac{s+5}{(s+3)\left[(s+2)^2+1^2\right]} = \frac{a}{s+3} + \frac{bs+c}{\left[(s+2)^2+1^2\right]} \tag{4.12}$$

Using Step 6 on Equation 4.12, obtain a common denominator and equate numerators yielding

$$s+5 = a\left[(s+2)^2+1^2\right] + (s+3)\,(bs+c) = (a+b)s^2 + (4a+3b+c)s + (5a+3c) \tag{4.13}$$

Solve for unknown coefficients in Equation 4.13 by equating terms with like powers of s:

$$0 = a+b$$
$$1 = 4a+3b+c \tag{4.14}$$
$$5 = 5a+3c$$

Solving Equation 4.14 yields

$$a=1, \quad b=-1, \quad c=0 \tag{4.15}$$

Substituting the coefficient values back into expanded partial fractions of Equation 4.12 yields

$$\frac{s+5}{(s+3)[(s+2)^2+1^2]} = \frac{1}{s+3} - \frac{s}{(s+2)^2+1^2} \tag{4.16}$$

Take inverse Laplace transforms of the linear combination of terms in Equation 4.15 using Theorem 1 in Table 4.2. Using Transform 4 from Table 4.1 on the first term of Equation 4.16 yields

$$\mathcal{L}^{-1}\left[\frac{1}{(s+3)}\right] = e^{-3t} \tag{4.17}$$

Expand the second term from Equation 4.16 appropriately so that the functions fit Transforms 14 and 15 from Table 4.1:

$$\frac{-s}{(s+2)^2+1^2} = \frac{-(s+2)}{(s+2)^2+1^2} + \frac{2}{(s+2)^2+1^2} \tag{4.18}$$

The inverse Laplace transform of the first term in Equation 4.18 yields

$$\mathcal{L}^{-1}\frac{[-(s+2)]}{(s+2)^2+1^2}=-e^{-2t}\cos t \qquad (4.19)$$

While the inverse Laplace transform of the second term in Equation 4.18 yields

$$\mathcal{L}^{-1}\frac{[2]}{(s+2)^2+1^2}=2e^{-2t}\sin t \qquad (4.20)$$

Combining Equations 4.17, 4.19, and 4.20 yields the final expression:

$$f(t) = e^{-3t} - e^{-2t}\cos t + 2e^{-2t}\sin t \qquad (4.21)$$

Example 4.2: Repeated Roots by the Residue Method

The initial Laplace function is

$$\frac{P(s)}{Q(s)} = \frac{s+2}{(s+1)^2} \qquad (4.22)$$

Using Step 4, expand Equation 4.22 as partial fractions, reaching Step 5:

$$\frac{s+2}{(s+1)^2} = \frac{a}{(s+1)} + \frac{b}{(s+1)^2} \qquad (4.23)$$

Using Step 9, multiply both sides of Equation 4.23 by $(s + 1)^2$ yielding

$$s+2 = a(s+1)+b \qquad (4.24)$$

Then using Step 8, evaluate at s = −1, yielding b = 1. Next using Step 10, take the derivative of Equation 4.24 with respect to s yields

$$\frac{d(s+2)}{ds} = 1 \qquad (4.25)$$

$$\frac{d[a(s+1)+b]}{ds} = a \qquad (4.26)$$

Equating Equations 4.25 and 4.26 yields a = 1. Then taking the inverse Laplace transform (Transforms 4 and 5 in Table 4.1) of Equation 4.23 yields the final transformed function:

$$\mathcal{L}^{-1}\left[\frac{1}{(s+1)}+\frac{1}{(s+1)^2}\right] = e^{-t} + te^{-t} = (t+1)e^{-t} \qquad (4.27)$$

4.1.2 Transfer Functions

The concept of a *transfer function* is important in characterizing the properties of a system such as a muscle or a reflex. The transfer function can be considered as a black box or operator that acts on an input function and transforms it into an output function. Thus, in a Laplace domain with all initial conditions set to zero, the ratio of the output, y(s), to the input, x(s), for that black box or system is defined as the transfer function, H(s):

$$x(s) \Rightarrow [\, H(s) \,] \Rightarrow y(s) \qquad \frac{y(s)}{x(s)} = H(s) \tag{4.28}$$

A special function, the *unit impulse* or *delta function*, $\delta(t)$, is used to better characterize system properties through the transfer function. The unit impulse could be considered as a pulse whose magnitude approaches infinite height as the width of the pulse approaches zero with an area remaining constant and equal to one. The unit impulse has some very useful mathematical properties. Using Theorem 2 from Table 4.2, the derivative or change of slope for a unit step becomes infinite or the unit impulse, and the corresponding Laplace transform of a unit impulse is simply one:

$$\mathcal{L}[\delta(t)] = \mathcal{L}\left[\frac{d(u(t))}{dt}\right] = sF(s) = s\left(\frac{1}{s}\right) = 1 \tag{4.29}$$

This property implies that by supplying a unit impulse forcing function to a system the output will simply be the transfer function of the system.

$$y(s) = H(s)\,x(s) = H(s) \tag{4.30}$$

Then by using an inverse transform, H(t), the *impulse response*, will describe system characteristics in a time domain. Obviously, such an input function cannot be realistically produced, although it is often used in an approximate mode to characterize some events occurring in mechanical systems. For example, the tendon tap in a patellar reflex could be considered as a unit impulse for modeling purposes. More details on Laplace transforms can be found in Kaplan (1962), Van Valkenburg (1964), or any other advanced calculus or network analysis textbook.

4.2 Viscoelastic Theory

Viscoelastic theory, introduced by Flügge (1975) and detailed by others including Christensen (1981), is the generalization of material or tissue elasticity and viscosity through the use of a variety of springs and dashpots. *Elasticity* is the property of a material, which enables it to recover from a deformation produced in the material by an external force. In a perfectly elastic material such as a spring, all deformation is recovered upon release of the external forces and stress is proportional to strain (see Figure 4.2a). This can be represented by a linear spring model (see Figure 4.2b) with

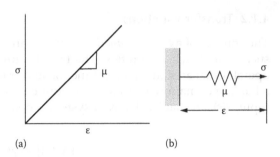

FIGURE 4.2
(a) Stress–strain characteristics of linear elastic spring. (b) Viscoelastic model of spring.

(a)   (b)

a characteristic equation known as Hooke's Law (named after the British physicist, Robert Hooke, 1635–1703):

$$\sigma = \mu\varepsilon \tag{4.31}$$

where
 σ is the stress or force per unit area
 ε is the strain or a change in length per original length, $(\ell - \ell_0)/\ell_0$
 μ is the spring constant

Note that in Section 2.3, when applied to materials, μ was termed Young's modulus of elasticity (named after the British physicist, Thomas Young, 1773–1829).

Viscosity is a property of a material or fluid that resists the force tending to make it flow. In a perfect fluid, the stress is proportional to the rate or velocity of flow (see Figure 4.3a) and can be represented by a dashpot (see Figure 4.3b) with its characteristic equation:

$$\sigma = \eta\frac{d\varepsilon}{dt} \tag{4.32}$$

where η is the dashpot constant.

These basic viscoelastic elements can be used in various combinations to model material behavior. The two simplest mechanical models are the Maxwell fluid (named after the Scottish physicist, James Maxwell, 1831–1879, see Figure 4.4a) and the Voigt solid (named after the German physicist Woldemar Voigt, 1850–1919, see Figure 4.4b)

In the Maxwell fluid under equilibrium conditions, the stress on the dashpot must equal the stress on the spring. Also, the total strain must be the sum of the individual strains for each component or element. We can express these relationships mathematically as

$$\varepsilon = \varepsilon_d + \varepsilon_s \tag{4.33}$$

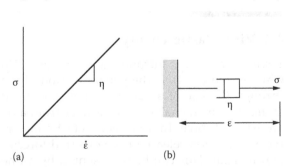

FIGURE 4.3
(a) Stress–strain rate characteristics of dashpot.
(b) Viscoelastic model of dashpot.

(a)   (b)

(a)   (b)

FIGURE 4.4
(a) Viscoelastic model of Maxwell fluid.
(b) Viscoelastic model of Voigt solid.

$$\sigma = \sigma_d = \sigma_s \tag{4.34}$$

where
  ε_d is the strain in the dashpot
  ε_s is the strain in the spring
  σ_d is the stress in the dashpot and equal to the expression in Equation 4.32
  σ_s is the stress in the spring and equal to the expression in Equation 4.31

The overall goal is to express the stress–strain relationship for the full Maxwell solid model. However, with more complicated models, combining the relationships expressed in Equations 4.33 and 4.34 could result in rather complex integrodifferential equations for $\sigma(t)$ in the time domain. A much easier approach is to use Laplace transforms to express the equations in the Laplace domain and then to use algebraic manipulations to arrive at the desired expressions (note that $\sigma(s)$ and $\varepsilon(s)$ will typically be simply expressed as σ and ε):

$$\mathcal{L}[\sigma_d(t)] = \mathcal{L}\left[\eta \frac{d\,\varepsilon_d(t)}{dt}\right] = \eta s\,\varepsilon_d(s) \tag{4.35}$$

$$\mathcal{L}[\sigma_s(t)] = \mu\,\varepsilon_s(s) \tag{4.36}$$

Rearranging Equations 4.35 and 4.36 and using a constant σ yields

$$\varepsilon_d = \frac{\sigma}{(\eta s)} \tag{4.37}$$

$$\varepsilon_s = \frac{\sigma}{\mu} \tag{4.38}$$

Substituting into Equations 4.37 and 4.38 in Equation 4.33 yields

$$\varepsilon = \frac{\sigma}{(\eta s)} + \frac{\sigma}{\mu} \tag{4.39}$$

Rearranging the expression yields either one of two forms, depending on whether stress or strain is considered as the input:

$$\varepsilon = \frac{\mu + \eta s}{\mu \eta s}\,\sigma \quad \text{or} \tag{4.40}$$

$$\sigma = \frac{\mu \eta s}{\mu + \eta s}\,\varepsilon \tag{4.41}$$

In either case, the polynomial expression in s is the transfer function. The choice of expression is typically constrained by the experimental set up in applying a forcing function or by the desired modeling objective.

The transfer function can be similarly established for the Voigt body. If a strain is applied to the body, then each element, since they are in parallel, should be experiencing the same strain but different stresses. Therefore, the total stress is the sum of the stresses for each element:

$$\sigma = \sigma_d + \sigma_s \tag{4.42}$$

$$\sigma = \eta s \varepsilon + \mu \varepsilon = (\eta s + \mu)\varepsilon \tag{4.43}$$

The resulting transfer function is $\eta s + \mu$.

Note the development of an interesting relationship that can be used in simplifying the derivation of a transfer function. The two elements, the dashpot and the spring, can be considered to act similarly to a capacitor in the simplification of a network circuit; the values add directly to obtain an equivalent component when the individual components are found in a parallel arrangement:

$$\mu_{eq} = \mu_1 + \mu_2 \tag{4.44}$$

where
  μ_{eq} is the equivalent spring
  μ_1, μ_2 is the parallel spring elements

When in series, the values are inverted, added and reinverted, i.e.,

$$\mu_{eq} = \left(\frac{1}{\mu_1} + \frac{1}{\mu_2} \right)^{-1} = \frac{\mu_1 \mu_2}{\mu_1 + \mu_2} \tag{4.45}$$

where
  μ_{eq} is the equivalent spring
  μ_1, μ_2 is the series spring elements

This relationship can be used in easily developing the transfer function for a Kelvin body (named after the English physicist and mathematician, William Kelvin, 1824–1907), which is the next more complicated viscoelastic model using three components (see Figure 4.5a). Note that, excluding the contractile element, the Kelvin body is identical to the muscle model developed by Hill (1938, 1970) (see Figure 3.21). The dashpot and the spring element in series combine to yield the equivalent component shown in Figure 4.5b with a value of

$$\mu_{eq} = \frac{\mu_1 \eta s}{\mu_1 + \eta s} \tag{4.46}$$

The equivalent component of Equation 4.46 and the spring element in parallel combine to yield the final transfer function:

$$\mu_{eq} = \frac{\mu_1 \eta s}{\mu_1 + \eta s} + \mu_2 \tag{4.47}$$

(a)

(b)

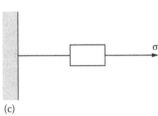

(c)

FIGURE 4.5
Derivation of the transfer function for the Kelvin model.

which rearranged, results in the final transfer function (see Figure 4.5c):

$$H(s) = \frac{(\mu_1+\mu_2)\eta s+\mu_1\mu_2}{\eta s+\mu_1} \tag{4.48}$$

The next step is to use in the transfer function on a specific input to determine the resulting output. This will allow the experimenter to compare actual material properties with model responses with the two most common properties being stress relaxation and strain retardation. *Stress relaxation* is the resulting stress-over-time curve for a unit step input of strain. *Strain retardation* is the resulting strain-over-time curve for a unit step input of stress, sometimes also termed as *creep*. This can be demonstrated quite nicely with the Voigt body and Equation 4.43 rearranged so that the input is stress and output is strain:

$$\varepsilon(s) = \frac{\sigma(s)}{(\eta s+\mu)} \tag{4.49}$$

Using a unit step input of $\sigma(t) = u(t)$ and its Laplace transform of $\sigma(s) = 1/s$, yields the expression:

$$\varepsilon(s) = \frac{1}{(\eta s+\mu)s} \tag{4.50}$$

Using the algebraic approach to the partial fraction expansion of Equation 4.50 yields

$$\frac{1}{\eta(s+\mu/\eta)s} = \frac{1}{\eta}\left[\frac{a}{s}+\frac{b}{(s+\mu/\eta)}\right] \tag{4.51}$$

Obtaining a common denominator for the right side of Equation 4.51 and equating numerators yields

$$1 = as+a\frac{\mu}{\eta}+bs \tag{4.52}$$

Equating common powers of s terms in Equation 4.52 yields two equations in two unknowns:

$$a+b = 0 \tag{4.53}$$

$$a\frac{\mu}{\eta} = 1 \tag{4.54}$$

Solving Equations 4.53 and 4.54 yields

$$a = \frac{\eta}{\mu} \quad b = \frac{-\eta}{\mu} \tag{4.55}$$

Substituting the above values into Equation 4.51 and taking the inverse Laplace transform yields

$$\varepsilon(t) = \frac{1}{\mu} \mathcal{L}^{-1} \left[\frac{1}{s} - \frac{1}{(s + \mu/\eta)} \right] \tag{4.56}$$

$$\varepsilon(t) = \frac{1}{\mu} (1 - e^{-\mu t/\eta}) \tag{4.57}$$

A plot of Equation 4.57 (see Figure 4.6) shows the characteristic creep that would be expected with a viscous damping element. As a constant stress is being continually applied to the Voigt material, the dashpot is continually yielding. However, with time the resulting increase in strain in the spring element has increased the internal stress, which ultimately will reach a value that resists the externally applied stress, stopping the creep process.

Similarly, we can examine the properties of a Maxwell fluid. Using Equation 4.41 and a unit step strain input, the resulting stress becomes

$$\sigma(s) = \frac{\mu \eta s}{(\mu + \eta s)s} \tag{4.58}$$

Canceling out one s term in the denominator and numerator, factoring out a μ, and taking the inverse Laplace transform yields

$$\sigma(t) = \mathcal{L}^{-1}[\sigma(s)] = \mathcal{L}^{-1} \mu \left\{ \frac{1}{(s + \mu/\eta)} \right\} = \mu e^{-\mu t/\eta} \tag{4.59}$$

and the resulting stress relaxation curve in Figure 4.7.

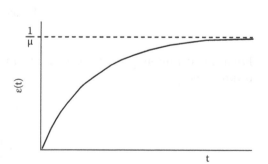

FIGURE 4.6
Strain retardation or creep in the Voigt solid.

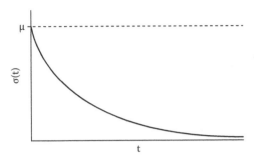

FIGURE 4.7
Stress relaxation in the Maxwell fluid.

Note that the calculation of a stress relaxation function for the Voigt body (Equation 4.43) results in an impulse function, which, although acceptable mathematically, is not realistic mechanically.

$$\mathcal{L}^{-1}[\sigma(s)] = \mathcal{L}^{-1}\left\{\frac{(\eta s + \mu)}{s}\right\} = \mathcal{L}^{-1}\left\{\eta + \frac{\mu}{s}\right\} = \eta\delta(t) + \mu\,u(t) \tag{4.60}$$

Example 4.3: Initial and Final Value Theorems

As the transfer functions become more complicated, the corresponding functions in time become more complicated to plot. In such cases, either the initial value theorem or the final value theorem will provide the critical and initial and final values of the time plot. The *initial-value theorem* is defined as

$$\lim_{t\to 0} f(t) = \lim_{s\to\infty} sF(s) \tag{4.61}$$

while the *final-value theorem* is defined as

$$\lim_{t\to\infty} f(t) = \lim_{s\to 0} sF(s) \tag{4.62}$$

Thus, the initial and final values, respectively, for the Voigt body creep function (Equation 4.57) can be found very simply from

$$\lim_{s\to\infty} sF(s) = \lim_{s\to\infty} \frac{s}{(\eta s + \mu)s} = 0 \tag{4.63}$$

$$\lim_{s\to 0} sF(s) = \lim_{s\to 0} \frac{s}{(\eta s + \mu)s} = \frac{1}{\mu} \tag{4.64}$$

4.3 Hill's Muscle Models

The basic mechanical properties, such as creep and stress relaxation, of Hill's three-element model (i.e., passive muscle with the contractile element removed) can be determined as follows. The isotonic after-loaded experiments of Fenn and Marsh (1935) led to the velocity–tension relationship developed in Section 3.7.3 and shown in Figure 3.18. In terms, of Hill's viscoelastic model, one can assume that initially the force on the parallel elastic

FIGURE 4.8
(a) Hill's three-element muscle model. (b) Simplified Hill's muscle model.

element is negligible because the dashpot cannot move instantaneously. Obviously, with increasing time, the dashpot slowly yields and strain increases. However, for low to moderate strains, Hill's model can be simplified to the model shown in Figure 4.8.

In this simplified model, the force on the dashpot is

$$T_0 - T = Bv \tag{4.65}$$

where
   T is the tension
   T_0 is the isometric or maximum tension
   v is the velocity

This relationship can then be used to approximate the initial slope (i.e., velocities close to zero or minimal strain) of the velocity–tension relationship. Or more importantly, this initial slope provides an approximate value for the dashpot parameter B.

One can reach the same result starting with Hill's equation for the velocity–tension relationship:

$$(T + a)\,(v + b) = (T_0 + a)\,b \tag{4.66}$$

Multiplying the factors and subtracting common terms yields

$$Tv + av + Tb = T_0 b \tag{4.67}$$

Rearranging the terms yields and adding/subtracting the term $T_0 v$ yields

$$T(v + b) = T_0 b - av + T_0 v - T_0 v \tag{4.68}$$

Rearranging terms again yields

$$T(v + b) = T_0(v + b) - (a + T_0)v \tag{4.69}$$

Now dividing both sides by (v + b) yields

$$T_0 - T = \frac{(a + T_0)}{(v + b)} v = Bv \tag{4.70}$$

where the term $(a + T_0)/(v + b)$ can be considered to be the initial slope of the velocity–tension relationship and an estimate of the dashpot parameter B.

From Hill's (1938) experiments on vertebrate muscles, the unknown constants a and b were found to be $T_0/4$ and $v_{max}/4$, respectively. Substituting these values into the expression for B from Equation 4.70, yields

$$B = \frac{(a + T_0)}{(v + b)} = \frac{1.25\,T_0}{v + v_{max}/4} \tag{4.71}$$

For values of velocity much less than $v_{max}/4$, B remains constant. Thus, again the initial slope of the velocity–tension curve can be used to estimate B. Data from Bawa et al. (1976) on the cat plantaris muscle have yielded values on the order of 4.6 g s/mm. K_{SE} can be determined from quick stretch experiments, in which a sudden pull is applied to a passive muscle at its resting length (see Figure 4.9). On a quick pull, the dashpot will not respond and all the strain will be absorbed in the series elastic element. Data from Jewell and Wilkie (1958) on the frog sartorius muscle, yield values for K_{SE} on the order of 85 g/mm (see Figure 4.10). Higher values of 380 g/mm for a cat plantaris muscle have reported by Bawa et al. (1976). This large variation is due to a variety of factors: the experimental procedures, masses and elasticities in the equipment, the type of muscle, and from which animal it was taken. In addition, the stress–strain relationship is not linear and can result in differing values for K_{SE} depending on the region of strain utilized.

K_{PE} is more difficult to determine and is typically done by looking at the second-order response to vibrations or other forcing functions. Bawa et al. (1976) indicate a value of 103 g/mm for a cat plantaris muscle. Note that K_{SE} is much stiffer than K_{PE}, which would seem reasonable considering that K_{SE} represents the tendon interface to the muscle, while K_{PE} represents the more elastic fascia separating bundles of muscle fibers.

4.3.1 Active Muscle Response

The active muscle response based on Hill's four-element model (see Figure 4.11) can be found most easily by developing the transfer function for muscle model. First, the equilibrium equations need to be determined as follows. The internally developed muscle force

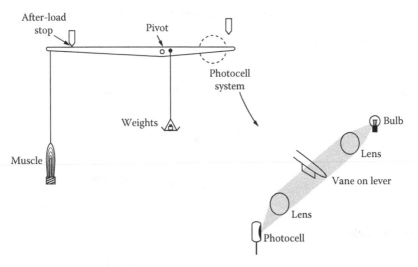

FIGURE 4.9
Quick stretch experiment for determining series elastic element. (Reproduced from Aidley, D.J., *The Physiology of Excitable Cells*, Cambridge University Press, Cambridge, U.K., 1985. With permission.)

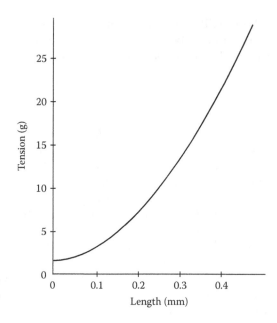

FIGURE 4.10
Length–tension relationship for a series elastic element. (Adapted from Jewell, B.R. and Wilkie, D.R., *J. Physiol.*, 143, 515, 1958.)

FIGURE 4.11
Hill's four-element active muscle model.

T_{CE} is modified by the viscous damping element and parallel elastic element to become the externally measured tension, T. In the process, it is also transferred through the series elastic element, resulting in two equilibrium equations:

$$T = T_{CE} + Bs\varepsilon_i + K_{PE}\varepsilon_i \qquad (4.72)$$

$$T = K_{SE}(\varepsilon - \varepsilon_i) \qquad (4.73)$$

Equating Equations 4.72 and 4.73 and rearranging results in

$$T_{CE} = K_{SE}\varepsilon - (Bs + K_{PE} + K_{SE})\varepsilon_i \qquad (4.74)$$

Solving Equation 4.73 for ε_i and substituting for ε_i into Equation 4.74 yields

$$\varepsilon_i = \varepsilon - \frac{T}{K_{SE}} \qquad (4.75)$$

$$T_{CE} = K_{SE}\varepsilon - (Bs + K_{PE} + K_{SE})\varepsilon + \frac{(Bs + K_{PE} + K_{SE})}{K_{SE}T} \qquad (4.76)$$

Rearrangement yields

$$T_{CE} = -(Bs + K_{PE})\varepsilon + \frac{(Bs + K_{PE} + K_{SE})}{K_{SE}T} \qquad (4.77)$$

Equation 4.77 can now be rearranged into two alternate forms: external muscle tension, T, as function of the active muscle contractile element tension, T_{CE}:

$$T = \frac{K_{SE}T_{CE}}{Bs + K_{PE} + K_{SE}} + \frac{K_{SE}(Bs + K_{PE})\varepsilon}{Bs + K_{PE} + K_{SE}} \qquad (4.78)$$

or strain, ε, in terms of the active muscle contractile element tension and external tension:

$$\varepsilon = \frac{(Bs + K_{PE} + K_{SE})T}{(Bs + K_{PE})K_{SE}} - \frac{T_{CE}}{Bs + K_{PE}} \qquad (4.79)$$

Note that both equations consist of two transfer functions, one for an external forcing function, either mechanical stress or strain, and the other for an internal forcing function from the contractile element.

4.3.2 Force Buildup

Consider an *isometric experiment*, in which both ends of a muscle are rigidly fixed so that it cannot shorten. Then, when stimulated it contracts isometrically and the resulting external tension can be measured with a force gage (see Figure 4.12). This case can be examined using Equation 4.80, but with the second term in ε eliminated, since the muscle is stimulated isometrically and no strain (at least externally) is possible. Assuming, a maximum tetanic stimulation, the input can be represented with a step function with magnitude T_{CE}. Using the Laplace transform of the step function, Equation 4.80 becomes

$$T = \frac{K_{SE}T_{CE}}{(Bs + K_{PE} + K_{SE})s} \qquad (4.80)$$

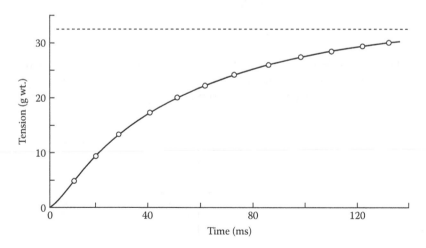

FIGURE 4.12
Tension buildup during isometric tetanus. (Adapted from Jewell, B.R. and Wilkie, D.R., *J. Physiol.*, 143, 515, 1958.)

Factoring constants and rearrangement yields

$$T = \frac{K_{SE}T_{CE}}{B} \left\{ \frac{1}{s + (K_{PE} + K_{SE})/B} \right\} \frac{1}{s} \tag{4.81}$$

A partial fraction expansion yields

$$T = \frac{K_{SE}T_{CE}}{B} \left\{ \frac{a}{s + (K_{PE} + K_{SE})/B} + \frac{b}{s} \right\} \tag{4.82}$$

Using residues to solve for a and b yields

$$a = \frac{1}{s}\bigg|_{s = -(K_{PE}+K_{SE})/B} = -\frac{B}{(K_{PE} + K_{SE})} \tag{4.83}$$

$$b = \frac{1}{s + (K_{PE} + K_{SE})/B}\bigg|_{s=0} = \frac{B}{(K_{PE} + K_{SE})} \tag{4.84}$$

Substituting the coefficients a and b back into Equation 4.82 yields

$$T = \frac{K_{SE}T_{CE}}{B} \left\{ \frac{-B/(K_{PE} + K_{SE})}{s + (K_{PE} + K_{SE})/B} + \frac{B/(K_{PE} + K_{SE})}{s} \right\} \tag{4.85}$$

Taking the inverse Laplace transform and simplifying yields

$$T(t) = \frac{K_{SE}T_{CE}}{K_{PE} + K_{SE}} \left\{ 1 - e^{-(K_{PE} + K_{SE})t/B} \right\} \tag{4.86}$$

The plot of Equation 4.86 (see Figure 4.13) corresponds nicely to the buildup of tension measured in the isometric experiment (see Figure 4.12). Note that active muscle contractile tension, T_{CE}, is not directly transferred to the force gage. Instead it is modified by the

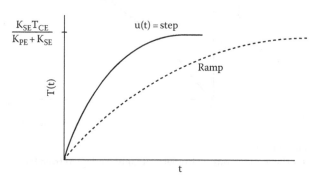

FIGURE 4.13
Calculated tension buildup using Hill's four-element model.

combination of the parallel and series elastic elements as a reduced value. Should the values of K_{PE} and K_{SE} be relatively equal, the tension reduction is almost 50%. If the values are quite unequal, as in the actual muscle, then the reduction is relatively small. Also, note that the tetanic stimulation is not truly a unit step. It is more likely to be a steady increase in tension until maximum tension is achieved, which is best simulated by a *ramp function*, f(t) = t. In that case, the resulting tension function would have an additional term in t and a slight modification in the slope or rise of tension.

4.3.3 Stress Relaxation

Consider a quick stretch experiment, in which the passive muscle undergoes a step strain input of magnitude ε_0. In such a case, T_{CE} is zero and the first term can be eliminated and the Laplace transform of a unit step is ε_0/s:

$$T = \frac{K_{SE}(Bs + K_{PE})}{Bs + K_{PE} + K_{SE}} \frac{\varepsilon_0}{s} \tag{4.87}$$

Rearrangement yields

$$T = K_{SE}\varepsilon_0 \frac{s + K_{PE}/B}{s\left[s + (K_{PE} + K_{SE})/B\right]} \tag{4.88}$$

A partial fraction expansion yields

$$T = K_{SE}\,\varepsilon_0\left\{\frac{a}{s + (K_{PE} + K_{SE})/B} + \frac{b}{s}\right\} \tag{4.89}$$

Using residues to solve for a and b yields

$$a = \frac{s + K_{PE}/B}{s}\bigg|_{s = -(K_{PE}+K_{SE})/B} = \frac{K_{SE}}{K_{PE} + K_{SE}} \tag{4.90}$$

$$b = \frac{s + K_{PE}/B}{s + (K_{PE} + K_{SE})/B}\bigg|_{s=0} = \frac{K_{PE}}{K_{PE} + K_{SE}} \tag{4.91}$$

Substituting the coefficients a and b back into Equation 4.89 yields

$$T = \frac{K_{SE}\varepsilon_0}{K_{PE} + K_{SE}}\left\{\frac{K_{SE}}{s + (K_{PE} + K_{SE})/B} + \frac{K_{PE}}{s}\right\} \tag{4.92}$$

Taking the inverse Laplace transform and simplifying yields the plot in Figure 4.14 and the function:

$$T(t) = \frac{K_{SE}\varepsilon_0}{K_{PE} + K_{SE}}\left\{K_{PE} + K_{SE}\,e^{-(K_{PE}+K_{SE})t/B}\right\} \tag{4.93}$$

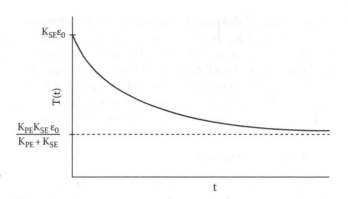

FIGURE 4.14
Calculated stress relaxation in Hill's
four-element model.

In this situation, the initial strain is all taken up in the series elastic element. However, the viscous damping element slowly yields, allowing the tension in the series elastic element to decrease to a point in which the tension between the two elastic elements is balanced. This phenomenon is termed stress relaxation and is observed in many tissues as well as engineering materials (Haddad, 1995).

4.3.4 Creep

The strain retardation or creep function for passive muscle can be generated in a similar manner to the stress relaxation of Section 4.3.3. Eliminate the active contractile component of T_{CE} From Equation 4.79, yielding

$$\varepsilon = \frac{(Bs + K_{PE} + K_{SE})T}{(Bs + K_{PE})K_{SE}} \tag{4.94}$$

Using a unit step input of external tension, and dividing the numerator and denominator by B yields

$$\varepsilon = \frac{s + (K_{PE} + K_{SE})/B}{K_{SE}(s + K_{PE}/B)s} \tag{4.95}$$

Using the partial fraction expansion yields

$$\varepsilon = \frac{1}{K_{SE}} \left\{ \frac{a}{s + K_{PE}/B} + \frac{b}{s} \right\} \tag{4.96}$$

Solving for a and b using residues yields

$$a = \left. \frac{s + (K_{PE} + K_{SE})/B}{s} \right|_{s = -K_{PE}/B} = \frac{-K_{SE}}{K_{PE}} \tag{4.97}$$

$$b = \left. \frac{s + (K_{PE} + K_{SE})/B}{s + K_{PE}/B} \right|_{s=0} = \frac{K_{PE} + K_{SE}}{K_{PE}} \tag{4.98}$$

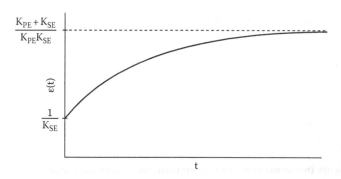

FIGURE 4.15
Calculated creep in Hill's four-element model.

Taking the inverse Laplace transform and rearranging yields the creep function plotted in Figure 4.15 and the equation:

$$\varepsilon(t) = \frac{K_{PE} + K_{SE}}{K_{PE}K_{SE}} - \frac{e^{-(K_{PE}/B)t}}{K_{PE}} \tag{4.99}$$

Note that in this situation, with the initial application of a unit stress, the damping element does not respond. However, the series elastic spring yields to the stress with a step jump of movement. Then, under continued loading the damping element begins to yield and allows the material to creep until the two elastic springs balance out the stress and the creep stops.

4.3.5 Time Constant

The creep rise (Equation 4.99) or stress-relaxation times (Equation 4.93) are determined by the exponent in the exponential term. This exponential term can also be formulated as $e^{-t/\tau}$, where τ is the termed the *time constant* and, in the case of active force buildup (Equation 4.86) and stress relaxation (Equation 4.93), is equal to

$$\tau = \frac{B}{(K_{PE} + K_{SE})} \tag{4.100}$$

The exponential function drops from $e^0 = 1.0$ to $e^{-1} = 0.37$ in one time constant and to $e^{-2} = 0.14$ in two time constants, etc. For active force buildup, the rise becomes 0.63 in one time constant and 0.86 in two time constants.

For Hill's muscle model, substituting experimentally determined values for the viscoelastic elements yields a time constant of

$$\frac{B}{(K_{PE} + K_{SE})} = \frac{5}{(103 + 380)} = 0.0103 \text{ s} \tag{4.101}$$

where from Bawa et al. (1976), $B = 5\,g\,s/mm$, $K_{PE} = 103\,g/mm$, and $K_{SE} = 380\,g/mm$.

Using a smaller value from Jewell and Wilkie (1958) of $K_{SE} = 85 \, g/mm$ with a correspondingly weaker $K_{PE} = 20 \, g/mm$, yields

$$\frac{B}{(K_{PE} + K_{SE})} = \frac{5}{(20 + 85)} = 0.0476 \, s \tag{4.102}$$

This means that the rise time for twitch tension ranges from 10.3 to 47.6 ms to reach 63% of the final value and 20.6–95.2 ms to reach 86% of the final value. Note that these times correspond relatively closely to the twitch times for fast- and slow-twitch muscle fibers given in Table 3.2.

Note also the relative relationship between the time constant for stress relaxation (or force buildup) and for the creep function. By taking the ratio of the two yields

$$\frac{\tau_{relax}}{\tau_{creep}} = \frac{B/(K_{PE} + K_{SE})}{B/K_{PE}} - \frac{K_{PE}}{K_{PE} + K_{SE}} \tag{4.103}$$

Given that K_{SE} is much stiffer than K_{PE}, then the time constant for stress relaxation is much smaller than the time constant for creep. This means that the muscle will relax much more quickly for stress than for strain changes.

4.4 Frequency Analysis

An alternate approach for muscle modeling and examining muscle properties is to consider the effects of a sinusoidal forcing function. Consider again the passive muscle from Equation 4.78, with T_{CE} set equal to zero:

$$T = \frac{K_{SE}(Bs + K_{PE})}{Bs + K_{PE} + K_{SE}} \varepsilon \tag{4.104}$$

From Table 4.1, a sinusoidal strain function:

$$\varepsilon(t) = \sin \omega t \tag{4.105}$$

would be transformed to the Laplace domain as

$$\varepsilon(s) = \frac{\omega}{(s^2 + \omega^2)} \tag{4.106}$$

Applying the transfer function of Equation 4.104 to a sinusoidal strain function of Equation 4.106 yields the muscle tension response in the Laplace domain:

$$T(s) = \frac{\omega \, K_{SE}(Bs + K_{PE})}{(Bs + K_{PE} + K_{SE})(s^2 + \omega^2)} \tag{4.107}$$

A partial fraction expansion yields

$$T(s) = \frac{a}{(Bs + K_{PE} + K_{SE})} + \frac{b}{(s^2 + \omega^2)} \tag{4.108}$$

Without further calculations, it can be seen from Equation 4.108 that the sinusoidal strain forcing function results in a transient response in stress of the form e^{-at}, which dies down to zero as time becomes large, and a sinusoidal steady-state response, which continues for large times. To examine Equation 4.108 for various times or various frequencies of sinusoids requires considerable effort. Therefore, a simpler approach is needed to examine the frequency response characteristics for muscle through a formalized frequency analysis.

4.4.1 Generalized Approach

It can be shown that for a system with transfer function H(t), a sinusoidal input of

$$x(t) = \sin \omega t \tag{4.109}$$

will result in a sinusoidal output that is similar to the sinusoidal input in that it has the same frequency, but the magnitude may be altered and the two sinusoidal functions may be out of phase. Consider the output represented as

$$y(t) = H(t)\,x(t) = M(\omega)\sin(\omega t + \varphi(\omega)) \tag{4.110}$$

where
  $M(\omega)$ is the magnitude
  $\varphi(\omega)$ is the phase angle

The magnitude $M(\omega)$ can be represented quite simply in the Laplace domain as the magnitude of the transfer function:

$$M(\omega) = \left|H(s)\right|_{s=j\omega} = \left|H(j\omega)\right| \tag{4.111}$$

while the phase angle $\varphi(\omega)$ can be represented as the phase angle of the transfer function or the argument of a complex variable, abbreviated as arg:

$$\varphi(\omega) = \arg H(s)\big|_{s=j\omega} = \arg H(j\omega) \tag{4.112}$$

For any complex variable $X(\omega) + jY(\omega)$ (where $X(\omega)$ is the real part, $Y(\omega)$ is the imaginary part, and $j = \sqrt{-1}$ or $j^2 = -1$), the magnitude then can be expressed as

$$M(\omega) = \left[X(\omega)^2 + Y(\omega)^2\right]^{\frac{1}{2}} \tag{4.113}$$

and the argument or phase angle as

$$\varphi(\omega) = \tan^{-1}\left[\frac{Y(\omega)}{X(\omega)}\right] \tag{4.114}$$

For a complete frequency-response analysis, the magnitude response of Equation 4.111 and phase angles of Equation 4.112 are plotted over the range of frequencies of interest.

4.4.2 Magnitude and Phase Angle in the Frequency Domain

Taking the Laplace transforms of Equations 4.109 and 4.110 yields Equation 4.111 with complex conjugate roots:

$$y(s) = \frac{H(s)\omega}{s^2 + \omega^2} = \frac{H(s)\omega}{(s+j\omega)(s-j\omega)} \tag{4.115}$$

Performing a partial fraction expansion yields the complex conjugate roots and other roots depending on the transfer function H(s):

$$y(s) = \frac{a}{(s+j\omega)} + \frac{b}{(s-j\omega)} \tag{4.116}$$

The constants a and b can be found using the residue method:

$$a = \frac{H(s)\omega}{(s-j\omega)}\bigg|_{s=-j\omega} = \frac{H(-j\omega)\omega}{-2j\omega} \tag{4.117}$$

$$b = \frac{H(s)\omega}{(s+j\omega)}\bigg|_{s=j\omega} = \frac{H(j\omega)\omega}{2j\omega} \tag{4.118}$$

Substituting the constants into Equation 4.116 and taking the inverse Laplace transform yield the solution in the time domain:

$$y(t) = \frac{H(-j\omega)\omega}{-2j\omega}e^{-j\omega t} + \frac{H(j\omega)\omega}{2j\omega}e^{j\omega t} \tag{4.119}$$

Canceling ωs and expanding H(jω) into its complex conjugate form yields

$$y(t) = \frac{[X(\omega) - jY(\omega)]e^{-j\omega t}}{-2j} + \frac{[X(\omega) + jY(\omega)]e^{j\omega t}}{2j} \tag{4.120}$$

Rearranging terms yields

$$y(t) = X(\omega)\frac{e^{j\omega t} - e^{-j\omega t}}{2j} + Y(\omega)\frac{e^{j\omega t+} + e^{-j\omega t}}{2} \tag{4.121}$$

From the Euler identities:

$$e^{j\omega} = \cos\omega + j\sin\omega \tag{4.122}$$

and

$$e^{-j\omega} = \cos\omega - j\sin\omega \tag{4.123}$$

$\sin \omega t$ can be expressed as

$$\sin \omega t = \frac{e^{j\omega t} - e^{-j\omega t}}{2j} \tag{4.124}$$

and $\cos \omega t$ as

$$\cos \omega t = \frac{e^{j\omega t} + e^{-j\omega t}}{2} \tag{4.125}$$

Substituting Equations 4.124 and 4.125 into Equation 4.121 yields the final solution in the time domain as

$$y(t) = X(\omega)\sin\omega t + Y(\omega)\cos\omega t \tag{4.126}$$

To find the magnitude and phase, Equation 4.126 needs to be manipulated into an alternate form. Multiply and divide Equation 4.126 by the same term $(X(\omega)^2 + Y(\omega)^2)^{1/2}$ yielding

$$y(t) = (X(\omega)^2 + Y(\omega)^2)^{1/2}\left\{\frac{X(\omega)\sin\omega t}{(X(\omega)^2 + Y(\omega)^2)^{1/2}} + \frac{Y(\omega)\cos\omega t}{(X(\omega)^2 + Y(\omega)^2)^{1/2}}\right\} \tag{4.127}$$

Note that based on a right triangle with sides X and Y:

$$\cos\varphi = \frac{X}{(X^2 + Y^2)^{1/2}} \quad \sin\varphi = \frac{Y}{(X^2 + Y^2)^{1/2}} \tag{4.128}$$

Substituting Equation 4.128 into 4.127 yields

$$y(t) = M(\omega)\{\sin\omega t\cos\varphi + \cos\omega t\sin\varphi\} \tag{4.129}$$

By trigonometric substitution, the alternate form of the solution in the time domain is

$$y(t) = M(\omega)\sin(\omega t + \varphi(\omega)) \tag{4.130}$$

where the magnitude, as indicated previously in Equation 4.113 is

$$M(\omega) = (X(\omega)^2 + Y(\omega)^2)^{1/2} \tag{4.131}$$

and the phase angle, as indicated in Equation 4.114 is

$$\varphi(\omega) = \tan^{-1}\frac{Y(\omega)}{X(\omega)} \tag{4.132}$$

Example 4.4: Calculation of Magnitude and Phase

Consider the simple transfer function:

$$H(s) = \frac{1}{s+1} \tag{4.133}$$

To find the magnitude and phase angle of H(s), substitute $s = j\omega$ and multiply numerator and denominator by the complex conjugate to form a complex variable of the form $X + jY$:

$$H(j\omega) = \frac{1}{1+j\omega}\frac{(1-j\omega)}{(1-j\omega)} = \frac{1-j\omega}{1+\omega^2} = \frac{1}{1+\omega^2} - \frac{j\omega}{1+\omega^2} \tag{4.134}$$

Note that only a pure imaginary component is used because of the Euler representation of sine and cosine functions in Equations 4.124 and 4.125. The magnitude is then

$$M = \left\{ \frac{1^2}{(1+\omega^2)^2} + \frac{\omega^2}{(1+\omega^2)^2} \right\}^{1/2} = \left\{ \frac{1}{1+\omega^2} \right\}^{1/2} \tag{4.135}$$

and the phase is

$$\varphi = \tan^{-1}\frac{-\omega/(1+\omega^2)}{1/(1+\omega^2)} = -\tan^{-1}\omega \tag{4.136}$$

Typically, these frequency responses are plotted on log–log scales (see Figure 4.16), so as to show the full range of possible frequencies. Also, on a log–log scale, several aspects of typical relationships are very much simplified. For very small ω, $\omega \ll 1$, the magnitude in Equation 4.135 is simply the value of 1 or a flat line for frequencies approaching $\omega = 1$ from the left-hand side. For very large ω, $\omega \gg 1$, the magnitude is essentially $1/\omega$, with the constant 1 in the denominator having little effect. On a log–log scale, $1/\omega$ is simply represented as line with a slope of −1. A critical point occurs at $\omega = 1$, which is known as a *break frequency*. There the two lines theoretically intersect, but the actual plot forms a curved connection. The actual magnitude at $\omega = 1$ is $1/\sqrt{2}$ or 0.707.

The phase angle is plotted in a similar manner although the ordinate for angles remains a linear scale. For very small angles, $\omega \ll 1$, $\tan^{-1}\omega = \omega$ and the phase angle is close to 0, but

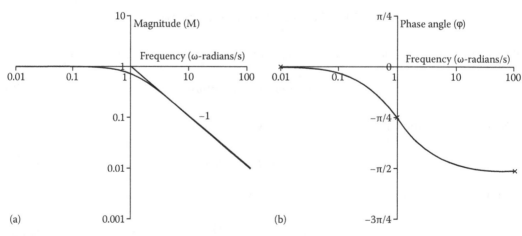

FIGURE 4.16
Magnitude (a) and phase angle (b) plots for H(s) = 1/(s + 1).

gradually decreasing (because of the minus sign) as ω becomes larger. For very large angles, as ω approaches ∞,– $\tan^{-1} \omega$ slowly approaches $-\pi/2$. At the break frequency of $\omega = 1$, the phase angle is $-\tan^{-1} 1$ which is equal to $-\pi/4$.

4.4.3 Magnitude and Phase Angle in the Laplace Domain

Frequency analysis can also be done in the Laplace or s-domain, in a more straight forward manner, as follows The transfer function, H(s) is put in a time constant format; i.e., the coefficient of s in each factor is put in the form of a time constant $(1 + s\tau)$, where $\tau = 1/\omega_i$, and ω_i is the break frequency.

The magnitude plot is examined in terms of frequency ranges. Wherever ω (or s notation as used in the Laplace domain) is less than ω_i, the slope of the plot will be zero for factors in the denominator. If the ω is larger than ω_i, then the slope is equal to -1. If there are two factors and ω is larger than both break frequencies, the slope becomes -2, etc. If there is an s factor in the numerator, similar rules apply, but the slopes are $+1$ or $+2$. This linearized approach for the magnitude is termed a *Bode plot* in electronics applications. In such cases the magnitude is typically expressed in terms of power with units of decibels.

The phase angle is determined by the simple relationship:

$$\varphi = \alpha \frac{\pi}{2} \tag{4.137}$$

where α = the average of the slopes of the magnitude plot for the immediately preceding and immediately following decade on either side of the frequency of interest. Further information on frequency plots and bode plots can be obtained from Schneck (1992), Van Valkenburg (1964), or any other electrical engineering textbook.

Example 4.5: Calculation of Magnitude and Phase in the s-Domain

Consider the transfer function:

$$H(s) = \frac{5(1 + s/1)(1 + s/10)}{(1 + s/0.1)(1 + s/100)} \tag{4.138}$$

and the logical reasoning as follows, with the corresponding points marked on the curves in Figure 4.17. First consider the magnitude plot of Figure 4.17a.

1. The first or smallest break frequency is 0.1. For $\omega \ll 0.1$, H(s) is approximately:

$$H(s) = \frac{5(1)(1)}{(1)(1)} = 5 \tag{4.139}$$

with slope 0.

2. The next largest break frequency is 1. For $0.1 < \omega < 1$, H(s) can be approximated as

$$H(s) = \frac{5(1)(1)}{(s/0.1)(1)} = \frac{0.5}{s} \tag{4.140}$$

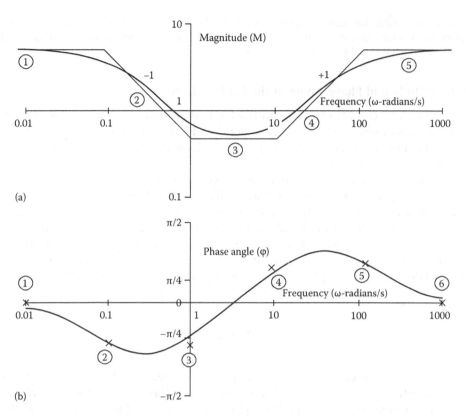

FIGURE 4.17
Magnitude (a) and phase angle (b) plots for H(s) = [5(1 + s/1)(1 + s/10)]/[(1 + s/0.1)(1 + s/100)].

or a downward sloping line with a slope of −1. Note that the +1 term has relatively little effect as compared to the s term.

3. The next break frequency is 10. For 1 < ω < 10, H(s) can be approximated as

$$H(s) = \frac{5(s/1)(1)}{(s/0.1)(1)} = \frac{0.5s}{s} = 0.5 \tag{4.141}$$

or simply a flat line with slope 0.

4. The last break frequency is 100. For 10 < ω < 100, H(s) can be approximated as

$$H(s) = \frac{5(s/1)(s/10)}{(s/0.1)(1)} = \frac{0.05s^2}{s} = 0.05s \tag{4.142}$$

or an upward sloping line with a slope of +1.

5. For ω ≫ 100, H(s) can be approximated as

$$H(s) = \frac{5(s/1)(s/10)}{(s/0.1)(s/100)} = \frac{5s^2}{s^2} = 5 \tag{4.143}$$

or simply a flat line again at a value of 5. Finally, the corners at the break frequencies are rounded to obtain a smooth curve.

The phase angle plot will simply use the above slopes input into Equation 4.137.

1. For $\omega \ll 0.1$, the adjacent slopes are 0 on the magnitude plot, yielding $\varphi = 0$.
2. At $\omega = 0.1$, the adjacent slopes are 0 and -1. The average value is $-1/2$, yielding $\varphi = -\pi/4$.
3. For $\omega = 1$, the adjacent slopes are -1 and 0. The average value is $-1/2$, yielding $\varphi = -\pi/4$.
4. For $\omega = 10$, the adjacent slopes are 0 and $+1$. The average value is $+1/2$, yielding $\varphi = +\pi/4$.
5. For $\omega = 100$, the adjacent slopes are $+1$ and 0. The average value is $+1/2$, yielding $\varphi = +\pi/4$.
6. For $\omega \gg 100$, the adjacent slopes are 0 and 0, yielding $\varphi = 0$.

Again, a smooth curve is drawn through all of the points, yielding the plot shown in Figure 4.17b.

4.5 Frequency Analysis of Passive Muscle

Consider a passive muscle subject to a sinusoidal forcing strain function. Setting the tension of the contractile element to zero in Equation 4.78 yields the transfer function:

$$H(s) = \frac{K_{SE}(Bs + K_{PE})}{Bs + K_{PE} + K_{SE}} \tag{4.144}$$

Rearranging the expression to obtain an $(s + a)$ format, multiplying by the complex conjugate of the denominator term, and substituting $s = j\omega$ yields

$$H(j\omega) = \frac{K_{SE}(K_{PE}/B + j\omega)[(K_{PE} + K_{SE})/B - j\omega]}{[(K_{PE} + K_{SE})/B + j\omega][(K_{PE} + K_{SE})/B - j\omega]} \tag{4.145}$$

Simplification yields the real and imaginary parts:

$$H(j\omega) = \frac{K_{SE}[\omega^2 + K_{PE}(K_{PE} + K_{SE})/B^2 + j\omega K_{SE}/B]}{\omega^2 + [(K_{PE} + K_{SE})^2/B^2]} \tag{4.146}$$

To simplify calculations and plots, assume a very stiff series elastic element with a ratio of $K_{SE}/K_{PE} = 10$ and a ratio of $K_{PE}/B = 1$. Correspondingly, K_{SE}/B becomes equal to 10. Then, Equation 4.146 becomes

$$H(j\omega) = \frac{K_{SE}(\omega^2 + 11 + j10\omega)}{\omega^2 + 121} \tag{4.147}$$

The magnitude of $H(j\omega)$ then becomes

$$M = K_{SE}\frac{[(\omega^2 + 11)^2 + 100\omega^2]^{1/2}}{\omega^2 + 121} = K_{SE}\frac{[\omega^4 + 122\omega^2 + 121]^{1/2}}{\omega^2 + 121} = K_{SE}\frac{[\omega^2 + 1]^{1/2}}{[\omega^2 + 121]^{1/2}} \tag{4.148}$$

while the phase angle is

$$\varphi = \tan^{-1}\frac{10\omega}{\omega^2 + 11} \tag{4.149}$$

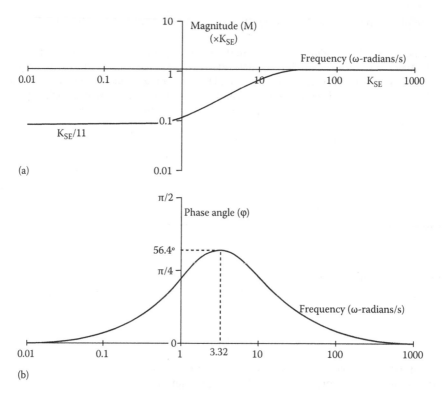

FIGURE 4.18
Magnitude (a) and phase angle (b) plots for $H(j\omega) = [K_{SE}(\omega^2 + 11 + j10\omega)]/[\omega^2 + 121]$.

To plot the magnitude, examine Equation 4.148 at small and large ω. For small ω, i.e., $\omega \ll 1$, the magnitude stays constant with a value of $K_{SE}/11$. For large ω, i.e., $\omega \gg 11$, the magnitude also remains constant at a value of K_{SE}. For values of ω around 11 the values change smoothly as an ogive curve from $K_{SE}/11$ to K_{SE}. The complete magnitude plot is shown in Figure 4.18.

The phase angle plot is similarly constructed from Equation 4.149. For small ω, the phase angle is roughly equal to $\tan^{-1} \omega$ or zero and increases very gradually for increasing values of ω. For large ω, the phase angle is roughly equal to $\tan^{-1} 10/\omega$ or also zero for large values of ω. For values of ω around the break frequency, the values of the phase angle first increase and then decrease. The critical break frequency can be inferred from the denominator as ω equal to $\sqrt{11}$ or calculated directly by finding the frequency at which point the phase angle reaches a maximum. This can be done by taking the derivative of Equation 4.149 with respect to ω and setting the resulting equation equal to zero:

$$\frac{d\varphi}{d\omega} = \frac{d}{d\omega}\left\{\tan^{-1}\frac{10\omega}{\omega^2 + 11}\right\} = 0 \tag{4.150}$$

Using the following identity with $u = 10\omega/(\omega^2 + 11)$ yields

$$\frac{d\tan^{-1}u}{d\omega} = \frac{du/d\omega}{1+u^2} \tag{4.151}$$

Only du/dω is critical and is set equal to zero:

$$\frac{du}{d\omega} = \frac{10}{\omega^2 + 11} - \frac{20\omega^2}{(\omega^2 + 11)^2} = 0 \tag{4.152}$$

yielding

$$(\omega^2 + 11)10 - 20\omega^2 = 10\omega^2 - 110 = \omega^2 - 11 = 0 \tag{4.153}$$

The critical break frequency is then $\sqrt{11} = 3.32$ and the maximum phase is then $\tan^{-1}(1.51)$ or $56.4°$. The complete phase angle plot is shown in Figure 4.18.

In terms of passive muscle, this means that at very low or high frequencies the forcing function and muscle response are practically in phase and elastically dominated by either the series elastic element (K_{SE}) for very high frequencies (i.e., the dashpot cannot respond sufficiently quickly, eliminating the parallel elastic element from the model) or by a combination of both elastic elements $K_{SE}/(K_{SE} + K_{PE})$ for very low frequencies (i.e., the dashpot responds, stretching the parallel elastic element with it). Around the critical break frequency the muscle is fully viscoelastic with the dashpot involved.

4.6 Hatze's Multielement Model

Hatze (1981) developed a muscle model considerably more complicated then Hill's four-element model (see Figure 4.19). It is termed a *distributed model* because it starts at the sarcomere level, modeling all of the individual structures rather than treating the complete muscle in a *lumped model* as done by Hill (1938). As with Hill's model, the purely contractile elements of the protein filaments are represented by CE_i. The parallel elastic elements of each sarcomere (PS_i) represent the surrounding fascia within muscle fibers such as the sarcolemna or endomysium, but not individually include a damping component, since the sarcolemna are firmly attached to the z-disks and do not allow appreciable movement. The damping element (DE) is contained in the fiber external structure and is thus placed parallel to the entire fiber. Similarly, the parallel elastic elements representing fascia are also placed parallel to the entire fiber. The series element is broken down into several components: a bridge element (BE_i) representing the elastic structures within the cross bridges and a series elastic element for the z-disk (SE_1). Finally, at both ends of each muscle fiber are lightly damped series elastic elements (SE_2) representing the tendinous parts of the fiber.

FIGURE 4.19
Distributed model of skeletal muscle. (Adapted from Hatze, H., *Myocybernetic Control Models of Skeletal Muscle*, University of South Africa, Pretoria, South Africa, 1981.)

FIGURE 4.20
Lumped model of skeletal muscle.

Obviously with hundreds and thousands of sarcomeres, such a distributed model for a complete muscle would be impossible to work with. Thus, a transition to a simple lumped model must be made. One justifiable assumption is that all the sarcomeres in a fiber are more or less identical and activated at approximately the same time. It follows then that all the SE_is for one fiber can be replaced by an equivalent single element SE. The same rationale can be applied to the elements CE_i, BE_i, and PS_i, resulting in the equivalent lumped elements of Figure 4.20.

A similar rationale can be used in lumping hundreds of muscle fibers into motor units and hundreds of motor units into a complete muscle. In general, although the motor unit fibers are distributed randomly over a certain volume of the muscle, all have similar morphological contractile and histochemical profiles. The motor units, however, vary in properties, and should perhaps be represented by separate models.

Certain assumptions allow a further reduction of the lumped model to simpler lumped model yet. The series elastic element SE and bridge element BE can be considered very stiff springs and eliminated completely. This contention is supported by Bawa et al. (1976), who found $K_{SE} = 380\,g/mm$ to be much larger than $K_{PE} = 103\,g/mm$. K_{BE} can be considered to be in a similar range with K_{SE}. Eliminating SE and BE results in a model with four parallel elements, two which are elastic and can be combined into one parallel elastic element. The final simplified model is given in Figure 4.21.

The total force developed by the simplified model of Figure 4.21 can now be expressed as

$$F = (f_{PE} + f_{CE} + f_{DE})F_{MAX} \tag{4.154}$$

Note that the each of the component elements are expressed as a fractional or relative force, which the final fraction to be scaled by the maximum force developed by the muscle F_{MAX}.

Each element within the model, needs further specification. Hill's model assumed simple linear properties which is not correct. For example, for the parallel elastic element (PE), extensive tests on the tensile properties of resting human sartorius muscle carried out by Yamada (1970) indicate an exponential force–strain function (see Figure 4.22):

$$f_{PE} = 0.00163(e^{7.66\varepsilon} - 1) \tag{4.155}$$

FIGURE 4.21
Simplified model of skeletal muscle.

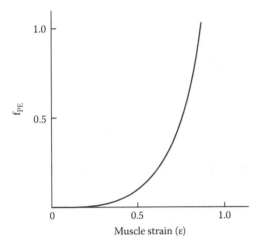

FIGURE 4.22
Force–strain function for the parallel elastic element of passive muscle.

The velocity dependence of the damping element (DE) was expressed previously as a simple dashpot. Alexander and Johnson (1965) separated the damping properties into a passive coefficient and the active force–velocity relationship, with the active component being 6.4 times larger than the passive component. Therefore, the Bawa et al. (1976) damping value for a cat plantaris muscle becomes 1.0 g s/mm, which when normalized to the plantaris resting length of 50 mm and maximum isometric tension of 245 g, yields a normalized slope of 0.2 F_{MAX}s/length. With maximum velocity for slow-twitch fibers reaching 2.9 muscle lengths/s, fairly significant viscous damping forces (0.6 F_{MAX} at maximum velocity) can be obtained (see Figure 4.23).

The contractile component can be modeled along its basic functions: the length–tension, velocity–tension, and active-state relationships. The first, as discussed previously, is determined by the number of active cross links and overlap of the thick and thin filaments and can be represented from the data of Gordon et al. (1966) by the function suggested by Hatze (1981):

$$f(\xi) = 0.32 + 0.71e^{-1.112(\xi-1)} \sin 3.722 \, (\xi - 0.656) \qquad (4.156)$$

FIGURE 4.23
Viscous characteristics for the damping element of passive muscle.

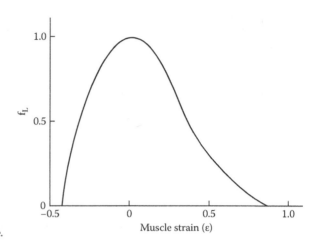

FIGURE 4.24
Length–tension relationship for active muscle.

where $f(\xi)$ is the normalized tension generation due to the length–tension relationship and ξ is ℓ/ℓ_0 with $0.58 \leq \ell \leq 1.8$. This relationship (see Figure 4.24) shows a fairly peaked response with more than a 20% reduction in force for less than ±20% changes in resting length.

The velocity–tension relationship is determined by the rate of breaking and reforming of cross bridges with higher rates producing less effective bonds. To account for the whole range of negative velocities (shortening or concentric contractions) as well as positive velocities (lengthening or eccentric contractions) Hatze (1981) has defined the following expression:

$$f(\dot{\eta}) = \frac{0.1433}{0.1074 + e^{-1.409\sinh(3.2\dot{\eta}+1.6)}} \qquad (4.157)$$

where
   $f(\dot{\eta})$ is the normalized tension due to the velocity–tension relationship
   $\dot{\eta}$ is the $= \dot{\varepsilon}/\dot{\varepsilon}_{MAX}$ or strain rate normalized to the maximum velocity of contraction

This relationship shows a rapid increase in force up to an asymptotic value 34% greater than the maximum isometric contraction level and a very rapid decrease in force down to zero for maximum concentric contractions (see Figure 4.25).

The active properties of the contractile element are also determined by the active-state function q(t). The relative force or tension due to the active state, f_q, is defined by the relative amount of calcium (Ca^{2+}) bound to troponin, the inhibitor of bonding between the myosin heads on the thick filament and globular actin on the thin filament. If the maximum number of potential interactive sites on the thin filament are exposed by the action of Ca^{2+}, then q = 1, while in a resting state q is very low, say q_0. Thus, the isometric tension developed by a muscle fiber at a given length ℓ_q is directly proportional to q(t) (Hatze, 1981, p. 33). The tension developed as a consequence of the active-state function can be defined as

$$f_q(t) = \frac{0.005 + 82.63v^2(1-e^{-mt})^2}{1 + 82.63v^2(1-e^{-mt})^2} \qquad (4.158)$$

with the value of m to be determined later. The complete details the led to development of this function, please refer to Example 4.6.

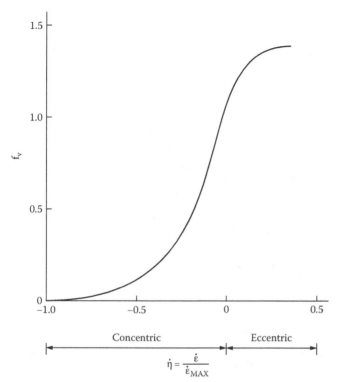

Concentric Eccentric

$$\dot{\eta} = \frac{\dot{\varepsilon}}{\dot{\varepsilon}_{MAX}}$$

FIGURE 4.25
Velocity–tension relationship for active muscle.

Example 4.6: Determination of the Active-State Tension Function

To find the active-state function q(t), define γ to be the difference between the free Ca^{2+} concentration γ_f and the free Ca^{2+} concentration γ_0 in the resting fiber. However, for practical purposes, since $\gamma_0 \ll \gamma_f$, γ and γ_f basically identical, let $\partial q/\partial \gamma$ denote the rate of change of the Ca^{2+} concentration during the active state q(t). The process of binding Ca^{2+} ions to the troponin sites is hypothesized by Hatze (1981) and supported by the experimental studies of Ebashi and Endo (1968) to be a function of the length ℓ of the contractile element and of the difference between the maximum and present value of q and is controlled by a negative feedback loop:

$$\frac{\partial p}{\partial \gamma} = \rho_1^2(\varepsilon)(1-q) - 2\rho_2(\varepsilon)\,\rho_1(\varepsilon)p \tag{4.159}$$

where p is defined as $\partial q/\partial \gamma$ and ρ_1 and ρ_2 are unknown functions to be determined. Note that Hatze's (1981) format has been changed by the substitution of standard strain ε for ξ where

$$\xi = \varepsilon + 1 \tag{4.160}$$

Solving the system of differential equations with initial conditions p(0) = 0 and q(0) = q_0 = 0.005, yields the normalized solution:

$$q(\varepsilon, \gamma) = 1 - \frac{(1-q_0)}{(m_1 - m_2)}\left\{m_1 e^{m_2\,\rho_1(\varepsilon)\gamma} - m_2 e^{m_1\,\rho_1(\varepsilon)\gamma}\right\} \tag{4.161}$$

where

$$m_{1,2} = -\rho_2(\varepsilon) \pm \left[\rho_2^{2}(\varepsilon) - 1\right]^{1/2} \quad \text{for } \rho_2 > 1 \tag{4.162}$$

Substituting experimentally found values Hatze (1981) found

$$\rho_1^{2}(\varepsilon) = 2.34 \times 10^{14} \left\{\frac{\varepsilon + 0.44}{\varepsilon + 1.0}\right\}^{1/2} \quad \text{for } -0.44 < \varepsilon < 0.8 \tag{4.163}$$

$$\rho_2(\varepsilon) = 1.05 \tag{4.164}$$

With appropriate simplification for mammalian muscle provided by Hatze (1981, p. 40) and substituting Equations 4.162, 4.163, and 4.164 into Equation 4.161 we find

$$q(\xi, \gamma) = \frac{q_0 + \rho^{2}(\varepsilon)\gamma^{2}}{1 + \rho^{2}(\varepsilon)\gamma^{2}} \tag{4.165}$$

where

$$\rho(\varepsilon) = 125{,}780 \frac{(\varepsilon + 1)}{(1.9 - \varepsilon)} \tag{4.166}$$

The function γ, the free Ca^{2+} ion concentration can be represented as a function of time t and the relative stimulation rate v by a trend function which represents the average behavior of γ in successive time intervals and which approaches a maximum value asymptotically and has the rate of increase proportional to the stimulation rate (Hatze, 1981, p. 39):

$$\frac{\partial \gamma}{\partial t} = m(1.373 \times 10^{-4}v - \gamma) \tag{4.167}$$

where v is the relative stimulation rate ranging between 0 and 1 and m is a constant to be determined later.

The rate of stimulation of motor units during voluntary contraction has been controversial. Several studies have found a fairly constant discharge frequency over a wide range of tension for individual motor units (Bigland and Lippold, 1954; Clamann, 1970), while others maintain that an increase in muscle tension is achieved in part by an increase in the stimulation rate and in part by an increase in the recruitment of motor units (Marsden et al., 1971; Person and Kudina, 1972; Milner-Brown et al., 1973). However, the rise in frequency with a rise in tension is associated with a high frequency close to the maximum stimulation rate (Tanji and Kato, 1973). Thus, it is fairly reasonable to assume a constant stimulation rate and, therefore, a constant relative stimulation rate.

Now solving Equation 4.167 with v constant yields

$$\gamma(t) = [\gamma(0) - 1.373 \times 10^{-4}v]e^{-mt} + 1.373 \times 10^{-4}v \tag{4.168}$$

where m is a unknown constant to be determined later. With $\gamma(0)$ much smaller than $1.373 \times 10^{-4}v$, Equation 4.168 reduces to

$$\gamma(t) = 1.373 \times 10^{-4} \, v \, [1 - e^{-mt}] \tag{4.169}$$

Substituting Equation 4.169 and Equation 4.166 with $\varepsilon = 0$ into Equation 4.165 yields the final active-state function and its resultant relative force or tension:

$$f_q(t) = \frac{0.005 + 82.63 \, v^2 (1 - e^{-mt})^2}{1 + 82.63 \, v^2 (1 - e^{-mt})^2} \tag{4.170}$$

Finally, f_{CE} can redefined as a combination of the three different component relationships:

$$f_{CE} = f_q(t) \, f_\ell(\varepsilon) \, f_v(\dot{\eta}) \tag{4.171}$$

An additional factor to consider is that the active-state function will vary depending on the type of motor units and relative stimulation rate. Although, the motor-unit properties such as the stimulation rate will vary continuously from very slow twitch to very fast twitch fibers, for modeling simplicity, the motor units can be considered as grouped into two distinct populations, type I or slow-twitch and type II or fast-twitch units. The total muscle tension output (Equation 4.154) now becomes the sum of the force output from N_I type I motor units and from N_{II} type II motor units:

$$F = (f_{PE} + f_{CEI} + f_{CEII} + f_{DE}) \, F_{MAX} \tag{4.172}$$

Also, the same total population of motor units can be subdivided into two other dynamically different populations: the N number of active motor units and the $\tilde{N}-N$ number of inactive or fatigued motor units, where $\tilde{N}$ is the total number of motor units in the muscle.

As mentioned previously, the motor units are recruited in a sequential order according to their size and twitch times. From Hatze (1981), the cumulative relative cross-sectional area u occupied by the recruited motor units increases by

$$u = u_0 \, e^{c(N-1)/\tilde{N}} \tag{4.173}$$

where u_0 is the relative cross-sectional area of the smallest motor unit and ranges from 0 to 1. c is a constant expressed as

$$c = -\ln u_0 \tag{4.174}$$

For N large, Equation 4.173 reduces to

$$u_n = u_0 \, e^{cN/\tilde{N}} = u_0^{(1-N/\tilde{N})} = u_0^{(1-n)} \tag{4.175}$$

where n is the fraction of recruited or active motor units or $N/\tilde{N}$. Examining the ratios of the smallest to the largest motor cross-sectional areas measured in muscle, allows estimates of u_0 to be made. Experimental values of u_0 range from 0.005 for the rectus femorus

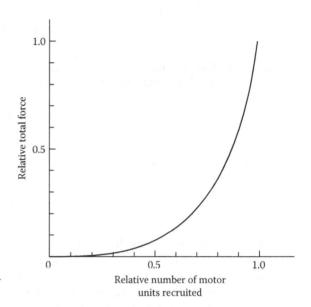

FIGURE 4.26
Muscle tension developed by orderly recruitment of motor units.

to 0.009 for the biceps (Hatze, 1979), with an average value of 0.00673. As the cross-sectional area increases exponentially, so also does the total muscle tension increase exponentially (see Figure 4.26).

Combining the two sets of overlapping population distributions of motor units yields two distinct cases:

1. $N < N_I$, only part of type I motor units are recruited and none of the type II are recruited because of the orderly recruitment pattern and
2. $N > N_I$, all type I motor units are recruited and some of the type II motor units are recruited, but none of the type I are inactive.

Additional appropriate motor unit properties are obtained from Henneman and Olson (1965). The contraction time t_c of a motor unit is a decreasing function of the fraction n of recruited motor units:

$$t_c = a - bn \tag{4.176}$$

For type I motor units, Equation 4.176 becomes

$$t_{cI} = a_I - b_I n \quad \text{for } 0 \le n \le n_I \tag{4.177}$$

and, for type II motor units, Equation 4.176 becomes

$$t_{cII} = a_{II} - b_{II} n \quad \text{for } n_I \le n \le 1 \tag{4.178}$$

The constants can be determined from experimental data. For n = 0, the value of t_c corresponds to the contraction time of the slowest type I motor unit in the muscle or approximately equal to 0.1 s; for n = n_I, the value of t_c corresponds to the fastest type I motor unit (and slowest type II unit) or approximately $0.045\,s$; and for $n = 1$, the value of t_c corresponds to the fastest type II motor unit or approximately $0.01\,s$ (Grimby and Hannerz, 1977). Substituting these values into Equations 4.172 and 4.173 and solving for the unknowns, yields

$$a_I = 0.1 \tag{4.179}$$

$$b_I = \frac{0.055}{n_I} \tag{4.180}$$

$$a_{II} = 0.01 + \frac{0.035}{(1 - n_I)} \tag{4.181}$$

$$b_{II} = \frac{0.035}{(1 - n_I)} \tag{4.182}$$

Equations 4.177 and 4.178 can now be expressed as

$$t_{cI} = 0.1 - 0.055\,\frac{n}{n_I} \tag{4.183}$$

$$t_{cII} = 0.01 + 0.035\,\frac{(1 - n)}{(1 - n_I)} \tag{4.184}$$

Close (1965) showed that for mammalian skeletal muscle, the maximum normalized speed of shortening is related to the contraction time of a muscle, consisting predominantly of one fiber type, by

$$\dot{\varepsilon}_{MAX} = \frac{0.297}{t_c} \tag{4.185}$$

This then indicates that the first or slowest motor unit at $n = 0$, has a relative contraction velocity of 2.97 lengths/s, while the last or fastest motor unit at $n = 1$ has a relative contraction velocity of 29.7 lengths/s. The value of $\dot{\varepsilon}_{MAX}$ is necessary for Equation 4.157.

The rate constant m in Equation 4.158 also depends on the contraction time:

$$m = \frac{0.372}{t_c} \tag{4.186}$$

For the slowest motor unit ($n = 0$) $m = 3.72$ while for the fastest motor unit ($n = 1$) $m = 37.2$. The relative force or tension, $f_q(t)$ developed during the active state is plotted in Figure 4.27 for pure type I and type II motor units, as well as for different relative stimulation rates. Now, finally, Equation 4.158 is completely determined. Further details on the simplified Hatze muscle model can be found in Freivalds and Kaleps (1984) and Freivalds (1985).

FIGURE 4.27
Muscle tension developed by the active state function for various conditions.

4.7 Applications of the Hatze Muscle Model

One important factor affecting the accuracy in modeling the neuromusculature for dynamic simulation such as the Articulated Total Body Model (Freivalds and Kaleps, 1984) is the accuracy of the placement of the musculature, i.e., the origins and insertions of the muscle being simulated. Specific data, in many cases, are obtained by measuring directly from anatomical scaled photographs (McMinn and Hutchings, 1977). Obviously, some human error is involved, especially in using two-dimensional photographs of three-dimensional structures. Thus, it was decided to simulate errors in muscle placement and compare the muscle forces developed through while "stimulating" the muscle.

The stimulation consisted of elbow flexion against a load with the three major elbow flexors: the biceps brachii, the brachialis, and the brachioradialis (see Figure 3.1). Using cross-sectional areas of 4.58, 4.63, and 1.37 cm² from Schumacher and Wolff (1966) and the maximum muscle force per area of 100 N/cm² from Hatze (1981), yielded maximum isometric tension values of 458, 463, and 137 N, respectively. Five different conditions were simulated. In Conditions 0 and 1, the origin of each muscle was displaced by ±10% of the insertion distance, respectively. In Condition 2, both the origin and insertion were shifted by 10%. In Condition 3, both the origin and insertion were shifted by 20%. Condition 4 was the control case with "true" origins and insertions. The simulation started with the hand holding a 270 N weight with the upper limb bent at 90° and the muscles stimulated for maximal contraction

FIGURE 4.28

Force developed by the biceps brachii (a) and brachioradialis (b) while holding a load of 270 N under five differ-ent conditions: 0, muscle origin displaced +10%; 1, muscle origin displaced –10%; 2, both origin and insertion displaced +10%; 3, both origin and insertion displaced +20%; 4, control case.

simultaneously. Since this weight exceeded the maximum weight that could be maintained by the elbow flexors, the muscles would necessarily be forced into eccentric contraction. This simulation corresponded closely in terms of muscle strength capabilities to the data of Wilkie (1950) who found his subjects could maintain a maximum of 196 N at the wrist.

The general pattern of the results shown in Figure 4.28 can be explained by the forces pro-duced by the various components of the muscle model. Initially, since the weight exceeded the resting tonus of the muscles, the muscles were forcibly extended in an eccentric con-traction, as exhibited by the rather sharp increase in force. As the arms are extended, the length–tension relationship contributes significantly in reducing the muscle force. The bra-chioradialis is affected the most because of its length, the biceps the least. However, for all four test conditions, there was a small deviation (average 3%, maximum 9%) from the control condition, indicating relatively low sensitivity for the location of the origins and insertions. Concentric contractions with smaller weights showed rapid decreases in muscle force due to the velocity–tension relationship. However, both simulations assumed maximal stimulation and recruitment to maximum force as in a ballistic movement. More commonly, movements are more controlled through the various feedback loops as well voluntarily control.

4.8 Control Theory and Motor Control

4.8.1 Basic Concepts

The musculoskeletal system, as any complex system, is composed of inputs, outputs, and either known or unknown (black box) components which act as transfer functions to modify the input to create the output. The action of the transfer function was discussed considerably in Section 4.1.2. It might be valuable at this time to distinguish between open-loop and closed-loop systems. A *closed-loop system* performs some action which requires continuous control in the form of some comparison between the system output and the command input. This means there is continual feedback of information about any error that should be taken into account for successful operation. Thus, these types of systems are often referred to as *feedback systems*.

At the physiological level the muscle spindle system is a feedback system for muscle length and the Golgi tendon organs act as feedback system for muscular tension. At a gross level, the tracking of cursor on a computer screen with a pointer is a feedback system that requires a variety of information including agonist muscle tension and length, antagonist muscle tension and length to be fed back and compared to the input.

An *open-loop system* is one in which the command input is independent of the system output. This type system, once activated, cannot be controlled any further, i.e., once the die is cast, fate is determined. While a guided missile is an example of a closed-loop system, a bullet from a rifle is an open-loop system. Such a system is sometimes termed a *feedforward system*. At the physiological level, e.g., when lifting a load, basic recruitment of α-efferent motor units at the cell body is an open-loop system. Either there is enough excitatory stimulation from the central nervous system or there is not. However, in the more complex sense, the muscle spindles will sense whether there is a stretching (i.e., the load is depressing the limb) and send feedback via the α-afferent pathway to provide further excitatory stimulation. At a gross level, a ballistic movement, such as throwing a ball, is theoretically an open-loop system, because once released the rock cannot be further controlled. However, there will be variety of control actions and feedback loops occurring during the recruitment of appropriate muscle to provide the appropriate limb movement.

Open-loop tasks performed by a human operator will have the following characteristics:

1. The task performance is automatic. The operator utilizes previous experience and training to provide the best command input for the best output.

2. Since there is no feedback, the final outcome (whether the ball hits the target) may or may not be acceptable depending on system disturbances (such as wind) that cannot be directly controlled by the operator. Obviously, the operator will alter the motion on a second throw to better hit the target.

3. The degree of accuracy in performing such an "open-loop" task is dependent on both operator's skill level and the presence of outside disturbances.

Closed-loop tasks performed by a human operator will have the following characteristics (as compared to an open-loop task):

1. The task performance requires continuous feedback of system output. For example, in the above tracking task, the location of the pointer with respect to the cursor must be continually observed for best performance.

2. Task performance increases with an increased ability to more precisely reproduce or control the command input, i.e., the pointer location.

3. System performance is less sensitive to external disturbances, since corrections can be or are made continually.

4. There is an increased tendency toward system oscillation and instability as will be described in more detail later.

4.8.2 First-Order System

Using Hill's four-element model, the external muscle tension was developed in Equation 4.78 as a function of the internal tension from the contractile element and the external strain:

$$T = \frac{K_{SE}T_{CE}}{Bs + K_{PE} + K_{SE}} + \frac{K_{SE}(Bs + K_{PE})}{Bs + K_{PE} + K_{SE}}\varepsilon \tag{4.187}$$

Typically, such linear lumped models give rise to transfer functions that have polynomials in s both in the numerator and denominator, where the power of s in the numerator should typically be lower than the power of s in the denominator for system stability (e.g., an impulse response would not be feasible). The *roots* of these polynomials are those values that make the polynomial equal to zero.

The roots of the denominator have a special significance because they characterize the exponential and/or sinusoidal terms of the impulse response. It is called the *characteristic function* of the system and its roots are called the *poles* of the system. The roots of the numerator affect the magnitude and phase of the response, but not its basic nature. They are called the *zeros* of the system.

Assuming an isometric contraction for the characteristic muscle function in Equation 4.187 yields the simpler form:

$$T = \frac{K_{SE}T_{CE}}{Bs + K_{PE} + K_{SE}} = \frac{K_{SE}T_{CE}/B}{s + 1/\tau} \tag{4.188}$$

where $1/\tau$ is the pole of the system and $\tau = B/(K_{PE} + K_{SE})$ is the time constant of the system. In a frequency analysis, the critical break frequency is $\omega = 1/\tau$. This basic system is known as a *first-order system* because there is only one pole or the power of s in the denominator is one. The step response and frequency analysis is shown in Figure 4.29.

4.8.3 Second-Order System

A *second-order system* has two poles or the power of s in the denominator (or the characteristic function) is two. This is probably the most common and most intuitive model of physical systems and is used to represent the mass-spring-dashpot system of Figure 4.30:

$$\frac{\varepsilon(s)}{\sigma(s)} = \frac{1}{Ms^2 + Bs + K} \tag{4.189}$$

where
   M is the mass of the object
   B is the damping constant
   K is the spring constant

Reorganizing Equation 4.189, yields the characteristic form of a second-order system:

$$\frac{\varepsilon(s)}{\sigma(s)} = \frac{\omega_n^2/K}{s^2 + 2\omega_n\zeta s + \omega_n^2} \tag{4.190}$$

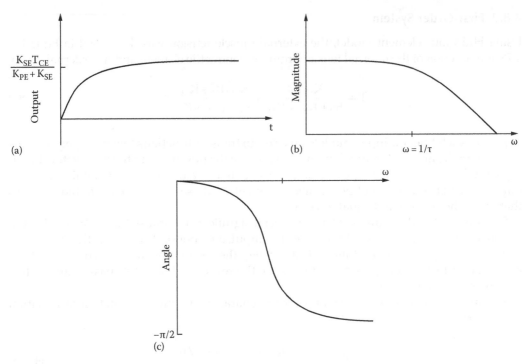

FIGURE 4.29
Step response (a) magnitude plot (b) and phase angle plot (c) for a first-order system. $T = (K_{SE}T_{CE})/(Bs + K_{PE} + K_{SE})$.

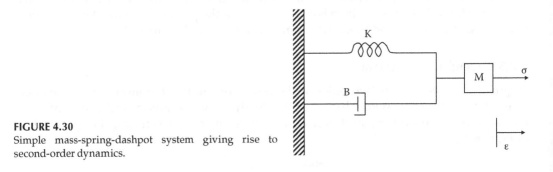

FIGURE 4.30
Simple mass-spring-dashpot system giving rise to second-order dynamics.

where ω_n is termed the undamped *natural frequency* and is the frequency at which the system would oscillate if the damping, B, were zero. It is defined as

$$\omega_n = \left(\frac{K}{M}\right)^{1/2} \tag{4.191}$$

ζ is termed the *damping ratio* and is defined as

$$\zeta = \frac{B}{2M\omega_n} \tag{4.192}$$

The frequency response of such a second-order system is obtained by replacing s with $j\omega$ in Equation 4.190, yielding

$$H(j\omega) = \frac{\omega_n^2/K}{-\omega^2 + 2j\omega_n\zeta\omega + \omega_n^2} = \frac{\omega_n^2}{K}\frac{1}{(\omega_n^2 - \omega^2) + 2j\zeta\omega_n\omega} \tag{4.193}$$

Multiplying the numerator and denominator the complex conjugate yields

$$H(\omega) = \frac{\omega_n^2}{K}\frac{(\omega_n^2 - \omega^2) - 2j\zeta\omega_n\omega}{(\omega_n^2 - \omega^2)^2 + 4\zeta^2\omega_n^2\omega^2} \tag{4.194}$$

The magnitude, as defined from Equation 4.113, is

$$M(\omega) = [X(\omega)^2 + Y(\omega)^2]^{1/2} = \frac{\omega_n^2}{K}\left[(\omega_n^2 - \omega^2)^2 + 4\zeta^2\omega_n^2\omega^2\right]^{-1/2} \tag{4.195}$$

For small ω, $\omega \ll \omega_n$, the magnitude is

$$M(\omega) = \frac{1}{K} \tag{4.196}$$

with a slope of zero on the magnitude plot. For large ω, $\omega \gg \omega_n$, the magnitude becomes

$$M(\omega) = \frac{Y\omega_n^2}{K\omega^2} \tag{4.197}$$

with a slope of −2 on the magnitude plot.
   The phase angle, from Equation 4.114, is defined as

$$\varphi(\omega) = \tan^{-1}\left[\frac{Y(\omega)}{X(\omega)}\right] = \tan^{-1}\frac{2\zeta\omega_n\omega}{(\omega_n^2 - \omega^2)} \tag{4.198}$$

For small ω, $\omega \ll \omega_n$, the phase angle is

$$\varphi(\omega) = \tan^{-1}\frac{2\zeta\omega}{\omega_n} \approx 0 \tag{4.199}$$

For large ω, $\omega \gg \omega_n$, the phase angle is

$$\varphi(\omega) = -\tan^{-1}2\zeta\frac{\omega_n}{\omega} \approx -\tan^{-1}\infty = -180° \tag{4.200}$$

The resulting magnitude and phase plots, for various values of ζ, are shown in Figure 4.31.
   For a larger range of values of ζ, the second-order system exhibits four distinct types of behavior. Figure 4.32 summarizes these responses in a *pole-zero diagram*. For $\zeta = 0$,

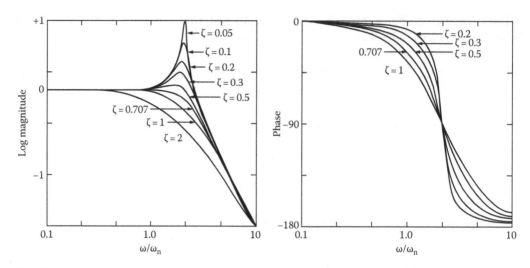

FIGURE 4.31
Magnitude and phase plots for a second-order system for various values of ζ. (From Milsum, J.H., *Biological Control Systems*, McGraw-Hill, New York, 1966. With permission.)

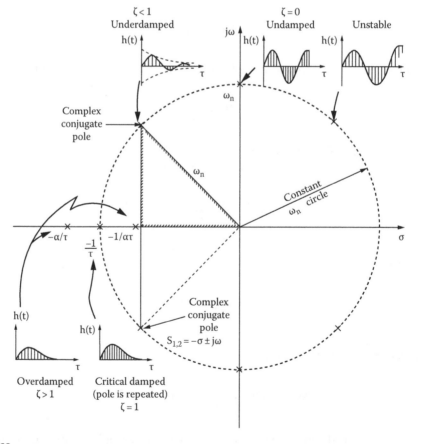

FIGURE 4.32
Impulse responses for a second-order system for various pole locations. (From Milsum, J.H., *Biological Control Systems*, McGraw-Hill, New York, 1966. With permission.)

the system is termed *undamped* and the impulse response will be a steady-state sinusoid of frequency ω_n. For $\zeta < 1$, the system is termed *underdamped* and sinusoids of ω_n will die out over time. For $\zeta = 1$, the system is termed *critically damped* and the impulse response rises and then dies out. Note that in this case the pole is repeated. For $\zeta > 1$, the system is termed *overdamped* and the impulse response dies out more quickly than for the critically damped case. Note that for poles on the positive side of the pole-zero diagram, the resulting exponential envelope for the sinusoids explodes. This is termed an unstable system will be discussed later. The transfer functions and step responses for these four cases are given in Table 4.3. Further details on such systems and response can be found in Milsum (1966), Melsa and Schultz (1969), and Stark (1968).

Example 4.7: Step Response of a Second-Order System

Assume a critically damped ($\varsigma = 1$) second-order system similar to the mass-spring-dashpot system of Equation 4.189, with a step-stress (e.g., muscle force) input. The resulting strain output (i.e., movement) is

$$\varepsilon(s) = \frac{\omega_n^2 / K}{\left(s^2 + 2\omega_n s + \omega_n^2\right)s} = \frac{\omega_n^2}{K}\frac{1}{(s+\omega_n)^2} \tag{4.201}$$

A partial fraction expansion of Equation 4.201 yields

$$\varepsilon(s) = \frac{a}{s} + \frac{b}{s+\omega_n} + \frac{c}{(s+\omega_n)^2} \tag{4.202}$$

Using the residue method the following solutions are obtained:

$$a = \left.\frac{\omega_n^2}{K(s+\omega_n)^2}\right|_{s=0} = \frac{1}{K} \tag{4.203}$$

$$c = \left.\frac{\omega_n^2}{Ks}\right|_{s=-\omega n} = \frac{-\omega_n}{K} \tag{4.204}$$

$$b = \left.\frac{\omega_n^2}{K}\frac{d(1/s)}{ds}\right|_{s=-\omega n} = \left.\frac{-\omega_n}{Ks^2}\right|_{s=-\omega n} = \frac{-1}{K} \tag{4.205}$$

Substituting Equations 4.203, 4.204, and 4.205 into 4.202 yields

$$\varepsilon(s) = \frac{1}{K}\left\{\frac{1}{s} - \frac{1}{s+\omega_n} - \frac{\omega_n}{(s+\omega_n)^2}\right\} \tag{4.206}$$

Taking the inverse Laplace transform yields the final solution as shown in Table 4.3:

$$\varepsilon(t) = \frac{1}{K}\left\{1 - (1+\omega_n t)e^{-\omega n t}\right\} \tag{4.207}$$

TABLE 4.3

Transfer Functions and Step Responses of Second-Order Systems

Damping Ratio	Type of Damping	Transfer Function	Frequency Domain Step Response	Time Domain Step Response
$\zeta = 0$	Undamped	$\dfrac{\omega_n^2}{s^2 + \omega_n^2}$	$\dfrac{\omega_n^2}{s\left(s^2 + \omega_n^2\right)}$	$1 - \cos \omega_n t$
$0 < \zeta < 1$	Underdamped	$\dfrac{\omega_n^2}{s^2 + 2\zeta\omega_n s + \omega_n^2}$	$\dfrac{\omega_n^2}{s\left(s^2 + 2\zeta\omega_n s + \omega_n^2\right)}$	$1 - \dfrac{e^{-\zeta\omega_n t}}{\sqrt{1-\zeta^2}}\sin\left(\omega_n\sqrt{1-\zeta^2}\,t + \tan^{-1}\sqrt{1-\zeta^2}/\zeta\right)$
$\zeta = 1$	Critically damped	$\dfrac{\omega_n^2}{(s+\omega_n)^2}$	$\dfrac{\omega_n^2}{s(s+\omega_n)^2}$	$1 - (1+\omega_n t)e^{-\omega_n t}$
$\zeta > 1$	Overdamped	$\dfrac{\omega_n^2}{(s+\omega_n/\alpha)(s+\alpha\omega_n)}$	$\dfrac{\omega_n^2}{s(s+\omega_n/\alpha)(s+\alpha\omega_n)}$	$1 - \dfrac{(e^{-\alpha\omega_n t} - a^2 e^{-\omega_n t/\alpha})}{\alpha^2 - 1}$

Source: Milsum, J.H., *Biological Control Systems*, McGraw-Hill, New York, 1966. With permission.

4.8.4 Human Information Processing and Control of Movements

One approach to modeling and understanding movement is to use information theory. *Information theory* measures information in bits, where a *bit* is the amount of information of information required to decide between two equally likely alternatives. The term bit came from the first and last part of the words *bi*nary dig*it* used in the computer and communication theory to express the on/off state of a chip or the polarized/reverse polarized position of small pieces of ferromagnetic core used in archaic computer memory. Mathematically, this can be expressed as

$$H = \log_2 n \tag{4.208}$$

where
  H is the amount of information
  n is the number of equally likely alternatives

With only two alternatives, such as the on/off state of a chip or the toss of an unweighted coin, there is one bit of information presented. With ten equally likely alternatives, such as the numbers from 0 to 9, 3.322 bits of information can be conveyed ($\log_2 10 = 3.322$). An easy way of calculating $\log_2$ is to use the following formula:

$$\log_2 n = 1.4427 \times \ln n \tag{4.209}$$

When the alternatives are not equally likely, the information conveyed is determined by

$$H = \sum p_i \times \log_2 \left(\frac{1}{p_i} \right) \tag{4.210}$$

where
  p_i is the probability of the ith event
  i is the alternatives from 1 to n

As an example, consider a weighted coin such that heads come up 90% of the time and tails only 10% of time. The amount of information conveyed in a coin toss becomes

$$H = 0.9 \times \log_2 \left(\frac{1}{0.9} \right) + 0.1 \times \log_2 \left(\frac{1}{0.1} \right) = 0.9 \times 0.152 + 0.1 \times 3.32 = 0.469 \text{ bits} \tag{4.211}$$

The amount of information that a human processes can be quantified through a *choice-reaction time* experiment, in which the operator responds to several stimuli with several appropriate responses. This can be considered as simple decision making, and based on the human information processing system, the response time should increase as the number of alternative stimuli increases. The response is nonlinear (see Figure 4.33a) but, when decision complexity is quantified in terms of the amount of information conveyed

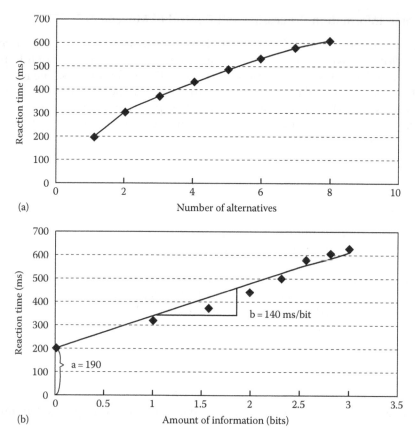

FIGURE 4.33
Hick–Hyman law illustrated with raw data (a) and information expressed in bits (b).

in bits, then the response becomes linear (see Figure 4.33b) and is referred to as the *Hick–Hyman Law* (Hick, 1952; Hyman, 1953):

$$RT = a + bH \qquad (4.212)$$

where
  RT is the response time (s)
  H is the amount of information (bits)
  a is the intercept
  b is the slope, sometimes referred to as the information processing rate

Note that when there is only one choice (e.g., when the light appears, press the button), H equals zero and the response time is equal to the intercept. This is known as *simple reaction time*. It can vary depending on the type of stimulus (auditory reaction times are about 40 ms faster than visual reaction times), the intensity of the stimulus, and preparedness for the signal.

Information theory was applied to the modeling of human movement by Fitts (1954) who developed the *index of difficulty* to predict movement time. The index of difficulty was defined as a function of the distance of movement and target size in a series of positioning movements to and from identical targets:

$$ID = \log_2\left(\frac{2D}{W}\right) \tag{4.213}$$

where
    ID is the index of difficulty (bits)
    D is the distance between target centers
    W is the target width

Movement time was found to follow the Hick–Hyman Law, now termed *Fitts' Law*:

$$MT = a + bID \tag{4.214}$$

where
    MT is the movement time (s)
    a is the intercept
    b is the slope

In a particularly successful application of Fitts' Law, Langolf et al. (1976) modeled human movement by different limbs across a wide range of distances, including very small targets visible only with the assistance of a microscope. Their results (see Figure 4.34) yielded slopes of 105 ms/bit for the arm, 45 ms/bit for the wrist, and 26 ms/ bit for the finger. The inverse of the slope is interpreted, according to information theory, as the motor system *bandwidth*. In this case, the bandwidths were 38 bits/s for the finger, 23 bits/s for the wrist, and 10 bits/s for the arm. This decrease in information processing

FIGURE 4.34
Fitts' Law illustrated arms, wrist, and finger movements. (Reproduced from Sanders, M.S. and McCormick, E.J., *Human Factors in Engineering and Design*, McGraw-Hill, New York, 1993. With permission.)

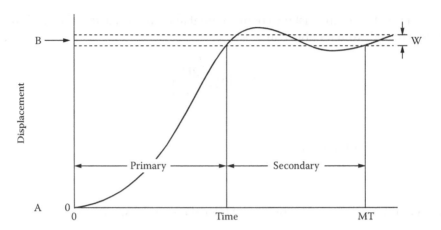

FIGURE 4.35
Typical movement response in target acquisition showing second-order control. (Adapted from Langolf, G., *J. Motor Behav.*, 8, 113, 1976.)

rates was explained as the result of added processing for the additional joints, muscles, motor units, receptors, etc.

Interestingly, Langolf et al. (1976) also showed that the typical human movement response to a unit-step input follows a second-order response. The desired input is a step change in displacement of the hand from a starting point A to a target or an ending point B with an arbitrary width W. The response shows the actual displacement of the hand plotted against time with two distinct phases (see Figure 4.35). The first or primary phase consists of acceleration and deceleration of the hand resulting in a relatively overall constant velocity. The second or secondary phase consists of homing into the target, with one or more overshoots and undershoots, thus showing the characteristic oscillation of an underdamped second-order control system. This is contrast to rapid, almost, ballistic type motions produced in a boxing punch or jab, which operates in an open-loop fashion with minimal or no feedback.

4.9 Root-Locus Approach to Muscle Modeling

4.9.1 Root-Locus Method

An open-loop system with no feedback can be simply represented as a black box for the plant with function G(s) (see Figure 4.36a). The *plant* can be considered as a simple transfer function or element that exerts control over the input, to transform it into the output. A closed-loop system has a feedback path, which may also have a transfer function element to it represented as H(s) (see Figure 4.36b). With more elements, the representation, termed a *block diagram*, may become more complicated. Therefore, there are several identities that may be useful for manipulating such block diagrams (see Figure 4.37). The most useful is Identity 6, which will typically be used to convert a feedback system to a simple transfer function for further manipulation or inverse transform calculation.

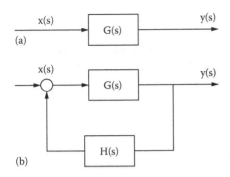

FIGURE 4.36
(a) Open-loop system. (b) Closed-loop system with feedback path.

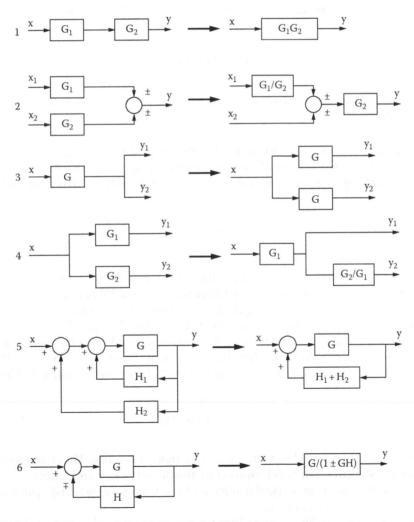

FIGURE 4.37
Block diagram identities.

Example 4.8: Derivation of Identity 6

The difference between the input x(s) and the feedback path can be defined as an error function, e(s), which is then operated on by the plant G(s) to yield the output:

$$y(s) = G(s)\,e(s) \tag{4.215}$$

This error function can be formally defined as

$$e(s) = x(s) - H(s)\,y(s) \tag{4.216}$$

Substituting Equation 4.215 into Equation 4.216 the yields

$$y(s) = G(s)\,[x(s) - H(s)\,y(s)] = G(s)\,x(s) - G(s)\,H(s)\,y(s) \tag{4.217}$$

Collating y(s) terms and dividing both sides by x(s) yields the final expression:

$$\frac{y(s)}{x(s)} = \frac{G(s)}{1 + G(s)\,H(s)} \tag{4.218}$$

Note that if it was a positive feedback system, then the plus sign in Equation 4.218 would become a minus sign.

For a real system to function properly, it must also be a stable system. There are several definitions of stability; however, they all apply to the steady-state response (i.e., as $t \to \infty$) rather than the transient response. The classic definition of stability is that G(t) is finite as defined by

$$\int_{0}^{\infty} |\,G(t)\,|\,dt < \infty \tag{4.219}$$

However, as shown previously, working in the time domain can be difficult. Therefore, in practice, the Laplace domain and an alternate definition of stability is used: the poles of the closed loop transfer function, y(s)/x(s), lie in the left half of the s-plane.

In the generalized representation of a control loop (see Figure 4.36b), G(s) is typically referred to as the plant, with an internal gain control K, and H(s) is the feedback element. One of the easiest aspects to controlling the stability of the system is to adjust the gain K of the controller as needed. The overall system transfer function (according to Identity 6) is

$$\frac{y(s)}{x(s)} = \frac{KG(s)}{1 + KG(s)H(s)} \tag{4.220}$$

This representation is referred to as the *closed-loop transfer function*. The characteristic function of this transfer function is determined by the denominator and, effectively, by KG(s) H(s). Consequently, the term KG(s)H(s), referred to as the *open-loop transfer function*, can be used to determine system stability.

There is a graphical analytical procedure for determining the location of the poles (and zeros) of this open loop transfer function as a function of certain systems parameters, most typically the controller gain K. This *root-locus* plots the poles or roots of the open-loop transfer function as a function of K using a structured procedure given as a set of 12 rules in Table 4.4 These are explained below in relation to the relatively simple open-loop transfer function:

$$KG(s)H(s) = \frac{K(s+2)}{s(s+6)} \tag{4.221}$$

Rule 1—Number of branches: The number of branches of the root-locus plot is equal to the number of poles of the open-loop transfer function. In Equation 4.221, there are two poles, s = 0 and s = −6, yielding two branches.

Rule 2—Starting points: The branches of the root locus start at the poles of the open-loop transfer function. In Equation 4.221, the branches start at s = 0 and s = −6. Note that for the system identified by Equation 4.221 to be stable, as s approaches the poles (in which case the denominator goes to zero and the transfer function goes to infinity), K must approach zero. Thus, K = 0 at the poles.

Rule 3—End points: The branches of the root locus terminate at the zeros of the open-loop transfer function. For the example in Equation 4.221, the branches terminate at s = −2. Another zero needs to be identified and will eventually be found somewhere at infinity. Note that the system identified by Equation 4.221 can be stable as s approaches the zero (in which case the numerator goes to zero) even if K approaches infinity. Thus, K = ∞ at the zeros.

Rule 4—Behavior on the real axis: A point on the real axis is part of the root locus if an odd number of poles and/or zeros lie to the right of this point. This means that for the system of Equation 4.221 the root locus exists between 0 and −2 and from −6 leftwards, as shown in Figure 4.38.

Rule 5—Value of gain: The value of the gain, K, can be determined at a given point, s = s′, on the root locus by evaluating the characteristic function of the closed loop transfer function:

$$1 + KG(s)H(s) = 0 \tag{4.222}$$

or in an alternate form:

$$KG(s)H(s) = |1| \tag{4.223}$$

at a phase angle of 180°. Consequently, the value of gain K is

$$K = \frac{1}{|G(s)H(s)|_{s=s'}} = \frac{s(s+6)}{(s+2)}\Bigg|_{s=s'} \tag{4.224}$$

For the system of Equation 4.221, the following values of gains can be calculated.

S	−0.1	−1.0	−1.5	−1.9
K	0.31	5.0	13.5	77.9

TABLE 4.4

Summary of Root-Locus Construction Rules

Rule 1	Number of branches	There is one branch for each pole of the open-loop transfer function $KG(s)H(s)$
Rule 2	Starting points ($K = 0$)	The branches of the root locus start at the poles of $KG(s)H(s)$
Rule 3	End points ($K = \infty$)	The branches of the root locus end at the zeroes of $KG(s)H(s)$
Rule 4	Behavior along the real axis	The root locus exists on the real axis at every point for which an odd number of poles and/or zeroes lie to the right
Rule 5	Gain determination	At a point s_1 on the root locus, the gain is given by $K = \left. \left\| \dfrac{1}{\|G(s)H(s)\|} \right\| \right\|_{s=s_1}$
Rule 6	Symmetry of locus	The root locus is always symmetric with respect to the real axis
Rule 7	Breakaway or reentry points	The root locus breaks away from the real axis at a point of relative maximum gain and returns to the real axis at a point of relative minimum gain
Rule 8	Breakaway or reentry angles	At points of breakaway or reentry, the branches of the root locus are separated by an angle of $180°/\alpha$ where α is the number of branches that intersect
Rule 9	Asymptotic behavior for large K	The asymptote angles are given by $\phi_{asy} = \dfrac{180° + k360°}{p - z}$ $k = 0, 1, 2, ..., p - z - 1$ and the origin of the asymptotes is $OA = \dfrac{\sum (\text{Pole locations}) - \sum (\text{Zero locations})}{p - z}$
Rule 10	Imaginary-axis crossing	The branches of the root locus cross the imaginary axis at points where the phase shift is $180°$
Rule 11	Sum of the closed-loop poles	If $p - z \geq 2$, the sum of the closed-loop poles is a constant
Rule 12	Angles of departure and arrival	The angles of departure and arrival at complex conjugate poles and zeroes are determined by satisfying the angle criterion near the pole or zero in question

Source: Melsa, J.L. and Schultz, D.G., *Linear Control Systems*, McGraw-Hill, New York, 1969.

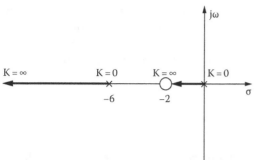

FIGURE 4.38
Root-locus plot for K(s + 2)/s(s + 6).

Rule 6—Symmetry: The root locus is symmetric with respect to the real or x-axis. If the poles of the open-loop transfer function happen to be complex conjugate roots, then these roots will lie equidistant above and below the real axis. This means that the root locus will necessarily deviate from the x-axis and may have breakaway and reentry points and angles to the real axis. However, for Equation 4.221, the root locus lies completely on the x-axis as shown in Figure 4.38.

For the rest of the rules, a slightly more elaborate root locus will be utilized. Its open-loop transfer function is defined as

$$KG(s)H(s) = \frac{K(s+6)}{s(s+2)} \tag{4.225}$$

The first six rules yield the following characteristics for the root locus. From Rule 1, there are two poles and, thus, two branches. From Rule 2, the starting points are the poles, s = 0 and s = −2. From Rule 3, the ending points are the one direct zero of s = −6 and another zero, implied at s = ∞. From Rule 4, the two branches of the root locus would start on the real axis at 0 and −2, head toward each other, then breakaway somewhere from the real axis and finally reenter the real axis beyond −6. Based on these rules and Rule 6 of symmetry, an approximate root locus for Equation 4.225 is given by Figure 4.39.

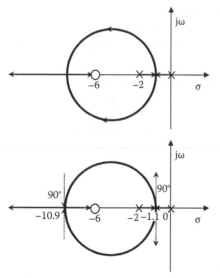

FIGURE 4.39
Step-by-step development of a root-locus plot for K(s + 6)/s(s + 2).

Rule 7—Breakaway or reentry points: The root locus breaks away from the real axis at a point of relative maximum gain and reenters the real axis at a point of relative minimum gain. The relative maximum and minimum points for a continuous function can be determined by taking the derivative of the function, setting it equal to zero and solving for the roots, i.e.,

$$\frac{d[G(s)H(s)]}{ds} = 0 \tag{4.226}$$

or

$$\frac{d}{ds}\left\{\frac{1}{G(s)H(s)}\right\} = 0 \tag{4.227}$$

depending on whichever form is easier to differentiate. In terms of the final solution, the form does not matter since one is the expression for K and the maximum, while the other is the expression for 1/K or the minimum. Differentiation of Equation 4.225 yields

$$\frac{d}{ds}\left\{\frac{s(s+2)}{s+6}\right\} = \frac{2s+2}{s+6} - \frac{(s^2+2s)}{(s+6)^2} = 0 \tag{4.228}$$

Simplification of Equation 4.228 yields

$$s^2 + 12s + 12 = 0 \tag{4.229}$$

Based on the quadratic formula, the roots for Equation 4.229 are

$$s = \frac{-b \pm (b^2 - 4ac)^{1/2}}{2a} = \frac{-12 \pm (12^2 - 4 \times 12)^{1/2}}{2} = -1.1 \text{ and } -10.9 \tag{4.230}$$

Therefore, without even calculating the exact value of gain, the root locus breaks away from the real axis at −1.1 and reenters at −10.9.

Rule 8—Breakaway and reentry angles: At the breakaway and reentry points, the angle of breakaway and reentry is determined by 180°/α where α is the number of branches intersecting at that point. For Equation 4.225, α = 2 and the breakaway and reentry angles are 180°/2 = 90°.

Rule 9—Asymptotic behavior: For cases in which the number of poles p exceeds the number of zeros z, there will an indirect zero at infinity with the root locus showing asymptotic behavior as it moves toward that indirect zero. Note that in such situations, the gain K will also be increasing in value. There will p − z number of asymptotes with the angle of the asymptote with respect to the real axis given by

$$\text{Angle} = \frac{\pm\pi}{(p-z)}, \frac{\pm 3\pi}{(p-z)}, \dots \tag{4.231}$$

Also, the origin of the asymptotes is given by the centroid equal to

$$\text{Origin} = \frac{\sum \text{poles} - \sum \text{zeros}}{(p-z)} \tag{4.232}$$

For Equation 4.225, p = 2, z = 1, and p − z = 1. Therefore, there is one asymptote with angle of −π. The origin of the asymptote is not critical in the case of just one asymptote, but will be in the case of two or more asymptotes.

The final root locus for the system as represented by Equation 4.225 is shown in Figure 4.39b. Note that although the transfer function appears to be quite similar to the transfer function of the system as represented by Equation 4.221, the resulting root loci are quite different.

Rule 10—Imaginary axis crossing: The branches of the root locus cross the imaginary axis at points where the phase shift is 180°. Consider a system represented by the following open-loop transfer function:

$$KG(s)H(s) = \frac{K(s + 2)}{s\,(s-1)\,(s + 6)} \tag{4.233}$$

From Rule 1, there are three poles and, thus, three branches of the root locus. From Rule 2, the starting points are the poles 0, +1, and −6. From Rule 3, the end points are the direct zero at −2 and two indirect zeros at infinity. From Rule 4, the root locus will exist on the real axis between 0 and +1 and between −6 and −2. From Rule 6, the root locus will be symmetrical. From Rule 7, the breakaway point can be determined from maximum relative gain. Rather than performing a difficult differentiation, it could be approximated as midway between 0 and +1. Substituting several values of s around +0.5 yields the following values of gain K and a maximum at +0.45, where K is

$$K = \frac{s(s-1)\,(s + 6)}{(s + 2)} \tag{4.234}$$

S	0.40	0.45	0.50	0.55
K	0.640	0.652	0.650	0.636

From Rule 8, there are two diverting branches and the breakaway angle is 180°/2 = 90°. From Rule 9, p = 3 and z = 1, and p − z = 2. The asymptote angles are given by 180°/2 = 90° and the centroid origin for the asymptotes is [0 − 6 + 1 − (−2)]/2 = −1.5.

Now, using Rule 10, one can find the imaginary axis crossing point by finding the phase angle of the transfer function and setting it equal to zero (i.e., tan 180° = 0).

$$G(j\omega)H(j\omega) = \frac{2 + j\omega}{-5\omega^2 - j(\omega^3 + 6\omega)} \tag{4.235}$$

Multiplying the numerator and denominator by the complex conjugate of the denominator yields

$$G(j\omega)H(j\omega) = \frac{(2 + j\omega)}{[-5\omega^2 - j(\omega^3 + 6\omega)]} \frac{[-5\omega^2 + j(\omega^3 + 6\omega)]}{[-5\omega^2 + j(\omega^3 + 6\omega)]} \tag{4.236}$$

This expression simplifies to

$$G(j\omega)H(j\omega) = \frac{-(\omega^4 + 16\omega^2) + j\,(-3\omega^3 + 12\omega)}{-25\omega^4 - \omega^2(6 + \omega^2)^2} \tag{4.237}$$

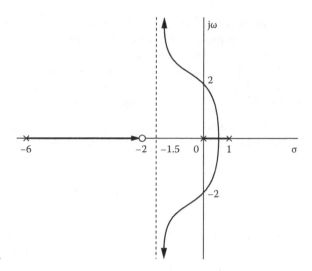

FIGURE 4.40
Root-locus plot for K(s + 2)/s(s − 1)(s + 6).

The phase angle is determined by the arc tangent of the imaginary part over the real part, which is equal to 180°. This also means that the ratio of the imaginary part over the real part equals zero, since the arc tangent of zero is 180°. Consequently, the imaginary part alone must also equal zero:

$$-3\omega^3 + 12\omega = 0 \tag{4.238}$$

The solution to the equation is ω either is equal to 0 or ± 2. Substituting in $\omega = 2$ into the expression for magnitude based on Equation 4.223, yields a value of K = 10 at the critical crossing point and the complete root locus is shown in Figure 4.40.

$$|G(j\omega)H(j\omega)| = \frac{[(\omega^4 + 16\omega^2)^2 + (-3\omega^3 + 12\omega)^2]^{1/2}}{25\omega^4 + \omega^2(6 + \omega^2)^2} \tag{4.239}$$

$$|G(j\omega)H(j\omega)| = \frac{[(2^4 + 16 \times 4)^2 + (-3 \times 2^3 + 12 \times 2)^2]^{1/2}}{25 \times 2^4 + 2^2(6 + 2^2)^2} = \frac{80}{800} = \frac{1}{K} \tag{4.240}$$

Thus, for all values of gain, K, ranging from the starting point with K = 0 up to K = 10, the roots will like on the right half of the s-plane and the system will be unstable. Note that the exact crossing point, $\omega = \pm 2$, yields a pure sinusoidal response in the time domain. Since the function does not expand to infinity, but also does not approach zero, it could be considered a form of limited stability.

There is also a graphical approach that can be much simpler for complicated expressions of s. It is based on the characteristic equation of Equation 4.222 exhibiting a phase angle relationship of 180° (Equation 4.223 or 4.224). Although, this relationship applies to any point on the root locus, it is very tedious to take random points on the s-plane and determine whether the phase angle criterion is true. However, there are a relatively limited number of points available for which the crossing of the imaginary axis will satisfy this criterion. At the critical crossing point, the total phase-angle contributions from each of the poles and zeros of the open-loop control system should add up to 180°.

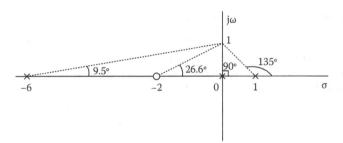

FIGURE 4.41
Graphical approach to finding imaginary axis crossing point.

In the format of Rule 9, the angles from each pole and zero to the critical crossing point summate to 180°:

$$\sum \text{pole angles} - \sum \text{zero angles} = 180° \tag{4.241}$$

For the system defined by Equation 4.234 and whose root locus is shown in Figure 4.40, the phase-angle relationship works as follows. Since the breakaway point on the right half of the s-plane is 0.45 and the asymptote line is −1.5, a rough estimate for the crossing point is relatively small ω, perhaps $\omega = 1$ (see Figure 4.41). Starting with the pole at −6, the phase angle at the crossing point is

$$\tan^{-1} \frac{1}{6} = 9.5° \tag{4.242}$$

For the zero at −2, the phase angle at the crossing point is

$$\tan^{-1} \frac{1}{2} = 26.6° \tag{4.243}$$

The pole at the origin creates a 90° phase angle. The pole at +1 yields a phase angle of

$$180° - \tan^{-1} \frac{1}{1} = 180° - 45° = 135° \tag{4.244}$$

The sum of all these phase angles according to Equation 4.241 is

$$9.5° + 90° + 135° - 26.6° = 207.9° \tag{4.245}$$

This sum is close but a bit larger than the required 180° angle. By increasing ω, the angle to the zero at −2 increases and the angle to the pole at +1 decreases, bringing the sum closer to 180°. At $\omega = 2$, the respective angles in Equation 4.241 become

$$18.4° + 90° + 116.6 - 45° = 180° \tag{4.246}$$

Note that the origin also satisfies the 180° phase-angle relationship, and, in a limited sense, is a crossing point. In this particular case, it is the pole at zero and a starting point for the root locus.

A third and final approach may also be used. For this Rule 11 is used.

Rule 11—Sum of the poles: If $p - z \geq 2$, the sum of the poles remains a constant independent of K. For the system defined by Equation 4.233, there are three poles and one zero, allowing Rule 11 to be used. The sum of the poles (with K = 0) is $-6 + 0 + 1 = -5$. Therefore at $s = -5$, the sum of the other two poles must be zero, indicating that they are complex conjugates on the imaginary axis. The value of K must be the same for which ever pole is used to calculate it. Thus, instead of using the complex conjugate roots, K can be calculated much quicker using the root or pole at $s = -5$.

$$K = \frac{s\,(s-1)(s+6)}{(s+2)} = \left|\frac{(-5)(-6)(1)}{(-3)}\right|_{s=-5} = 10 \tag{4.247}$$

Rule 12—Complex poles and zeros: The angles of departure from complex poles and the angle of arrival at complex zeros are determined by the 180° phase angle criterion.

Consider a system represented by the following open-loop transfer function:

$$KG(s)H(s) = \frac{K}{s^2 + 2s + 2} \tag{4.248}$$

The denominator is partitioned into two complex conjugate roots:

$$KG(s)H(s) = \frac{K}{(s+1+j)(s+1-j)} \tag{4.249}$$

From Rule 1, there are two poles and, thus, two branches of the root locus. From Rule 2, the starting points are the poles $-1 - j$ and $-1 + j$. From Rule 3, the end points are two indirect zeros at infinity. From Rule 4, the root locus cannot exist on the real axis because there can never be an odd number of roots. From Rule 5, the root locus will be symmetrical. From Rule 9, the asymptote angles are $\pm 180°/2 = \pm 90°$. From Rule 12, the angles of departure are determined as follows. For the top pole $(-1 + j)$, the angle of departure plus the angle to bottom pole (90°) must sum to 180°. Therefore, the departure angle is 90°. From Rule 5 and symmetry, the angle of departure for the bottom pole is $-90°$ and the final complete root locus is shown in Figure 4.42.

The root-locus plots and frequency-analysis magnitude and phase-angle plots for a variety of different simple transfer functions are given in Table 4.5. These will be useful in helping to identify the transfer functions and develop models based experimentally observed data for different physiological entities. Further details on root-locus plots can be found in Melsa and Schultz (1969) or other textbooks on linear control systems.

4.9.2 Muscle Spindle Model

Since the muscle spindle consists of intrafusal muscle fibers in the pole region and the elastic annulospiral element in the nuclear bag region, it would be reasonable to use the Hill's four-element model to also represent the muscle spindle (see Figure 4.43). The pole region would then be represented by a dashpot B in parallel with a parallel elastic element, K_{PE} and the contractile element. Input from the gamma neurons is assumed to control the force level generated by the contractile element. The series elastic element of the intrafusal fibers is combined with the elastic element of the annulospiral element for a combined K_{SE}. Obviously, the values of the muscle spindle parameters will be different than the values for Hill's muscle model.

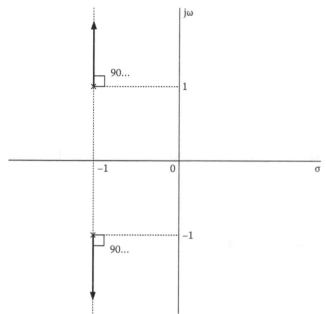

FIGURE 4.42
Root-locus plot for $K/(s^2 + 2s + 2)$ showing complex poles.

In principle, the spindle provides information not only on length but also on the rate of change of length. Upon an instantaneous stretch, the dashpot element cannot change its length instantaneously. Therefore, all of the stretch is initially taken up by the series elastic element, K_{SE}, and there is a large increase in the firing rate of the α afferent neuron proportional to the stretch ε_0. If the amount of stretch is increased, the initial amount of firing is also increased (see Figure 3.28). After the initial stretch is over, the dashpot slowly extends, allowing K_{PE} to take up some of the increased length, so that the firing rate drops to a steady level substantially below the initial peak.

Should the gamma system not be activated, this drop in the firing rate can be modeled very similarly to passive muscle in a quick stretch experiment. Consider Equation 4.78 and step stretch of the muscle spindle.

$$\Upsilon = \frac{K_{SE}(Bs + K_{PE})}{Bs + K_{PE} + K_{SE}} \frac{\varepsilon_0}{s} \tag{4.250}$$

A partial fraction expansion yields

$$T = \frac{K_{SE}\varepsilon_0}{K_{PE} + K_{SE}} \left\{ \frac{K_{SE}}{s + (K_{PE} + K_{SE})/B} + \frac{K_{PE}}{s} \right\} \tag{4.251}$$

Taking the inverse Laplace transform, simplifying, and using numerical data on muscle (not the spindle) from Bawa et al. (1976) of $B = 5\,g\,s/mm$, and from Jewel and Wilkie (1958) of $K_{SE} = 80\,g/mm$ and the weaker $K_{PE} = 20\,g/mm$, yields $\tau = B/(K_{PE} + K_{SE}) = 5/(20 + 80) = 0.05\,s$ and the response in the time domain of

$$T(t) = \frac{K_{SE}\varepsilon_0}{K_{PE} + K_{SE}} \left\{ K_{PE} + K_{SE}\, e^{-(K_{PE} + K_{SE})t/B} \right\} = 16\varepsilon_0(1 + 4e^{-t/0.05}) \tag{4.252}$$

Assuming $\varepsilon_0 = 1$, Equation 4.251 yields the resultant plot shown in Figure 4.44a.

TABLE 4.5

Summary of Root-Locus, Magnitude, and Phase Angle Plots for Several Simple Transfer Functions

Tranfer Function	Frequency Analysis			Transfer Function		Frequency Analysis	
	Root Locus	Magnitude	Phase Angle (φ)		Root Locus	Magnitude	Phase Angle (φ)
$\dfrac{1}{s}$ (a) Integrator				$\dfrac{1}{s^2}$ (f) Inertial system			
$\dfrac{1}{s+1}$ (b) Single lag				$\dfrac{1}{s(s+1)}$ (g) Integrator with lag			
$\dfrac{s}{s+1}$ (c) Derivative with lag				$\dfrac{1}{(s+1)(s+T)}, T>1$ (h) Double lag			
$\dfrac{1}{T}\times\dfrac{s+T}{s+1}, T<1$ (d) Phase lead				$\dfrac{1}{s^2+2\zeta s+1}, \zeta>1$ (i) Damped oscillator			
$\dfrac{1}{T}\times\dfrac{s+T}{s+1}, T>1$ (e) Phase lag							

FIGURE 4.43
Schematic model of a muscle spindle. (Adapted from McMahon, T.A., *Muscles, Reflexes, and Locomotion*, Princeton University Press, Princeton, NJ, 1984.)

FIGURE 4.44
Calculated muscle spindle response to a step input (a) and ramp input (b).

Experimentally instantaneous stretches are not realistic. In practice, the application of the stretch becomes more of a steep ramp function, which can be also modeled using Laplace transforms. In this particular case, assume a ramp, $20t$, reaching the value of 1 in one time constant of $0.05\,s$. The response then becomes

$$T = \frac{K_{SE}(Bs + K_{PE})}{Bs + K_{PE} + K_{SE}} \frac{20\varepsilon_0}{s^2} \tag{4.253}$$

Rearrangement and a partial fraction expansion yields

$$T = 20\,K_{SE}\,\varepsilon_0 \left\{ \frac{a}{s + (K_{PE} + K_{SE})/B} + \frac{b}{s^2} + \frac{c}{s} \right\} \tag{4.254}$$

Using residues to solve for a and b yields

$$a = \frac{s + K_{PE}/B}{s^2}\bigg|_{s=-(K_{PE}+K_{SE})/B} = \frac{-K_{SE}B}{(K_{PE}+K_{SE})^2} \qquad (4.255)$$

$$b = \frac{s + K_{PE}/B}{s + (K_{PE}+K_{SE})/B}\bigg|_{s=0} = \frac{K_{PE}}{K_{PE}+K_{SE}} \qquad (4.256)$$

$$c = \frac{d}{ds}\left\{\frac{s + K_{PE}/B}{s + (K_{PE}+K_{SE})/B}\right\}\bigg|_{s=0} = \frac{K_{SE}B}{(K_{PE}+K_{SE})^2} \qquad (4.257)$$

Substituting the coefficients a, b, and c back into Equation 4.254, taking the inverse Laplace transform, and simplifying yields

$$T(t) = \frac{20K_{SE}^2\varepsilon_0}{(K_{PE}+K_{SE})^2}\left\{1 - e^{-(K_{PE}+K_{SE})t/B} + \frac{K_{PE}(K_{PE}+K_{SE})}{K_{SE}B}t\right\} = 64\varepsilon_0(1 - e^{-t/0.05} + 5t) \qquad (4.258)$$

The resulting plot (see Figure 4.44b) for a sluggish stretch input (i.e., not a true step input, but a very steep ramp, reaching the value of 1 in one time constant of 0.05 s) shows a sluggish rise in the firing frequency, reaching a peak level lower than for a true step input, and then a fall to a steady-state firing rate. This plot also corresponds very nicely to data observed by Bessou et al. (1965) shown in Figure 4.45.

4.9.3 Time Delays

Time delays in a neuromuscular system can occur because of synaptic crossing times, neural conduction times and times for the calcium ions to release from the sarcoplasmic

FIGURE 4.45
Muscle spindle response (afferent firing frequency) to a stretch of constant velocity (i.e., ramp function). (Reproduced from Bessou, P. et al., *J. Physiol.*, 180, 649, 1965. With permission.)

FIGURE 4.46
Closed-loop system with a time delay of 1 s in the feedback path.

reticulum and diffuse into the surrounding muscle tissue. In an engineering control system, time delays in a negative feedback system can result in oscillatory behavior of the output even though the input is steady. This can obviously cause problems with stability.

An example of a pure time delay in a negative-feedback loop is shown in Figure 4.46. The Laplace transform of a pure time delay corresponds to a time-shift transform from Table 4.1:

$$\mathcal{L}[f(t-a)] = e^{-as}\mathcal{L}[f(t)] = e^{-as} \tag{4.259}$$

Using the Laplace transform of the closed-loop response from Equation 4.218 and assuming a simple plant with a gain of 1 yields the final closed-loop transfer function:

$$\frac{y(s)}{x(s)} = \frac{1}{1+e^{-as}} \tag{4.260}$$

Using a unit step input with Laplace transform of $1/s$ yields an output response of

$$y(s) = \frac{1}{s(1+e^{-as})} \tag{4.261}$$

The inverse transform (from a detailed mathematics handbook such as Selby, 1970) is

$$y(t) = \frac{1}{2}[1-(-1)^n] \quad n-1 < t < n \tag{4.262}$$

The input step and output square wave responses are plotted in Figure 4.47. Although the output response is a stylized response, it still supports the principle of time delays in a negative-feedback system causing oscillatory behavior. This phenomenon was particularly observed by Lippold (1970) who elicited tremor in an extended finger with a small initial mechanical perturbation. These oscillations were found to be in phase with groups of muscle action potentials recorded from the extensor digitorum communis muscle (see Figure 4.48) and were thought to originate due to time delays in the neuromuscular loops as described in Chapter 3, particularly when the loop gain is greater than one.

An alternate approach is to examine the system in Figure 4.46 directly. The error, $e(t)$, is the difference between the input $x(t)$ and the feedback path, which is $y(t-1)$, i.e., the output delayed by 1 s. Note, also, that in this case, $y(t) = e(t)$, since there is only a gain of one in the direct open-loop path. At $t = 0$, the input jumps to value of 1, which is also the output for up to $t = 1$, since the feedback path is delaying the output signal for 1 s. At $t = 1$, the feedback passes its value of 1 to the junction and, being a negative feedback, is subtracted from 1, yielding an output of 0 for the next second, up to $t = 2$. At $t = 2$, the previous value 0 is

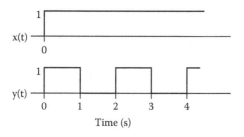

FIGURE 4.47
Output of a closed-loop system with a time delay of 1 s to a unit step input.

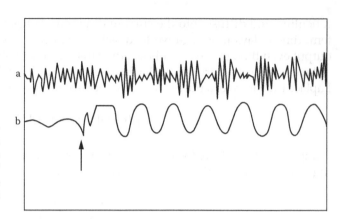

FIGURE 4.48
(a) EMG from extensor digitorum communis. (b) Self-sustained oscillations in the middle finger elicited from a small tap at the arrow (seven oscillations over 600ms). (Reproduced from Lippold, O.C.J., *J. Physiol.*, 206, 359, 1970. With permission.)

passed through the feedback loop which has no effect on the input, which passed through unchanged to the output which jumps to 1. This square wave continues *ad infinitum* as a form of oscillatory behavior and a destabilizing factor in motor control.

In engineering systems, the system may be stabilized by introducing an attenuator into the feedback loop, such that the loop gain is less than 1. Therefore, consider an attenuator of 1/2 in the feedback path (see Figure 4.49). Now reexamine the system flow directly. At $t = 0$, the input jumps to value of 1, which is also the output for up to $t = 1$, since the feedback path is delaying the output signal for 1s. At $t = 1$, the feedback passes its attenuated value of 1/2 to the junction and, being a negative feedback, is subtracted from 1, yielding an output of 1/2 for the next second, up to $t = 2$. At $t = 2$, the previous value of 1/2 is passed through the feedback loop, reduced to 1/4 and subtracted from the input value of 1, yielding an output value of 3/4. This value is reduced to 3/8 in the next cycle and subtracted from 1, yielding an output value of 5/8, etc. The oscillations are decreasing (see Figure 4.50) and the final converging value can be calculated from the closed-loop transfer function:

$$\frac{y(s)}{x(s)} = \frac{G(s)}{1 + G(s)H(s)} = \frac{1}{1 + 1(1/2)} = \frac{2}{3} \tag{4.263}$$

This is comparable to the experience of hearing the loud, screech of public address systems, whose microphone happens to pick up sound from its own speaker and through the

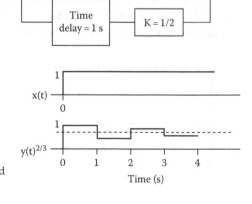

FIGURE 4.49
Closed-loop system with a time delay of 1s and attenuator of 1/2 in the feedback path.

FIGURE 4.50
Output of a closed-loop system with a time delay of 1s and attenuator of 1/2 in the feedback path.

FIGURE 4.51
Undamped pendulum defined in terms of displacement.

amplification creates oscillations. The screech goes away when the gain on the amplifier is decreased. Similarly, Lippold (1970) showed that tremor could be decreased by inflating a blood pressure cuff on the oscillating limb. This reduced the blood flow to the neuromuscular system and most likely decreased the gain in the feedback loop.

4.9.4 Velocity Control

Consider an undamped pendulum that is released from an angle θ_0 (see Figure 4.51). With no damping, the pendulum will swing past center, reach an identical angle θ_0 on the other side, and continue back and forth in a pure harmonic oscillation. The torque acting to restore the pendulum to the center position depends on the horizontal component of the angle θ and balances the moment of inertia for the pendulum:

$$ml^2\ddot{\theta} = -mg\,l\sin\theta \tag{4.264}$$

which for small angles, when $\sin\theta \approx \theta$, becomes

$$\ddot{\theta} + \frac{g}{l}\theta = 0 \tag{4.265}$$

FIGURE 4.52
Undamped pendulum defined in terms of velocity control.

The solution to this is similar to the undamped mass-spring-dashpot system equation:

$$s^2 + \omega_n^2 = 0 \tag{4.266}$$

The future position of the pendulum can be predicted by an angle θ^+ which defined by the present angle θ (see Figure 4.52) and a change in position determined by the velocity of movement:

$$\theta^+ = \theta + k\dot{\theta} \tag{4.267}$$

Note that the velocity is negative, i.e., restoring the pendulum back to center. If the restoring force is proportional to α rather than θ, then substituting Equation 4.267 back into Equation 4.260, in the Laplace domain, yields

$$\dot{\theta} + \frac{g}{l}(\theta + k\dot{\theta}) = \left(s^2 + g\frac{k}{l}s + \frac{g}{l}\right)\theta = 0 \tag{4.268}$$

The pendulum can be considered analogous to muscle force in the stretch reflex. If muscle force is proportional to stretch only, one would get pure oscillations only. But when the stretch receptors are sensitive to both displacement and velocity, the velocity term contributes a damping and stabilizing effect to the reflex (McMahon, 1984).

4.9.5 Reflex Stiffness

Motor control and maintenance of muscle stiffness was generally thought to be solely due to muscle spindles, either directly through the α afferent and α efferent pathways or through greater control of the γ efferent pathway. However, more recent studies have shown the influence of lower level feedback also from Golgi tendon organs, which were once thought to respond only to excessive forces as in the clasp-knife reflex (Stuart et al., 1972).

FIGURE 4.53
Muscle stiffness with and without reflexes
present. (Reproduced from Hoffer, J.A. and
Andreassen, S., *J. Neurophysiol.*, 45, 267, 1981.)

Furthermore, neither muscle length nor force may be regulated as individual variables, but
may be a combination of force changes in ration to length changes in the form of stiffness
(Houk, 1979).

Detailed studies of a decerebrate cat soleus, using incremental applications of muscle
stretch show increases in muscle force from which the reflex stiffness of the muscle can
be calculated (Hoffner and Andreassen, 1981). The effects for the initial small increases
in force show corresponding increase in muscle stiffness (see Figure 4.53). However, as
the muscle force levels increase, the stiffness plateaus. When the soleus nerve is cut, the
response is very different with a continual increase in stiffness, indicating that the reflex
maintenance of stiffness has been lost.

In human experiments (Greene and McMahon, 1979), male subjects stood on a beam
with knees flexed at a constant angle (see Figure 4.54). Slight vertical bouncing motions
at appropriate frequencies (as determined by the natural frequency of a second-order
damped system for the appropriate masses) produced resonant bouncing deflections in
the beam. The range of frequencies for which this resonance was very narrow, indicating
a fine level of tuning. Using second-order system calculations the stiffness of the leg muscles could be calculated. Interestingly, a doubling of the body weight (by holding weights)
caused less than 10% increase in muscle stiffness, indicating a reflex response in maintaining constant muscle stiffness over a wide range of conditions.

Many of the various modeling techniques presented in Chapter 4, especially related
to the muscle–tendon complex and Hill's Model, are covered in considerable detail in a
review paper by Zajac (1989).

FIGURE 4.54
Measurement of in vivo reflex stiffness
by natural frequency. (Adapted from
Greene, P.R. and McMahon, T.A., *J.
Biomech.*, 12, 881, 1979.)

Example 4.9: Development of Model for Parkinson Tremor

Frequency analysis data on normal and Parkinson's patients (Stark, 1968) was used to develop a transfer function model (see Figure 4.55). Many pathological types of tremor are caused by lesions in the brain as opposed to perturbations of the normal stretch reflex as performed by Lippold (1970). Parkinson's disease is one example in which arteriosclerotic changes in the basal ganglia, especially in the elderly, cause large-amplitude tremors of low frequency (2–3 Hz, much lower than normal tremor of 10–11 Hz) and rigidity of movements.

In this particular example, the transfer function for normal subjects will be derived. Based on the magnitude plot of Figure 4.55a, a breakpoint at approximately 2 Hz can be identified. This corresponds to a frequency of $2\pi \times 2$ or 12.5 radians. At this point the slope drops off at

$$\frac{\Delta y}{\Delta x} = \frac{\log(1) - \log(0.1)}{\log(2) - \log(6)} = -2 \tag{4.269}$$

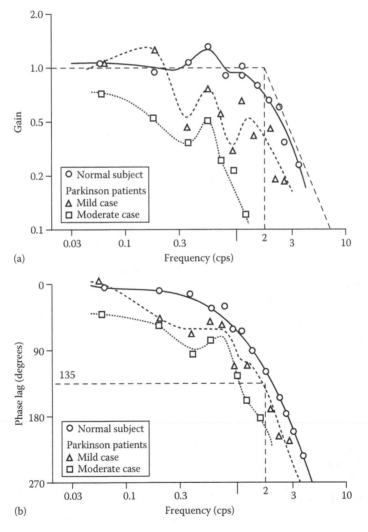

FIGURE 4.55
Magnitude (a) and phase angle (b) plots for normals and Parkinson patients. (Reproduced from Stark, L., *Neurological Control Systems*, Plenum Press, New York, 1968. With permission.)

From Table 4.5 (f), this indicates a double pole and a transfer function of the form of

$$\frac{y(s)}{x(s)} = \frac{K}{(s+12.5)^2} \tag{4.270}$$

A double pole should yield a −90° phase lag at the critical frequency of 2 Hz on the phase plot (see Figure 4.55b). However, the actual phase lag is −135°, which indicates that the additional −45° of phase lag must be due to a time lag. From the Laplace representation of a pure time delay in Equation 4.259 and the Euler identity in Equation 4.122, the phase lag of a time delay is found to be

$$\theta = \tan^{-1}\frac{-\sin a\omega}{\cos a\omega} = -a\omega \tag{4.271}$$

A 45° angle is equal to $2\pi \times 45°/360°$ or 0.78 radians. Substituting 0.78 radians into Equation 4.271 yields a time constant at the critical frequency of

$$a = \frac{0.78}{\omega} = \frac{0.78}{12.5} = 0.06\,s \tag{4.272}$$

The revised form of the transfer function now becomes

$$\frac{y(s)}{x(s)} = \frac{Ke^{-0.06s}}{(s+12.5)^2} \tag{4.273}$$

The value of gain K can be determined by finding the magnitude of the transfer function in Equation 4.273 and setting it equal to 1. This is a fairly difficult process but can be simplified if one realizes that the gain of 1 occurs as frequency approaches 0. Substituting s = 0 into Equation 4.273 yields a K of 156 and the final form of the transfer function of

$$\frac{y(s)}{x(s)} = \frac{156e^{-0.06s}}{(s+12.5)^2} \tag{4.274}$$

The response for Parkinson patients is more difficult to model, deviating considerably from the normal second-order feedback system. It almost appears that the opposing agonist and antagonist feedback systems are permanently switched on, counteracting typical feedback and leading to permanent contraction of muscles and rigidity in the muscles. Much of this is due to the lesions in the basal ganglia and consequent interference in the normal functioning of the γ-loop feedback systems.

Questions

1. What is the purpose of using Laplace transforms in biomechanical modeling?
2. What are the tradeoffs of using the algebraic and residue approaches in partial fraction expansions?
3. What is a transfer function?
4. Given that a unit impulse is not a realistic function, what purpose does an impulse response provide?
5. Compare and contrast the two basic elements in viscoelastic theory.

6. What is a stress-relaxation function?

7. What is creep?

8. How do the time constants for the stress relaxation and creep functions compare in Hill's three-element model?

9. What are the frequency characteristics of passive muscle?

10. What is the difference between a distributed and a lumped model?

11. Compare and contrast open- and closed-loop systems.

12. What are the differences between first- and second-order systems?

13. What are poles and zeroes?

14. What purpose do the roots of the characteristic function serve?

15. What is natural frequency and how does it relate to motor control?

16. What is a bit?

17. Explain the Hick–Hyman Law in terms of information processing.

18. What is the index of difficulty?

19. Explain the Fitts' Law in terms of motor control.

20. What is system bandwidth?

21. What is the difference between an open-loop and a closed-loop transfer function? What useful purpose does each provide?

22. What effect does a time lag in a feedback loop have on system performance? How can it be controlled?

Problems

1. Find entry 3 in the Laplace transform table (Table 4.1) from entry 1.

2. Find entry 4 from entry 1.

3. Find entry 10 from entry 9.

4. Find the Laplace transform of $\sin^2 t$.

5. Find the Laplace transform of $te^{2t}u(t-1)$.

6. Find the inverse Laplace transform of $3s/(s^2 + 1)(s^2 + 4)$.

7. Find the inverse Laplace transform of $(s + 1)/(s^2 + 2s)$.

8. Find the inverse Laplace transform of $1/(s + 1)(s + 2)^2$.

9. Find the transfer function, $H(s)$, for this model.

10. Compare these two viscoelastic models.

a. Find the transfer function $H(s) = \varepsilon(s)/\sigma(s)$ for both models.

b. Find the strain for an impulse and step stress input for Model 1.

c. How are the parameters of the two models related? (Hint: they are alternate ways of representing the same Hill's passive three-element muscle model!)

11. The ratio of peak twitch tension generated from a single stimulus to tetanic tension generated from tetanic stimulation is termed the twitch/tetanus ratio. Research shows that it is higher in fast-twitch muscles than slow-twitch muscles. Use Hill's four-element active muscle model to calculate the twitch/tetanus ratio for slow- and fast-twitch muscles. Assume isometric tension.

12. Find the magnitude and phase plots for $10/s(10 + s)$.

13. Find the magnitude and phase plots for $10(s + 1)/s(s + 10)^2$.

14. Consider a new viscoelastic element called a "slipshot," which can be represented in the Laplace domain as $1/(s + 2)$. A more complex gel-like element can be created by putting a dashpot (with coefficient of one) in series with the slipshot.

a. Find the gel's transfer function $H(s) = \sigma(s)/\varepsilon(s)$.

b. What are the gel's stress relaxation and creep functions?

c. What is the frequency response for the gel?

15. a. Simplify the following block diagram to a basic closed-loop feedback system.

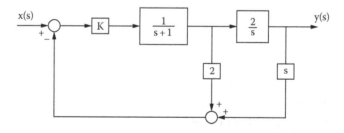

b. Find the overall transfer function.

c. Calculate a step response for $K = 1$.

d. Find the root-locus plot.

16. Find the root-locus plot for $10K/(s^3 + 12s^2 + 20s)$. For what K is the system stable?

17. Find the root-locus plot for $K(s + 2)/(s^2 + 2s + 2)$. For what K is the system stable?

18. a. Consider three different cases of muscle contraction: normal taught cable to the force dial, a spring, with spring constant of 400 g/mm, inserted between the wrist attachment

and force dial (as shown below), and a dashpot, with a value of 5g/mm/s, inserted in place of the spring. The subject is told to "pull as hard as possible" and hold that force for 5 s. Using Hill's model, with values $K_{PE} = 100\,g/mm$, $K_{SE} = 400\,g/mm$, and $B = 5\,g/mm/s$, show the force dial reading as a function of time for each of the three cases. Compare carefully in terms of peak tension and rise times.

b. Suppose the subject is asked to fluctuate the force reading as quickly as possible between 0 and maximum. Which case would yield the worst response? Verify quantitatively. (Hint: perform frequency analysis.)

References

Aidley, D.J. (1985). *The Physiology of Excitable Cells*, 2nd edn, Cambridge, U.K.: Cambridge University Press.

Alexander, R.S. and Johnson, P.D. (1965). Muscle stretch and theories of contraction. *American Journal of Physiology* 208:412–416.

Bawa, P., Mannard, A., and Stein, R.B. (1976). Predictions and experimental tests of a viscoelastic muscle model using elastic and inertial loads. *Biological Cybernetics* 22:139–145.

Bessou, P., Emonet-Dénand, F., and Laporte, Y. (1965). Motor fibres innervating extrafusal and intrafusal muscle fibres in the cat. *Journal of Physiology* 180:649–672.

Bigland, B. and Lippold, O.C.J. (1954). Motor unit activity in the voluntary contraction of human muscle. *Journal of Physiology* 125:322–225.

Christensen, R.M. (1981). *Theory of Viscoelasticity: An Introduction*, 2nd edn, New York: Academic Press.

Clamann, H.P. (1970). Activity of single motor units during isometric tension. *Neurology* 20:254–260.

Close, R.I. (1965). The relation between intrinsic speed of shortening and duration of the active state of muscle. *Journal of Physiology* 180:542–559.

Ebashi, S. and Endo, M. (1968). Calcium ion and muscular contraction. *Progress in Biophysics and Molecular Biology* 18:125–183.

Fenn, W.O. and Marsh, B.S. (1935). Muscle force at different speeds of shortening. *Journal of Physiology* 85:277–297.

Fitts, P. (1954). The information capacity of the human motor system in controlling the amplitude of movement. *Journal of Experimental Psychology* 47:381–391.

Flügge, W. (1975). *Viscoelasticity*, 2nd edn, Berlin, Germany: Springer-Verlag.

Freivalds, A. (1985). *Incorporation of Active Elements into the Articulated Total Body Model*, AAMRL-TR-85–061. Wright-Patterson Air Force Base, OH: Armstrong Aerospace Medical Research Laboratory.

Freivalds, A. and Kaleps, I. (1984). Computer-aided strength prediction using the Articulated Total Body Model. *Computers & Industrial Engineering* 8:107–118.

Gordon, A.M., Huxley, A.F., and Julian, F.J. (1966). The variation in isometric tension with sarcomere length in vertebrate muscle fibers. *Journal of Physiology* 184:170–192.

Greene, P.R. and McMahon, T.A. (1979). Reflex stiffness of man's antigravity muscles during knee-bends while carrying extra weights. *Journal of Biomechanics* 12:881–891.

Grimby, L. and Hannerz, J. (1977). Firing rate and recruitment order of toe extensor motor units in different modes of voluntary contraction. *Journal of Physiology* 264:864–879.

Haddad, Y.M. (1995). *Viscoelasticity of Engineering Materials*. New York: Chapman & Hall.

Hatze, H. (1979). A teleological explanation of Weber's law and the motor unit size law. *Bulletin of Mathematical Biology* 41:407–425.

Hatze, H. (1981). *Myocybernetic Control Models of Skeletal Muscle*. Pretoria, South Africa: University of South Africa.

Henneman, E. and Olson, C.B. (1965). Relations between structure and function in the design of skeletal muscle. *Journal of Neurophysiology* 28:581–598.

Hick, W.E. (1952). On the rate of gain of information. *Quarterly Journal of Experimental Psychology* 4:11–26.

Hill, A.V. (1938). The heat of shortening and the dynamic constants of muscle. *Proceedings of the Royal Society* 126B:136–195.

Hill, A.V. (1970). *First and Last Experiments in Muscle Mechanics*. Cambridge, U.K.: University Press.

Hoffer, J.A. and Andreassen, S. (1981). Regulation of soleus muscle stiffness in premamillary cats: Intrinsic and reflex components. *Journal of Neurophysiology* 45:267–285.

Houk, J. (1979). Regulation of stiffness by skeletomotor reflexes. *Annual Review of Physiology* 41:99–114.

Hyman, R. (1953). Stimulus information as a determinant of reaction time. *Journal of Experimental Psychology* 45:423–432.

Jewell, B.R. and Wilkie, D.R. (1958). An analysis of the mechanical components in frog's striated muscle. *Journal of Physiology* 143:515–540.

Kaplan, W. (1962). *Operational Methods for Linear Systems*. Reading, MA: Addison Wesley.

Langolf, G., Chaffin, D., and Foulke, J. (1976). An investigation of Fitts' law using a wide range of movement amplitudes. *Journal of Motor Behavior* 8:113–128.

Lippold, O.C.J. (1970). Oscillation in the stretch reflex arc and the origin of the rhythmical, 8–12 c/s component of physiological tremor. *Journal of Physiology* 206:359–382.

Marsden, C.D., Meadows, J.C., and Merton, P.A. (1971). Isolated single motor units in human muscle and their rate of discharge during maximal voluntary effort. *Journal of Physiology* 217:12P–13P.

McMahon, T.A. (1984). *Muscles, Reflexes, and Locomotion*. Princeton, NJ: Princeton University Press.

McMinn, R.M.H. and Hutchings, R.T. (1977). *Color Atlas of Human Anatomy*. Chicago, IL: Yearbook Medical Publishers.

Melsa, J.L. and Schultz, D.G. (1969). *Linear Control Systems*. New York: McGraw-Hill.

Milner-Brown, H.S., Stein, R.B., and Yemm, R. (1973). Changes in firing rates of human motor units during linearly changing voluntary contractions. *Journal of Physiology* 230:371–390.

Milsum, J.H. (1966). *Biological Control Systems*. New York: McGraw-Hill.

Person, R. and Kudina, L.P. (1972). Discharge frequency and discharge pattern of human motor units during voluntary contraction of muscle. *Electroencephalography and Clinical Neurophysiology* 32:471–483.

Sanders, M.S. and McCormick, E.J. (1993). *Human Factors in Engineering and Design*, 7th edn, New York: McGraw-Hill.

Schneck, D. (1992). *Mechanics of Muscle*, 2nd edn, New York: New York University Press.

Schumacher, G.H. and Wolff, E. (1966). Trockengewicht and physiologischer Querschnitt der menschlichen skelettmuskulatur, II. Physiologischer querschnitte, (Dry weight and physiological cross section of human skeletal muscle, II. Physiological cross section). *Anatomischer Anzeiger* 119:259–269.

Selby, S.M., ed. (1970). *CRC Standard Mathematical Tables*, 18th edn, Cleveland, OH: Chemical Rubber Company.

Stark, L. (1968). *Neurological Control Systems*. New York: Plenum Press.

Stuart, D.G., Mosher, C.G., and Gerlach, R.L. (1972). Properties and central connections of Golgi tendon organs with special reference to locomotion. In: B.Q. Banker, R.J. Prybylski, J.P. Van Der Meulen, and M. Victor (eds), *Research in Muscle Development and the Muscle Spindle*. Amsterdam, the Netherlands: Excerpta Medica, pp. 437–464.

Tanji, J. and Kato, M. (1973). Firing rate of individual motor units in voluntary contraction in abductor digital minimi muscle in man. *Experimental Neurology* 40:771–783.

Van Valkenburg, M.E. (1964). *Network Analysis*, 2nd edn, Englewood Cliffs, NJ: Prentice-Hall, Inc.

Wilkie, D.R. (1950). Relation between force and velocity in human muscle. *Journal of Physiology* 110:249–280.

Yamada, H. (1970). *Strength of Biological Materials*. Baltimore, MD: Williams & Wilkins.

Zajac, F.E. (1989). Muscle and tendon: Properties, models, scaling, and application to biomechanics and motor control. *Critical Reviews in Biomedical Engineering* 17:359–411.

5

Models of the Upper Limbs

5.1 Anatomy of the Hand and Wrist

5.1.1 Bones of the Hand and Wrist

The human hand has 27 bones divided into three groups: 8 carpal bones in the wrist, 5 *metacarpal* bones, and 14 phalanges of the fingers. The *carpal* bones are arranged in two rows and have names reflecting their shapes (see Figure 5.1). The bones of the distal row, from the lateral side to the medial side, include the *trapezium* (four sided with two parallel sides), *the trapezoid* (four sided), the *capitate* (the central bone), and the *hamate* (hook shaped). These four bones fit together, tightly bound by interosseous ligaments to form a relatively immobile unit that articulates with the metacarpals to form the *carpometacarpal* (CMC) joint. The bones of the proximal row include the *scaphoid* (boat shaped), the *lunate* (half-moon shaped), *the triquetrum* (triangle shaped), and the *pisiform* (pea shaped). The proximal surfaces of the scaphoid, lunate, and triquetrum form a biconvex elliptical surface which articulates with the biconcave surface of the distal extremity of the radius. The articulation between the proximal and distal rows is called the midcarpal joint while articulations between adjacent bones are called intercarpal joints.

The five metacarpal bones are cylindrical in shape and articulate proximally with the distal carpal bones and distally with the proximal phalanges of the digits. The base of the metacarpal bones of the index and middle fingers are linked together tightly and articulate little with the trapezoid and the capitate bones in the CMC joint. On the other hand, the CMC joint for metacarpals of the ring and little fingers with the hamate allow up to 10°–15° and 20°–30° of flexion/extension, respectively. The arched shafts of the metacarpal bones form the palm and the distal ends are spherical in shape, allowing articulation with the base of the corresponding phalanges. Interosseous muscles and extensor tendons run along the concave side and the large and smooth dorsal surface of the shaft, respectively, while the distal ends have a grooved volar surface for the flexor tendons (Nordin and Frankel, 2001).

There are three phalanges for each digit and two for the thumb with a total of 14 bones. They are labeled proximal, middle, and distal phalanges (with the middle one missing in the thumb), according to their positions and become progressively smaller. The heads of the proximal and middle phalanges are bicondylar, facilitating flexion and extension and circumduction. The shafts are semicircular in cross section (the palmar surface being almost flat), as opposed to the cylindrical metacarpals. The axes of the distal phalanges of the index, ring, and little fingers are, respectively, deviated ulnarly, radially, and radially from the axes of the middle phalanges (Gigis and Kuczynski, 1982).

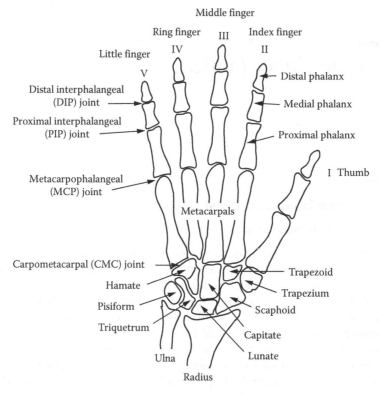

FIGURE 5.1
Bones and joints of the right hand (palmar view). (Modified from Spence, A.P., *Basic Human Anatomy*, 3rd edn., Benjamin/Cummings Pub. Co., Redwood City, CA, 1990.)

5.1.2 Joints of the Hand

There are four joints in each finger, in sequence from the proximal to distal: carpometacarpal (CMC), *metacarpophalangeal* (MCP), proximal *interphalangeal* (PIP), and distal interphalangeal (DIP) joints (see Figure 5.1). As mentioned in Section 5.1.1, the CMC joints are formed by the bases of the four metacarpals and the distal carpal bones and are stabilized by interosseous ligaments to form a relatively immobile joint. However, a major function of the CMC joint is to form the hollow of the palm and allow the hand and digits to conform to the shape of the object being handled (Norkin and Levangie, 1992).

The MCP joints are composed of the convex metacarpal head and the concave base of the proximal phalanx and stabilized by a joint capsule and ligaments. Flexion of 90° and extension of 20°–30° from neutral take place in the sagittal plane. The range of flexion differs among fingers (and individuals), with the index finger having the smallest flexion angle of 70° and the little finger showing the largest angle of 95° (Batmanabane and Malathi, 1985). Radial and ulnar deviation of approximately 40°–60° occurs in the frontal plane, with the index finger showing up to 60° abduction and adduction, middle and ring fingers up to 45°, and the little finger about 50° of mostly abduction (Steindler, 1955). The range of motion at the MCP joint decreases as the flexion angle increases because of the bicondylar metacarpal structure (Youm et al., 1978; Schultz et al., 1987). There is also some axial rotation of the fingers from a pronated to a supinated position as the fingers are extended. In the reverse motion, the fingers crowd together as they go into flexion (Steindler, 1955).

The IP joints, being hinge joints, exhibit only flexion and extension. Each finger has two IP joints, the PIP joint and the DIP joint, except the thumb, which has only one. Volar and collateral ligaments, connected with expansion sheets of the extensor tendons, prevent any side-to-side motion. The largest flexion range of 100°–110° is found in the PIP joints, while a smaller flexion range of 60°–70° is found in the DIP joints. Hyperextension or extension beyond the neutral position, due to ligament laxity, can also be found in both DIP and PIP joints (Steindler, 1955).

5.1.3 Muscles of the Forearm, Wrist, and Hand

The muscles producing movement of the fingers are divided into two groups: extrinsic and intrinsic, based on the origin of the muscles. The *extrinsic* muscles originate primarily in the forearm, while the *intrinsic* muscle originates primarily in the hand. Therefore, the extrinsic muscles are large and provide strength, while the intrinsic muscles are small and provide precise coordination for the fingers. Each finger is innervated by both sets of muscles, requiring good coordination for hand movement.

The extrinsic muscles are divided into flexors found primarily on the anterior forearm (see Figure 5.2) and extensors found primarily on the posterior forearm (see Figure 5.3). Most of the flexors originate from the medial epicondyle of the humerus while most of extensors originate from the lateral epicondyle of the humerus. Both sets of muscles insert on the carpal bones, metacarpals, or phalanges. Each group can be further divided into superficial and deep groups of muscles as categorized in greater detail in Table 5.1.

The intrinsic muscles are divided into three groups: the thenar, the hypothenar, and the midpalmar muscle groups. The *thenar* group acts on the thumb and comprises the thenar eminence at the base of the thumb. The *hypothenar* group acts on the little finger and comprises the hypothenar eminence at the base of the medial palm. The midpalmar muscles act on all of the phalanges except the thumb. Primarily located on the palmar side, these intrinsic muscles allow for the independent flexion/extension and abduction/adduction of each of the phalanges giving rise to precise finger movements. These muscles are shown in Figure 5.4 and categorized in Table 5.2.

5.1.4 Flexor Digitorum Profundus and Flexor Digitorum Superficialis

The *flexor digitorum profundus* (FDP) and *flexor digitorum superficialis* (FDS) are the main finger flexor muscles and are involved in most repetitive work. Using EMG, Long et al. (1970) identified the FDP as the muscle performing most of the unloaded finger flexion, while the FDS came into play when additional strength was needed, with the FDP comprising about 12% of the total muscle capability below the elbow. There are significant variations in the force contributions of the FDS tendons for each finger (0.9%–3.4%) while the FDP tendons provide a relatively constant force contribution to each finger (2.7%–3.4%). This results in a relatively large range of force ratios, from 1.5 to 3. Average FDP resting tendon fiber length is slightly shorter than that for the average FDS tendon. Table 5.3 provides a summary of the general mechanical characteristics of the FDP and FDS tendons for each finger.

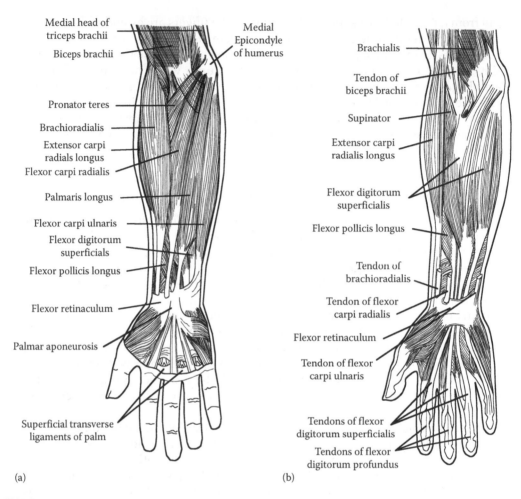

FIGURE 5.2
Anterior muscles of the right hand: (a) superficial layer and (b) middle layer. (Modified from Spence, A.P., *Basic Human Anatomy*, 3rd edn., Benjamin/Cummings Pub. Co., Redwood City, CA, 1990.)

The FDP originates from the proximal anterior and medial surface of the ulna and inserts into the base of the distal phalanx (see Figure 5.5). In the midforearm, the muscle divides into two bellies: the radial and the ulnar. The radial part inserts into the index finger, while the ulnar part inserts into middle, ring, and little fingers. Consequently, the latter three fingers tend to move together, while the index finger can function independently of the others. The FDP tendon passes along the finger through a series of pulleys, which maintain a reasonably constant moment arm for flexing or extending the finger. Before inserting into the distal phalanx, the FDP passes through a split in the FDS tendon (Fahrer, 1971; Steinberg, 1992; Brand and Hollister, 1993).

5.1.5 Flexor Tendon Sheath Pulley Systems

The tendon sheath is a double-walled tube, surrounding the tendons and containing synovial fluid. The synovial sheath provides both a low-friction gliding as well as a nutritional environment for the flexor tendon. The flexor tendon sheath, sometimes

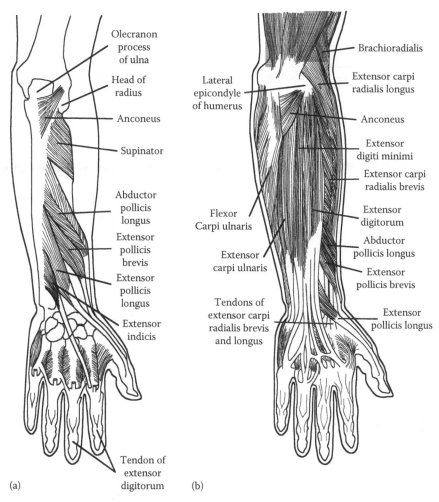

Olecranon
process
of ulna

Head of
radius

Anconeus

Supinator

Abductor
pollicis
longus

Extensor
pollicis
brevis

Extensor
pollicis
longus

Extensor
indicis

Tendon of
extensor
digitorum

(a)

Lateral
epicondyle
of humerus

Flexor
Carpi ulnaris

Extensor
carpi ulnaris

Tendons of
extensor carpi
radialis brevis
and longus

(b)

Brachioradialis

Extensor carpi
radialis longus

Anconeus

Extensor
digiti minimi

Extensor carpi
radialis brevis

Extensor
digitorum

Abductor
pollicis longus

Extensor
pollicis brevis

Extensor
pollicis longus

FIGURE 5.3
Posterior muscles of the right hand: (a) deep layer and (b) superficial layer. (Modified from Spence, A.P., *Basic Human Anatomy*, 3rd edn., Benjamin/Cummings Pub. Co., Redwood City, CA, 1990.)

termed the fibrosseous tunnel, begins at the neck of the metacarpal bone, ends at the DIP joint, and is held against the phalanges by pulleys. These pulleys primarily act to prevent tendon bowstringing across the joints during flexion but also maintain a relatively constant moment arm.

The pulleys can be divided into three types based on their locations: a palmar aponeurosis pulley, five annular (ring-shaped) pulleys (A1, A2, A3, A4, and A5), and three cruciate (cross-like) pulleys (C1, C2, and C3). The A2 and A4 pulleys are located on the proximal and middle phalanges, while the A1, A3, and A5 pulleys are located at the palmar surface of the MCP, PIP, and DIP joints (see Figure 5.6). The A2 and A4 pulleys are most important for normal function and a stable joint, with the A3 and other pulleys coming into play when the A2 and A4 have been damaged (Manske and Lesker, 1977; Idler, 1985; Lin et al., 1990). Such damage to the pulleys can occur in extreme activities, in which much of the body weight is supported by the fingers, such as rock climbing.

TABLE 5.1

Extrinsic Muscles of the Hand and Wrist

Group	Layer	Name	Nerve	Function
Anterior	Superficial	Flexor carpi radialis	Median	Flexes and adducts hand; aids in flexion/pronation of forearm
		Palmaris longus	Median	Flexes hand
		Flexor carpi ulnaris	Ulnar	Flexes and adducts hand
	Middle	Flexor digitorum superficialis	Median	Flexes phalanges and hand
	Deep	Flexor digitorum profundus	Median, ulnar	Flexes phalanges and hand
Posterior	Superficial	Extensor carpi radialis longus	Radial	Extends and abducts hand
		Extensor carpi radialis brevis	Radial	Extends hand
		Extensor digitorum	Radial	Extends little finger
		Extensor digiti minimi	Radial	Extends little finger
		Extensor carpi ulnaris	Radial	Extends and adducts hand
	Deep	Abductor pollicis longus	Radial	Abducts thumb and hand
		Extensor pollicis brevis	Radial	Extends thumb
		Extensor pollicis longus	Radial	Extends thumb
		Extensor indicis	Radial	Extends index finger

Source: Adapted from Spence, A.P., *Basic Human Anatomy*, 3rd edn., Benjamin/Cummings Pub. Co., Redwood City, CA, 1990; Tubiana, R., *The Hand*, Saunders, Philadelphia, PA, 1981.

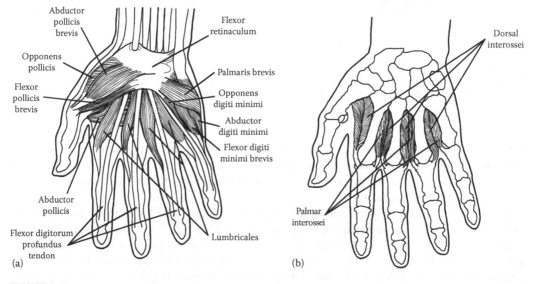

FIGURE 5.4

Intrinsic muscles of the hand: (a) palmar view and (b) dorsal view. (Modified from Spence, A.P., *Basic Human Anatomy*, 3rd edn., Benjamin/Cummings Pub. Co., Redwood City, CA, 1990.)

TABLE 5.2

Intrinsic Muscles of the Hand and Wrist

Group	Name	Nerve	Function
Thenar muscles	Abductor pollicis brevis	Median	Abducts thumb
	Opponens pollicis	Median	Pulls thumb toward little finger
	Flexor pollicis brevis	Median	Flexes thumb
	Adductor pollicis	Ulnar	Adducts thumb
Hypothenar muscles	Palmaris brevis	Ulnar	Folds skin on ulnar side of palm
	Abductor digiti minimi	Ulnar	Abducts little finger
	Flexor digiti minimi	Ulnar	Flexes little finger
	Opponens digiti minimi	Ulnar	Pulls little finger toward thumb
Midpalmar muscles	Lumbricales	Median, ulnar	Flex proximal phalanges
	Dorsal interossei	Ulnar	Abduct fingers
	Palmar inerossei	Ulnar	Adduct fingers

Source: Adapted from Spence, A.P., *Basic Human Anatomy*, 3rd edn., Benjamin/Cummings Pub. Co., Redwood City, CA, 1990; Tubiana, R., *The Hand*, Saunders, Philadelphia, PA, 1981.

TABLE 5.3

General Characteristics of the FDP and FDS Tendons

	Resting Fiber Length (cm)[a]		Moment Arm (cm)[b]						Relative Force of Finger Flexors (%)[c]		
			DIP Join		PIP Joint		MCP Joint				
Finger	FDP	FDS	FDP	FDS	FDP	FDS	FDP	FDS	FDP	FDS	FDP/FDS
Index	6.6	7.2	0.65	—	0.98	0.83	1.01	1.21	2.7	2.0	1.35
Middle	6.6	7.0	0.70	—	1.07	0.87	1.16	1.40	3.4	3.4	1.00
Ring	6.8	7.3	0.68	—	1.04	0.85	1.04	1.30	3.0	2.0	1.50
Little	6.2	7.0	0.60	—	0.85	0.74	0.89	0.98	2.8	0.90	3.11

[a] Brand et al. (1981).
[b] Ketchum et al. (1978).
[c] Brand and Hollister (1993).

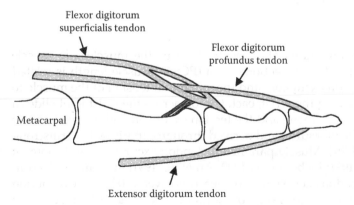

Flexor digitorum superficialis tendon

Flexor digitorum profundus tendon

Metacarpal

Extensor digitorum tendon

FIGURE 5.5
FDP and FDS tendons of a typical digit. (Modified from Thompson, J.S., *Core Textbook of Anatomy*, J.B. Lippincott Co., Philadelphia, PA, 1977.)

FIGURE 5.6
Pulley structure of the finger: A, annular; C, cruciate. (Modified from Nordin, M. and Frankel, V.H., *Basic Biomechanics of the Musculoskeletal System*, 3rd edn., Lippincott Williams & Wilkins, Philadelphia, PA, 2001.)

Although, the A3 pulley is relatively weaker and closer to the PIP joint, it is more flexible and stretches, transferring the load to the A2 and A4 pulleys, which then fail first (Marco et al., 1998).

5.1.6 Wrist Mechanics

The seven main muscles involved in wrist and hand motion are flexor carpi radialis (FCR), flexor carpi ulnaris (FCU), flexor digitorum profundus (FDP), flexor digitorum superficialis (FDS), extensor carpi radialis brevis (ECRB), extensor carpi radialis longus (ECRL), and extensor carpi ulnaris (ECU) (Garcia-Elias et al., 1991). The primary function FCR, FCU, ECRB, ECRL, and ECU is to move the wrist, while FDP and FDS are secondary wrist movers. FDP's and FDS's primary function is to flex and extend the fingers and secondarily to rotate the wrist. The FDP and FDS pass through the carpal tunnel. The primary muscles and tendons involved with wrist movements of flexion, extension, radial and ulnar deviation planes are listed below (An et al., 1981):

    Flexion: FCR and FCU

    Extension: ECRB, ECRL, and ECU

    Radial deviation: FCR, ECRB, and ECRL

    Ulnar deviation: FCU and ECU

The parameters that have been commonly used to describe the muscles are muscle fiber length (FL) and physiological cross sectional area (PCSA). Muscle length is related to mechanical potential for tendon excursion, and the maximum tension of the muscle to its PCSA (An et al., 1991). In moving the wrist, each tendon across the wrist joint slides a certain distance to execute the movement, and the tendon excursion and moment arm at various wrist joint angles can be measured and derived through experiments (Armstrong and Chaffin, 1978; An et al., 1991). Muscle parameters, tendon excursions, and moment arms at wrist joint (An et al., 1981; Lieber et al., 1990; An et al., 1991) are summarized in Table 5.4. The magnitudes of tendon excursion were measured over a 100° range of motion in the flexion–extension plane and a 50° range of motion in the radial–ulnar deviation plane in forearm neutral position.

TABLE 5.4

Physiological and Mechanical Properties of Wrist Joint Muscles and Tendons

Muscle and Tendon	Physiological Size		Tendon Excursion (mm)		Moment Arm (mm)[a]	
	Length (cm)	PCSA (cm²)	F/E Plane	R/U Plane	F/E Plane	R/U Plane
FCR	10.9–12.4	2.0	25 ± 4	7 ± 1	+15 ± 3	+8 ± 2
FCU	15.2–15.4	3.2–3.4	28 ± 4	12 ± 3	+16 ± 3	−14 ± 3
ECRB	13.8–15.8	2.7–2.9	20 ± 3	11 ± 1	−12 ± 2	+13 ± 2
ECRL	11.8–18.3	1.5–2.4	12 ± 3	17 ± 1	−7 ± 2	+19 ± 2
ECU	13.6–14.9	2.6–3.4	10 ± 2	16 ± 2	−6 ± 1	−17 ± 3

Source: Adapted from An, K.N. et al., *J. Biomech.*, 14, 659, 1981; An, K.N. et al., *Biomechanics of the Wrist Joint*, Springer Verlag, New York, 1991; Lieber, R.L. et al., *J. Hand Surg.*, 15, 244, 1990.

[a] Plus denotes flexion and radial deviation and minus denotes extension and ulnar deviation.

TABLE 5.5

Phalange Lengths as Percent of Hand Length for Males and Females

Phalanx	Proximal	Medial	Distal
Thumb	17.1	—	12.1
Index	21.8	14.1	8.6
Middle	24.5	15.8	9.8
Ring	22.2	15.3	9.7
Little	17.7	10.8	8.6

Source: Adapted from Davidoff, N.A., The development of a graphic model of a human hand, MS thesis, The Pennsylvania State University, University Park, PA, 1990; Davidoff, N.A. and Freivalds, A., *Int. J. Industrial Ergon.*, 12, 255, 1993.

Table 5.4 reveals that the FCR, FCU, and ECRB provide larger tendon excursion during flexion and extension movement than ECRL and ECU, while ECRL and ECU have greater tendon excursion during radial and ulnar deviation movement. The results also demonstrate that the FCR and FCU are prime muscles for flexion, ECRB for extension, ECRL for radial deviation, and ECU for ulnar deviation. In spite of the three-dimensional orientation of the wrist tendons to the rotation axes and the complexity of carpal bone motion, Table 5.5 indicates that the moment arms of wrist motion are maintained fairly consistently and correspond well with the anatomical location of the tendons. According to An et al. (1991), these findings are related to the anatomical considerations; the extensor retinaculum ensures a consistent relationship of the wrist extensors (ECRB, ECBL, and ECU) to the rotation axes, while the FCR is firmly fixed in the fibroosseous groove, and the FCU is fixed on the pisiform.

5.1.7 Select Finger Anthropometry Data

As discussed in Section 1.6, for any sort of biomechanical modeling using static equilibrium analyses, it is necessary to have a variety of key anthropometric properties,

TABLE 5.6

Interphalangeal Joint Dimensions—Mean and (Standard Deviations) in mm

	Breadth		Thickness	
Joint	Male	Female	Male	Female
IP (I)	22.9 (3.8)	19.1 (1.3)	20.1 (1.5)	16.8 (1.0)
PIP (II)	21.3 (1.3)	18.3 (1.0)	19.6 (1.3)	16.3 (1.0)
DIP (II)	18.3 (1.3)	15.5 (1.0)	15.5 (1.3)	13.0 (1.0)
PIP (III)	21.8 (1.3)	18.3 (1.0)	20.1 (1.5)	16.8 (1.0)
DIP (III)	18.3 (1.3)	15.2 (1.0)	16.0 (1.3)	13.2 (1.0)
PIP (IV)	20.1 (1.3)	18.3 (1.0)	18.8 (1.3)	15.8 (1.0)
DIP (IV)	17.3 (1.0)	14.5 (0.8)	15.2 (1.3)	12.5 (0.8)
PIP (V)	17.8 (1.5)	14.5 (0.8)	16.8 (1.3)	14.0 (1.0)
DIP (V)	15.8 (1.3)	13.2 (0.8)	13.7 (1.3)	11.4 (0.8)

Source: Adapted from Garrett, J.W., *Anthropometry of the Air Force Female Hand*, AMRL-TR-69-26, Aerospace Medical Research Laboratory, Wright-Patterson AFB, OH, 1970a; Garrett, J.W., *Anthropometry of the Hands of Male Air Force Flight Personnel*, AMRL-TR-69-42, Aerospace Medical Research Laboratory, Wright-Patterson AFB, OH, 1970b; Garrett, J.W., *Human Factors*, 13, 117, 1971.

Note: I, thumb; II, index finger; III, middle; IV, ring; V, little finger.

such as segment link lengths, segment weights, the location of the center of gravity, the location of the center of joint rotation, the range of motion for each joint, and muscle insertion points. Not all of this information has been measured or documented at the level of individual phalanges, but the following tables may provide some useful data: Table 5.5—phalange lengths, Table 5.6—interphalangeal joint dimensions, Table 5.7—interphalangeal joint flexion and extension ranges, Table 5.8—joint center locations, and Table 5.9—tendon insertion points. The latter two tables were adapted from the data of An et al. (1979) based on three separate coordinate systems located at the center of joint rotation for each phalanx as shown in Figure 5.7. Note the x-axis is in the axial direction of the phalanx, with the positive direction pointing proximally. The y-axis is perpendicular with the positive direction pointing dorsally. The positive z-axis points radially for the right hand. However, any deviations in the z-direction were generally minimal and were omitted for simplicity. The tendon insertion points of the Table 5.9 correspond approximately to the location of the five annular pulleys described in Section 5.1.5. This still allows for adequate modeling of finger flexion in the x–y plane. Other anthropometric data on the hand can be found in Garrett (1971), Greiner (1992), and Rogers et al. (2008) and detailed data on muscle moment arms and tendon excursions for the index finger can be found in An et al. (1983).

TABLE 5.7

Location of Finger Joint Centers from Distal End of Phalanx

Finger	DIP	PIP	MCP
Index	18	13	20
Middle	15	12	20
Ring	13	12	19
Little	17	14	24

Source: Adapted from An, K.W. et al., *J. Biomech.*, 12, 775, 1979.

Note: DIP distances as percentage of medial phalanx length, PIP and MCP distances as percentage of proximal phalanx length.

TABLE 5.8

Interphalangeal Joint Flexion and Extension Ranges—Means
and (Standard Deviations) in Degrees

Joint	Flexion		Extension	
	Male	Female	Male	Female
MCP (I)	56.3 (21.8)	60.0 (14.5)	3.7 (7.4)	11.2 (13.2)
IP (I)	62.3 (22.2)	67.2 (16.9)	21.5 (22.8)	21.5 (23.6)
MCP (II)	85.2 (7.4)	84.7 (7.8)	15.1 (10.7)	20.9 (8.0)
PIP (II)	94.8 (13.7)	103.8 (5.0)	0.3 (1.3)	0.0
DIP (II)	77.5 (13.0)	81.0 (5.4)	1.3 (3.5)	0.9 (3.6)
MCP (III)	86.7 (6.7)	89.1 (7.6)	13.5 (10.0)	19.7 (7.2)
PIP (III)	88.8 (23.8)	102.2 (5.0)	0.0	0.3 (5.7)
DIP (III)	80.2 (12.0)	83.5 (7.0)	0.0	0.9 (3.6)
MCP (IV)	86.0 (5.1)	87.4 (6.4)	13.5 (10.0)	19.4 (8.3)
PIP (IV)	93.2 (13.4)	100.9 (6.4)	0.0	0.0
DIP (IV)	79.1 (12.8)	80.0 (8.5)	0.0	0.9 (3.6)
MCP (V)	83.7 (7.9)	86.5 (6.8)	14.1 (8.3)	21.5 (6.8)
PIP (V)	90.5 (13.4)	96.6 (6.9)	0.0	0.0
DIP (V)	77.8 (11.5)	78.5 (10.7)	0.7 (2.6)	1.2 (3.8)

Source: Adapted from Davidoff, N.A. and Freivalds, A., *Int. J. Industrial Ergon.*,
12, 255, 1993.

5.2 Static Tendon-Pulley Models

Landsmeer (1960, 1962) developed three biomechanical models for finger flexor tendon
displacements, in which the tendon–joint displacement relationships are determined by
the spatial relationships between the tendons and joints. In Model I (see Figure 5.8a), he
assumed that the tendon is held securely against the curved articular surface of the proximal bone of the joint, and the proximal articular surface can be described as a trochlea.
Such a model is particularly useful in describing extensor muscles. The tendon displacement relationship is described by

$$x = r\theta \tag{5.1}$$

where
  x is the tendon displacement
  r is the distance from the joint center to the tendon
  θ is the joint rotation angle

However, if the tendon is not held securely, it may be displaced from the joint when the
joint is flexed and will settle in a position along the bisection of the joint angle (see Figure
5.8b). Model II is useful for describing tendon displacement in intrinsic muscles as

$$x = 2r \sin\left(\frac{\theta}{2}\right) \tag{5.2}$$

TABLE 5.9

Representative Tendon Insertion Distances for Each Finger with Respect to That Joint's Center Coordinate System

| | | Index Finger | | | | Middle Finger | | | | Ring Finger | | | | Little Finger | | | |
| | | Distal | | Proximal | | Distal | | Proximal | | Distal | | Proximal | | Distal | | Proximal | |
Joint	Muscle	x	y	x	y	x	y	x	y	x	y	x	y	x	y	x	y
DIP	FDP	-18	-13	25	-22	-19	-12	26	-22	-19	-13	26	-22	-18	-15	2	-20
PIP	FDP	-22	-14	18	-17	-27	-15	22	-14	-28	-16	23	-16	-24	-15	20	-18
	FDS	-22	-11	18	-13	-27	-11	22	-12	-28	-13	23	-13	-24	-13	20	-15
MCP	FDP	-24	-17	13	-27	-30	-18	16	-26	-31	-16	17	-26	-27	-20	15	-28
	FDS	-24	-22	13	-31	-30	-18	16	-31	-31	-19	17	-29	-27	-24	15	-32

Source: Adapted from An, K.W. et al., *J. Biomech.*, 12, 775, 1979.

Note: See Figure 5.7 DIP distances as percentage medial phalanx length, PIP and MCP distances as percentage of proximal phalanx length.

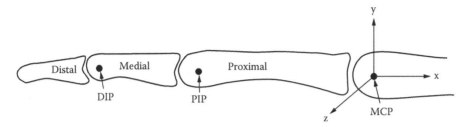

FIGURE 5.7
Finger coordinate system. (Modified from An, K.W. et al., *J. Biomech.*, 12, 775, 1979.)

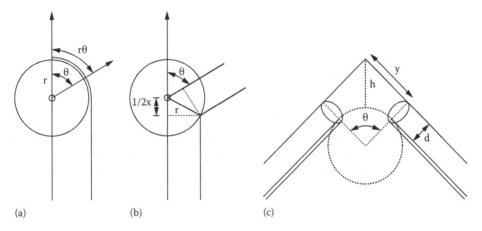

FIGURE 5.8
Landsmeer's tendon models: (a) Model I, (b) Model II, (c) Model III. (Modified from Landsmeer, J.M.F., *Ann. Rheum. Dis.*, 21, 164, 1962.)

Landsmeer's (1960) Model III depicts a tendon running through a tendon sheath held securely against the bone, which allows the tendon to curve smoothly around the joint (see Figure 5.8c). The tendon displacement is described by

$$x = 2\left[y + \frac{1}{2}\theta\left(\frac{d - y}{\tan\frac{1}{2}\theta} \right) \right]$$

(5.3)

where
  y is the tendon length to joint axis measured along long axis of bone
  d is the distance of tendon to the long axis of bone

For small angles of flexion ($\theta < 20°$), $\tan\theta$ is almost equal to θ, and Equation 5.3 simplifies to

$$x = d\theta$$

(5.4)

Armstrong and Chaffin (1979) proposed a static model for the wrist based on Landsmeer's (1962) tendon Model I and LeVeau's (1977) pulley-friction concepts (see Figure 5.9). Armstrong and Chaffin (1978) found that, when the wrist is flexed, the flexor tendons are supported by *flexor retinaculum* on the volar side of the carpal tunnel. When the wrist is extended, the

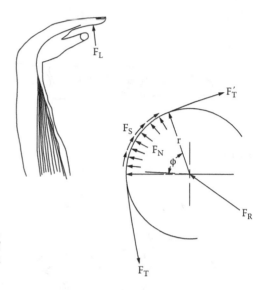

FIGURE 5.9
Armstrong tendon-pulley model for the wrist. (Reproduced from Chaffin, D.B. et al., *Occupational Biomechanics*, John Wiley & Sons, New York, 1999. With permission.)

flexor tendons are supported by the carpal bones. Thus, deviation of the wrist from neutral position causes the tendons to be displaced against and past the adjacent walls of the carpal tunnel. They assumed that a tendon sliding over a curved surface is analogous to a belt incurring friction forces while wrapped around a pulley as described in Section 1.7. The radial reaction force on the ligament or the carpal bones, F_R, can be characterized as follows:

$$F_R = 2F_T e^{\mu\Theta} \sin\left(\frac{\theta}{2}\right) \tag{5.5}$$

where
  F_R is the radial reaction force
  F_T is the tendon force or belt tension
  μ is the coefficient of friction between tendon and supporting tissues
  θ is the wrist deviation angle (in radians)

The resulting normal forces on the tendon exerted by the pulley surface can be expressed per unit arc length as

$$F_N = \frac{2F_T e^{\mu\Theta} \sin(\theta/2)}{r\theta} \tag{5.6}$$

where
  F_N is the normal forces exerted on tendon
  r is the radius of curvature around supporting tissues

For small coefficient of frictions, comparable to what is found in joints ($\mu < 0.04$) and for small angles of θ, Equation 5.6 reduces to the simple expression:

$$F_N = \frac{F_T}{r} \tag{5.7}$$

Thus, F_N is a function of only the tendon force and the radius of curvature. As the tendon force increases or the radius of curvature decreases (e.g., small wrists), the normal supporting force exerted on tendon increases. F_R, on the other hand, is independent of radius of curvature but is dependent on the wrist deviation angle.

An interesting variation on tendon-pulley modeling was presented by Roloff et al. (2006). They modeled the specific placement of the A2 and A4 pulleys (Figure 5.6) with respect to their effect on FDP and FDS normal (to the pulley) tendon forces for the optimization of surgical grafting of pulleys. The normal tendon forces are at a minimum in a position in which both pulleys are as close as possible to the center of rotation of the PIP joint. Increasing the distance of the pulleys from the PIP joint, dramatically increases the normal forces, until approximately 1/3 the phalanx length, at which point the forces start leveling off.

These tendon-pulley model provides a relatively simple mechanism for calculating the normal supporting force exerted on tendons that are a major factor in WRMSDs. However, this model does not include the dynamic components of wrist movements such as angular velocity and acceleration, which might be risk factors in work-related musculoskeletal disorders.

5.3 Dynamic Tendon-Pulley Models

Schoenmarklin and Marras's (1990) dynamic biomechanical model extended Armstrong and Chaffin's (1979) static model to include dynamic component of angular acceleration (see Figure 5.10). The dynamic model is two dimensional in that only the forces in flexion and extension plane are analyzed. This model investigates the effects of maximum angular acceleration on the resultant reaction force that the wrist ligaments and carpal bones exert on tendons and their sheaths.

Key forces and movements in the model include the reaction force at the center of the wrist (W_x and W_y), the couple or moment (M_w) required to flex and extend the wrist, and the inertial force ($M \times A_n$ and $M \times A_t$) and inertial moment ($I \times \ddot{\Theta}$) acting around the hand's center of mass. For equilibrium, the magnitude of moment around the wrist in the

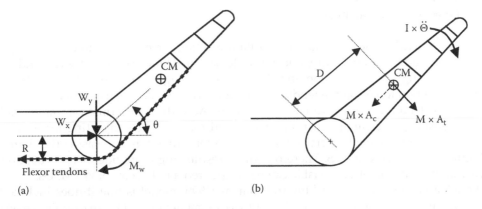

(a) (b)

FIGURE 5.10
Dynamic tendon-pulley model for the wrist: (a) free-body diagram and (b) mass × acceleration diagram. (Modified from Schoenmarklin, R.W. and Marras, W.P., *Proceedings of the Human Factors Society 34th Annual Meeting*, Human Factors Society, Santa Monica, CA, 1990.)

free-body diagram must equal the magnitude of moment acting around the hand's center of mass in the moment acceleration diagram:

$$F_t \times R = (M \times A_t + M \times A_c) \times D + I \times \ddot{\Theta} \tag{5.8}$$

where
  M is the mass
  A_t is the tangential acceleration
  A_c is the centripetal acceleration
  F_t is the tendon force
  I is the moment of inertia of the hand in flexion and extension
  $\ddot{\Theta}$ is the angular acceleration

Thus, the hand is assumed to accelerate from a stationary posture, so, the angular velocity is theoretically zero, resulted in zero centripetal force ($A_c = V^2/R = 0$). Then,

$$F_t \times R = (M \times A_t) \times D + I \times \ddot{\Theta} \tag{5.9}$$

$$F_t \times R = (M \times D \times \ddot{\Theta}) \times D + I \times \ddot{\Theta} \tag{5.10}$$

$$F_t = \frac{(M \times D^2 + I) \times \ddot{\Theta}}{R} \tag{5.11}$$

$$F_R = 2 \times \left(\frac{(M \times D^2 + I) \times \ddot{\Theta}}{R} \right) \times \sin\left(\frac{\theta}{2}\right) \tag{5.12}$$

where
  R is the radius of curvature of the tendon
  D is the distance between the center of mass of hand and wrist
  M is the weight of hand
  θ is the wrist deviation angle

The above equations indicate that the resultant reaction force, F_R, is a function of angular acceleration, radius of curvature, and wrist deviation. Thus, exertion of wrist and hand with greatly angular acceleration and deviated wrist angle would result in greater total resultant reaction forces on the tendons and supporting tissues than exertions with small angular acceleration and neutral wrist position. According to Armstrong and Chaffin (1979), increases in resultant reaction force would increase the supporting force that the carpal bones and ligaments exert on the flexor tendons, therefore, increasing the chance of inflammation and risk of CTS. Therefore, these results might provide theoretical support to why angular acceleration variable can be considered a risk factor of WRMSDs.

The advantage of Schoenmarklin and Marras (1990) model is that it does include the dynamic variable of angular acceleration into assessment of resultant reaction force on the tendons. But the model is two dimensional, and it does not consider the coactivation of antagonistic muscles in wrist joint motions. There is need for further model development to account for additional physiological factors.

5.4 Complex Tendon Models

Any model that incorporates more than the one muscle–tendon unit of the above models, all of a sudden, becomes much more complicated, due to the fact that the number of unknown muscle forces exceeds the number of equilibrium or constraint equations. This is known as the statically indeterminate problem. The two main approaches utilized in solving this problem are reduction methods and optimization methods.

5.4.1 Reduction Methods

The main objective of the reduction method is to reduce the number of excessive variables until the number of unknown forces is equal to the number of required equilibrium equations eliminating static indeterminacy.

Smith et al. (1964) initiated mathematical analyses of the finger tendon forces to find the effects of the flexor tendons acting on metacarpal phalangeal (MCP) joint deformed by rheumatoid arthritis. They used a two-dimensional model to analyze the MCP joint and muscle forces of the index finger during tip pinch. To reduce the number of unknown muscle forces, the following assumptions were applied: (1) the sum of the interosseous (I) forces is treated as a single force 2I; (2) half of the interosseous forces of I act at the PIP joint and the other half act at the DIP joint; (3) the lumbrical (L) is much smaller than the interosseous (I), as much as 1/3 I. They solved the three moment equations using these assumptions and anthropometrical data of the index finger obtained from a cadaver hand in a tip pinch position. They reported the tendon forces normalized to the external force F, as 3.8F, 2.5F, 0.9F, and 0.3F for the FDP, FDS, I, and L, respectively. They also found a value of 7.5F for the MCP joint force. The results indicate that the flexor tendons are dominant and the forces are many times larger than the intrinsic muscle forces during tip pinch.

Chao et al. (1976) presented a comprehensive analysis of the three-dimensional tendon and joint forces of the fingers in pinch and power grip functions. Kirschner wires (K-wires) were drilled through the phalanges to fix the finger configuration in the desired position and different surgical wires were inserted into the tendon and muscles of hand specimens of the cadaver to identify different tendons on x-ray film. The exact orientations of finger digits and the locations of the tendons were defined by biplanar x-ray analysis. Through a free-body analysis, 19 independent equations were obtained for 23 unknown joint and tendon forces. Using the permutation–combination principle of setting any four of the nine tendon forces equal to zero solved the indeterminate problem. The selection of these tendons was based primarily on electromyographic responses (EMG) and physiological assessment. They found that high constraint forces and moments at the DIP and PIP joints were found during pinches, whereas large magnitudes of constraint forces at the MCP joint were found during power grips. The total of the intrinsic muscles (RI, UI, and LI) produced a greater force than the total of the flexor tendons (FDP and FDS) in both pinch and power grip actions.

5.4.2 Optimization Methods

An alternate method using a typical optimization technique was suggested by Seireg and Arvikar (1973) and Penrod et al. (1974). In this approach, force equilibrium equations and anatomical constraint relationships were used for the equality constraints and the physiological limits on the tendon, muscle, and joint forces were applied as the inequality constraints. In addition, the most important factor in this method is optimal criteria that correspond to the objective function of the formulation. The possible solutions can vary based on the optimal criteria selected.

Chao and An (1978a) studied the middle finger during tip pinch and power grip actions, with an aid of three-dimensional analysis. They analyzed the same problem using the optimization and linear programming (LP) technique of Chao et al. (1976) instead of the previously described EMG and permutation–combination method. The predicted middle finger muscle and joint forces were very similar to those of the previous study (Penrod et al., 1974), except for the intrinsic muscle forces whose predicted values were considerably lower. They found that the highest joint contact forces for all three joints occurred for pinch grip rather than power grip. They also found that the main flexors (FDP and FDS) were most active in both pinch and power grip functions, whereas the intrinsic muscles were less active in power grip than in pinch.

An et al. (1985) also applied LP optimization techniques to solve the indeterminate problem of a three-dimensional analytic hand model. The ranges of muscle forces of the index finger under isometric hand functions, such as tip pinch, lateral key pinch, power grip, and other functional activities were analyzed. FDP and FDS carried high tendon forces compared with other muscles in most hand functions, although the predicted FDS force was zero in a pinch grip. The long extensors (LE) and two intrinsic muscles contributed large forces in the key pinch. The large force of these intrinsic muscles in pinch action can be explained by the role of these muscles maintaining balance and stabilization of the MCP joint. The joint constraint forces for each finger were also studied. The Chao et al. (1976) study showed a trend for joint constraint forces in which the DIP joint had the lowest force and the force progressively increased for the PIP joint and was largest at the MCP joint. An et al. (1985) showed the same trend in lateral pinch functions.

5.4.3 Combined Approaches

Chao and An (1978b) used a graphical presentation with a combined permutation–combination and optimization technique to solve the statically indeterminate tendon force problem. They analyzed the maximum tip pinch force of the index finger as a function of external force directions (0°, 30°, and 45°) and the DIP joint flexion angles (10°–50°). The results showed that the pinch strength relied on the direction of applied external force as well as the finger joint configuration. The tendon forces of the index finger were also studied with the same finger posture as that in Chao et al. (1976) study, but only one angle (45°) of the external force was assumed. Also, the predicted extrinsic extensor tendon force was considerably larger than in their previous studies.

Weightman and Amis (1982) presented a good critical review for the previously published studies and applied their two-dimensional finger model to the analysis of resultant joint forces and muscle tensions in various pinch actions. To create a statically determinate problem, all joints were assumed to be pin joints with a fixed center of rotation during flexion. The relationships of the intrinsic muscle forces were assumed identical to those of Chao and An (1978a), except that the long extensor muscles forces dropped to zero. They also used the physiological cross-sectional area (PCSA) of the muscles to define the force distributions in the intrinsic muscles. Their results compared to other previously published studies with a good correlation of both muscle and joint force predictions. Based on these comparisons, they verified that a two-dimensional finger model could be valid for analyzing two-dimensional finger actions, even though realistically any finger motion is still three dimensional.

5.5 Two-Dimensional Hand Model

From a biomechanical perspective, the extrinsic finger flexors, flexor digitorum profundus (FDP) and flexor digitorum superficialis (FDS) comprise the main sources of power for finger flexion in grasping type motions, especially the power grip. Also, since most of the tendon-pulley attachments are in line with the long axis (i.e., x-axis) of the phalanges (see Section 5.1.7) and there are small lateral force components (i.e., along the z-axis), only two axes, the x and y, need to be defined. Therefore, a simple two-dimensional model utilizing those two tendons should be sufficient for most applications.

To further define the model, several other assumptions need to be made. These are as follows:

1. The effects of intrinsic muscles and extensors on the finger flexion can be neglected since these muscles will typically be in a relaxed state during the normal range of motion for a power grip (Armstrong, 1976; Cailliet, 1994).

2. All of the interphalangeal and metacarpal joints (DIP, PIP, and MP joints) are assumed to be pure hinge joints, allowing only flexion and extension.

3. Anatomic analysis shows that the FDS is inserted by two slips to either side of the proximal end of the middle phalanx (Steinberg, 1992; Cailliet, 1994). It is assumed that each FDS tendon is inserted to the palmar side of the proximal end of the middle phalange, parallel to the long axis. In a two-dimensional biomechanical model, the effect of having two splits inserted along the sides of the bone is the same as having one tendon inserted on the palmar side of the proximal end of the middle phalange.

4. Tendons and tendon sheaths are modeled as frictionless cable and pulley system. Therefore, a single tendon passing through several joints maintains the same tensile force (Chao et al., 1976).

5. The externally applied forces are assumed to be a single unit-force exerted at the mid-point pulp of a distal phalange for pinch or by three unit forces applied normally at the mid-point of each phalange and metacarpal bone for grasp as shown in Figure 5.10. The direction of the force is assumed to be perpendicular to the long axis of the bone.

6. The weight of the bones together with other soft tissues on the hand is assumed to be negligible.

7. Due to indeterminacy, the tendon force ratio of FDP to FDS at the each phalange is assumed to be 3:1, i.e., is $\alpha = 0.333$ (Marco et al., 1998).

8. FDP and FDS tendon moment arms (in mm) are estimated for DIP, PIP, and MCP joints of different thickness equations from the equations of Armstrong (1976):

$$PR_{ik} = 6.19 - 1.66X_1 - 4.03X_2 + 0.225X_3 \tag{5.13}$$

$$SR_{ik} = 6.42 + 0.10X_1 - 4.03X_2 + 0.225X_3 \tag{5.14}$$

where
   PR_{ik} is the FDP moment arm for the ith finger and kth joints
   SR_{ik} is the FDS moment arm for the ith finger and kth joints
   X_1 is the 1 for PIP and 0 for all others
   X_2 is the 1 for DIP and 0 for all others
   X_3 is the joint thickness (mm) from Table 5.5

Consequently, the pertinent equations are as follows:

$$PR_{DIP} = 2.16 + 0.225X_3 \tag{5.15}$$

$$PR_{PIP} = 4.53 + 0.225X_3 \tag{5.16}$$

$$SR_{PIP} = 6.52 + 0.225X_3 \tag{5.17}$$

$$PR_{MCP} = 6.19 + 0.225X_3 \tag{5.18}$$

$$SR_{MCP} = 6.42 + 0.225X_3 \tag{5.19}$$

Four Cartesian coordinate systems are established to define the locations and orientations of the tendons and to describe the joint configuration (see Figure 5.11). There are two coordinate systems for both the middle and proximal phalanges and only one system for the distal and metacarpal phalanges. The y-axis is defined along the long axis of the each phalanx, from the proximal end to the distal end. The x-axis is defined as perpendicular to the long axis of each phalanx and in the palmar–dorsal plane, from the palmar side to the dorsal side of the finger bone. Both x- and y-axes have their origins at the center of the proximal end of phalanx. Note that these definitions are different from that used by An et al. (1979) in Figure 5.7 and Tables 5.8 and 5.9.

In terms of notation, subscript i refers to fingers, with 1–4 for the index, middle, ring, and little finger, respectively, subscript j refers to joints, with 1–4 for the DIP, PIP, MP, and wrist joints, respectively, while subscript k refers to phalanges, with 1–4 for the distal, middle, proximal phalanges, and the metacarpal bone, respectively.

In terms of model input values, the external force on each phalange of each finger is indicated by F(i, k). The finger joint flexion angles, measured with reference to straight fingers as the hand is lying flat, are indicated by (i, θ_j). The length of each phalanx for each finger is indicated by L(i, k).

For the model output variables, the FDP tendon force for each phalanx of each finger is indicated by TP(i, k). The FDS tendon force for each phalanx of each finger is

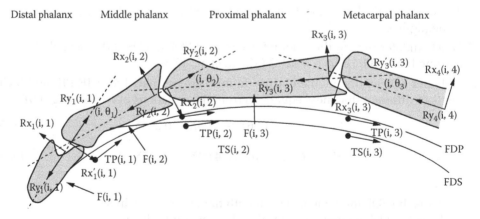

FIGURE 5.11
Free-body diagram for a two-dimensional hand model. For symbols and notation, see text. (Reproduced from Kong, Y.K., Optimum design of handle shape through biomechanical modeling of hand tendon forces, PhD dissertation, The Pennsylvania State University, University Park, PA, 2001. With permission.)

indicated by TS(i, k). Finally, joint constraint forces along the X_k and Y_k axes are indicated by $Rx_k(i,j)$ and $Ry_k(i,j)$, respectively.

To solve for the above unknown model output variables, a static equilibrium analysis (per Section 1.5) of each phalanx must be performed. Specifically, the summation of forces acting on each phalanx in the x-and y-axes must be zero. Similarly, the summation of all moments acting on each phalanx must also be equal to zero. The resulting equations for the distal phalanx are

$$TP(i,1) = \frac{0.5L(i,1)\,F(i,1)}{PR(i,1)} \tag{5.20}$$

$$Ry_1(i,1) = TP(i,1)\cos(i,\theta_1) \tag{5.21}$$

$$Rx_1(i,1) = TP(i,1)\sin(i,\theta_1) - F(i,1) \tag{5.22}$$

For the middle phalanx, they are

$$TP(i,2) = \left[\frac{0.5F(i,2) - Rx_1(i,1)\cos(i,\theta_1) + Ry_1(i,1)\sin(i,\theta_1)}{\alpha SR(i,2) + PR(i,2)}\right]L(i,2) \tag{5.23}$$

$$TS(i,2) = \alpha TP(i,2) \tag{5.24}$$

$$Ry_2(i,2) = Rx_1(i,1)\sin(i,\theta_1) + Ry_1(i,1)\cos(i,\theta_1) + (\alpha+1)TP(i,2)\cos(i,\theta_2) \tag{5.25}$$

$$Rx_2(i,2) = Rx_1(i,1)\cos(i,\theta_1) - Ry_1(i,1)\sin(i,\theta_1) + (\alpha+1)TP(i,2)\sin(i,\theta_2) - F(i,2) \tag{5.26}$$

For the proximal phalanx, they are

$$TP(i,3) = \left[\frac{0.5F(i,3) - Rx_2(i,2)\cos(i,\theta_2) + Ry_2(i,2)\sin(i,\theta_2)}{\alpha SR(i,3) + PR(i,3)}\right]L(i,3) \tag{5.27}$$

$$TS(i,3) = \alpha TP(i,3) \tag{5.28}$$

$$Ry_3(i,3) = Rx_2(i,2)\sin(i,\theta_2) + Ry_2(i,2)\cos(i,\theta_2) + (\alpha+1)TP(i,3)\cos(i,\theta_3) \tag{5.29}$$

$$Rx_3(i,3) = Rx_2(i,2)\cos(i,\theta_2) - Ry_2(i,2)\sin(i,\theta_2) + (\alpha+1)TP(i,3)\sin(i,\theta_3) - F(i,3) \tag{5.30}$$

One interesting application of such a biomechanical hand model is to identify the optimum handle size for gripping so as to minimize tendon forces. However, in a typical power grip, there are two alternate ways in which the geometry of a cylindrical handle surface and phalange contacts can be defined. In Grip I (see Figure 5.12), the point of contact between the distal phalange (L_1) and a handle is assumed to be at the middle point of the distal phalange; i.e., the distal phalange is divided into two equal lengths ($L_1/2$). The

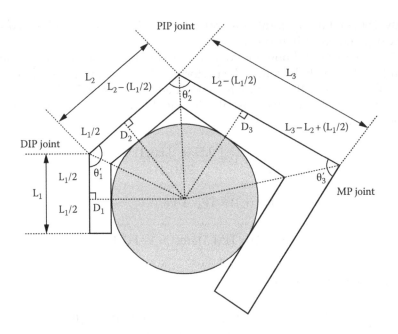

FIGURE 5.12
Schematic diagram of Grip I. (Reproduced from Kong, Y.K., Optimum design of handle shape through biome-chanical modeling of hand tendon forces, PhD dissertation, The Pennsylvania State University, University Park, PA, 2001. With permission.)

bisector of the DIP angle establishes a right triangle with the distal phalanx as the base and the altitude pass through the contact point to the center of handle. Through trigonometry, the DIP joint angle then becomes:

$$\theta_1' = 2\tan^{-1}\left[\frac{2(R + D_1)}{L_1}\right] \tag{5.31}$$

where
   θ_1' is the DIP joint angle
   R is the radius of the cylindrical handle
   D_1 is the thickness of distal phalanx

The second contact point (between the middle phalange (L_2) and the handle) divides the middle phalange into two unequal lengths, one being $L_1/2$ (due to the DIP bisector) and the other being (($L_2 - L_1$)/2). The bisector of the PIP angle establishes a right triangle with the medial phalanx as the base and the altitude again passing through the contact point to the center of handle. Through trigonometry, the PIP joint angle then becomes

$$\theta_2' = 2\tan^{-1}\frac{2(R + D_2)}{2L_2 - L_1} \tag{5.32}$$

where
   θ_2' is the PIP joint angle
   D_2 is the thickness of medial phalanx

The third contact point with the handle also divides the proximal phalange (L_3) into two parts, one being the same length as the proximal part of middle phalange (($L_2 - L_1$)/2) and the other being (($L_3 - L_2 + L_1$)/2). The bisector of the MP angle established another right triangle as previously leasing to

$$\theta_3' = 2\tan^{-1}\frac{2(R+D_3)}{2L_3 - 2L_2 + L_1} \tag{5.33}$$

where θ_3' is the MP joint angle.

In the case of Grip II (see Figure 5.13), the second contact point is assumed to divide the medial phalanx into two equal lengths ($L_2/2$). The perpendicular bisector of the medial phalanx forms two identical right triangles, yielding equal DIP and PIP joint angles (θ_1' and θ_2'):

$$\theta_1' = \theta_2' = 2\tan^{-1}\left[\frac{2(R+D_2)}{L_2}\right] \tag{5.34}$$

The third contact point divides the proximal phalange into two unequal lengths. One is $L_2/2$ while the other is (($L_3 - L_2$)/2). The MP joint angle (θ_3') can then be estimated as

$$\theta_3' = 2\tan^{-1}\frac{2(R+D_3)}{2L_3 - L_2} \tag{5.35}$$

Based on this biomechanical hand model, tendon forces for each finger and in total were calculated for both types of grip and for eleven cylindrical handles with diameters ranging from 10 to 60 mm. For Grip I, tendon force were minimized at 30–35, 38–43, 40–45,

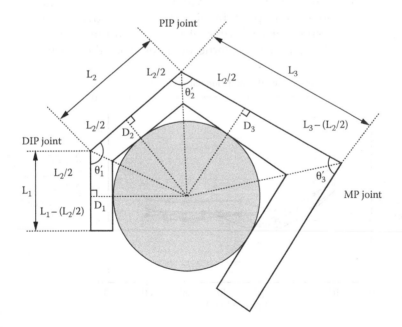

FIGURE 5.13
Schematic diagram of Grip II. (Reproduced from Kong, Y.K., Optimum design of handle shape through biomechanical modeling of hand tendon forces, PhD dissertation, The Pennsylvania State University, University Park, PA, 2001. With permission.)

FIGURE 5.14
Finger tendon forces for Grip I. (Reproduced from Kong, Y.K., Optimum design of handle shape through biomechanical modeling of hand tendon forces, PhD dissertation, The Pennsylvania State University, University Park, PA, 2001. With permission.)

and 25–30 mm for index, middle, ring, and little fingers, respectively. The total of tendon force for all fingers was minimized for an approximately 40 mm cylindrical handle (see Figure 5.14). As the size of the handle deviated above or below 40 mm, the total tendon forces increased.

For Grip II, tendon force were minimized at 23–28, 28–33, 28–33, and 20–25 mm for index, middle, ring, and little fingers, respectively. The total of tendon force for all fingers was minimized for an approximately 28 mm cylindrical handle (see Figure 5.15). The combined results for each type of grip are summarized in Table 5.10. As noted previously, as the size of the handle deviates from the optimum size, tendon

FIGURE 5.15
Finger tendon forces for Grip II. (Reproduced from Kong, Y.K., Optimum design of handle shape through biomechanical modeling of hand tendon forces, PhD dissertation, The Pennsylvania State University, University Park, PA, 2001. With permission.)

TABLE 5.10

Summary of Optimal Cylindrical Handle Sizes

Finger	Grip I	Grip II	Combined Grip
Index	30	25	25–30
Middle	40	30	30–40
Ring	40	30	30–40
Little	25	20	20–25

forces increase. This is an important principle that should be utilized in the design of hand tools (see Section 9.3.2). Also, in either type of grip, the optimal handle size depends greatly on which finger is considered. Therefore, a purely traditional cylindrical handle cannot provide optimality for all fingers simultaneously and alternate handle shapes need to be considered (see Section 9.3.3). Further details can be found in Kong (2001) and Kong et al. (2004), with applications to meat hook handles in Kong and Freivalds (2003).

5.6 Direct Measurement Validation Studies

Directly measured tendon forces under isometric finger function were first reported by Bright and Urbaniak (1976). They developed a strain gauge to measure the tendon forces in both tip pinch and power grip actions during operative procedures. Flexor tendon forces were found to be in the range of 40–200 N and 12.5–150 N for the FDP and FDS, respectively, in power grip action, and 25–125 N for the FDP and 10–75 N for the FDS in pinch action. Since they directly measured the tendon forces only, they did not report the actual applied pinch and power grip force and the ratio of tendon force to the externally applied force.

Schuind et al. (1992) directly measured the flexor tendons (Flexor Pollicis Longus [FPL], FDP, and FDS) during various finger functions. They developed an s-shaped tendon force transducer and measured the flexor tendon forces in pinch and power grip functions. Also, a pinch dynamometer was used to record the applied loads in pinch action. The tendon forces showed proportionality to the externally applied forces. To compare their results with the previously published mathematical finger models, they normalized their tendon forces, as a ratio of the tendon force to the applied forces. In tip pinch, the ratios were 3.6F, 7.92F, and 1.73F, for the externally applied force F, for the FPL, FDP, and FDS, respectively. In lateral pinches, the ratios were 3.05F, 2.9F, and 0.71F for the FPL, FDP, and FDS, respectively. Although the FDP and FPL showed high forces during tip and lateral pinch, the maximal values recorded are probably on the lower side of the potential forces and it could be explained by the significantly weaker pinch and power grip forces during carpal tunnel surgery due to the denervation or partial anesthesia of the sensory area of the median nerve. However, the magnitude of tendon forces was similar to values reported by Bright and Urbaniak (1976), although direct comparison is not possible since the applied force was not recorded in their study.

In another in vivo tendon force measurement study, Dennerlein et al. (1998) measured only the FDS tendon forces of the middle finger at three finger postures, which ranged from extended to flexed pinch postures, using a gas-sterilized tendon force transducer (Dennerlein et al., 1997) and a single axis load cell. The investigation was centered upon the average ratio of the FDS tendon tension to the externally applied force. The average ratio ranged from 1.7F to 5.8F, with a mean of 3.3F, in the study. Tip pinches with the DIP joint flexed were also studied with the tendon-to-tip force ratio being 2.4F. These ratios were compared with the results of their own three finger models as well as other contemporarily published isometric tendon force models. These ratios were larger than those of other studies. The average values were also slightly higher than that (1.73F) of Schuind et al.'s (1992) in vivo tendon force measurement study. It was found that the tendon force ratios and muscle strength varied substantially from individual to individual, although the ratio of force from tendon to tendon was relatively constant within the same limb for all studies (Ketchum et al., 1978; Brand et al., 1981; Dennerlein et al., 1998). A more recent study by Kursa et al. (2005) also found mean FDP to fingertip force ratio of 2.4 and mean FDS to fingertip ratio of 1.5, with the ratios remaining constant over a range of loading rates. A summary of these tendon force models is given in Table 5.11.

More recently, Park et al. (2009) studied tendon forces in vivo using forearm specimens from cadavers. He built a neuromuscular grip simulator consisting of five components: (1) an aluminum frame supporting the specimen, (2) a motion delivery unit with stepper motors applying force to the FDP and FDS tendons, (3) a data acquisition unit for force transducers measuring tendon forces, (4) camera system measuring finger joint angles, and (5) an operating system to control the complete simulator (Figure 5.16). This was basically an extension of Valero-Cuevas et al. (2000) cadaver set up, but instead of extension springs supplying tendon forces, stepper motors provided a higher level of tension control. Of special necessity were an adjustable fixation system (Wristjack®, Hand Biomechanics Lab, http://www.handbiolab.com/) and the use of freeze clamps with liquid nitrogen (Sharkey et al., 1995) to insure a tight bond between the slippery tendons and the force delivery system. Further details on the interactive

TABLE 5.11

Summary of Tendon Force Models

Model		References	Key Features
Static		Landsmeer (1960, 1962)	Simplest tendon-pulley model
		Armstrong and Chaffin (1978, 1979)	Pulley model with tendon force
Dynamic		Schoenmarklin and Marras (1990)	Pulley model with acceleration
Complex tendon forces	Reduction	Smith et al. (1964)	Two dimensional, scaled tendon forces
		Smith et al. (1964)	Three dimensional, some forces set equal to zero
	Optimization	Seireg and Arvikar (1973)	Objective function with constraints
		Penrod et al. (1974)	Objective function with constraints
		Chao and An (1978a)	Three dimensional, linear programming
		An et al. (1985)	Three dimensional, linear programming
	Combined	Chao and An (1978b)	Graphical, optimization
		Weightman and Amis (1982)	Some F = 0, some F ∝ muscle area
In vivo studies		Bright and Urbaniak (1976)	Strain gauge
		Schuind et al. (1992)	S-shape tendon force transducer
		Dennerlein et al. (1998)	Gas-sterilized tendon force transducer

FIGURE 5.16
Schematic drawing of the integrated neuromuscular gripper.

neuromuscular gripper system (sometimes facetiously referred to as the Thing, from the 1960s TV show *The Addams Family*) can be found in Park (2009).

Key experimental factors varied were five different diameter handles and the ratio of FDP to FDS tendon forces from 1:10 to 10:1 (which typically has been assumed to be 3:1 by Marco et al. (1998) and Kong et al. (2004). This latter factor was very critical in changing the gripping forces and the gripping dynamics as evidenced by varying finger joint angles, shown in Figure 5.17. In general, there was an inverse relationship of handle size and grip force, with a 3:2 ratio giving the largest gripping force for each of the fingers (Figure 5.18). Internal tendon forces averaged 6.2 times the external forces and the cadaver simulations produced very similar results to those predicted by Kong et al. (2004) (Figure 5.19). Note, that the cadaver tendon forces were kept at relatively low levels (factor of 4 or 5 lower than predicted from Kong et al., 2004) producing external gripping forces of only 10%–20% of maximum voluntary human grip exertions. This was done so as to avoid tissue failures as the cadaver specimens slowly deteriorated.

FIGURE 5.17
Finger joint angles for five handle diameters (in mm) and selected % FDS contributions.

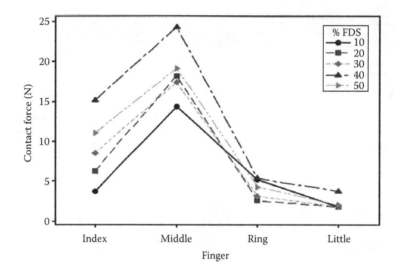

FIGURE 5.18
Finger contact forces for selected % FDS contributions.

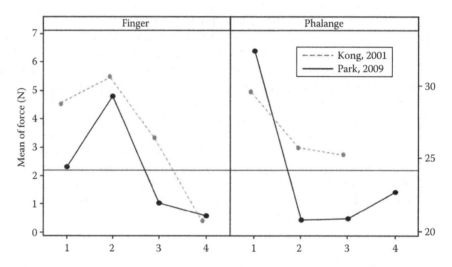

FIGURE 5.19
Comparison of Park (2009) cadaver tendon forces with Kong et al. (2004) model predictions for selected fingers and phalanges.

5.7 Critical Evaluation of Modeling Approaches

Although the intrinsic muscles are more active in pinch action than in power grip action, the relative magnitudes of the main flexor tendon forces (such as FDP and FDS) are usually high in both actions. These in vivo tendon forces of the flexors are presented in Table 5.12 based on the previous studies. In general, these averages and ranges of tendon forces are very similar with a few exceptions. Schuind et al. (1992) showed lower FDS tendon forces in power grip action than those of other types of grips. The tendon force ranges of Brand et al. (1981) show similar magnitudes with Bright and Urbaniak (1976) power

TABLE 5.12

In Vivo FDP and FDS Tendon Forces (in kg)

Study	Finger Configuration	FDP	FDS
Brand et al. (1981)	—	14.9[a] (13.5–17.0)	10.4[a] (4.5–17)
Ketchum et al. (1978)	MCP joint flexion	5.7[a] (5.27–6.18)	6.12[a] (3.73–7.63)
Bright and Urbaniak (1976)	Tip Pinch	2.5–12.5	1.0–7.5
	Power grip	4.0–20.0	1.25–15.0
Schuind et al. (1992)	Tip pinch	8.3 (2.0–12.0)	1.9 (0.3–3.5)
	Power grip	4.0 (1.9–6.4)	0.6 (0.0–0.9)

[a] Average tendon forces for all fingers.

grips. Ketchum et al. (1978) and Bright and Urbaniak (1976) tip pinch action also show the similar ranges of tendon forces. Schuind et al. (1992) represented the significant differences between FDP and FDS tendon forces in both pinch and power grip, whereas the others showed that the force of FDP tendon was only slightly larger than that of the FDS tendon. These discrepancies can be explained by the different finger postures utilized in each study, since each finger could have various functional muscle capacities depending upon its joint configuration (Chao and An, 1978b).

In all these in vivo tendon force studies, the muscle and tendon forces were proportional to the externally applied forces. However, these predicted maximum tendon forces are probably lower than the true potential forces because these experiments were performed during carpal tunnel surgery under local anesthesia in the median nerve innervation area. In such case, the muscles are partially inactive and produce lower pinch and power grip forces. To normalize these tendon forces, the ratios of the tendon force to the applied force, FDP to FDS, and joint forces were studied for both pinch and power grip functions (Tables 5.13 and 5.14).

Average ratios of tendon forces to the applied forces in the tendon force prediction models were, for an external force of F, 3.5F, 1.8F, and 3.67F, respectively, for the FDP, FDS, and I (intrinsic) tendons in pinch, while 3.14F, 3.48F, and 11.4F were for FDP, FDS, and I tendons in power grip, respectively. Generally, all data agreed with high contributions of flexor tendons (FDP and FDS) for both pinch and power grip actions, although intrinsic tendons showed high variations among those data. The average ratios of FDP to FDS were also obtained, 2.92:1 and 0.93:1 for pinch and power grip, respectively. These data showed the significant strength contribution of the FDP tendon to the pinch, as opposed to the fairly equal contributions of these two flexors to the overall power grips.

Although they did not measure the externally applied force with the tendon forces in a power grip, Schuind et al. (1992) attempted to validate these mathematical solutions experimentally. They only used the pinch dynamometer for measuring the amount of the applied force for pinch functions. Thus, the mean tendon forces were applied for validating power grip functions in this study.

In pinch studies, Schuind et al. (1992) reported the higher ratio of FDP to the applied force (7.92F) than the result (3.5F) of mathematical tendon force prediction models. The FDS ratio to the applied force (1.73F), however, was fairly similar to the average ratio (1.8F) in the finger model studies. Because of the large force measurement for the FDP tendon, a higher ratio of FDP/FDS (4.6F) was presented in their study than that of finger model studies. Dennerlein et al. (1998) also found higher ratios of the FDS tendon to the applied force (3.3F) than those of mathematical finger model studies.

TABLE 5.13

Tendon and Joint Forces during Pinch (Normalized to External Force)

Study	Pinch Type	Muscle Force				Joint Force		
		FDP	FDS	FDP/FDS	I	DIP	PIP	MCP
Bright and Urbaniak (1976)	Tip	2.50–12.5 kg[a]	1.0–7.5 kg[a]					
Schuind et al. (1992)	Tip	7.92	1.73	4.60				
	Lateral	2.90	0.71	4.08				
Dennerlein et al. (1998)	Tip	—	3.30 (1.7–5.8)					
Smith et al. (1964)	Tip	3.80	2.50	1.52	2.10			7.50
Chao et al. (1976)	Tip, radial, ulnar	4.32	0.73	5.90	7.05	5.60	6.00	8.80
Chao and An (1978a)	Tip[b]	3.30	3.10	1.06	2.41	4.68	8.29	8.51
Chao and An (1978a)	Tip	3.97	0.82	4.84	3.11			
Weightman and Amis (1982)	Tip	2.40[c]	1.85[c]	1.30				
An et al. (1985)	Tip	1.93–2.08	1.75–2.16		0–0.99	2.40	4.40	3.50

[a] Tendon force.
[b] Middle finger tip pinch.
[c] Average value for various finger configurations.

TABLE 5.14

Tendon and Joint Forces in Power Grip (Normalized to External Force)

Study	Finger	Tendon Force				Joint Force		
		FDP	FDS	FDP/FDS	I	DIP	PIP	MCP
Bright and Urbaniak (1976)		4.0–20.0[a]	1.25–15.0[a]					
Schuind et al. (1992)		4.0[b]	0.6[b]	6.67				
Chao et al. (1976)	Index	2.77	2.53	1.09	15.76	3.09	4.35	12.70
	Middle	3.05	4.23	0.72	13.10	3.17	7.11	13.90
	Little	3.37	3.40	0.99	15.21	3.31	6.02	14.50
Chao and An (1978a)	Middle	3.37	3.75	0.90	1.64	3.89	6.80	5.18
An et al. (1985)	Index	3.17–3.47	1.51–2.14		0.1–1.19	2.8–3.4	4.5–5.3	3.2–3.7

[a] Tendon force, unit: kg.
[b] Mean tendon forces, unit: kg.

In power grip studies, there are few in vivo tendon force to externally applied force ratio data. Thus, only the FDP:FDS ratio of direct measurement study can be used for the comparison with finger model studies. Schuind et al. (1992) presented a 6.67:1 ratio based on their mean tendon forces of FDP and FDS. The force of FDP was significantly larger than that of FDS in direct measurement studies (see Table 5.12). DP and FDS showed similar contributions to power grip (3.14F for FDP and 3.48F for FDS; Kong, 2001) and a FDP/FDS ratio of 0.93:1 was also calculated in finger force prediction models. The variability of these results may be expected since all researchers did not use the same finger characteristics: moment arms, finger configurations, and angles of the applied forces to the finger tip regarding the function of intrinsic versus flexor muscles during pinch and power grips. Based on the solutions from the three moment equations, Smith et al. (1964) found that flexor tendons usually carry larger forces than other intrinsic muscles during tip pinch. Chao and An (1978b) also supported this result in their study. They showed the flexors were most active and produced high tendon forces in both pinch and power grip actions. However, Chao et al. (1976) and An et al. (1985) suggested contradictory results for the contributions of intrinsic muscles in finger actions. They presented higher contributions of intrinsic muscles than those of flexors did in pinch and power grip functions. In general, although the magnitude of the intrinsic muscle force was less than that of the flexors, the intrinsic muscles were more active in pinches than in power grip. An et al. (1985) also agreed with high intrinsic muscle forces in pinches and explained it by the need for these intrinsic muscles to balance and stabilize the large MCP joint forces.

Most of these studies showed similar trends for joint forces. Small constraint forces and moments were seen at both the DIP and PIP joints, while the constraint forces and moments were considerably higher at the MCP joint in both actions. DIP- and PIP-joint forces of the power grip actions were relatively lower than those of the pinch actions. It may be explained by why hands are more adaptable in performing powerful grip actions rather than with pinches since it is more difficult to maintain the proper stability requirements at the distal joints (Chao et al., 1976).

Questions

1. Describe the structural anatomy of the hand and wrist.

2. Describe the musculature needed to produce a gripping action.

3. What are the major differences between extrinsic and intrinsic muscles?

4. Compare and contrast the flexor digitorum profundus and flexor digitorum superficialis.

5. Describe the flexor tendon-pulley systems.

6. What is bowstringing?

7. Compare and contrast the three Landsmeer pulley models.

8. What is the reasoning behind the development of tendon strain and tendinitis in repeated manual exertions?

9. What is the reasoning behind the development of tendon strain and tendinitis in hand motions with extreme deviations?

10. What is it thought that individuals with small wrist may be more susceptible to injuries than those with large wrists?

11. How do dynamics affects modify the static tendon-pulley models?

12. How can static indeterminacy problems be handled in hand/wrist models?

13. In a model of a power grip, what are the two major approaches or assumptions needed to begin the modeling process?

14. Compared to the external forces, what are the ranges of tendon forces predicted by modeling and reported by direct measurement? What are differences between a power and pinch grip?

Problems

1. Complete the development of Landsmeer's Model III; i.e., derive Equation 5.3.

2. Compare the differences in tendon forces predicted by the three Landsmeer models.

3. What is the relative difference in tendon forces resulting between the two different assumptions used in modeling a power grip (i.e., Kong's Grip I and Grip II).

4. Estimate the normal tendon forces incurred in a neutral wrist position, with minimal tendon friction ($\mu = 0.01$), as opposed to a wrist flexed at 20° in a worker with CTS symptoms and higher friction ($\mu = 0.08$). Assume the radius of the virtual wrist pulley at 15 cm.

5. Using Kong's (2001) model, estimate the tendon forces (normalized to external force) required for pressing down with an extended finger (e.g., pressing a button).

References

An, K.W., Chao, E.Y., Cooney, W.P., and Linscheid, R.L. (1979). Normative model of human hand for biomechanical analysis. *Journal of Biomechanics* 12:775–788.

An, K.N., Hui, F.C., Morrey, B.F., Linscheid, R.L., and Chao, E.Y.S. (1981). Muscle across the elbow joint: A biomechanical analysis. *Journal of Biomechanics* 14:659–669.

An, K.N., Ueba, Y., Chao, E.Y., Cooney, W.P., and Linscheid, R.L. (1983). Tendon excursion and moment arm of index finger muscles. *Journal of Biomechanics* 16:419–425.

An, K.N., Chao, E.Y., Cooney, W.P., and Linscheid, R.L. (1985). Forces in the normal and abnormal hand. *Journal of Orthopaedic Research* 3:202–211.

An, K.N., Horii, E., and Ryu, J. (1991). Muscle function. In: K.N. An, R.A. Berger, and W.P. Cooney (eds), *Biomechanics of the Wrist Joint*. NewYork: Springer Verlag, pp. 157–169.

Armstrong, T.J. (1976). Circulatory and local muscle responses to static manual work. PhD dissertation. Ann Arbor, MI: University of Michigan.

Armstrong, T.J. and Chaffin, D.B. (1978). An investigation of the relationship between displacements of the finger and wrist joints and the extrinsic finger flexor tendons. *Journal of Biomechanics* 11:119–128.

Armstrong, T.J. and Chaffin, D.B. (1979). Some biomechanical aspects of the carpal tunnel. *Journal of Biomechanics* 12:567–570.

Batmanabane, M. and Malathi, S. (1985). Movements at the carpometacarpal and metacarpophalangeal joints of the hand and their effect on the dimensions of the articular ends of the metacarpal bones. *Anatomical Record* 213:102–110.

Brand, P.W. and Hollister, A. (1993). *Clinical Mechanics of the Hand*, 2nd edn, St. Louis, MO: Mosby-Year Book, Inc.

Brand, P.W., Beach, R.B., and Thompson, D.E. (1981). Relative tension and potential excursion of muscles in the forearm and hand. *Journal of Hand Surgery* 6:209–218.

Bright, D.S. and Urbaniak, J.S. (1976). Direct measurements of flexor tendon tension during active and passive digit motion and its application to flexor tendon surgery. *Transactions 22nd Annual Orthopedic Research Society*, 240.

Cailliet, R. (1994). *Hand Pain and Impairment*, 3rd edn, Philadelphia, PA: Davis.

Chaffin, D.B., Andersson, G.B.J., and Martin, B.J. (1999). *Occupational Biomechanics*, 3rd edn, New York: John Wiley & Sons.

Chao, E.Y.S. and An, K.N. (1978a). Determination of internal forces in human hand. *Journal of Engineering Mechanics Division ASCE* 104:255–272.

Chao, E.Y.S. and An, K.N. (1978b). Graphical interpretation of the solution to the redundant problem in biomechanics. *Journal of Biomechanics* 11:159–167.

Chao, E.Y.S., Opgrande, J.D., and Axmear, F.E. (1976). Three-dimensional force analysis of finger joints in selected isometric hand functions. *Journal of Biomechanics* 9:387–396.

Davidoff, N.A. (1990). The development of a graphic model of a human hand. MS thesis. University Park, PA: The Pennsylvania State University.

Davidoff, N.A. and Freivalds, A. (1993). A graphic model of the human hand using CATIA. *International Journal of Industrial Ergonomics* 12:255–264.

Dennerlein, J.T, Miller, J., Mote, C.D. Jr., and Rempel, D.M. (1997). A low profile human tendon force transducer: The influence of tendon thickness on calibration. *Journal of Biomechanics* 30:395–397.

Dennerlein, J.T, Diao, E., Mote, C.D. Jr., and Rempel, D.M. (1998). Tensions of the flexor digitorum superficialis are higher than a current model predicts. *Journal of Biomechanics* 31:295–301.

Fahrer, M. (1971). Considerations on functional anatomy of the flexor digitorum profundus. *Annales de Chirurgie* 25:945.

Garcia-Elias, M., Horii, E., and Berger, R.A. (1991). Individual carpal bone motion. In: K.-N. An, R.A. Berger, and W.P. Cooney (eds), *Biomechanics of the Wrist Joint*. New York: Springer-Verlag, pp. 61–75.

Garrett, J.W. (1970a). *Anthropometry of the Air Force Female Hand*, AMRL-TR-69-26. Wright-Patterson AFB, OH: Aerospace Medical Research Laboratory.

Garrett, J.W. (1970b). *Anthropometry of the Hands of Male Air Force Flight Personnel*, AMRL-TR-69-42. Wright-Patterson AFB, OH: Aerospace Medical Research Laboratory.

Garrett, J.W. (1971). The adult human hand: Some anthropometric and biomechanical considerations. *Human Factors* 13:117–131.

Gigis, P.I. and Kuczynski, K. (1982). The distal interphalangeal joints of the human fingers. *Journal of Hand Surgery* 7:176–182.

Greiner, T.M. (1992). *Hand Anthropometry of the U.S. Army Personnel*, NATICK/TR-92/011. Natick, MA: U.S. Army Natick Research, Development & Engineering Center.

Idler, R.S. (1985). Anatomy and biomechanics of the digital flexor tendons. *Hand Clinic* 1:3–12.

Ketchum, L.D., Thompson, D., Pocock, G., La, C., and Wallingford, D. (1978). A clinical study of forces generated by the intrinsic muscles of the index finger and the extrinsic flexor and extensor muscles of the hand. *The Journal of Hand Surgery* 3:571–578.

Kong, Y.K. (2001). Optimum design of handle shape through biomechanical modeling of hand tendon forces. PhD dissertation. University Park, PA: The Pennsylvania State University.

Kong, Y.K. and Freivalds, A. (2003). Evaluation of meat hook handle shapes. *International Journal of Industrial Ergonomics* 32:13–23.

Kong, Y., Freivalds, A., and Kim, S.E. (2004). Evaluation of handles in a maximum gripping task. *Ergonomics* 47:1350–1364.

Kursa, K., Diao, E., Lattanza, L., and Rempel, D. (2005). *In vivo* forces generated by finger flexor muscles do not depend on the rate of fingertip loading during an isometric task. *Journal of Biomechanics* 38:2288–2293.

Landsmeer, J.M.F. (1960). Studies in the anatomy of articulation. *Acta Morphologica Nederlands* 3–4:287–303.

Landsmeer, J.M.F. (1962). Power grip and precision handling. *Annals of Rheumatoid Diseases* 21:164–170.

LeVeau, B. (1977). *William and Lissner Biomechanics of Human Motion*. Philadelphia, PA: W.B. Saunders.

Lieber, R.L., Fazeli, B.M., and Botte, M.J. (1990). Architecture of selected wrist flexor and extensor muscles. *Journal of Hand Surgery* 15:244–250.

Lin, G.T., Cooney, W.P., Amadio, P.C., and An, K.N. (1990). Mechanical properties of human pulleys. *Journal of Hand Surgery* 15B:429–434.

Long, C., Conrad, P.W., Hall, E.A., and Furler, S.L. (1970). Intrinsic-extrinsic muscle control of the hand in power grip and precision handling: An electromyographic study. *Journal of Bone and Joint Surgery* 52A:853–867.

Manske, P.R. and Lesker, P.A. (1977). Strength of human pulleys. *Hand* 9:147–152.

Marco, R.A.W., Sharkey, N.A., and Smith, T.S. (1998). Pathomechanics of closed rupture of the flexor tendon pulleys in rock climbers. *The Journal of Bone and Joint Surgery* 80A:1012–1019.

Nordin, M. and Frankel, V.H. (2001). *Basic Biomechanics of the Musculoskeletal System*, 3rd edn, Philadelphia, PA: Lippincott Williams & Wilkins.

Norkin, C.C. and Levangie, P.K. (1992). *Joint Structure & Function: A Comprehensive Analysis*. Philadelphia, PA: Davis.

Park, S. (2009). Biomechanical analysis of hand grip motion of hand grip motion for optimal handle design: Using a cadaver model. PhD dissertation. University Park, PA: The Pennsylvania State University.

Park, S., Freivalds, A., Sharkey, N., and Lowe, B. (2009). A new device for measuring flexor tendon forces and grip force: A cadaver model. *The Annual Meeting of the American Society of Biomechanics*, University Park, PA.

Penrod, D.D., Davy, D.T., and Singh, D.P. (1974). An optimization approach to tendon force analysis. *Journal of Biomechanics* 7:123–129.

Rogers, M.S., Barr, A.B., Kasemsontitum, B., and Rempel, D.M. (2008). A three-dimensional anthropometric solid model of the hand based on landmark measurements. *Ergonomics* 51:511–526.

Roloff, I., Schöffl, V.R., Vigouroux, L., and Quaine, F. (2006). Biomechanical model for the determination of the forces acting on the finger pulley system. *Journal of Biomechanics* 39:915–923.

Schoenmarklin, R.W. and Marras, W.P. (1990). A dynamic biomechanical model of the wrist joint. *Proceedings of the Human Factors Society 34th Annual Meeting*. Santa Monica, CA: Human Factors Society, pp. 805–809.

Schuind, F., Garcia-Elias, M., Cooney W.P. III, and An, K.N. (1992). Flexor tendon forces: In vivo measurements. *The Journal of Hand Surgery* 17A:291–298.

Schultz, R.B., Stroave, A., and Krishnamurthy, S. (1987). Metacarpophalangeal joint motion and the role of the collateral ligaments. *International Orthopaedics* 11:149–155.

Seireg, A. and Arvikar, R.B. (1973). A mathematical model for evaluation of forces in lower extremities of musculoskeletal system. *Journal of Biomechanics* 6:313–326.

Sharkey, N.A., Smith, T.S., and Lundmark, D.C. (1995). Freeze clamping musculotendinous junctions for *in vitro* simulations of joint mechanics. *Journal of Biomechanics* 28:631–635.

Smith, E.M., Juvenile, R.B., Bender, L.F., and Pearson, J.R. (1964). Role of the finger flexors in rheumatoid deformities of the metacarpophalangeal joints. *Arthritis and Rheumatism* 7:467–480.

Spence, A.P. (1990). *Basic Human Anatomy*, 3rd edn, Redwood City, CA: Benjamin/Cummings Pub. Co.

Steinberg, D.R. (1992). Acute flexor tendon injuries. *Orthopaedics Clinics of North America* 23:125–140.

Steindler, A. (1955). *Kinesiology of the Human Body under Normal and Pathological Conditions*. Springfield, IL: Thomas.

Thompson, J.S. (1977). *Core Textbook of Anatomy*. Philadelphia, PA: J.B. Lippincott Co.

Tubiana, R., ed. (1981). *The Hand*, Vol. 1. Philadelphia, PA: Saunders.

Valero-Cuevas, F.J., Towles, J.D., and Hentz, V.R. (2000). Quantification of fingertip force reduction in the forefinger following simulated paralysis of extensor and intrinsic muscles. *Journal of Biomechanics* 33:1601–1609.

Weightman, B. and Amis, A.A. (1982). Finger joint force predictions related to design of joint replacements. *Journal of Biomedical Engineering* 4:197–205.

Youm, Y., McMurty, R.Y., Flatt, A.E., and Gillespie, T.E. (1978). Kinematics of the wrist. *Journal of Bone and Joint Surgery* 60A:424–431.

6

Musculoskeletal Disorders and Risk Factors

6.1 Extent of the Problem

There are six major surveys that have estimated the magnitude of the musculoskeletal disorders (MSDs) in the general U.S. population: the National Health and Nutrition Examination Survey from 1976 to 1988, the National Ambulatory Medical Care Survey of 1989, the National Health Interview Surveys of 1988 and 1995, the Health and Retirement Survey from 1992 to 1994, and the Social Security Supplemental Security Income survey of 1998. Unfortunately, all of these are based on individual self-reports and not on medical diagnosis and none identify the work-relatedness aspect, if any, of these disorders. Given that the vast majority of adults are in the active workforce, there would be difficulty in finding comprehensive data on an occupationally unexposed group, which, by definition, would be unrepresentative of the U.S. adult population.

In terms of overall musculoskeletal disorders, the 1988 National Health Interview Survey found a prevalence of almost 15% for the U.S. population (Lawrence et al., 1998), which stayed relatively constant at 13.9% for the 1995 survey (Praemer et al., 1999). However, the Social Security Supplemental Security Income survey of 1998 did indicate a noticeable increase in prevalence with age, 16.9% for those 50–59 and 23.9% for those 60–65. In terms of upper limb musculoskeletal disorders, the 1988 National Health Interview Survey found a prevalence of 9.4% in the hand or wrist, with 1.5% being specifically carpal tunnel syndrome (CTS) and 0.4% being tendinitis (Tanaka, 1995). Interestingly, when based on reported symptoms, the prevalence for CTS can be as high as 14.4%, but when referred for a clinical diagnosis the prevalence drops to 2.7% (Atroshi et al., 1999).

Information about the work-related nature of musculoskeletal disorders is again difficult to obtain, there not being one central comprehensive surveillance data system. Perhaps, the best source of data is the Annual Survey of Occupational Injuries and Illnesses survey, produced by the U.S. Department of Labor's Bureau of Labor Statistics (BLS). It covers the private industry but excludes self-employed, small farms, and federal, state, and local government agencies, or about 25% of the total workforce, collected primarily from the injury and illness data reports required by the Occupational Safety and Health Administration (OSHA Form 300). One category subset is labeled "disorders associated with repeated trauma" and provides a historical trend in musculoskeletal disorders. The number of cases was relatively steady from 1976 to 1982 at around 22,000 and then increased sharply to 332,100 by 1994, at which point there was a gradual reduction to 246,700 by 1999 (see Figure 6.1). This recent decline was speculated to have occurred as a result of a better recognition of such musculoskeletal disorders and the implementation of industrial health and safety programs (Conway and Svenson, 1998).

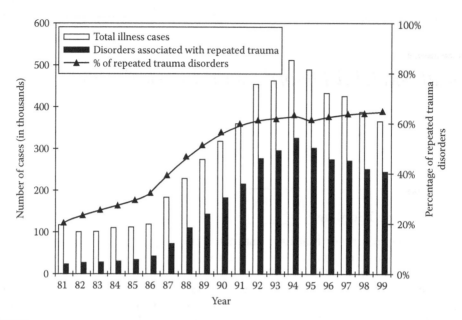

FIGURE 6.1
Incidence of disorders primarily associated with repeated trauma in private industry, 1982–1999. (Courtesy of Bureau of Labor Statistics, Washington, DC, http://www.bls.gov/iif)

Further evidence for the work-relatedness of these types of musculoskeletal injuries can be found from the survey data of Tanaka et al. (1995, 1997). Of the 1.87 million reporting having symptoms of CTS, a third were diagnosed as having the condition by the health care provider and over one half believed these were work related. Of the nearly 600,000 reporting having tendinitis symptoms, 28% were labeled as work related by the health care provider. In summary, all of these surveys and studies indicate a large-scale work-related problem that had a rapid growth in the 1980s and early 1990s with a slight decline in the recent years.

6.2 Common Musculoskeletal Disorders and Their Etiology

There are a large variety of musculoskeletal disorders that have some commonality both in the physiological or anatomical characteristics and in the general location of the problem (see Figure 6.2). For introducing and describing common musculoskeletal disorders, it is best to categorize them by the anatomical characteristics, while later, in providing more detailed scientific evidence for risk factors, it is best to categorize them by joint. It would not be unusual for a complaining worker or the medically untrained ergonomist lump medically different disorders into one collective "shoulder" disorder, since, probably, neither can identify the disorder more specifically. From the anatomical viewpoint, musculoskeletal disorders can be classified into six basic types: tendon, muscle, nerve, vascular, bursa, and bone/cartilage.

6.2.1 Tendon Disorders

The tendon, as described previously in Chapter 2, is the part of the muscle and the surrounding fascia transmitting force from the muscle that attach to the bone and produce

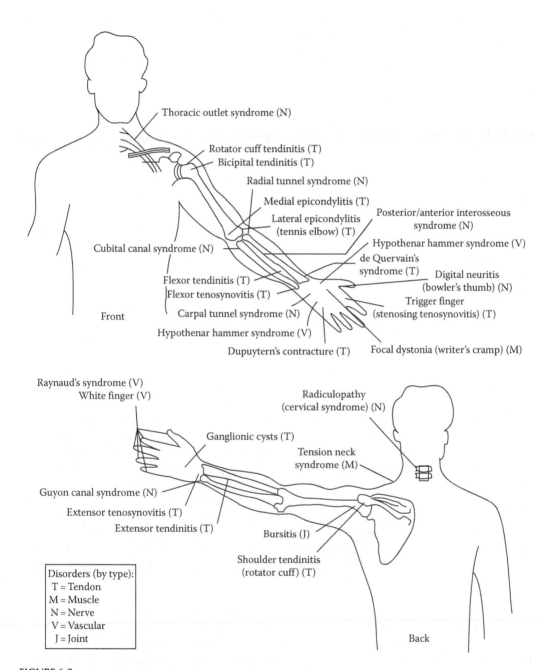

FIGURE 6.2
Examples of musculoskeletal disorders, which may be work related. (Reproduced from Kuorinka, I. and Forcier, L., *Work Related Musculoskeletal Disorders (WMSDs): A Reference Book for Prevention*, Taylor & Francis, London, U.K., 1995. With permission.)

joint motion. In places where there is a great deal of movement (e.g., fingers, wrist, shoulder), the tendon may pass through a sheath that protects and lubricates the tendon to reduce friction. When this sheath and the tendon within become inflamed, it is termed *tenosynovitis*. When a tendon without the sheath becomes inflamed, it is termed *tendinitis*. This inflammation can progress to the point of having microtrauma or even visible fraying of the tendon fibers. Sometimes, cases are further identified as to sublevel where found on the tendon. *Enthesopathy* or insertional tendinitis occurs at the tendon–bone interface with relatively little inflammation. A common one is enthesopathy of the extensor carpi radialis brevis from the lateral epicondyle, resulting from forceful, twisting motions, which then is referred to as *lateral epicondylitis*, or more commonly as *tennis elbow*. *Peritendinitis* refers to the inflammation of the tendon proper, where there is no tendon sheath, while the inflammation of the muscle–tendon interface is termed *myotendinitis*. Technically, these are all different disorders but they are often found together and exhibit similar symptoms of localized pain and tenderness and are typically collectively referred to as tendinitis. Two common examples of tendinitis are *bicipital tendinitis*, or inflammation of the long head of the biceps tendon as it passes over the head of the humerus through the bicipital groove caused by hyperabducting the elbow or forceful contractions of the biceps, and *rotator cuff tendinitis*, inflammation of tendons of various muscles around the shoulder (supraspinatus, infraspinatus, teres minor) caused from abducted arms or arms raised above the shoulders.

Acute cases of tenosynovitis may develop localized swelling, a narrowing or *stenosing* of the sheath, and even the formation of a nodule on the tendon, causing the tendon to be become temporarily entrapped or *triggered* as it attempts to slide through the sheath. If this occurs in the index finger, typically used in repeatedly and forcefully activating a power tool, it is colloquially termed *trigger finger*. Many times, upon attempting to straighten the finger and stretching the tendon, the tendon will crackle or crepitate leading to the more complete term of *stenosing tenosynovitis crepitans*. Other examples of tenosynovitis in the hand include *DeQuervain's disease* with inflammation of the tendons of the abductor pollicis longus and extensor pollicis brevis of the thumb. Repetitive forceful motions of the thumb in a variety of tasks, even games, lead to such problems and also to names popularized in the media referring back to those tasks, e.g., *Atari* or *Nintendo thumb* (Reinstein, 1983). *Dupuytren's contracture* is the formation of nodules in the palmar fascia, an extension of the tendon of the palmaris longus muscle, leading to triggering of the ring and little fingers. Tenosynovitis of the flexor tendons (carpi, digitorum profundus, and superficialias) within the wrist from repeated forceful wrist motion may lead to CTS. Similarly, repeated opening of scissors or other tools may lead to tenosynovitis in the extensor tendons in the fingers. A by-product of tenosynovitis is the excess release of synovial fluid which may collect and form fluid filled *ganglionic cysts* that appear as nodules under the skin on the surface of the hand.

The mechanism of injury for tendon disorders depends on a variety of factors, some of which have been studied in animal studies. Exercise with controlled conditions can have positive long-term effects by increasing tendon cross-sectional area and strength. Remodeling of the tendon can occur with the laying down of additional fibrocartilaginous tissue (Woo et al., 1980). However, when the exercise becomes excessive (high rates of loading in rabbits), there are degenerative changes in the tendon with increased number of capillaries, inflammatory cells, edema, microtears, and separation of fibers consistent with pathology of tendinosis in humans. Elevated temperatures and hypoxia in the core of the tendon may play a role in these degenerative changes (Backman et al., 1990). When a tendon experiences compressive loading in addition to tension, e.g., curving around a bone or ligament as in the Armstrong and Chaffin (1978) tendon-pulley model, the tendon becomes transformed from linear bands of collagen fascicles into irregular patterned fibrocartilage with changes in the proteoglycans (Malaviya et al., 2000). Coincidentally, tendon strength, at least in rats, decreases with age (Simonsen et al., 1995).

6.2.2 Muscle Disorders

Muscle disorders start as simple muscle soreness or pain, termed *myalgia*, in workers, both old and especially new, performing unaccustomed strenuous or repetitive work. The affected area will be sore and tender to touch because of microstrain and inflammation of the tissue, termed *myositis*. If the work is soon stopped (e.g., a one-time job or a weekend activity), relief will occur in several days. If the work is continued a gradual manner (i.e., a break-in period), generally, a conditioning process occurs, the muscle heals, becomes accustomed to task, and becomes more resistant to injury. However, if the work is continued in an excessive manner (i.e., few rest periods and frequent overtime), the muscle strain and myalgia become chronic and the disorder becomes *myofascial pain syndrome*. The muscle may spasm, dysfunction, and temporary disability may result. In chronic stages, the disorder is characterized by chronically painful spastic muscles, tingling sensations, nervousness, and sleeplessness and is termed *fibromyalgia* or *fibrositis*. It is aggravated by both repeated activities and also, paradoxically, by rest; it may be worse upon rising in the morning. Another characteristic of fibromyalgia is the presence of *trigger points*, small areas of spastic muscle that is tender to touch surrounded by unaffected muscle. Pressure on these trigger points will often result in pain shooting up or down the extremity. Details on trigger points and treatments of these disorders can be found in Travell and Simons (1983).

One specific and rather common myofascial syndrome is the *tension-neck syndrome*, characterized by pain and tenderness in the shoulder and neck region for clerical workers and small-parts assemblers, who typically are slightly hunched forward for better visibility and have contracted the upper back (trapezius) and neck muscles (Kuorinka and Forcier, 1995). More active and excessive muscle contraction may lead to a writer's *cramp* or *focal dystonia*. It was first noticed in Victorian England in scriveners who were responsible for copying contracts by hand using quills gripped firmly. The resulting spasms were first described in detail by Wilks (1878) and later by others (Sheehy and Marsden, 1982) as resulting from the repetitive forceful contractions of the hand with complications induced by co-contractions of the forearm flexors and extensors. The problem is that individuals tend to over grip tools or other objects by as much as a factor of 5. The problem is further exacerbated by CTS or other neurological disorders which reduce sensory feedback and increase overgripping to a factor of 10 (Lowe and Freivalds, 1999).

The mechanism of injury for muscle disorders is quite different from tendon disorders. Typically, muscle injury occurs as the result of excessive external forces on the passive structures, mainly connective tissue, rather than from overuse. Excessive muscle use will result in muscle fatigue limiting contractile capability before cellular damage can occur. This fatigue is due to intramuscular pressure exceeding capillary pressure (about 30 mm Hg) causing ischemia and hypoxia to the active muscle fibers (Sjøgaard and Søgaard, 1998), which then may contribute to alterations in the intracellular pH, lactic acid, calcium, and potassium concentrations and may upset overall homeostasis (Sjøgaard and Jensen, 1997). Eccentric contractions, in which external loads cause the sarcomeres to length during active cross-bridging, are also likely to cause structural damage, inflammation, hemorrhaging, and loss of force-generating capacity (McCully and Faulkner, 1985; McComas, 1996). Based on an exponential relationship exists between stress and the number of cycles, with greater stress requiring fewer cycles, there should be a theoretical stress limit, below which injury could be avoided (Warren et al., 1993). However, no such value has been derived for human muscle. There are also indications that passive stretch (Noonan et al., 1994) and vibration (Necking et al., 1966) contribute to muscle injury. As for tendons, there are age-related changes in skeletal muscle, with a gradual decrease in strength starting at age 40 and increasing more dramatically after age 65 (Faulkner et al., 1990). Although, most of this is related to inactivity, some 20% of the decrease cannot be prevented with exercise (Faulkner and Brooks, 1995).

6.2.3 Nerve Disorders

Nerve entrapment occurs between two different tissues, muscles, bones, ligaments, or other structures, and may be due to a variety of diseases, such as hyperthyroidism or arthritis, vascular disorders or edema, in addition to chronic work-related trauma. During entrapment, pressure on the nerve will impair blood flow and oxygenation of the Schwann cells and the myelin sheath with consequent affects on axonal transport system and production of action potentials. If the pressure is high enough, mechanical blocking of the depolarization process will occur (Lundborg, 1988). A complicating factor is that entrapment at one location of the nerve (which may be up to 1 m in length) increases the susceptibility to further injury at points either distal or proximal to the first location, due to impairment of the axonal flows of ions. This multiple entrapment, known as the *double crush syndrome*, makes it even more important that ergonomists consider the whole extremity when analyzing a job and diagnosing potential problems.

The most common nerve entrapment of the upper limbs is CTS. The *carpal tunnel* is formed by eight carpal bones on the dorsal side and the transverse carpal ligament (flexor retinaculum, which serves to prevent bowstringing) on the palmar side of the wrist (see Figure 6.3). Through this tunnel, in a tight fit, pass various blood vessels, flexor tendons, and the median nerve, which innervates the index and middle fingers and parts of the thumb and ring finger. Any additional increase in the contents of the tunnel will increase the pressure on the median nerve with consequent disruption of nerve conduction. This may occur in pregnant females when additional water retention results in swelling of the contents of carpal tunnel (Punnett et al., 1985) or in clerical, assembly, garment, and food processing workers from forceful repetitive wrist flexions/extensions or ulnar/radial deviations. The resulting friction of the tendons when sliding through their sheaths wrapped around the carpal tunnel bones or ligaments in the Armstrong and Chaffin (1978) tendon-pulley model (presented in Section 5.2) is compensated by additional secretions of synovial fluid. This causes swelling, increases resting carpal canal pressures by up to a factor of 3 (Okutsu et al., 1989), and compresses the median nerve resulting in shooting pains, especially at night, tingling and numbness, and loss of fine motor control to the above-mentioned fingers.

Two other nerves, ulnar and radial, pass through the wrist area, although, not through the carpal tunnel. The ulnar nerve enters the hand at Guyon's canal on the medial (little finger) side, innervating the little finger and part of the ring finger. Sometimes the ulnar nerve is entrapped leading to the *Guyon canal syndrome* with tingling and numbness of the associated fingers. The ulnar nerve may also be trapped further back in either the ulnar groove or the cubital tunnel formed by the two heads of the flexor carpi ulnaris near the elbow in the *cubital tunnel syndrome* as a result of direct pressure on the area from resting the elbows on sharp table edges or twisting motions at the elbow. Symptoms include pain and soreness at the medial elbow and tingling and numbness in the associated fingers. An acute blow to the ulnar nerve at the ulnar groove results in the funny bone sensation.

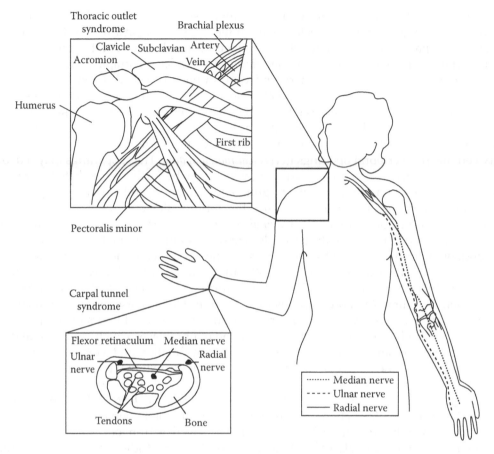

FIGURE 6.3
Carpal tunnel and thoracic outlet syndromes. (Reproduced from Kuorinka, I. and Forcier, L., *Work Related Musculoskeletal Disorders (WMSDs): A Reference Book for Prevention*, Taylor & Francis, London, U.K., 1995. With permission.)

The radial nerve also passes into the forearm just below the lateral epicondyle near the head of the radius. Compression of the nerve due to a contracted muscle or bones will result in localized pain and tenderness and tingling and numbness in the thumb, termed the *radial tunnel syndrome*. A similar effect will result from an entrapment of a deep branch of the radial nerve (interosseous) within the supinator muscles of the forearm in the Arcade of Frohse in the *posterior interosseous syndrome*. This condition will also show a weakness in extensor muscles for the wrist and little finger.

The median nerve can similarly be trapped both at the elbow, in the *pronator teres syndrome*, and in the forearm, in the *anterior interosseous syndrome*. In the first case, the median nerve is trapped beneath the two heads of the pronator teres muscle, due to inflammation and swelling of muscle from constant pronation as in the classic clothes-wringing motion. Symptoms include spasm and tightness of the pronator teres muscle resulting in pain on the palm side of forearm and symptoms distally that are similar to those of CTS and may result in misdiagnosis. The only difference is that the palmar cutaneous branch of median nerve branches off before the carpal tunnel. Therefore, it will produce impaired sensations in the palm in the pronator teres syndrome but not the CTS (Parker and Imbus, 1992). In the second case, the anterior interosseus branch of the median nerve can be compressed by the deep anterior forearm muscles from overuse. Since the nerve innervates muscles in mid-forearm and the flexor pollicis longus, symptoms include pain in the front of the forearm and difficulty producing an O-shaped pattern in a thumb–index finger tip pinch (Parker and Imbus, 1992).

Further back on the upper limb, the *thoracic outlet syndrome* is entrapment of the brachial plexus (and also the subclavian artery and vein) in one or more different sites: the scalenus muscles in the neck, between the clavicle and first rib and between the chest wall and the pectoralis minor muscle (see Figure 6.3). Symptoms include numbness or tingling and pain in the arm and hand, especially on the ulnar side. Even the spinal nerve roots that form the brachial plexus (cervical vertebrae C5, C6, C7, and C8) may be compressed between the intervertebral openings in *cervical radiculopathy*. These openings may narrow due to degenerative disc disease or arthritis, which may be further exacerbated by repetitive neck motions. Symptoms include tingling and numbness and pain radiating to various locales determined by the innervation of the appropriate nerve root.

In a different type of nerve disorder, *digital neuritis*, direct pressure while grasping tools (e.g., scissors) or other items with sharp edges may result in inflammation and swelling of the underlying nerve and eventual numbness in the associated digit. Again the aggravating task or item may lead to descriptive colloquial names such as *bowler's thumb* (Howell and Leach, 1970; Dunham et al., 1972) or *cherry pitter's thumb* (Viegas and Torres, 1989).

Extraneural compression pressures as low as 30 mm Hg decrease intraneural flow and impair axonal transport within peripheral neurons. After several hours of compression, inflammation leads to fibrin deposits, proliferation of fibroblasts, which after several days leads to growth of fibrous tissues. After a week, demyelination and axonal degeneration are observed, with the degree of injury correlated with the external pressure (Dyck et al., 1990). Chronic nerve compression in rats shows a similar etiologic pattern ending in nerve fiber degeneration (Sommer et al., 1993; Mosconi and Kruger, 1996). Vibration exposure shows similar edema formation, demyelination, and ultimately nerve degeneration both experimentally induced in rats (Chang et al., 1994) as well as from occupational exposure in humans (Strömberg et al., 1997). Although experimental studies on spinal nerve root compression are much less common than for peripheral nerves, the injury mechanisms appear to be similar. Direct acute mechanical compression leads to intraneural edema and subsequent fibrosis (Rydevik et al., 1976). Chronic nerve compression may be less severe with changes evolving gradually, allowing for adaptation of the axons and vasculature. On the other hand, the compression leads to an increase in neurotransmitters that stimulate pain transmission (Cornefjord et al., 1997).

6.2.4 Vascular Disorders

In vascular disorders, one or more of three different factors, vibration, cold temperatures, and direct pressure, cause ischemia of the blood supply to nerves and muscle resulting in hypoxia to the tissue with tingling, numbness and loss of fine control. In the *hand–arm vibration syndrome*, (HAVS) vibration (e.g., from power tools) activates the smooth muscle surrounding arterioles causing a clamping action and loss of blood flow (*ischemia*) to the hand resulting in a blanching or the colloquial *white finger syndrome*. This will also result in numbness and an inability to perform precision work. Cold temperatures have a very similar ischemic effect on the arterioles through a local vasoconstrictor reflex. However, some individuals, especially women in northern climates, have an especially pronounced response leading to painful sensations, termed *Raynaud's syndrome*. The prevalence for HAVS increases markedly when there is a combination of vibration from power tool usage in cold environments, e.g., railroad work (Yu et al., 1986), stone cutting (Taylor et al., 1984), mining (Hedlund, 1989), and forestry work (Olsen and Nielsen, 1988). Vibration also happens to be a major factor in CTS (see Section 6.5.6).

Direct pressure on the circulatory vessels can also cause ischemia and loss of fine motor control, effects similar to vibration or cold. This can occur in the thoracic outlet syndrome, where the subclavian vessels are in close proximity to the brachial plexus and are similarly entrapped within the shoulder area, or in the *hypothenar hammer syndrome*, where the ulnar artery is compressed against the hypothenar eminence (muscle below the little and ring fingers) during hand hammering.

6.2.5 Bursa Disorders

Bursitis is inflammation of *bursae*, closed sacs filled with synovial fluid. Bursae are usually located in areas with potential for friction and help facilitate the motion of tendons and muscles over bone protuberances, especially around joints. Bursitis may be caused by friction, trauma, inflammatory diseases such as rheumatoid arthritis, and by bacteria. In the upper limbs, it is found at the elbow (olecranon bursa) and the shoulder (subacromial bursitis), the latter developing as part of the degeneration of the rotator cuff tendons. The most common occupationally induced bursitis, however, is in the knee (prepatellar bursitis) found in carpet layers due to the kneeling posture and use of the knee kicker (Thun et al., 1987).

6.2.6 Bone and Cartilage Disorders

Arthritis can be of two forms: *rheumatoid arthritis*, which is a generalized inflammatory process associated with diseases such as gout, and *osteoarathritis*, which is a degenerative process of joint cartilage. Despite an increase in cartilage water content and increased synthesis of proteoglycans, the cartilage decreases in thickness, with increased trauma to subchondral bone resulting in sclerosis. How the process begins is quite unclear. Many cases are idiopathic, having no clear predisposing factors, while other cases may occur as a result of specific trauma or injury to the joint. There is some evidence that repetitive work such as lifting may contributed to osteoarthritis severity in the shoulder joint (Stenlund et al., 1992).

The above MSDs, for convenience purposes, have been summarized in Table 6.1. Further details on specific types of MSDs can be found in Parker and Imbus (1992) and Kuorinka and Forcier (1995).

6.2.7 Myofascial Pain and Trigger Points

Although not considered WRSMDs, myofascial pain and trigger points need to be addressed as confounding symptoms of WRMSDs. *Myofascial pain* is a chronic form of muscle pain that may be centered at certain spots in the muscles termed *trigger points*. The nature and origins of myofascial pain (sometimes termed *myalgia*) were first described in detail by Travell et al. (1942) with the concept of the pain-spasm reflex. In this hypothesis, pain is the result of a sustained muscle spasm, which causes further pain and reflexively causes more spasms in a never-ending cycle. They recommended intramuscular injections of an anesthetic so as to relax the muscle and break the vicious cycle. Although supported by many researchers (Cobb et al., 1975; review by Roland, 1986) and commonly referred to by physical therapists, athletic trainers (http://www.sportsinjuryclinic.net/cybertherapist/back/backlowerleg/tightcalfs.htm), and pharmaceutical companies for tension headaches (http://www.drugs.com/cg/tension-headache.html), there are equally many, if not more,

TABLE 6.1

Common MSDs by Tissue Type and Their Associated Features

Tissue	General Injury	Common Specific Injuries (Colloquial Terms)	Occupational Risk Factors	Characteristic Features
Tendons	Tendinitis	Lateral epicondylitis (tennis elbow)	Repetitive forceful supination with wrist extension	Microtears in fibers, fraying of tendon, localized pain, tenderness, limited motion
		Medial epicondylitis (golfer's elbow)	Repetitive forceful pronation with wrist flexion	
		Bicipital tendinitis (shoulder pain)	Reaching overhead	
		Supraspinatus tendinitis (rotator cuff)	Outward shoulder rotations	
	Tenosynovitis	Flexor tenosynovitis in index finger (trigger finger)	Repetitive finger flexion	Thickening of synovial sheath, swelling, narrowing of space for tendon, resulting in localized pain and tenderness, triggering, and crackling sounds
		DeQuervain's disease (Nintendo thumb)	Repetitive thumb flexion	
		Dupuytren's contracture (ring/little fingers)	Repetitive forceful gripping	
		Flexor tenosynovitis in wrist	Repetitive wrist motions (precursor to CTS)	
		Extensor tenosynovitis in fingers	Repetitive finger extension	
		Ganglionic cysts	Repetitive joint motions (by-product of tenosynovitis)	Fluid-filled sacs that may form bumps on skin
Muscles	Acute strain	Myalgia	Overuse of muscle	Muscle pain from microstrains
	Chronic strain	Myositis, myofascial syndromes, fibromyalgia, fibrositis, in various areas	Overuse of muscle	Chronic myalgia from inflammation of muscle and surrounding fibrous tissue, presence of trigger points or tender areas, commonly idiopathic
		Tension neck syndrome (stiff neck)	Static neck flexion	
	Cramping	Focal dystonia (in finger = writer's cramp)	Excessive gripping	Cramping, pain, limited motion

Category	Type	Disorder	Risk factors	Description
Nerve related	Nerve entrapment	CTS	Repetitive forceful wrist motion	Median nerve entrapment at wrist, pain and tingling in index and middle fingers
		Guyon canal syndrome	Repetitive wrist flexion/extension, hand hammering, pressure on wrist	Ulnar nerve entrapment near wrist, pain/tingling in little finger
		Cubital tunnel syndrome	Repetitive elbow flexion with wrist extension, pressure on elbow	Ulnar nerve entrapment in the ulnar groove or cubital tunnel at the elbow, pain and tingling in little finger
		Posterior interosseous syndrome	Repetitive wrist extension	Radial nerve entrapment in the forearm, pain in forearm and thumb
		Anterior interosseous syndrome	Repetitive wrist motions	Median nerve entrapment in the forearm, pain in midforearm
		Radial tunnel syndrome	Repetitive forearm rotation, wrist flexion with pronation, wrist extension with supination	Radial nerve entrapment at the elbow, pain on palm side of forearm
		Pronator teres syndrome	Repetitive pronation with finger flexion (gripping)	Median nerve entrapment at the elbow
		Thoracic outlet syndrome	Reaching above shoulders, repetitive use of shoulders	Entrapment of brachial plexus in shoulder area, pain in the arm, headaches
		Cervical syndrome or radiculopathy	Repetitive neck motions	Compression of spinal nerve roots in the neck, pain radiating down arm
	Direct compression	Digital neuritis (bowler's thumb)	Gripping object with sharp edges	Pain, tingling, and loss of fine control in the fingers
Vascular	Ischemia	HAVS (white fingers)	Vibration	Ischemia of ulnar artery, tingling, numbness, loss of fine control in hand
		Hypothenar hammer syndrome	Hand hammering	
		Thoracic outlet syndrome	Reaching above shoulders, repetitive use of shoulders	Ischemia of subclavian vessels, tingling, numbness in the arm
		Raynaud's syndrome (white fingers)	Cold temperatures	Idiopathic ischemia of blood supply due to cold
Joints	Bursitis	Subacromial bursitis, adhesive capsulitis (frozen shoulder)	Repetitive should motions, lifting	Thickening of bursa, pain, limited motion
	Arthritis	Inflammatory, rheumatoid	Systemic disease, not work related	Inflammation and thickening of synovial tissues
		Osteoarthritis, degenerative	Repetitive joint motions	Thinning of cartilage, symptoms confused with other MSDs

Note: In many cases, several types of disorders may occur simultaneously and the symptoms can be quite broad, nonspecific, and overlapping.

researchers who argue against this concept primarily because of the simple physiological observation that motor reflexes are completed in under 100 ms (Section 3.10.2) and do not cause pain. Although the nociceptive input may be painful (touching a hot stove), there is no pain in the flexor muscles, which quickly contract to move the limb away from the stimulus (Mense and Simons, 2000). Even more convincingly, there was no significant increase in EMG activity recorded during tension headaches (Jensen, 1996), even when induced artificially (Jensen and Olesen, 1996). Johnson (1989), as editor, wrote a strong editorial condemning such terminology and deplored physicians prescribing muscle relaxants as a simple solution for complaining patients with relatively nonspecific pain.

An alternative theory for myofascial pain is that it is caused by hyperirritable spots located in the muscle termed trigger points. It is thought that irritability arises from neuromuscular dysfunction at the motor endplate of extrafusal skeletal muscle fibers, characterized internally by spontaneous electrical activity and externally by tender, palpable nodules thought to be extremely contracted sarcomeres (Simons and Travell, 1983; Mense and Simons, 2000). More recent studies (Mense et al., 2003; Kuan, 2009) seem to indicate excessive acetylcholine leakage as the cause for both the increased electrical activity and contracted knots. Muscle stretching, deep-stroking massage, ultrasound, and injections of lidocaine and botulinum toxin have all been recommended as potential treatments (Mense and Simons, 2000). In any case, the physician and ergonomists need to separate symptoms of myofascial pain from the symptoms of true WRMSDs.

6.2.8 Theories for MSD Causation

There are a variety of theories for the causation of MSDs, focusing on the disruption of the mechanical order of the body with its individual components and their individual mechanical properties. However, most of these can be grouped into four basic categories as nicely summarized by Kumar (2001). The first is the multivariate interaction theory which opines that a combination of factors, including individual genetic makeup, morphological characteristics, psychosocial characteristics, and occupational stressors, all lead to injury development. The second is differential fatigue theory in which unbalanced and asymmetric work and daily-life activities create differential loading and fatigue on the body and its components leading to injury causation.

The third is the cumulative loading model with a multivariate threshold of force loading, motion range, and repetition, which when exceeded results in tissue degradation and injury development. The fourth is the overexertion model, which is similar to the previous cumulative loading model, except that the former is cumulative over time, while the latter is acute or rather momentary in time. All of these include multiple causation factors on the disruption of the normal order of the body.

6.3 Medical Diagnosis and Treatment of MSDs

If a worker reports musculoskeletal pain, the physician will perform a physical examination with a series of steps to identify the disorder. The first is a general inspection of the patient, looking for asymmetry between the two sides of the body or for other visible irregularities like ganglionic cysts or swelling. The second part involves a series of range of motion (ROM) maneuvers. These include passive, resisted, and active motions. In a passive ROM, the patient

FIGURE 6.4
Resisted range of motion maneuvers as a diagnosis for MSDs. (Reproduced from Putz-Anderson, V., *Cumulative Trauma Disorders: A Manual for Musculoskeletal Diseases of the Upper Limbs*, Taylor & Francis, London, U.K., 1994. With permission.)

is told to relax and the physician moves the patient's limb through a set of positions. Since the muscles and tendons surrounding the joint are generally relaxed, any pain or stress may be more of joint problem. However, if there is tightness or limited range of motion there may be a case of tenosynovitis. In resisted ROM, the patient attempts to move the limb while the physician holds the limb steady (Figure 6.4). Since the muscles and tendons are contracting without the joint moving, problems in the former may be better identified. However, any muscle weakness may also be due to nerve entrapment. In active ROM tests, the patient voluntarily moves the limb and all aspects of the musculoskeletal system are examined.

In the third step, the physician may check for localized pain, tenderness, and trigger points by palpating or pressing with the fingers against various parts of the body. This will help identify the most inflamed parts of the body. However, pain can be generalized or even referred, with respect to nerves, and, therefore, one needs to be careful not to draw misleading conclusions.

In the fourth step, a series of specific diagnostic tests may be performed to isolate specific MSDs. In *Finkelstein's test* (Figure 6.5), the patient wraps the fingers around the thumb and deviates the wrist in the ulnar direction (Finkelstein, 1939). If pain occurs at the radial styloid at the wrist and along the thumb extensor tendon, there may be the possibility of DeQuervain's disease. Note, however, that there may be a possibility of a false-positive error, because somewhere over the years, physicians may have misdefined Finkelstein's test (Elliott, 1992).

In *Phalen's test* (Figure 6.5), the patient holds the wrist in hyperflexion for 1 min. Pain, tingling, or numbness radiating distally throughout the median distribution of the hand is positive sign that CTS may be present (Phalen, 1966; Gellman et al., 1986). A reverse Phalen's test involves wrist and finger extension held for minute. The consequent wrist extension may cause larger increases in carpal canal pressure then for wrist flexion in the normal Phalen's test and the resulting pain and tingling symptoms are again a positive sign of CTS (Robert et al., 1994).

Similar positive signs may be found in *Tinel's test*, in which the median nerve at the wrist is tapped (Tine, 1915; Steward and Eisen, 1978; Buch-Jaeger, and Foucher, 1994). In *Adson's*

FIGURE 6.5
Finkelstein's and Phalen's tests for diagnosing wrist MSDs. (Reproduced from Putz-Anderson, V., *Cumulative Trauma Disorders: A Manual for Musculoskeletal Diseases of the Upper Limbs,* Taylor & Francis, London, U.K., 1994. With permission.)

test, the patient is seated with the head extended and turned to the affected side. If on raising the affected arm and taking a deep breath, the pulse at the wrist becomes weaker, thoracic outlet syndrome may be present (Adson and Coffey, 1927).

Each of the above diagnostic tests for evaluating CTS evokes a subjective response from the patient with varying sensitivity and specificity (see Chapter 8). Their sensitivity varies widely from 32% to 89% and the specificity from 72% to 84% (Ghavnini and Haghighat, 1998). As such, they should not be interpreted as an unequivocal diagnoses but as part of a set of tools the lead to final diagnosis.

More complete or accurate diagnosis of the specific nerve disorder may fall to specialized laboratory tests. For example, if some of the above signs indicate CTS, further diagnostic tests can be one to identify the impaired nerve is truly the median nerve. The three main nerves innervating the hand, the radial, median, and ulnar nerves have separate and distinct innervation areas (Figure 6.6). The affected area may have tingling or numbness or decreased sensation which may be evaluated by a *two-point discrimination test.* Impaired individuals may only be able to distinguish two points from a single point when they are at least 5 mm apart (Dellon and Kallman, 1983; Shurr et al., 1986). Similarly, reduced sensitivity to vibration at various frequencies and intensities (Dellon, 1983; Lundborg et al., 1986), to standardized pressures (Bell, 1990), and to temperatures (Arezzo et al., 1986) are further indications of innervation problems. Other potential diagnostic tests include grip and pinch strength compared to normative data (Mathiowetz et al., 1985) and efficiency of muscular contraction (Chaffin et al., 1980). Of course, all of these procedures require an honest cooperation by the patient.

A direct measurement of nerve conduction velocities and resultant slowing (discussed in detail in Chapter 7) is considered by many as the gold standard in clearly diagnosing

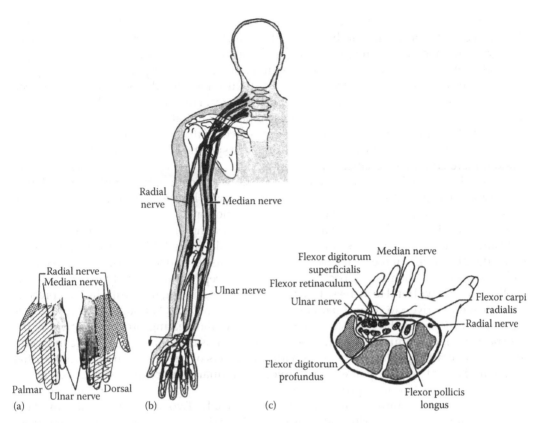

FIGURE 6.6
Median, radial, and ulnar nerve innervation patterns. (Reproduced from Armstrong, T.J., *An Ergonomics Guide to Carpal Tunnel Syndrome*, American Industrial Hygiene Association, Akron, OH, 1983. With permission.)

the appropriate nerve disorder. By measuring the velocity of median nerve and comparing it to the velocity of the ulnar nerve a more rigorous diagnosis can be made. Note, however, that all of the median nerve entrapment syndromes (carpal tunnel, anterior interosseous, pronator teres, cubital tunnel) show quite similar nerve response and palpation may be required to further isolate the specific disorder.

Electromyographic (EMG) techniques can also be used to assess muscle activity while x-rays and dye-induced arthrograms can be used to examine bones and joints. Similarly, magnetic resonance imaging (MRI) can be used to provide images, based on the realignment hydrogen atoms to the energy supplied by specific radio-frequency waves, of soft tissues such as tendons and ligaments. Even though expensive, the idea is to provide as much diagnostic information in localizing the specific disorder as possible, so as to avoid unneeded surgery. Further details on medical diagnosis and various testing procedures can be found in Parker and Imbus (1992) or Putz-Anderson (1994).

The basic medical treatment philosophy should be to assist the patient with the most effective treatment plan at minimal cost, side effects, and disruption of life, and allowing the patient to return to work and normal life as quickly as possible and with minimal pain. Therefore, the treatment strategy should follow a plan using the simplest approaches first, termed conservative treatments, and progressing toward more elaborate treatments with surgery as the last resort. Conservative treatments include the restriction of motion and splinting, applying heat and/or cold, medications and injections, and special exercises.

The purpose to restriction of motions is to avoid the activities that cause pain or stress the injured body part. This can be achieved by work restrictions, avoiding specific tasks on a job or, perhaps, changing the job altogether, in being placed on an alternate or a light-duty job. Splints may be used to restrict extreme motions or support specific body parts in a neutral posture of lower stress. This will reduce pain for the worker and, in effect, decrease inflammation and swelling for the critical area. For example, in CTS, wrist splints may be used to maintain the wrist in a neutral posture but allow the fingers and thumbs to move. Splints are perhaps best used at night, to avoid falling asleep with a deviated posture. During the working day, if the job has not been specifically redesigned for the injured worker, there could be a chance for more stress and greater injury, if the worker tries to fight the splint in performing the typically large range of motions required on assembly or other types of jobs. Furthermore, extended splinting with limited muscle or joint inactivity could result in loss of muscle tone or joint range of motion.

Heat and cold are used to relieve and facilitate the healing process. Ice, if applied immediately after an acute injury or overuse strain, reduces pain and swelling. Heat should be only used after 24 or 48h, to increase the blood flow to the muscles and tendons in the injured area. It can be superficial, such as heat packs or hot baths, or deep heating from ultrasound. If heat is applied earlier, it will tend to increase bleeding and swelling and aggravate the healing process.

Medication is given to reduce pain and fight inflammation. Although, inflammation is a natural response of the body to injury, it can slow the healing process. Aspirin is the cheapest and most common drug that serves this purpose. Unfortunately, some individuals do not tolerate high doses of aspirin with side effects of heartburn and gastrointestinal problems. Several, relatively new non-steroidal anti-inflammatory drugs have been developed as an alternative to aspirin. Unfortunately, most require a prescription, are quite costly, and may not eliminate the side effects completely. Two are now available over the counter, ibuprofen (e.g., Motrin) and naproxen sodium (i.e., Aleve). Injections of even stronger corticosteroids into the inflamed site offer the most effective relief, but are limited in the number of times they can be used. Injections of lidocaine or botulism may be useful in blocking of selected pathways for various focal dystonias (Kaji, 2000).

Although, somewhat counterintuitive, special exercise programs with stretching, tend to promote increased circulation, increased range of motion, and decreased muscle tension. These programs are most effective in recovering from shoulder injuries and will also tend to prevent further muscle strains. For hand and wrist disorders, care should be taken, since exercise may aggravate the existing condition. Note that these conservative approaches are most beneficial when pursued in parallel with an effective job-redesign program.

6.4 Epidemiologic Approach to MSDs

6.4.1 Introduction to Epidemiology

Epidemiology, in the traditional sense, is the branch of medicine that studies epidemic diseases. Normally, this would not be of concern to the industrial ergonomist; however, to identify, understand, and control occupational risk factors leading to the development of workplace musculoskeletal disorders (which can be considered a form of disease and is sometimes termed *morbidity*), it is important to understand and utilize epidemiological techniques. Epidemiological studies can be of many forms with many different variables: directionality of exposure to the risk factors, types of data collection methods, timing of data collection, types and availability of subjects, number of observations made, etc. Two basic factors, manipulation and randomization, determine the design of the research approach. Manipulation of the study factor means that the experimenter can control exposure. In a traditional study, rats may be exposed to specific levels and durations of a carcinogen. In a workplace study, this may be more difficult to control. Randomization of the study subjects is a process in which the chance (e.g., random number tables) is used to assign subjects to exposure conditions. Again, this is easy to do for rats being exposed to a toxin, but is much more difficult to do in an industrial environment, given worker choice, seniority, and union requirements.

The various permutations of the two factors produce three different general study types: experimental, quasi-experimental, and observational studies (see Table 6.2). Experimental studies have the greatest control over both the factor of interest and the subjects involved. Since this factor can be directly manipulated, these are also called *intervention studies* and because they commonly involve testing new drugs or therapies in a medical environment, they are also referred to as *clinical trials*. As shown in Figure 6.7, the procedures for clinical trials include screening a sample population for eligibility with a pretest to eliminate those individuals already having the outcome. Then individuals are randomly assigned to one of two study groups: an intervention group and a control group. Finally, the outcome of interest is measured in both groups to see the efficacy of the intervention. However, as mentioned previously, because of cost and ethical issues (e.g., people cannot be forced to be exposed to a risk factor), these types of studies may not be possible for the industrial ergonomist.

Quasi-experimental studies involve the manipulation of the study factor but not randomization of study subjects (see Figure 6.8). These typically are community interventions oriented toward education and behavioral changes at the population level, and, at best, the communities may be randomly assigned or not assigned to the intervention. Thus, study factors may involve control of alcohol use, cessation of smoking, driver safety, or control of dietary behavior. The interventions may be focused on targeted populations, i.e., individuals at risk for heart attacks, young teens at risk for drug use or may be mandated by state law, i.e., seat-belt use, driver blood-alcohol levels, etc. However, the populations may not be well controlled, i.e., not all individuals follow the suggested procedures or all states do not follow the same levels of exposure, etc., and, thus, the quasi-experimental nature.

As a first observation, the above experimental types of studies may not seem an option for the industrial ergonomist. However, in practice, ergonomists do perform intervention studies, either in the mode of a clinical trial or a community trial. If a true randomization of subjects to either study group is restricted or completely lacking, the study then assumes the form of a community trial. For example, it is not uncommon that one plant is willing to undergo an intervention, e.g., an ergonomics program or an exercise program, while another plant is not. However, the plants or communities may not truly be randomly assigned treatments either and the validity of the results is confounded with other factors. In terms of analysis purposes, the study then assumes the shape of a prospective/cohort study discussed shortly.

Observational studies make careful measurements of patterns of exposure of musculoskeletal injuries in given populations to draw inferences about *etiology* or the development of the injury. There are three main types of observational studies, all based on the 2 × 2 contingency table shown in Table 6.3. This table cross-classifies exposure states and outcome status and allows one to tabulate individuals in various categories. Note that the outcome status is either having a musculoskeletal disorder or not having the

TABLE 6.2

Types of Epidemiological Studies

General Type	M	R	Experimental Unit/Design	Rigor (Precision)	Time Duration	Cost	Specific Type (Analysis)	Best For	Worst For
Experimental (intervention)	Yes	Yes	Selected individuals	Tight	Relatively short (days, weeks)	High	Clinical trials (many)	Statistical rigor Intervention control	Cost and effort Ethical concerns
Quasi-experimental (intervention)	Yes	No	Population subsets	Less tight	Long (months)	Medium	Community studies (see cohort)	Large database Public education	Time and effort Loss of subjects
Observational	No	No	Individuals in two groups (with and without exposure)	Less tight	Long (several observations, longitudinal)	Medium	Cohort studies = prospective (RR, IR)	Clear cause and effect Accurate risk and exposure data	Time and effort Loss of subjects
			Individuals in two groups (with and without outcome)	Loose (unless well matched)	One observation (surveys and records)	Low	Case-control (OR?)	Rare disorders Small groups	Selection bias Risk and exposure estimates
			Individuals sorted into four groups	Very loose	One observation (survey)	Very low	Cross-sectional (p, OR?)	Quick, simple study Identifying risk factors	Temporality, validity survivor bias

Note: M, manipulation; R, randomization; RR, risk ratio; IR, incidence rate; OR, odds ratio; p, prevalence.

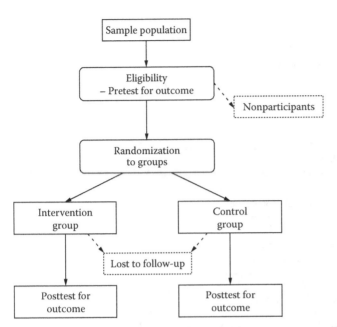

FIGURE 6.7
Schematic diagram of a clinical trial intervention study.

disorder. Out of a total number of n subjects, a have been exposed to a particular risk factor and have shown signs of the disorder, c have been exposed but are still healthy, b have not been exposed but have the disorder, and d have not been exposed and are healthy. A total of a + b have the disorder while c + d can be considered healthy, or at least are not yet showing signs of the disorder. A total of a + c have been exposed while b + d have not been exposed. These four values are known as *marginal totals* and will permit calculation of various probabilities and risk values. This table also serves as a point of reference in classifying the various types of observational studies.

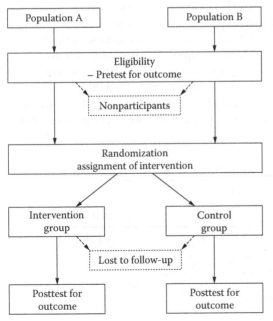

FIGURE 6.8
Schematic diagram of a community trial intervention study.

TABLE 6.3

The 2×2 Contingency Table

Outcome Status	Exposure to Risk Factors		
	Yes	No	Total
Yes	a	b	$r_1 = a + b$
No	c	d	$r_2 = c + d$
Total	$c_1 = a + c$	$c_2 = b + d$	$n = a + b + c + d$

Note: r, row; c, column.

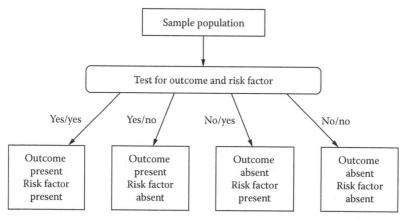

FIGURE 6.9
Schematic diagram of a cross-sectional study.

In a *cross-sectional study*, or *prevalence study*, the ergonomist starts by selecting a sample of subjects (n) and then determining their distribution in terms of exposures and outcomes (see Figure 6.9 and Table 6.4). This is most typically done as a survey of individuals in a single observation, i.e., a snapshot of time. Since exposure and outcome histories are collected simultaneously, one depends on the recall of the subjects to establish which of the risk factor exposures or outcomes came first. This is frequently unreliable due to a long time lag and lack of specialized knowledge of the part of the subject. Consequently, cross-sectional studies are most useful in identifying risk factors or in establishing prevalence of a relatively frequent disorder with a long duration or of one that is not often reported, such as is the case for WRMSDs. It can thus be considered as a fishing expedition on which

TABLE 6.4

The 2×2 Contingency Table Leading to a Cross-Sectional Study

Outcome Status	Exposure to Risk Factor		
	Yes	No	Total
Yes (cases)	a	b	$r_1 = a + b$
No (noncases)	c	d	$r_2 = c + d$
Total	$c_1 = a + c$	$c_2 = b + d$	$n = a + b + c + d$

Note: Subject selection $\rightarrow \rightarrow$.

to base more rigorous studies. Another problem is that only a small subset of the total population is examined, which is typically based on convenience of the ergonomist or the willingness to participate. Therefore, the results may not be valid for the full population. A better approach would be use a *stratified sampling* approach, in which the population is divided into mutually exclusive strata with random sampling performed within each stratum. However, practically, in an industrial setting, this might be quite difficult to accomplish, with individuals refusing to participate.

In a *case-control study*, the ergonomist uses the basic premise that a disorder does not occur randomly but in a logical pattern that reflects the underlying etiology. Therefore, two groups are selected: *cases*, in which everyone has the disorder (a+b), and *controls*, a comparable group in which everyone is free of the disorder (c+d) (see Figure 6.10 and Table 6.5).

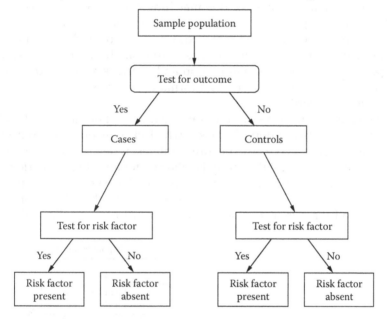

FIGURE 6.10
Schematic diagram of a retrospective case-control study.

TABLE 6.5

The 2 × 2 Contingency Table Leading to a Case-Control Study

Outcome Status	Exposure to Risk Factor		
	Yes	No	Total
Yes (cases)	a	b	$r_1 = a + b$
No (controls)	c	d	$r_2 = c + d$
Total	$c_1 = a + c$	$c_2 = b + d$	$n = a + b + c + d$

Note: Outcome-based selection →→.

The ergonomist then seeks to identify possible causes of the disorder by finding out how the two groups differ. Because the disorder most likely does not occur randomly, the case group must have been exposed to some occupational risk factor that the control group was not exposed to. Therefore, one is progressing from effect to a possible cause. However, this causality cannot be definitely established because of the lack of time sequence. Among some of the other potential problems is the determination of cases. If the criteria are too broad, some individuals of the case group may not truly have the disorder. If the criteria are too restrictive, there may be too few cases to statistically analyze.

The selection of controls, termed *matching*, is similarly, if not more, critical. The closer the control group is to the case group in terms of age, gender, education, fitness, working skills, job titles, etc., the more likely one is to ascribe differences in disorder status to the exposure of interest. The closeness of this matching can easily be checked through the use of *t*-tests. If the two groups are not statistically different in various characteristics, then they should be reasonably well matched. Case-control studies are most useful for evaluating rarely occurring disorders or ones with a small number of cases. Similar to cross-sectional studies, the unit of observation and analyses are the individual and data collection can be survey or more in-depth information sources such as employee, health-insurance, or medical records.

To eliminate the problems of recall and examine the effect of causality directly, a *cohort study* is used. It starts with a group of subjects who lack a history of the outcome but still are at risk for it (see Figure 6.11). The exposure of interest is determined for each individual of the group, i.e., the cohort, and the group is followed for an extended period of time into the future to document the incidence of the outcome in the exposed and nonexposed individuals (a+c and b+d in Table 6.6). Because of this, it can be thought of going from cause to effect and is good for demonstrating causation, the direct opposite of the progression

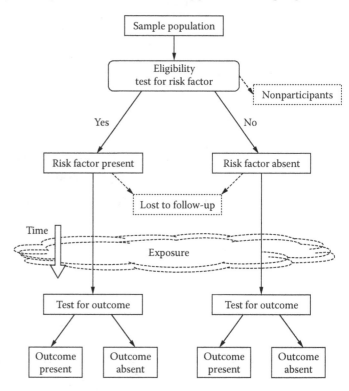

FIGURE 6.11
Schematic diagram of a prospective cohort study.

TABLE 6.6

The 2×2 Contingency Table Leading to a Cohort Study

Outcome Status	Exposure to Risk Factor		
	Yes	No	Total
Yes (cases)	a	b	$r_1 = a + b$
No (noncases)	c ②	② d	$r_2 = c + d$
Total	$c_1 = a + c$	$c_2 = b + d$ ①	(n) $= a + b + c + d$

Note: Sample selection → ①, finding effect from cause ⋯→ ②.

in the case-control study. Because of the progression in time, is also referred to as a *prospective* or *longitudinal study*. Another distinguishing feature of a cohort study is that at least two observations are made: an initial one to determine exposure status and eligibility into the group and a second one to determine the number of incident cases of the outcome that develop over the given time period (① and ② in Table 6.6). In this case, it is a one-sample cohort study, with the proportion being exposed determined upon analysis of the first observation point. In a multisample cohort study, two or more select subgroups are chosen, an exposed cohort (a + c) and a nonexposed, comparison cohort (b + d). However, because of the selection procedure, the frequency of exposure in the population cannot be determined. Also, cohort studies are not suitable for rare disorders or ones with a long latency, because of the need for a large baseline sample or for a long study period. As in the case-control study, the cohort groups should be as matched as possible and the unit of observation and analyses is the individual. Data collection can involve both surveys and other secondary data sources.

Sometimes cohort studies can be *retrospective* or historical. In a retrospective study, the investigation starts after both the exposure and outcome have occurred, as opposed to a prospective study, in which the outcome occurs after the exposure is measured. Typically, a retrospective study would examine the medical records of two similar working populations, one of which has the outcome, while the other does not, over the course of several years to find differences in exposure between the two groups. The advantage is that all the exposures have already occurred and the conclusions can be drawn more rapidly than in a prospective study.

Although, classically intervention studies are experimental, in practice, intervention studies also refer to prospective cohort studies that investigate the course of a control action on the development, or more likely, the reduction, of a musculoskeletal disorder. Workers are assigned to the intervention group at random and then followed to determine the proportion of those exposed who develop the outcome as compared to the proportion of those unexposed, the nonintervention group. Unfortunately, there are several issues that can confound the demonstration of the potential benefits of intervention studies, especially in an industrial setting. As aptly pointed out by Dempsey (2007), industrial ergonomists may be less conscious of performing appropriate statistical power tests and may end up with an inconclusive study because of too low of power. Similarly, it may be difficult to find large enough groups of workers with sufficiently long consistent exposure conditions. Finally, cost

TABLE 6.7

Detailed Comparison of the Three Types of
Observational Studies

Feature	Cohort	Case-Control	Cross-Sectional
Survivor bias	+	−	−
Selection bias	+	+	−
Recall bias	+	−	−
Loss to follow-up	−	+	+
Temporality	+	−	−
Time and effort	−	+	+
Cost	−	+	+

Note: +, strength; −, weakness.

justification during economic downturns and pressures to increase productivity may reduce any potential benefits to be gained from ergonomic interventions.

Further details on epidemiological studies can be found in Sorock and Courtney (1996), Friis and Sellers (1996), Greenberg et al. (1996), and Woodward (1999). The ergonomist may also find the summary of the different features for each type of observational study in Table 6.7 useful for selecting the appropriate approach.

6.4.2 Statistical Analyses

The statistical analyses and inferences based on the contingency table in Table 6.2 are basically the same for cross-sectional and case-control studies except for the interpretation of the results in view of the higher potential for bias in cross-sectional studies. For added interest and a practical application of the following statistical analyses, consider the injury data from a plant using power tools shown in Table 6.8. The hypothesis or association of interest is whether vibration is a risk factor for developing WRMSDs.

Considering the data as that from a cross-sectional study, the simplest statistics to calculate are various measures of *prevalence*, where p_a and p_b are the proportions of existing number of MSD cases in the exposed and unexposed groups, respectively. The samples estimates of p_a and p_b are obtained from

$$p_a = \frac{a}{c_1} \quad \text{and} \quad p_b = \frac{b}{c_2} \tag{6.1}$$

The prevalence difference (PD) for exposed versus unexposed groups is

$$PD = p_a - p_b \tag{6.2}$$

TABLE 6.8

Association of Musculoskeletal Injuries and Exposure
to Vibration from Power Tools

Musculoskeletal Injuries	Exposure to Vibration		
	Yes	No	Total
Yes (cases)	9	39	48
No (non-cases)	14	134	148
Total	23	173	196

The above being only point estimates, don't allow for testing of significance. For that, some form of interval estimation, such as a confidence interval, is needed. The simplest calculation of the confidence interval is based on the standard error (SE) approach, in which a $100(1 - \alpha)\%$ confidence interval for PD is defined by

$$p_a - p_b \pm z_{\alpha/2} \left[\frac{p_a(1-p_a)}{c_1} + \frac{p_b(1-p_b)}{c_2} \right]^{\frac{1}{2}} \tag{6.3}$$

Other commonly used approaches for developing a confidence interval are described in Sahai and Khurshid (1996).

For the above vibration example in Table 6.8, the prevalence values are

$$p_a = \frac{9}{23} = 0.39 \quad \text{and} \quad p_b = \frac{39}{173} = 0.23 \tag{6.4}$$

while the prevalence difference is

$$PD = 0.39 - 0.23 = 0.16 \tag{6.5}$$

The 95% confidence interval (given that $z_{0.025}$ is 1.96) is

$$0.16 \pm 1.96 \left[\frac{0.39 \times 0.61}{23} + \frac{0.23 \times 0.77}{173} \right]^{\frac{1}{2}} = 0.16 \pm 0.21 = (-0.05, 0.37) \tag{6.6}$$

Since the confidence interval overlaps 0, the difference in prevalence of MSDs between exposed and unexposed is not significant (at least not at an α of 5%) and vibration does not appear to be a risk factor.

One can also calculate the prevalence *odds ratio* (OR) which is the ratio of the prevalence odds for exposed and unexposed groups, defined as

$$OR = \frac{p_a/(1-p_a)}{p_b/(1-p_b)} = \frac{0.39/0.61}{0.23/0.77} = 2.21 \tag{6.7a}$$

Or equivalently:

$$OR = \frac{ad}{bc} = \frac{9 \times 134}{39 \times 14} = 2.21 \tag{6.7b}$$

Another traditional analysis approach for contingency tables is the *chi-square* (χ^2) in which the summation of difference between observed and expected values is calculated:

$$\chi^2 = \sum \frac{(o_i - e_i)^2}{e_i} \tag{6.8}$$

where
   o_i is the observed value
   e_i is the expected value

If the calculated value is larger than the test statistic $\chi^2_{\alpha/2}$ with

$$v = (r - 1)(c - 1) \tag{6.9}$$

degrees of freedom, then there is a significant difference between observed and expected values and significant association between outcome and exposure. Note that this is the Pearson or ordinary chi-square. Many epidemiologists use the Mantel–Haenszel (1959) chi-square, especially for large sample approximation.

The expected values are calculated from the product of the intersecting column and row marginal probabilities × the total number of subjects:

$$e_a = \frac{c_1}{n} \times \frac{r_1}{n} \times n = \frac{c_1 r_1}{n} \tag{6.10}$$

Similarly:

$$e_b = \frac{c_2 r_1}{n} \tag{6.11}$$

$$e_c = \frac{c_1 r_2}{n} \tag{6.12}$$

$$e_d = \frac{c_2 r_2}{n} \tag{6.13}$$

Substituting these expressions into Equation 6.8 and simplifying yields

$$\chi^2 = \frac{n(ad - bc)^2}{c_1 c_2 r_1 r_2} \tag{6.14}$$

For this example, the value of chi-square is

$$\chi^2 = \frac{196(9 \times 134 - 39 \times 14)^2}{23 \times 173 \times 48 \times 148} = 3.02 \tag{6.15}$$

and there are

$$v = (2 - 1)(2 - 1) = 1 \tag{6.16}$$

degree of freedom. The test statistic for an α of 5% is

$$\chi^2_{0.025} = 3.84 \tag{6.17}$$

Since, the calculated value is less than the test statistic, then the association is not significant. Note, however, that if the number of subjects was doubled (e.g., more subjects were studied), then from Equation 6.14, the calculated chi-square is 6.04 and becomes significant. This implies that chi-square is an excellent measure of the significance of the association, but not at all useful as a measure of the degree of association.

One measure of the degree of association is the *phi coefficient*:

$$\varphi = \left(\frac{\chi^2}{n} \right)^{\frac{1}{2}} \tag{6.18}$$

In this example, the value of the phi coefficient is

$$= \left(\frac{3.08}{196} \right)^{\bullet} = 0.124 \tag{6.19}$$

It can be interpreted as a correlation coefficient with values ranging between 0 and 1. Values below 0.4 or so, as a rule of thumb, are considered as having poor association.

For the more controlled cohort studies, there are several measures of quantifying risk for incurring the disorder. Since in this type of study there are two groups of individuals, one of which will incur the disorder in the future and the other which will not incur the disorder, the calculation of risk is of interest. The first measure is the *risk ratio* or *relative risk* (RR), which relates the risks for MSDs for exposed and unexposed groups in a cohort study (since that is the design and direction of a cohort study as shown in Table 6.6). Among exposed individuals, the risk of a MSD is defined as

$$R_{exposed} = \frac{\text{exposed individuals incurring disorder}}{\text{all exposed individuals}} = \frac{a}{a+c} \tag{6.20}$$

Among unexposed individuals, the risk of a MSD is defined as

$$R_{unexposed} = \frac{\text{unexposed individuals incurring disorder}}{\text{all unexposed individuals}} = \frac{b}{b+d} \tag{6.21}$$

The risk ratio then becomes

$$RR = \frac{R_{exposed}}{R_{unexposed}} = \frac{a(b+d)}{b(a+c)} \tag{6.22}$$

The ratio assumes a value between 0 and ∞. A value greater than 1 indicates that the risk (or odds) is greater with exposure, a value of 1 indicates that the risk is the same for both groups, and a value less than 1 indicates that risk is less with exposure. Table 6.9 provides some general guidelines for interpreting the strength of association between exposure and the resulting disorder, but the true evaluation comes from a statistical analysis with the corresponding confidence interval.

TABLE 6.9

Guidelines for the Interpretation of Risk
Ratios and ORs

Value	Effect of Exposure
0.00–0.39	Strong benefit
0.40–0.59	Moderate benefit
0.60–0.89	Weak benefit
0.90–1.19	No benefit or effect
1.20–1.69	Weak hazard
1.70–2.59	Moderate hazard
≥2.60	Strong hazard

Source: Adapted from Greenberg, R.S., Prospective studies, in S. Kotz and N.L. Johnson (eds), *Encyclopedia of Statistical Sciences*, Vol. 7, John Wiley & Sons, New York, 1986.

Sometimes the risk ratio is converted to *attributable risk* (AR, also termed *etiologic fraction*):

$$AR = \frac{(RR - 1)}{RR} \tag{6.23}$$

This estimates the proportion by which the rate of the outcome among the exposed would be reduced if the exposure were eliminated. Note that in many cases, a variety of factors may contribute to the total outcome, so that the removal of one exposure does not reduce the outcome rate to zero. Rather, it provides a guide to the relative importance of the various study factors in reducing the outcomes.

The $100(1 - \alpha)\%$ confidence interval around the above point estimate of risk ratio can be calculated from the SE of the risk ratio based on a Taylor series approximation (Sahai and Khurshid, 1996):

$$RR \exp(\pm z_{\alpha/2} SE) \tag{6.24}$$

Where SE is defined by

$$SE = \left\{ \frac{c}{a(a+c)} + \frac{d}{b(b+d)} \right\}^{\frac{1}{2}} \tag{6.25}$$

The other commonly used test-based and exact approaches for developing a confidence interval are described in Sahai and Khurshid (1996).

For the vibration example, the risk ratio is

$$RR = \frac{9 \times 173}{39 \times 23} = 1.74 \tag{6.26}$$

and the SE is

$$SE = \left\{ \frac{14}{9 \times 23} + \frac{134}{39 \times 173} \right\}^{\frac{1}{2}} = 0.296 \tag{6.27}$$

The 95% confidence interval then becomes

$$1.74 \exp(\pm 1.96 \times 0.296) = (0.97, 3.11) \tag{6.28}$$

Although the risk ratio value of 1.74, at first glance, seems to indicate a moderate hazard, the confidence interval encompasses the value of 1.0. Therefore, the risk ratio is not statistically significant and the risks to the exposed and unexposed groups are not significantly different.

Since, the cohort study collects data prospectively, exposure time is available, from which an *incidence rate* (IR) can be calculated. An incidence rate reflects the number of new cases with respect to exposure time (t) in person hours or person days:

$$IR = \frac{a}{t} \tag{6.29}$$

It is somewhat similar to prevalence which measures existing cases within a population. Given that the incidence rate is constant over time, the incidence rate is related to prevalence by the following relationship:

$$IR = \frac{p}{(1-p)d} \tag{6.30}$$

where d is the duration of the disorder.

In a case-control or in a retrospective study, the RR calculation would theoretically measure the risk of exposure to an antecedent risk, given the presence or absence of a disorder. However, this does not make logical sense, since the disease did not cause the risk. Therefore, the RR is usually not of interest for case-control studies and the OR is a more useful measure of risk. The probability that the outcome of interest or a case was exposed to the risk factor can be expressed as the case exposure probability:

$$p_a = \frac{\text{exposed cases}}{\text{total cases}} = \frac{a}{a+b} \tag{6.31}$$

The probability for a case with no exposure is

$$p_b = \frac{\text{unexposed cases}}{\text{total cases}} = \frac{b}{a+b} \tag{6.32}$$

The overall odds of obtaining the outcome when the risk factor is present is then estimated by

$$\frac{p_a}{p_b} = \frac{a}{b} \tag{6.33}$$

Similarly, the odds of exposure among controls or those not having the outcome is

$$\frac{p_c}{p_d} = \frac{c}{d} \tag{6.34}$$

The OR is then the odds of exposure for cases divided by odds of exposure for controls:

$$OR = \frac{a/b}{c/d} = \frac{ad}{bc} \qquad (6.35)$$

The $100(1 - \alpha)\%$ confidence interval around the above point estimate can be calculated from the SE of the OR based on a Taylor series approximation (Sahai and Khurshid, 1996):

$$OR \exp(\pm z_{\alpha/2}SE) \qquad (6.36)$$

Where SE is defined by

$$SE = \left(1/a + 1/b + 1/c + 1/d\right)^{\frac{1}{2}} \qquad (6.37)$$

The other commonly used test-based and exact approaches for developing a confidence interval are described in Sahai and Khurshid (1996).

Using the vibration exposure data of Table 6.8, the OR is

$$OR = \frac{ad}{bc} = \frac{9 \times 134}{39 \times 14} = 2.21 \qquad (6.38)$$

This value measures the association between the two characteristics of the study, MSDs and vibration, and can be interpreted to mean that the odds for a group of workers using power tools with vibration exposure to incur some type of MSD is over twice as great as group workers not similarly exposed. Note that it is identical terms and value (except for round off errors) to the prevalence OR previously presented for a cross-sectional study (Equation 6.7).

An argument has also been made that the OR can be used as estimate of the incidence rate ratio, since both case and control groups only include only newly diagnosed or "incident" cases. Subjects can be queried to exclude those who already had the disorder before the study period (Greenberg et al., 1996).

The SE and 95% confidence interval around the point estimate of OR is

$$SE = \left(1/a + 1/b + 1/c + 1/d\right)^{\frac{1}{2}} = \left(1/9 + 1/39 + 1/14 + 1/134\right)^{\frac{1}{2}} = 0.464 \qquad (6.39)$$

$$OR \exp(\pm z_{\alpha/2}SE) = 2.21 \exp(\pm 1.96 \times 0.464) = (0.89, 5.49) \qquad (6.40)$$

Since the confidence interval overlaps 1.0, the association could have possibly occurred by chance alone and the association is not statistically significant.

Note that since cohort groups eventually either incur the outcome or remain outcome free, the same line of reasoning and OR analysis as described above for case-control studies can also be utilized in cohort studies. The question then arises about the relationship between the OR and risk ratio for cohort studies, since both measure the association between the two characteristics of interest. Comparing the definitions of the OR and risk ratio:

$$OR = \frac{ad}{bc} \approx \frac{a(b+d)}{b(a+c)} = RR \qquad (6.41)$$

the two expressions will be mathematically very similar if the values of a and b are very small compared to c and d, respectively, i.e., the prevalence of the outcome is very low or its is a very rare disorder. For the vibration example of Table 6.8, OR was 2.1 and the risk ratio was 1.74. These values are similar but not that close, because the corresponding prevalences ($p_a = 0.39$ and $p_b = 0.23$) were not that close to zero. This will typically be the case with WRMSDs, which in certain industries are actually quite prevalent.

There also has been some criticism of ORs, in that by taking the ratio as a measure of association, the base level of cases is lost. Thus, a large OR for a small number of cases (e.g., an OR of 10 for 1000 cases) versus a small OR for a large number of cases (e.g., an OR of 2 for 1,000,000 cases) would obscure the real problem that there over million individuals suffering from some undesirable outcome. Several measures to correct this disparity are discussed in Fleiss (1981).

In summary, there are several common measures used in epidemiological studies: risk, prevalence, and incidence. However, there are variations in the units, interpretation, and applications of these measures. Incidence rates have units per time, whereas prevalence and risk have no units. Incidence rates and risk describe new occurrences of a disorder, whereas prevalence reflects existing cases of an already occurring disorder. Risk is most useful in predicting the proportion of a population that will incur the disorder over a specified period of time and thus can be used as an estimate of incidence rates. Incidence rates are preferred in predicting the rapidity of arising new cases while prevalence is preferred for quantifying the proportion of existing cases within a given population. Further information on various statistical techniques for epidemiological studies can be found in Fleiss (1981), Sahai and Khurshid (1996), and Woodward (1999). Again, Tables 6.2 and 6.7 might be useful in sorting out these differences.

6.4.3 Multivariate Modeling

In epidemiological studies, the ergonomist is most concerned with finding which and how risk factors are related to the musculoskeletal disorder. Since there are more than likely several risk factors contributing to the disorder with potentially confounding effects, multivariate models permit the simultaneous evaluation of these risk factors with greatest computational and statistical efficiency. Implicitly, the risk factors are the independent x variables, which are potentially causing the negative outcome or the disorder, which is then the dependent y variable. The classical modeling approach would be to use a linear model of the form:

$$y = \beta_0 + \beta_1 x_1 + \beta_2 x_2 + \cdots + \beta_n x_n + \varepsilon \tag{6.42}$$

where
β is the linear regression coefficients
ε is the random error term

Although, mathematically, it is possible to use the above linear-regression model for epidemiological analysis, there are several major problems with this approach. All are related to the basic fact that the independent outcome variable is typically either a binary variable with a value of 0 if no outcome occurs or a value of 1 if the outcome is present, or a proportion, representing a risk with a value in the range of 0–1. Therefore, the y–x relationship will most likely not be linear and the error distribution will not be the standard normal distribution. Proportions will typically arise from a binomial distribution.

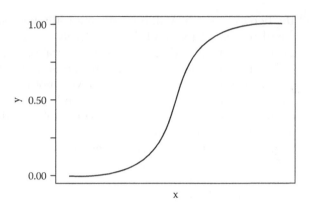

FIGURE 6.12
The logistic function.

One remedial measure to linearize the regression and stabilize the error term variance is to transform the data. The arcsine square root is one suggestion (Woodward, 1999). However, this approach is only an approximation.

The best approach for binary variables is to use a *logistic* or *logit function* of the form:

$$y = [1 + \exp - (\beta_0 + \beta_1 x_1)]^{-1} \qquad (6.43)$$

Its S-shape matches well both the binary or proportional form of the data (see Figure 6.12). Equation 6.43 can be manipulated to the alternate form:

$$\ln\left[\frac{p}{(1-p)}\right] = \beta_0 + \beta_1 x_1 \qquad (6.44)$$

Note that the left-hand side is the natural logarithm of the odds for a disorder, with probability p substituted for y. Thus, the logistic function forms a direct relationship between the logarithm of the odds of a disorder and the corresponding risk factors (Christensen, 1997).

As in linear-regression analysis, the regression coefficients can be tested for statistical significance, under the hypothesis that $\beta_i = 0$, using the *Wald statistic* (W):

$$W = \frac{\beta_i}{SE(\beta_i)} \qquad (6.45)$$

The Wald statistic follows the standard normal distribution and the null hypothesis can be rejected for either large positive or negative values of the test statistic (Hosmer and Jennings, 1986; Lemeshow, 1989).

The traditional approach to statistical model building is to seek the most parsimonious model that still explains the variability of the data. The inclusion of too many variables may cause confounding of variables and overfitting the model (i.e., too many variables as compared to the size of the data), resulting in unrealistically large coefficient estimates and correspondingly large SEs. Furthermore, logistic regression with a large number of variables requires considerable amount of computational time due to the iterations of the maximum likelihood function.

Therefore, a typical approach is to first conduct a multiple logistic regression concentrating on a single factor of interest. Termed "pseudo" univariate logistic regression, this allows one to find a smaller set of competent candidate variables for the final model. These variables are entered into full multiple logistic-regression model through a forward stepwise algorithm, using specified inclusion level for the Wald statistic. Once included, all variables are examined again to check if the one with largest probability (i.e., smallest z or W) should be removed at a specified exclusion level. Hosmer and Lemeshow (1989) recommend values in the range of 0.15–0.20 for inclusion to prevent excluding important variables from the model.

Once the model is complete (i.e., no more variables can be entered into the model), a goodness-of-fit test should be performed using one of several different measures. The Hosmer–Lemeshow (1989) statistic, H_c, based on a $2 \times m$ contingency table and the Pearson chi-square statistic in Equation 6.8, is perhaps easiest. An arbitrary number of groups, m, are chosen. Typically, m equals 10, corresponding to deciles of risk. The groups are defined by probabilities corresponding to values of $k/10$, with $k = 1, 2, \ldots, 10$ and the groups contain all subjects with estimated probabilities between adjacent cutpoints. Thus, the first group contains all subjects whose probability is ≤ 0.1, while the tenth group contains all those subjects whose probability is >0.9. Each group has two rows, corresponding to the outcome and or to the lack of outcome. The observed values are the actual subject counts in the appropriate groupings. Estimates of the expected values are obtained by summing the estimated probabilities over all subjects in the outcome row in a group. For the lack of outcome row, the estimated expected value is obtained by summing, over all subjects in that group, one minus the estimated probability. The average expected value for each case is found by dividing the sums by the number of responses. The final calculation of the chi-square statistic in Equation 6.8 would have 20 entries for $m = 10$ and would be compared to the χ^2 with $m -2$ or 8 degrees of freedom.

Now, the model terms can be interpreted to make inferences about the study populations and occupational risk factors. For example, consider the simple model in Equation 6.44. Assume that the two populations are defined by the influence of one risk factor x_1. The control population was not exposed and x_1 is zero. Substituting into Equation 6.44 yields

$$\ln\left[\frac{p}{(1-p)}\right] = \beta_0 \tag{6.46}$$

By taking the antilog of both sides, the odds for the control population to incur the disorder becomes

$$\frac{p}{(1-p)} = \exp \beta_0 \tag{6.47}$$

The case population is exposed to the risk factor and x_1 is one. Substituting into Equation 6.44 yields

$$\ln\left[\frac{p}{(1-p)}\right] = \beta_0 + \beta_1 \tag{6.48}$$

Again taking the antilog of both sides yields the odds for the case population to incur the disorder:

$$\frac{p}{(1-p)} = \exp(\beta_0 + \beta_1) = \exp\beta_0 \times \exp\beta_1 \qquad (6.49)$$

The OR for the case population as compared to the control population with regards to the risk factor, becomes the ratio of Equations 6.47 and 6.49 and is simply

$$OR = \exp\beta_1 \qquad (6.50)$$

Thus, the OR for any given risk factor can be found by taking the antilog of the corresponding coefficient. The $100(1 - \alpha)\%$ confidence interval for the OR can be calculated using the SE of the corresponding risk factor coefficient (Woodward, 1999):

$$\exp\left[\beta_1 \pm z_{\alpha/2}SE(\beta_1)\right] \qquad (6.51)$$

As an example, consider You's (1999) case-control study of CTS. The most significant risk factors were age, wrist ratio, musculoskeletal disorder history, and exposure of the hands to cold temperatures. The model coefficients β_i (all significant at $p < .05$) were 0.08, 0.32, 2.76, and 2.86, respectively, with corresponding SEs of 0.042, 0.106, 0.933, and 1.193. The ORs for the cold temperature risk factor can be calculated simply from

$$\exp(2.86) = 17.5 \qquad (6.52)$$

The 95% confidence interval is

$$\exp(2.86 \pm 1.96 \times 1.193) = (1.68, 181.0) \qquad (6.53)$$

Since the confidence interval does not include the value of 1.0, the OR is significant, and one can conclude that workers exposed to cold temperatures will be considerably more likely (17.5 times, to be exact) to incur CTS as compared to unexposed workers. The ORs for the first three risk factors compute to values of 1.08, 1.37, and 15.76.

Since, there are several other variables in the model and there could be possible interactions between the different risk factors also as confounding effects. Also, the specific odds (rather than ORs) and confidence intervals for the odds can be calculated. However, this is a much more difficult procedure involving the variance–covariance matrix. Details for the above techniques can be found in Woodward (1999).

Other statistical techniques can be used to further ascertain the sensitivity, specificity, and validity of the model. These concepts will be discussed in greater detail in Section 8.4.1 as the appropriateness, meaningfulness, or usefulness of a model or test to predict or quantify the actual risk that is incurred for a given individual while performing a given task in a given work environment. The plotting of *sensitivity* as a function of (1-*specificity*) in a *receiver-operating characteristic* (ROC) plot (see Figure 6.13) can demonstrate that the models have a high power of discriminating cases from controls. The further the ROC curve deviates from the diagonal line, the more discriminating the test is. A test having a curve on the diagonal has equal chances of making a correct or incorrect decision. A perfect

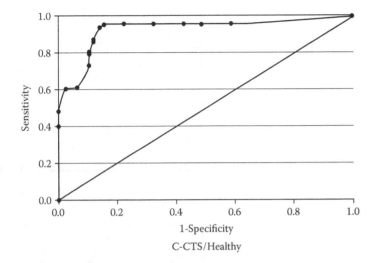

FIGURE 6.13
ROC curves of CTS risk assessment model. (Reproduced from You, H. The development of a risk assessment model for carpal tunnel syndrome, Unpublished PhD thesis, Penn State University, University Park, PA, 1999. With permission.)

test would have an ROC curve going up the y-axis to a sensitivity of 1 and then go straight across parallel to the x-axis. The model plotted in Figure 6.13 shows a high level of discriminability, although not perfect. The actual value of discriminability, identified as d′, of the ROC curve can be computed by adding the two z-scores corresponding to the sensitivity and specificity at a specific cut-off criterion probability p_c. In this particular example, d′ equals 2.51. It can vary from 0 to ∞, with larger values best (You, 1999; You et al., 2004).

A p_c is established to classify an individual into one of the two groups—if the probability of an individual belonging to the case group is greater than p_c, then the individual is classified to the case group; if less than p_c, then the individual is classified to the control group. For this particular study, the determination of p_c was determined by the intersection of the specificity and sensitivity curves at roughly 0.50 (see Figure 6.14). Note that for the overall model, the sensitivity is 87%, specificity is 88%, and accuracy is 88%.

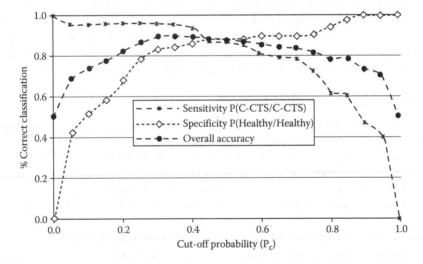

FIGURE 6.14
Classification performance of CTS risk assessment model. (Reproduced from You, H. The development of a risk assessment model for carpal tunnel syndrome, Unpublished PhD thesis, Penn State University, University Park, PA, 1999. With permission.)

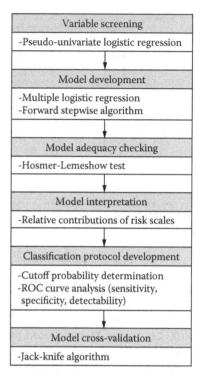

FIGURE 6.15
The development and validation procedure for a multivariate CTS risk assessment model. (Reproduced from You, H. The development of a risk assessment model for carpal tunnel syndrome, Unpublished PhD thesis, Penn State University, University Park, PA, 1999. With permission.)

The final step in model assessment is cross validation to determine the classification accuracy of the model. In lieu of selecting a new subject pool, the jack-knife method by Afifi and Clark (1996) creates an half-sized data set by choosing subject data elements randomly from both cases and controls in proportion to their original set size. Then, each of the above-selected subjects is removed one at a time from the original data set upon which a new multiple logistic-regression model is created. A probability is estimated for each excluded participant using the corresponding logistic-regression model and a classification is made for that excluded participant based on the new p_c. This new classification, as well as new sensitivity and specificity values, is compared to the original model. Obviously, this procedure requires considerable effort and computing resources. Figure 6.15 summarizes the various procedures and techniques used in the development of a multivariate model.

6.4.4 Quality of Epidemiological Research

For any study to adequately determine the work-relatedness of musculoskeletal disorders, several key criteria have to be fulfilled. First, the study must show that there is an exposure, i.e., workers were being exposed to vibration while using power tools. Second, the study must show that the outcome of interest occurred, i.e., CTS has been diagnosed. Third and most importantly, *causality* or a direct association between exposure and the outcome must be shown. This association depends on several factors (Campbell and Stanley, 1966):

1. *Temporality*, or having the exposure precede the outcome in time
2. *Temporal contiguity*, or the timeliness of the precedence. The more temporally remote an exposure the more likely other factors may affect the outcome.
3. Exposure and outcome *covary*, i.e., a reduction in the exposure should result in a reduction of the outcome.

4. *Congruity* of exposure and outcome. The direct association between levels of exposure and the levels of outcome is typically expressed as a *dose–response relationship*. In a linear relationship, a doubling of the dose would result in a doubling of the response. However, not all relationships are linear.

5. *Plausibility*, or the likelihood that an association is compatible with a physiological mechanism, or that there is not some other plausible explanation or a confounding variable that is associated with both the exposure and outcome.

The strength of this association can be evaluated by various measures discussed already: the OR or relative risk ratio, consistency of the association across various subgroups, specificity of the association, and quantitative dose–response values.

More specifically, the general criteria mentioned above, reflect in the following details to define a quality study:

1. In cohort studies, the inclusion or exclusion criteria for both exposed and nonexposed groups should be clearly defined. In case-control studies, the criteria for defining a case versus a control must also be clearly defined. Similar criteria need to be identified for subdividing cases into work-related and non-work-related cases. This is will increase statistical power and population validity.

2. Participation rates for groups or subgroups must exceed 70% or more. This will limit selection bias in the study.

3. Health outcome must be defined both by symptoms and a physical examination. The use of objective measures will limit the unreliability found in self-reports.

4. The investigators were blinded to health status when assessing exposure status, or vice versa. This will again limit selection bias.

5. The exposure measures were well defined and assessed independently. Again self-reports tend to be less reliable than direct observations or actual measurements.

Unfortunately, not all the studies reviewed here fulfilled all of the criteria. In fact, generally, few did. Typically, most studies were cross sectional, the simplest to implement, but having the least validity. However, these also tended to have large subject pools, which is good from a representative sample of the population standpoint. On the other hand, they tended to use less costly but more subjective approaches, job titles, or self-reports, to evaluate exposures. In general, these studies were not rejected because that would have eliminated a large proportion of studies. Also, many studies were not that rigorous in having high participation rates or using objective measures to evaluate outcomes. Therefore, so long as a study provided quantitative results (i.e., an OR, RR, or AR value) and fulfilled either the participation rate or outcome evaluation criteria, they were retained for further analyses.

These studies are summarized in Tables 6.10 through 6.16 for neck MSD, shoulder MSD, elbow MSD, hand/wrist CTS, hand/wrist tendinitis, and hand/wrist vibration syndrome cases, with as much quantitative information as could be gleaned from the published information. Note that the AR fraction was calculated with the OR as an estimate for the relative risk. As mentioned in Section 6.4.2, this approximation will be fairly accurate when the prevalence low, roughly below 20%–30%. A complete listing of all relevant MSD research studies with specialized categorizations can be found in the very detailed compendiums by NIOSH (1995), Kourinka and Forcier (1995), NIOSH (1997), and National Research Council (2001).

TABLE 6.10

Summary to Epidemiological Studies Examining Neck MSDs

Reference	Number of Subjects	Type of Study	Study Population	Participation Rate > 70%	Physical Exam	Risk Factor	Risk Estimate (OR, RR)	AR (%)	Exposure Assessment
Andersen and Gaardboe (1993a)	1,482	CS	Sewing machine operators	Yes	No	F, R	4.6*	78	Job titles
Andersen and Gaardboe (1993b)	107	CS	Sewing machine operators	Yes	Yes	F, R	6.8*	85	Job titles
Baron et al. (1991)	281	CS	Grocery scanners	No	Yes	F, R	2.00	—	Job titles
Bergqvist et al. (1995a)	260	CS	Office workers	Yes	No	P	4.4*	77	Observed
Bergqvist et al. (1995b)	322	CS	Office workers	Yes	Yes	R, C	6.9*	86	Self-reports
Bernard et al. (1994)	973	CS	Office workers	Yes	No	P, R	1.4*	29	Self-reports
Ekberg et al. (1994)	746	CC	Physician patients	Yes	No	P R	4.8* 15.6*	79 94	Self-reports Self-reports
Ekberg et al. (1995)	687	CS	General population	Yes	No	R	1.2*	17	Self-reports
Hales and Fine (1989)	112	CS	Poultry processors	Yes	Yes	F, R	1.60	—	Job titles
Hales et al. (1994)	518	CS	Office workers	Yes	Yes	C	3.8*	74	Self-reports
Holmström et al. (1992)	1,773	CS	Construction workers	Yes	No	P	1.4–2.0*	29–50	Self-reports
Hünting et al. (1981)	295	CS	Office workers	NR	Yes	P, R	9.9*	90	Observed
Kamwendo et al. (1991)	420	CS	Office workers	Yes	No	C	1.6*	39	Self-reports
Kiken et al. (1990)	294	CS	Poultry processors	Yes	Yes	F, R	1.30	—	Job titles
Kukkonen et al. (1983)	161	CS	Office workers	NR	Yes	P, C	2.3*	57	Self-reports
Kuorinka and Koskinen (1979)	206	CS	Manufacturing	Yes	Yes	P, C	4.1*	76	Job titles

Study	Type of study	Number of subjects	Population			Risk factor	Risk estimate	Participation rate	Assessment
Linton and Kamwendo (1989)	CS	22,180	Industrial workers	Yes	No	C	3.5*	71	Self-reports
Luopajärvi et al. (1979)	CS	285	Assembly workers	Yes	Yes	F, R	1.60	—	Observed
Milerad and Ekenvall (1990)	CS	199	Dentists	Yes	No	P, R	2.1*	52	Self-reports
Ohlsson et al. (1995)	CS	214	Manufacturing	Yes	Yes	P, R	3.6*	72	Observed
Punnett et al. (1991)	CS	254	Meat packers	Yes	No	F, R	1.8 (males)	—	Observed
Rossignol et al. (1987)	CS	191	Office workers	Yes	No	R	4.6*	78	Self-reports
Schibye et al. (1995)	C	303	Sewing machine operators	Yes	No	C	3.3*	70	Self-reports
Tola et al. (1988)	CS	2,143	Machine operators	Yes	No	P	1.8*	44	Self-reports
Veiersted and Westgaard (1994)	C	30	Manufacturing	No	Yes	F / P	6.7* / 7.2*	85 / 86	Measured
Viikari-Juntura et al. (1991b)	C	154	General population	Yes	Yes	P	1.50*	—	Self-reports
Viikari-Juntura et al. (1994)	C	1,832	Machine operators	Yes	No	C	4.2*	76	Job titles
			Carpenters	Yes	No	C	3.0*	67	
Welch et al. (1995)	CS	47	Sheet metal workers	Yes	No	P	7.50*	—	Self-reports
Wells et al. (1983)	CS	399	Mail carriers	Yes	No	F, P	2.6*	61	Self-reports
Yu and Wong (1995)	CS	151	Office workers	Yes	No	R	28.9*	97	Self-reports

Notes: Some studies did not separate neck and shoulder disorders. Type of study: C, cohort; CC, case-control; CS, cross-sectional. Number of subjects: Total of study population and referents or controls. Risk factor: C, combination or many; F, force; P, posture; R, repetition; V, vibration. Participation rate: NR, not reported. Risk estimate: OR, odds ratio; RR, relative risk.

* $p \leq .05$.

TABLE 6.11

Summary of Tables 6.10 through 6.16 Showing Strength of Evidence for Contributory Risk Factors to MSDs

| Upper Limb Area | Contributory Risk Factors | | | | | | | | | | Conclusions Regarding Association of Risk Factors and MSDs |
| | Repetition | | Posture | | Force | | Vibration | | Combination | | |
	Sign	OR	Sign	OR	Sign	OR	Sign	OR	Sign	OR	
Neck	4/4	1.2–29	5/7	1.4–7.2	1/1	6.7	15/20	—	1.4–9.9	1.4–9.9	Repetition, posture, force, and combinations thereof show positive associations
Shoulder	1/1	1.6	4/4	2.4–18	3/3	1.8–18	7/7	—	1.7–7.3	1.7–7.3	Combinations of repetition, posture, and force show strong positive associations
Elbow	1/1	2.8	2/2	4–37	1/2	6.7	5/9	4.9	1.7–6.7	1.7–6.7	Most individual and combinations of factors show positive associations
Hand/Wrist — CTS	4/9	1.9–5.5	2/2	5.4–8.7	3/5	1.5–2.0	4/5	1.9–21	2.3–8.3	2.3–8.3	Vibration shows a very strong association, the combination of factors is also strong
Tendinitis	0/1	—	1/1	3.7–6.2	0/0	—	5/5	—	2.5–17	2.5–17	The combination of risk factors shows strong positive associations
Vibration syndrome	—	—	—	—	—	—	—	3.4–85	—	—	Vibration shows a very strong positive association

Notes: Sign is the number of studies showing significant results out of the total number studies in the given category. OR, Odds ratios for the statistically significant studies.

TABLE 6.12

Summary of Epidemiological Studies Examining Shoulder MSDs

Reference	Type of Study	Number of Subjects	Study Population	Participation Rate >70%	Physical Exam	Risk Factor	Risk Estimate (OR, RR)	AR (%)	Exposure Assessment
Andersen and Gaardboe (1993a)	CS	1294	Sewing machine operators	Yes	No	C	7.3*	86	Job titles
Baron et al. (1991)	CS	281	Grocery scanners	No	Yes	F, R	3.9*	74	Job titles
Bjelle et al. (1979)	CC	51	Industrial workers	NR	Yes	P	10.6*	91	Measured
Chiang et al. (1993)	CS	207	Fish processors	Yes	Yes	F / R	1.8* / 1.6*	44 / 38	Measured
English et al. (1995)	CC	1576	General population	Yes	Yes	R, P	2.3*	57	Self-reports
Herberts et al. (1981)	CS	188	Shipyard welders, clerks	NR	Yes	P	18.3*	95	Job titles
Herberts et al. (1984)	CS	188	Shipyard welders, clerks	NR	Yes	F	18.3*	95	Job titles
		188	Plate workers	NR	Yes	F	16.2*	94	Job titles
Hoekstra et al. (1994)	CS	108	Office workers	Yes	No	P	5.1*	80	Self-reports
Milerad and Ekenvall (1990)	CS	199	Dentists	Yes	No	P	2.4*	58	Self-reports
Ohlsson et al. (1994)	CS	736	Fish processors	Yes	Yes	C	2.9–3.5*	66–71	Observed
Ohlsson et al. (1995)	CS	214	Manufacturing	Yes	Yes	P, R	5.0*	80	Observed
Sakakibara et al. (1995)	CS	52	Fruit pickers	Yes	Yes	P, R	1.7*	41	Observed
Stenlund et al. (1992)	CS	110	Rock blasters	Yes	Yes	F, V	2.2*	55	Self-reports
		109	Bricklayers	Yes	Yes	F, V	4.0*	75	Self-reports
Wells et al. (1983)	CS	399	Mail carriers	Yes	No	F	3.3–5.7*	70–82	Self-reports

Notes: Type of study: C, cohort; CC, case-control; CS, cross-sectional. Number of subjects: Total of study population and referents or controls. Risk factor: C, combination or many; F, force; P, posture; R, repetition; V, vibration. Participation rate: NR, not reported. Risk estimate: OR, odds ratio; RR, relative risk.

* $p \leq .05$.

TABLE 6.13

Summary of Epidemiological Studies Examining Elbow MSDs

Reference	Type of Study	Number of Subjects	Study Population	Participation Rate >70%	Physical Exam	Risk Factor	Risk Estimate (OR, RR)	Attributable Risk (%)	Exposure Assessment
Andersen and Gaardboe (1993a)	CS	1,205	Sewing machine operators	Yes	No	F, R	1.7	—	Job titles
Baron et al. (1991)	CS	270	Grocery scanners	No	Yes	F, R	2.3	—	Job titles
Bovenzi et al. (1991)	CS	96	Chain saw operators	NR	Yes	V	4.9*	80	Measured
Burt et al. (1990)	CS	836	Newspaper employees	Yes	No	R	2.8*	64	Observed
Byström et al. (1995)	CS	385	Auto assembly workers	Yes	Yes	C	0.7	—	Self-reports
Chiang et al. (1993)	CS	207	Fish processors	Yes	Yes	F, R	6.7* (males)	85	Measured
							1.4 (females)	—	
Hoekstra et al. (1994)	CS	108	Office workers	Yes	No	P	4.0*	75	Self-reports
Hughes et al. (1997)	CS	211	Smelter workers	No	Yes	P	37.0*	97	Observed
Kurppa et al. (1981)	C	862	Meat processors	Yes	Yes	F	6.7*	85	Observed
Luopajärvi et al. (1979)	CS	285	Food packers	Yes	Yes	C	2.7	—	Observed
Moore and Garg (1994)	CS	230	Pork processors	Yes	Yes	F, R	5.5*	82	Observed
Punnett et al. (1985)	CS	238	Garment workers	No	No	C	2.4*	58	Self-reports
Ritz (1995)	CS	290	Gas and water workers	NR	Yes	C	1.7–2.2*	41–55	Observed
Roto and Kivi (1984)	CS	162	Meatpackers	Yes	Yes	C	6.4*	84	Job titles
Viikari-Juntura et al. (1991a)	CS	709	Meatpackers	Yes	Yes	F	0.9	—	Observed

Notes: Type of study: C, cohort; CC, case-control; CS, cross-sectional. Number of subjects: Total of study population and referents or controls. Risk factor: C, combination or many; F, force; P, posture; R, repetition; V, vibration. Participation rate: NR = not reported. Risk estimate: OR, odds ratio; RR, relative risk.

* $p \leq .05$.

TABLE 6.14

Summary of Epidemiological Studies Examining Hand/Wrist CTS Cases

Reference	Type of Study	Number of Subjects	Study Population	Participation Rate >70%	Physical Exam	Risk Factor	Risk Estimate (OR, RR)	Attributable Risk (%)	Exposure Assessment
Barnhart et al. (1991)	CS	173	Ski fabricators	No	Yes	R	1.9–3.9*	47–75	Observed
Baron et al. (1991)	CS	175	Grocery scanners	No	Yes	F	3.7	—	Job titles
Bovenzi et al. (1991)	CS	96	Chain saw operators	NR	Yes	V	21.3*	95	Measured
Bovenzi (1994)	CS	1,148	Rock drillers and cutters	Yes	Yes	V	3.4*	71	Measured
Cannon et al. (1981)	CC	120	Aircraft engine workers	NR	Yes	V	7.0*	86	Measured
Chattarjee (1992)	CC	31	Rock drillers	Yes	Yes	V	10.9*	91	Measured
Chiang et al. (1990)	CS	207	Frozen food workers	Yes	Yes	Cold R	1.9* 1.9*	46 47	Measured
Chiang et al. (1993)	CS	207	Fish processors	Yes	Yes	F R	1.8* 1.1	44 —	Measured
deKrom et al. (1990)	CC	629	Hospital patients	Yes	Yes	P	5.4–8.7*	81–89	Self-reports
English et al. (1995)	CC	1,167	Hospital patients	Yes	Yes	P R	1.8* 0.4	44 —	Self-reports
Feldman et al. (1987)	CS	586	Electronics workers	Yes	No	P, R	2.3*	56	Observed
Moore and Garg (1994)	CS	230	Pork processors	Yes	Yes	C	2.8	—	Observed

(continued)

TABLE 6.14 (continued)

Summary of Epidemiological Studies Examining Hand/Wrist CTS Cases

Reference	Type of Study	Number of Subjects	Study Population	Participation Rate >70%	Physical Exam	Risk Factor	Risk Estimate (OR, RR)	Attributable Risk (%)	Exposure Assessment
Morgenstern et al. (1991)	CS	1,058	Grocery workers	Yes	No	R	1.9	—	Self-reports
Nathan et al. (1988)	CS	471	Industrial workers	NR	Yes	F R	1.7–2.0* 1.0	41–50 —	Self-reports
Nathan et al. (1992)	C	315	Industrial workers	No	Yes	F R	1.5* 1.1	33 —	Self-reports
Osorio et al. (1994)	CS	56	Supermarket workers	Yes	No	F, R	8.3*	88	Observed
Punnett et al. (1985)	CS	238	Garment workers	No	Yes	C	2.7*	63	Self-reports
Schottland et al. (1991)	CS	178	Poultry processors	NR	Yes	C	1.7 LH 2.9* RH	— 65	Job titles
Silverstein et al. (1987)	CS	652	Industrial workers	Yes	Yes	F R	2.9 5.5*	— 82	Measured
Tanaka et al. (1997)	CS	44,233	General population	Yes	No	P V	5.5* 1.9*	82 47	Self-reports
Wieslander et al. (1989)	CC	177	Hospital patients	Yes	Yes	F R V	1.8* 2.7* 6.1*	44 63 84	Self-reports

Notes: Type of study: C, cohort; CC, case-control; CS, cross-sectional. Number of subjects: Total of study population and referents or controls. Risk factor: C, combination or many; F, force; P, posture; R, repetition; V, vibration. Participation rate, Physical exam: NR, not reported. Risk estimate: OR, odds ratio; RR, relative risk. LH, left hand; RH, right hand.

* p ≤ .05.

TABLE 6.15

Summary of Epidemiological Studies Examining Hand/Wrist Tendinitis Cases

Reference	Type of Study	No. of Subjects	Study Population	Participation Rate >70%	Physical Exam	Risk Factor	Risk Estimate (OR, RR)	Attributable Risk (%)	Exposure Assessment
Amano et al. (1988)	CS	204	Assembly line workers	NR	Yes	P	3.7–6.2*	73–84	Observed
Armstrong et al. (1987)	CS	652	Industrial workers	Yes	Yes	F, R	17.0*	94	Measured
Byström et al. (1995)	CS	385	Auto assembly workers	Yes	Yes	C	2.5*	60	Self-reports
Kuorinka and Koskinen (1979)	CS	236	Scissor makers	Yes	Yes	R	1.4	—	Observed
Kurppa et al. (1991)	C	765	Meat processors	Yes	Yes	C	14–38.5*	93–97	Observed
Luopajärvi et al. (1979)	CS	285	Food packers	Yes	Yes	C	4.1*	76	Observed
Roto and Kivi (1984)	CS	162	Meatpackers	Yes	Yes	C	3.1*	68	Job titles

Notes: Type of study: C, cohort; CC, case-control; CS, cross-sectional. Number of subjects: Total of study population and referents or controls. Risk factor: C, combination or many; F, force; P, posture; R, repetition; V, vibration. Participation rate: NR, not reported. Risk estimate: OR, odds ratio; RR, relative risk.

* $p \le .05$.

TABLE 6.16

Summary of Epidemiological Studies Examining Hand/Wrist Vibration Syndrome Cases

Reference	Type of Study	No. of Subjects	Study Population	Participation Rate >70%	Physical Exam	Risk Factor	Risk Estimate (OR, RR)	Attributable Risk (%)	Exposure Assessment
Bovenzi et al. (1988)	CS	136	Rock drillers and cutters	NR	Yes	V	6.1*	83	Measured
Bovenzi (1994)	CS	855	Rock drillers and cutters	Yes	Yes	V	9.3*	89	Measured
Bovenzi et al. (1995)	CS	427	Forestry workers	Yes	Yes	V	6.2–32.3*	84–97	Measured
Kivekäs et al. (1994)	C	353	Lumberjacks	Yes	Yes	V	3.4–6.5*	71–85	Self-reports
Letz et al. (1992)	CS	271	Shipyard workers	Yes	No	V	5.0–40.6*	80–98	Self-reports
McKenna et al. (1993)	CS	92	Riveters	NR	Yes	V	24.0*	96	Self-reports
Mirbod et al. (1994)	CS	2,979	Dental, industrial workers	NR	No	V	3.8*	73	Measured
Nagata et al. (1993)	CS	384	Chain-saw operators	NR	Yes	V	7.1*	86	Self-reports
Nilsson et al. (1989)	CS	150	Platers	Yes	Yes	V	14–85*	93–99	Measured

Notes: Type of study: C, cohort; CC, case-control; CS, cross-sectional. Number of subjects: Total of study population and referents or controls. Risk factor: C, combination or many; F, force; P, posture; R, repetition; V, vibration. Participation rate, physical exam: NR = not reported. Risk estimate: OR = odds ratio, RR = relative risk. LH, left hand; RH, right hand.

* $p \le .05$.

6.5 Scientific Research and Evidence for Occupational Risk Factors

6.5.1 Neck Disorders

With regards to neck MSDs, studies from the United States have generally separated neck from shoulder disorders, whereas Scandinavian and Japanese studies have tended to lump the two together. This was based on the anatomical reasoning that many muscles act simultaneously on both the shoulder girdle and upper spine. For the present discussions, both categories were combined. Overall prevalence ranges from 1.4% when diagnosed by physical findings to 4.9% when defined simply by symptoms alone (Hagberg and Wegman, 1987). Of the 30 studies examined and shown in Table 6.10, 23 found statistically significant effects for one or more contributory risk factors. With regards to repetition, defined as repetitive neck movements or repeated arm or shoulder motions, all four studies that could identify repetition as a separate factor, found a significant positive association, with ORs ranging from 1.2 to 28.9 that accounted for an average of 72% of AR. Twelve more studies examined repetition but in conjunction with other variables. Seven of these found statistically significant positive associations. Unfortunately, many studies primarily utilize hand/arm exposure assessments without specifically identifying neck or shoulder assessments. This gives rise to the possibility of misclassification errors. Also, since in most cases, the studies were cross-sectional, temporality cannot be determined. However, several studies (Kiken et al., 1990; Baron et al., 1991; Hales et al., 1994) defined outcome definition by excluding persons reporting symptoms prior to the job, insuring that exposure preceded MSD occurrence. There were no studies that showed a clear dose–response relationship between repetition and neck MSDs. Plausibility of repetition being a risk factor for injury is found in sports injuries whereby low-load forces with high repetition result in a gradual deterioration of tissue strength from stress/strain deformation fatigue (Nicholas, 1990).

Posture, as a risk factor, has been generally defined either as an external load or as an internal force. Five of seven studies that could isolate force from other risk factors found a significant positive association, with ORs ranging from 1.4 to 7.2, that accounted for 56% of the AR (see Table 6.11). If the two studies with nonsignificant effects are added in, then the AR would drop to 42%. Four more studies examined posture but in conjunction with other variables and all four found statistically significant positive associations. Temporality is most apparent in the prospective study of Veiersted and Westgaard (1994), in which workers developed MSDs within 6–51 weeks of staring work. Several studies (Rossignol et al., 1987; Andersen and Gaardboe, 1993a,b) found a dose–response relationship with prevalence or symptoms increasing with increased number of hours spent on task or the number of years at work, controlling for age. Plausibility for posture, indirectly through force, since the two are related, as a risk factor has been established by studies showing decreased blood, increased metabolite concentrations, and potential injury in nearly maximally contracted muscles (Larsson et al., 1990).

Most studies examined force in conjunction with other variables; in fact, only one study found a significant positive association with force as a single factor. Eight more studies examined force in combination, but only three of these found statistically significant positive associations. However, the combination of posture and force, especially in the form of static posture or static loading in extreme postures, causes an especially positive association with MSDs accounting for up to 80% of AR (Veiersted and Westgaard, 1994). Similar to repetition, there was no clear demonstration of temporality or a dose–response relationship. There was also no evidence for vibration to have a positive association with neck MSDs.

Overall, one can conclude, from Table 6.10 or the summary in Table 6.11, that there is evidence for positive association between repetition, posture, and force, individually, and neck-related MSDs. Interestingly, of the seven studies with nonsignificant associations, five relied on job titles or self-reports to assess exposure, while four of six studies that used direct observations or quantitative measurements to evaluate exposure had statistically significant positive associations between risk factors and MSDs. Therefore, one can conclude that the more objective the exposure assessment, the more likely a significant positive association can be found. Such associations are more easily visible for the neck as opposed to the other joints because the large number of available studies performed.

6.5.2 Shoulder Disorders

For shoulder-related MSDs, repetition was defined by the number of predefined shoulder movements, the number of pieces handled per unit time, or some generalized characterization of repetitive work with the arm. The number of studies that examined repetition, or other risk factors individually, was rather limited (see Table 6.12). However, repetition in combination with other risk factors showed an especially strong positive association with MSDs, with all five such studies showing statistically significant ORs ranging from 1.6 to 5.0 that accounted for and average AR of 58%. Several studies of a cross-sectional design limited the number cases in which the MSD was already present during exposure in order to suggest some temporality (Chiang et al., 1993; Ohlsson et al., 1994, 1995). For a dose–response relationship, Chiang et al. (1993) found a significant increasing prevalences with increased repetition and Ohlsson et al. (1995) found increased MSDs with increased number of arm elevations and abductions. Plausibility is evidenced by Herberts et al. (1984) findings of fatigue in the supra- and infraspinatus muscles. This leads to the hypothesis that the rotator cuff muscles may develop high intramuscular pressures leading to impaired circulation in the muscles and tendons. The latter effect may also lead to inflammation and consequent tendinitis.

Four studies isolated posture from other risk factors and all found a significant positive association with ORs ranging from 2.4 to 18.3 and accounting for 81% of the AR (see Table 6.11). Three other studies found posture in combination with repetition to have statistically significant positive associations. In spite of the cross-sectional design of studies, elimination of workers with preexisting symptoms will improve the ability to detect temporality (Baron et al., 1991). Four studies found some evidence of a dose–response relationship, typically a higher OR for shoulder MSDs for individuals working longer hours (Bjelle et al., 1979; Baron et al., 1991; Ohlsson et al., 1994, 1995). Plausibility follows the same line of reasoning as for repetition (and force, next), a more abducted arms place more pressure on the tendon and other tissues causing inflammation, microtrauma, and further problems.

Three studies isolated force from other risk factors and all found a significant positive association with ORs ranging from 1.8 to 18.3 and accounting for 72% of the AR. Two other studies found force in combination with other variables to have statistically significant positive associations. Wells et al. (1983) found some evidence of temporality of carrying increased loads having shoulder disorders in mail carriers. For those carriers who experienced a weight increase as compared to the control group, the OR was 5.7 (p < .05) demonstrating a dose–response effect. Similarly Stenlund et al. (1992) found that for the left shoulder, ORs increased with level of lifetime load lifted. This latter study was also the only one that examined the effects of vibration (in combination with force) on MSDs, finding a significant positive association. Overall, one can conclude from Table 6.12 or the summary in Table 6.11 that there is evidence for a positive association between repetition, posture, and force and shoulder-related MSDs.

6.5.3 Elbow Disorders

There are relatively few studies examining risk factors and elbow MSDs (primarily epicondylitis). Repetition was typically defined by the number of cyclical elbow flexions/extensions, elbow pronations/supinations, or wrist motions that led to changes in the elbow region. Only one study for each of the risk factors (repetition, force, vibration) showed a significant positive association with MSDs (see Table 6.13). There were two such studies for posture. However, nine studies showed combinations of risk factors to have positive associations with MSDs, five of which yielded statistically significant results with ORs ranging from 1.7 to 6.4 that accounted for 40% of the AR (see Table 6.11). Since almost all of the studies were cross sectional, temporality cannot be easily determined. However, some dose–response relationship was shown by Baron et al. (1991) for number of hours worked per week, by Moore and Garg (1994) with respect to increasing strain on jobs, and Ritz (1995) with duration of exposure to stressful tasks. Plausibility is consistent with earlier clinical case studies and parallel sports research studies. Repetitive contractions of forearm extensors produce a force that is transmitted to the origin of the tendon on the lateral epicondyle. A chronic overload on the bone–tendon junction leads to microtrauma and inflammation. The lack of significance in many, especially cross sectional, studies may result from a *survivor bias*. Only workers who are resistant to injury stay on the high-exposure jobs, while those with MSDs shift to less stressful jobs. Overall, the majority of epidemiological studies support the hypothesis of repetitive, forceful work or repetitive flexions, extensions, pronations, or supinations leading to an increased risk of epicondylitis.

6.5.4 Hand/Wrist: Carpal Tunnel Syndrome

Vibration, as an individual risk factor, shows the strongest association with CTS cases, with all six studies showing statistically significant ORs ranging from 1.9 to 21.3 that accounted for an average of 80% of the AR (see Tables 6.11 and 6.14). Since all studies used a dichotomous classification any dose–response relationship is difficult to determine. Also, there were no longitudinal studies to show temporality. The exact physiological mechanism for the development of CTS from vibration is not known because of the confounding factors of repetitive, forceful exertions typically found while using vibrating power tools. However, Taylor (1982) speculates that vibration either directly injures peripheral nerves reducing tactile sensitivity or indirectly, through the arterial vasoconstriction and the resulting ischemia of nerve tissue. The other three factors, repetition, posture, and force, individually show some evidence for a positive association with CTS. Four of nine studies found repetition individually to have a significant positive association with CTS. The lack of more significant results is again probably due to a survivor bias. In fact, Nathan et al. (1992) found that the highest risk group had a decrease in CTS prevalence over time. This could only occur as workers dropped out (and did not return) from the high-risk group as they incurred injuries. The expected temporality was reported by Feldman et al. (1987) who found increased median nerve motor latencies over time. For posture, individually, only two studies found significant positive associations with ORs ranging from 5.4 to 8.7. However, one study (English et al., 1995) confounded other upper limb joints with the wrist, while the second (Tanaka et al., 1997) was based purely on self-reports, which may limit the strength of the association. A dose–response effect was shown by deKrom et al. (1990) when workers suffered increased CTS with reportedly increased working hours.

In terms of force as risk factor, three of five studies found a significant positive association with ORs ranging from 1.5 to 2.0 and accounting for 42% of the AR. However, in these and other studies, force was typically combined with other exposure variables (repetition or awkward postures). Temporality is again difficult to ascertain from the cross-sectional nature of the studies. A dose–response relationship was shown individually only in Chiang et al. (1993) but more definitely when combined with repetition in Silverstein et al. (1987), Wieslander et al. (1989), and Osorio et al. (1994). The first study found an OR of 15.5 (or 94% AR) for the combined effect. Plausibility is established by Rempel (1995) who found increased pressure in the carpal tunnel due to tendon forces from repetitive forceful exertions. This pressure in turn may reduce compress venules (which have weaker walls than arterioles) which causes an increasing capillary pressure and greater edema. If the edema becomes chronic, it may trigger fibrosis of nerve tissue. This hypothesis is supported by observations during CTS surgery for of greater edema and vascular sclerosis and fibrosis (Rempel, 1995). Deviated or flexed wrist postures only further exacerbate the problem by potentially reducing the cross-sectional area of the tunnel and further increasing carpal pressure (Skie et al., 1990).

6.5.5 Hand/Wrist: Tendinitis

There were only seven epidemiological studies that examined physical risk factors on hand/wrist tendinitis. While force, repetition, and posture, individually, showed little evidence for a positive association with the incidence hand/wrist tendinitis case, the combination of these risk factors showed a very positive association. All five studies in the combination category (see Tables 6.11 and 6.15) showed statistically significant ORs ranging from 2.5 to 17.0, with an average of 79% AR. The only prospective study by Kurppa et al. (1991) showed a significant increase in risk for injury with increasing time on the job indicating direct temporality. Armstrong et al. (1987) demonstrated strong evidence for a dose–response relationship in that the high-force, high-repetition group had a 17 times greater risk than the low-force, low-repetition group. However, somewhat contrary to the proportional role of stressors in CTS, the response of muscles and tendons to repetitive activity may be more like a U-shaped curve. Too little or too much activity may be harmful, but intermediate levels may be beneficial. These tissues have the ability to repair themselves, within reason. The difficulty is finding the threshold at which point overuse exceeds the ability of the tissue repair the damage (Hart et al., 1995).

6.5.6 Hand/Arm: Vibration Syndrome

There is strong evidence of vibration showing a positive association with hand/arm vibration syndrome (HAVS). All nine studies (see Tables 6.11 and 6.16) showed statistically significant ORs from 3.4 to 85 with an average AR of 87%. Although most of the studies are cross sectional with a high possibility of recall bias and weakening temporality, many studies have indicated information about the latency period between initial exposure and the development of symptoms. This latency ranged from 0.7 to 17 years with a mean of 6.3 years. The one prospective study (Kivekäs et al., 1994) clearly showed an increased incidence rate of 14.7% in Finnish lumberjacks as compared to an incidence rate of only 2.3% in the referent group. In terms of a dose–response relationship (NIOSH 1989), took data of 23 cross-sectional studies and found a statistically significant linear relationship between vibration acceleration levels and prevalence of symptoms ($r = 0.67$, $p < .01$). As mentioned previously, plausibility has been established by many experts in that vibration either directly injures peripheral nerves reducing tactile sensitivity or indirectly, through the arterial vasoconstriction and the resulting ischemia of nerve tissue. Furthermore, if the blood vessels are damaged, they may become less sensitive to the reverse process vasodilation further exacerbating recovery from cold working conditions. In fact, there is some evidence that wall of digital blood vessels may become permanently thickened in HAVS patients (Takeuchi et al., 1986).

6.6 Scientific Research and Evidence for Psychosocial Risk Factors

Psychosocial risk factors for upper limb MSDs have been studied less frequently than occupational risk factors, partly because there are fewer good objective measures of exposure and/or risk and, partly, because psychosocial factors are measured at an individual level rather than a group level as for occupational factors, which limits the accuracy or precision of the measurements. Typically, psychosocial factors are separated into three subcategories. The first includes job and work-environment factors that are not strictly physical and includes factors related to (1) job content, e.g., work load, control over the job, rest breaks and other cyclical aspects; (2) work organization, e.g., supervision, interpersonal relationships, prestige, status, office hierarchy; and (3) financial aspects, e.g., pay, benefits, vacation, equity issues. The second category includes activities outside the work environment, e.g., exercise, a second job, family, child care issues. The third category is individual characteristics such as genetic, e.g., gender, race, intelligence and anatomical; social, e.g., social class, cultural background, educational level, and individual personality, i.e., attitudes toward work, attitudes toward life, susceptibility to stress and pain, etc., (Hurrell and Murphy, 1992).

Of the 19 studies that roughly fit previously discussed quality issues and included quantitative information (OR values and statistical calculations), most focused primarily on the work-environment factors rather than individual factors (see Table 6.17). High workload, in a variety of forms including job pressures and lack of rest breaks, was the one factor that was most consistently associated with upper limb MSDs. Twelve of the 19 studies found statistically significant positive associations. Somewhat, counter intuitively, low workload in the form of monotonous work, was also found to be a significant factor for MSDs in 5 of the 19 studies. Lack of control over the job was another factor that had significant positive associations with MSDs in 10 of the 19 studies.

Gender and age were the most common individual characteristics showing positive associations with MSDs, with females and older workers being typically more at risk. Outside-of-work factors showed few significant associations, perhaps due to the overlapping, confounding effects of many of these factors or due to the fact that outside work situations may be exacerbated by work conditions (Sauter and Swanson, 1996). Positive associations were found for all types of MSDs, depending on which questions were asked of which type of symptoms. However, twice as many studies found significant positive associations with neck and shoulder disorders rather than with elbow, wrist, or hand disorders.

There is not a clear link between psychosocial factors and the etiology of MSDs. Some of the hypothesized explanations are as follows. An increased awareness of the problem leads to an increased perception and increased reporting. Increased muscle tension may lead to increased muscle strain or may exacerbate existing muscle strain, which may then develop into pain spasm cycles and a chronic problem (Bergkvist, 1984; Bongers et al., 1993; Sauter, and Swanson, 1996). The key would then be to break the cycle so that the initial pain and discomfort can be relieved. Finally, in a perverse way, the present system

TABLE 6.17

Summary of Epidemiological Studies Examining Psychosocial Factors and MSDs in the Upper Limbs

| Reference | Type of Study | No. of Subjects | Study Population (Workers) | MSD Outcome Assessment | Associations with Upper Limb Outcomes (OR) | | | | | | | |
| | | | | | Job and Work Environment | | | | | Individual | | |
					Job Dissatis-faction	High Workload	Monot-onous Work	Low Job Control	Low Social Support	Sex	Age	Other
Bergqvist et al. (1995a,b)	CS	260	VDT	Survey, exam		U2.7* N7.4*		S3.2*	H4.5*	S7.1*	N2.1* H2.4	N4.0* glasses N6.4* children
Bernard et al. (1994)	CS	973	Newspaper	Survey		S1.5* Z1.4*		S1.6* Z1.4*				
Ekberg et al. (1994)	CC	746	General	MD exam		U3.8*		U16.5*		U16*		U3.7* smoker
Hales et al. (1994)	CS	553	Telecommuni-cations	MD exam		Z2.3* N3.0* E2.4*	N4.2* E2.8*	S2.7* N3.5* E2.9*				E2.4* race
Houtman et al. (1994)	CS	5865	General	Survey		M1.3*	M1.3*	M1.0		M1.6*	M4.0*	
Kamwendo et al. (1991)	CS	420	Clerical	Survey	U1.9*							
Karasek et al. (1987)	CS	8700	White collar	Survey		M1.2*		M1.1*			M1.3*	
Kvarnström (1983)	CC	224	Fabrication	Medical records		S5.2*	S4.0*					S5* married
Lagerström et al. (1995)	CS	668	Female nurses	Survey		S1.7*	H1.6*	S1.7*				

Study	Type	N	Population	Method						
Leclerc et al. (1998)	CS	1006	Industrial	MD exam	W1.4*		W1.6*		W2.2*	W2.3* well-being
Lemasters et al. (1998)	CS	552	Carpenters	Interview		S1.5 E1.4 Z1.5*	S1.9* E1.6 Z1.6*			
Magnavita et al. (1999)	CS	2041	Sonographers	Survey						
Marcus and Gerr (1996)	CS	449	Female clerical	Survey		U2.5* EZ2*	U2.2*			
Pocekay et al. (1995)	CS	3175	Semiconductor	Survey	O1.5*					O1.8* stress
Roquelaure et al. (1997)	CC	130	Blue-collar	Survey		O6.3*				
Silverstein et al. (1987)	CS	136	Casting	Interview				O4.8*		
Tola et al. (1988)	CS	3221	Machinists, carpenters, clerical	Survey	U1.2*			U1.6*		
Toomingas et al. (1997)	CS	358	Male MMH Female clerical	Survey		S2.2* Z1.5	S3.2* Z1.8*			

Notes: Type of study: C, cohort; CC, case-control; CS, cross-sectional. Number of subjects: Total of study population and referents or controls. E, elbow; H, hand; M, overall muscle pains; O, overall MSDs; N, neck; S, shoulder; U, neck/shoulder combined; W, wrist; Z, hand/wrist combined. Vast majority used self-reporting for exposure assessment. +, positive but not significant.

* $p \leq .05$.

of workers compensation may be a form of incentive that encourages workers to overreport symptoms (Frank et al., 1995).

Primarily because of the ease of administration of a survey as a snapshot in time, all but one study (Kvarnström, 1983) was cross-sectional. This, to some degree, does limit the usefulness of the data and conclusions. Ideally, there should be more cohort (prospective) studies to truly identify the critical risk factors. Most studies used surveys or past medical records to establish the assessment of MSD outcome. Again, a worker's recall or subjective evaluation of pain or discomfort is not equivalent to a medically verified MSD. Finally, a wide variety of questionnaires or evaluations were used to classify psychosocial exposures. Ideally, only a few consistent measures should be used such that comparisons can be made between studies or data combined across studies to establish more significant conclusions. Nevertheless, there is still a clear positive association between psychosocial risk factors and MSDs in the upper limbs. This indicates the importance of not only modifying work-related physical sources of job stress but also the non-work-related sources of stress.

6.7 Iatrogenesis: A Contrarian View

Iatrogenesis refers to the argument, advocated by a small but vocal group of medical and public health researchers, that work-related musculoskeletal disorders (WRMSDs) are merely an iatrogenic labeling of everyday pains. Iatrogenic is medically defined as resulting from the course of the professional activities of a physician, implying autosuggestion from discussions, examinations, or treatments. In practice, iatrogenesis refers to the discounting of physical occupational risk factors in the development of MSDs, in favor of extraneous, sociological, or individual factors. Iatrogenesis was first proposed Ferguson (1971a,b, 1973) as a form of "craft neuroses" or occupational disorders with considerable amount of anxiety and other behavioral issues specific to a craft. The term first appeared in articles by Ferguson (1987) and Cleland (1987) to explain the rapid, almost epidemic-like, increase in RSIs (repetition strain injury, the Australian term for WRMSDs) in the telecommunications industry in Australia in the early 1980s, which consequently even earned the derogatory term "kangaroo paw" (Awerbuch, 1985). The same concept was soon appropriated and advanced in the United States by Hadler (1986, 1990, 1993).

Their basic arguments are multifold and fault a wide range of parties, including the medical establishment. In the current medical system, patients expect to be healthy; if not there must be a specific reason for the illness or disorder. For lack of finding a specific cause or subjecting patients to endless and costly tests and rather than attempting to explain that the patient may have to endure nonspecific pain or discomfort for some time, the physician will assign a syndrome label. Next the Worker's Compensation system is indicted for requiring structured responses (when they might not be easily available), encouraging over reporting, and extending disability periods (which may also be the case for back pain—Hadler, 1986; Frank et al., 1995). It is also an adversarial system, in which if the condition is not improving rapidly, the claimant cannot back out easily without casting doubt on their original claims and symptoms. The worker is indicted partially for being gullible and succumbing to general rumors or media alarms and partially for being greedy and seeking easy compensation. Ergonomists and other researchers are faulted for methodological problems in cross-sectional studies (which are the vast majority in the epidemiological studies cited in Section 6.5) in which prevalence or morbidity depends on reporting recall, volunteer biases, and difficulty in distinguishing between etiological and forecasting factors (Sackett, 1979). There are also sociological aspects such as sustained media interest and sensationalism, strong union support for "empowering the dispossessed," and, sometimes, an almost Luddite reaction to high-technology advancements (Arksey, 1998).

Similar to the "nature versus nurture" concept in child development, there is probably some truth to the iatrogenic concept. Many of the above arguments can be found to occur, especially in extremes cases. Also, anecdotally (and from personal experience) there seems to be an increase in the reporting of MSDs upon completion of a symptom survey or participation in an ergonomics awareness program. This is only natural. Worker awareness has been increased and the person realizes there is a cause for the discomfort or pain that the person is already experiencing, making it easier for that person to go the plant nurse and report the problem. However, this increase in incidence rates is typically only a spike, which then should decrease below previous levels, once an ergonomics program has been implemented or, in the worst case, return to preexisting levels, once work returns to the status quo.

There are undoubtedly overlapping and confounding psychosocial and individual factors that exacerbate the development of MSDs by amplifying already existing strains and pains that normally result with many jobs. Unhappiness with the job, the supervision, pay, etc., were all shown to be contributory factors to MSDs. The key, however, is existing strains and pains. It would be unreasonable to expect that job unhappiness in itself would lead to MSDs. There has to be some underlying physical cause first. To completely eliminate the physical occupational stressors, seems foolhardy at the least and potentially very costly, both to the company and to the individual workers. On the other hand, equal attention should be also given to the mental well-being of the worker. The company may be pleasantly surprised by increased productivity through increased worker motivation and the *Hawthorne effect* (Freivalds, 2009).

6.8 Legal Issues

Ergonomists may also need to be aware of some the legal issues involved with WRMSDs. Owen (1994) provided a nice summary of some of these issues. Most WRMSDs arise from the interaction of a person's upper limbs while using a tool, device, or some other manufactured product. Since this product is entered into the stream of commerce by the manufacturer, they then could be exposed to product liability litigation. The manufacturer has a duty to produce and distribute safe products. If the product causes an injury, then the manufacturer could be held liable due to *negligence* through breach of duty. One key issue of negligence is proof that the product caused this injury.

This is not as simple as it may seem, since WRMSDs can be brought about by many causes and can be aggravated by other diseases such as diabetes or arthritis and by the time factor typical in cumulative injuries. In addition to negligence, *proximate causation* (the two events are closely, legally related) must be shown. This may also be difficult. A worker may be exposed to repetitive wrist motions with the manufacturer's product. However, the worker may also be stressing the wrist by motions using other products off the work site. Epidemiological studies may not be so precise so as to separate the two potential stressors.

In addition to negligence, the other key issue in legal proceedings is *liability* on the part of the manufacturer. As part of *strict liability*, two questions need to be answered: (1) Would the user of the product be expected to know of its dangers? (2) Is the risk in providing the product balanced by the benefit the user derives from using it? For example, if a manufacturer produced a product that was dangerous regardless of how well designed and how covered by warnings, the manufacturer would still be held strictly liable.

In a product liability case, the product manufacturer could use any of the common defenses: denying the allegations, claiming contributory negligence, and claiming assumption of risk. For the first, regardless of what the manufacturer does, there may always be some risk that cannot be completely avoided. Also, a particular product, e.g., a shovel, has had its design, shape, and function semi-standardized over many years through normal usage and user preferences. Essentially, the product is state of the art. Negligent use or misuse of the product by the user could be considered contributory negligence and used as a possible defense. This second issue overlaps with the third one, assumption of risk. If a user chose a particular product to use, e.g., a normal straight knife as opposed to a more ergonomically designed, but more expensive, bent-handled knife, then the user assumed the risk and the manufacturer may have some defense.

Other potential legal issues include: regulatory violations (e.g., OSHA standards), unfair labor practices, medical malpractice, and Worker Compensation. Although, Worker Compensation was meant to be a no-fault way of handling injury claims and compensation, there are some pitfalls for companies. It is not unusual for companies to "buy" a Workers Comp case. A recent hiree may have worked for many years on a stressful job at another company, recently switched to a better paying job at the current company (which presumably may also have deeper pockets), and only then files a claim. From the author's experience, it is difficult for the current company to avoid the Workers Comp claim, although better preemployment evaluation may help. In addition, companies need to be aware of individuals who attempt to "game" the system and continue filing claims to obtain benefits without working. Again, companies may mitigate such problem cases, by utilizing physicians who have occupational disorder experience (and may have even visited the plant) and assigning such workers to light-duty jobs.

In summary, the legal implications of WRMSDs are not simple and straightforward. There are many gray areas with complex interpretations of the law. But, in general, the more a company or a product manufacturer does to promote ergonomics and safety within the company, should benefit both the workers and consumers and also tend to mitigate unexpected legal problems. Further information on product liability can be obtained from Hammer (1993) and Owen (1994).

Questions

1. Describe the etiology of tendon-related disorders.

2. What are some of the common tendon-related disorders?

3. Name several muscle disorders.

4. What is the etiology of muscle disorders? How are they different from tendon disorders?

5. What is a trigger point?

6. What are some of the possible causes of nerve disorders?

7. What is the carpal tunnel? What is the purpose of the flexor retinaculum?

8. What are some of the common nerve disorders?

9. What is the white finger syndrome? How is it related to Raynaud's syndrome?

10. What is bursitis? What occupation is typically associated with bursitis in the knee?

11. Compare and contrast rheumatoid arthritis and osteoarthritis.

12. Describe some of the medical tests used to diagnose WRMSDs in the upper limbs? What is the gold standard for such diagnostic tests?

13. What are some of the medical remedies used for treating WRMSDs?

14. What are the two key issues that affect the effectiveness of an epidemiological study?

15. What are the three main types of epidemiological studies? What are the tradeoffs between these studies?

16. What is an intervention study? Why or why not may a cohort study be considered an intervention study?

17. What are the positive aspects and also limitations of a cohort study?

18. What factor in a cohort study changes it from a retrospective to a prospective study? Give an example that could be used for WRMSDs in an industrial situation.

19. Compare and contrast case-control and cross-sectional studies. What is the key difference?

20. Which of the observational studies is best for showing causality? Why?

21. What is prevalence? How is statistical significance established for prevalence?

22. What is the basis for a chi-square analysis?

23. What is a risk ratio and for what type of studies is it an appropriate analysis tool?

24. What is an OR and for what type of studies is it an appropriate analysis tool?

25. How is statistical significance established for an OR?

26. Compare and contrast a risk ratio to an OR? How may they be similar?

27. What is AR?

28. What is an incidence rate? How is it related to prevalence?

29. What is a logit function? What purpose does it serve in epidemiological studies?

30. What are some of the problems of multivariate modeling in epidemiological studies?

31. What are some of the ways of establishing the adequacy and validity of multivariate models?

32. What factors can be used define causality in epidemiological research?

33. What are the occupational WRMSD risk factors that appear consistently across most epidemiological studies? For each explain plausibility.

34. Which psychosocial and individual factors may contribute to upper limb WRMSDs? Explain plausibility for each of these.

35. What is iatrogenesis? Why may this be a factor in the reporting of WRMSDs?

36. How may the Hawthorne effect enter into the control of WRMSDs?

Problems

1. Show that Equations 6.8 and 6.14 are equivalent expressions.
2. A matched case-control study of power tool usage in an automotive assembly plant indicated that 190 of 320 workers using powers experienced some sort of WRMSD symptoms, while only 10 of 70 unexposed workers showed similar symptoms.
   a. What is the OR for power tool usage for WRMSD symptoms?
   b. Is this a statistically significant result?
3. A case-control study of indicated that 15 of 100 workers exposed to high forces on the job exhibited WRMSD symptoms, while only 10 of 200 unexposed workers showed similar symptoms.
   a. What is the OR for exposure?
   b. Is this a statistically significant result?
4. The Cool T-shirt Co. decided to evaluate the effects of an ergonomics program, which also included job rotation, rest breaks, and the elimination of its incentive program. After 2 years, in Plant A, with the ergonomics program, only 43 of 345 of sewers showed WRMSD symptoms, while, in Plant B, without an ergonomics program, 42 of 122 sewers showed WRMSD symptoms.
   a. What type of epidemiological study was utilized?
   b. What is risk ratio for exposure?
   c. Is this a statistically significant result?
5. A survey of 50 workers in a meatpacking plant regarding their working conditions (i.e., exposure to cold) and symptoms for white fingers yielded the following information:
   - 11 workers were exposed to cold and had symptoms for white fingers
   - 13 workers were exposed to cold but had no symptoms for white fingers
   - 3 workers were not exposed to cold but had symptoms for white fingers
   - 23 workers were not exposed to cold and had no symptoms for white fingers
     a. What type of epidemiological study was used in the plant?
     b. What are implications (i.e., limitations) for this type of a study?
     c. What is the prevalence of white fingers in workers exposed to cold?
     d. What is the prevalence of white fingers in workers not exposed to cold?
     e. What is the OR for incurring white fingers due to exposure to cold?
     f. Is this a statistically significant result? Use $\alpha = 0.05$.
     g. What does a chi-square analysis indicate?
     h. What is your overall conclusion regarding this plant?
6. Many workers in an electronics assembly plant have been reporting tingling sensations in the hand, which, in many cases, has been diagnosed as CTS. Initial observations indicate the use of high levels of pinch forces to insert wires into connectors. An ergonomist has suggested measuring the grip force ratio (force used divided by minimum force required) on a tracking task as a screening tool for CTS (the median nerve innervates the index finger) in addition to diagnostic testing of CTS by a physician.

Seven workers with strong symptoms of CTS are evaluated on the tracking task. Seven relatively similar symptom-free workers are also evaluated on the tracking task. The jobs of both sets of workers are studied for evidence of high-pinch forces. The following data are obtained:

CTS	Gender	Age	Wrist Circumference (mm)	Grip Force Ratio	Exposure to High Forces
Yes	M	35	184	7.4	Yes
Yes	F	35	168	7.7	Yes
Yes	F	57	156	10.0	Yes
Yes	F	45	187	6.0	Yes
Yes	F	56	193	4.0	No
Yes	F	29	145	5.6	No
Yes	M	43	189	7.2	Yes
No	M	31	168	5.0	No
No	F	40	159	4.6	No
No	F	62	161	5.0	Yes
No	F	45	153	4.6	No
No	F	47	151	5.4	Yes
No	F	33	166	3.8	No
No	M	45	174	3.2	No

a. What type of epidemiological study was used in the plant?

b. What are the implications (i.e., limitations) for this type of study?

c. Are the groups well matched? (*Hint:* Perform t-test on various characteristics.)

d. What is the prevalence of CTS in workers exposed to high-pinch forces?

e. What is the prevalence of CTS in workers not exposed to high-pinch forces?

f. What is the OR for incurring CTS due to exposure of high-pinch forces?

g. Is this a statistically significant result? Use $\alpha = 0.05$.

h. What does a chi-square analysis indicate?

i. Is the grip force ratio a good screening tools for CTS? Consider a ratio over 6 to be excessive.

j. Does it appear that any of the individual characteristics (age, gender, wrist circumference, grip force ratio) may predispose one to CTS? (Hint: Perform OR s on a binary breakdown for each characteristic. For example, consider 45 years as a dividing line between young and old workers.)

k. What are your overall conclusions regarding this plant and study.

7. Develop a multiple logistic-regression model for the data presented in Problem 6. Calculate the OR s and the respective confidence intervals for the significant factors.

8. A survey of 60 workers in a meatpacking plant regarding their working conditions and symptoms for "trigger finger" yielded the following information: (i) out of 20 workers using meat hooks, 14 had symptoms for trigger finger while 6 had no symptoms, and (ii) out of 40 workers not using meat hooks, 2 had symptoms for trigger finger while 38 had no symptoms.

a. What type of epidemiological study was used in the plant? What are the implications (i.e., limitations and/or advantages) for this type of a study?

b. What is the prevalence of trigger finger in workers using meat hooks? What is the prevalence of trigger finger in workers not using meat hooks?

c. What is the OR for incurring trigger finger due to using meat hooks? Is this a statistically significant result? Use $\alpha = 0.05$.

References

Adson, A.W. and Coffey, J.R. (1927). Cervical rib: A method of anterior approach for relief of symptom by division of the scalenus anticus. *Annals of Surgery* 85:839–857.

Afifi, A.A. and Clark, V. (1996). *Computer-Aided Multivariate Analysis*, 3rd edn, New York: Chapman & Hall.

Amano, M., Gensyo, U., Nakajima, H., and Yatsuki, K. (1988). Characteristics of work actions of shoe manufacturing assembly line workers and a cross-sectional factor-control study on occupational cervico-brachial disorders. *Japanese Journal of Industrial Health* 30:3–12.

Andersen, J.H. and Gaardboe, O. (1993a). Musculoskeletal disorders of the neck and upper limb among sewing machine operators: A clinical investigation. *American Journal of Industrial Medicine* 24:689–700.

Andersen, J.H. and Gaardboe, O. (1993b). Prevalence of persistent neck and upper limb pain in a historical cohort of sewing machine operators. *American Journal of Industrial Medicine* 24:677–687.

Arezzo, J.C., Shumburg, H.H., and Laudadio, C. (1986). Thermal sensitivity tester/device for quantitative assessment of thermal sense in diabetic neuropathy. *Diabetes* 35:590–592.

Arksey, H. (1998). *RSI and the Experts, the Construction of Medical Knowledge*. London, U.K.: UCL Press/Taylor & Francis.

Armstrong, T.J. (1983). *An Ergonomics Guide to Carpal Tunnel Syndrome*. Akron, OH: American Industrial Hygiene Association.

Armstrong, T.J. and Chaffin, D.B. (1978). An investigation of the relationship between displacements of the finger and wrist joints and the extrinsic finger flexor tendons. *Journal of Biomechanics* 11:119–128.

Armstrong, T.J., Fine, L.J., Goldstein, S.A., Lifshitz, Y.R., and Silverstein, B.A. (1987). Ergonomic considerations in hand and wrist tendonitis. *Journal of Hand Surgery* 12A:830–837.

Atroshi, I., Gummesson, C., Johnsson, R., Ornstein, E., Ranstam, J., and Rosen, I. (1999). Prevalence of carpal tunnel syndrome in a general population. *Journal of the American Medical Association* 282:153–158.

Awerbuch, M. (1985). RSI or "Kangaroo paw." *Medical Journal of Australia* 142:237–238.

Backman, C., Boquist, L., Friden, J., Lorentzon, R., and Toolanen, G. (1990). Chronic achilles paratenonitis with tendinosis: An experimental model in the rabbit. *Journal of Orthopaedic Research* 8:541–547.

Barnhart, S., Demers, P.A., Miller, M., Longstreth, W.T. Jr., and Rosenstock, L. (1991). Carpal tunnel syndrome among ski manufacturing workers. *Scandinavian Journal of Work, Environment & Health* 17:46–52.

Baron, S., Milliron, M., Habes, D., and Fidler, A. (1991). Hazard evaluation and technical assistance report: Shoprite supermarkets, NJ, NY. NIOSH Report No. HHE 88-344-2092. Cincinnati, OH: U.S. Department of Health and Human Services, National Institute for Occupational Health and Safety.

Bell, J.A. (1990). Light touch—Deep pressure testing using Semmes-Weinstein monofilaments. In: J.M. Hunter, E.J. Mackin, and A.D. Callahan (eds), *Rehabilitation of the Hand*. St. Louis: C.V. Mosby, pp. 585–593.

Bergkvist, U. (1984). Video display terminals and health. *Scandinavian Journal of Work, Environment & Health* 10:68–77.

Bergqvist, U., Wolfgast, E., Nilsson, B., and Voss, M. (1995a). Musculoskeletal disorders among visual display terminal workers: Individual, ergonomic, and work organizational factors. *Ergonomics* 38:763–776.

Bergqvist, U., Wolfgast, E., Nilsson, B., and Voss, M. (1995b). The influence of VDT work on musculoskeletal disorders. *Ergonomics* 38:754–762.

Bernard, B., Sauter, S., Fine, L.J., Petersen, M., and Hales, T. (1994). Job task and psychosocial risk factors for work-related musculoskeletal disorders among newspaper employees. *Scandinavian Journal of Work, Environment & Health* 20:417–426.

Bjelle, A., Hagberg, M., and Michaelsson, G. (1979). Clinical and ergonomic factors in prolonged shoulder pain among industrial workers. *Scandinavian Journal of Work, Environment & Health* 5:205–210.

Bongers, P.M., de Winter, C.R., Kompier, M.A.J., and Hildebrandt, V.H. (1993). Psychosocial factors at work and musculoskeletal disease. *Scandinavian Journal of Work, Environment & Health* 19:297–312.

Bovenzi, M. (1994). Hand-arm vibration syndrome and dose-response relation for vibration-induced white finger among quarry drillers and stonecarvers. Italian Study Group on Physical Hazards in the Stone Industry. *Occupational and Environmental Medicine* 51:603–611.

Bovenzi, M., Franzinelli, A., and Strambi, F. (1988). Prevalence of vibration-induced white finger and assessment of vibration exposure among travertine workers in Italy. *International Archives of Occupational and Environmental Health.* 61:25–34.

Bovenzi, M., Franzinelli, A., Mancini, R., Cannava, M.G., Maiorano, M., and Ceccarelli, F. (1995). Dose-response relation for vascular disorders induced by vibration in the fingers of forestry workers. *Occupational and Environmental Medicine* 52:722–730.

Bovenzi, M., Zadini, A., Franzinelli, A., and Borgogni, F. (1991). Occupational musculoskeletal disorders in the neck and upper limbs of forestry workers exposed to hand-arm vibration. *Ergonomics* 34:547–62.

Buch-Jaeger, N. and Foucher, G. (1994). Correlation of clinical signs with nerve conduction tests in the diagnosis of carpal tunnel syndrome. *Journal of Hand Surgery (Br).* 19:720–724.

Burt, S., Hornung, R., and Fine, L. (1990). Hazard evaluation and technical assistance report: Newsday, Inc., Melville, N.Y. NIOSH Report No. HHE 89-250-2046. Cincinnati, OH: U.S. Department of Health and Human Services, National Institute for Occupational Health and Safety.

Byström, S., Hall, C., Welander, T., and Kilbom, Å. (1995). Clinical disorders and pressure-pain threshold of the forearm and hand among automobile assembly line workers. *Journal of Hand Surgery* 20:782–790.

Campbell, D.T. and Stanley, J.C. (1966). *Experimental and Quasi-experimental Designs for Research.* Chicago, IL: Rand McNally.

Cannon, L.J., Bernacki, E.J., and Walter, S.D. (1981). Personal and occupational factors associated with carpal tunnel syndrome. *Journal of Occupational Medicine* 23:255–258.

Chaffin, D.B., Lee, M.W., and Freivalds, A. (1980). Muscle strength assessment from EMG analysis. *Medicine and Science in Sports and Exercise* 12:205–211.

Chang, K.Y., Ho, S.T., and Yu, H.S. (1994). Vibration induced neurophysiological and electron microscopical changes in rat peripheral nerves. *Occupational and Environmental Medicine* 51:130–135.

Chattarjee, D. (1992). Workplace upper limb disorders: A prospective study with intervention. *Journal of Occupational Medicine* 42:129–136.

Chiang, H., Chen, S., Yu, H., and Ko, Y. (1990). The occurrence of carpal tunnel syndrome in frozen food factory employees. *Kaohsiung Journal of Medical Sciences* 6:73–80.

Chiang, H., Ko, Y., Chen, S., Yu, H., Wu, T., and Chang, P. (1993). Prevalence of shoulder and upper-limb disorders among workers in the fish-processing industry. *Scandinavian Journal of Work, Environment& Health* 19:126–131.

Christensen, R. (1997). *Log-linear Models and Logistic Regression.* New York: Springer.

Cleland, L.G. (1987). "RSI", a model of social iatrogenesis. *Medical Journal of Australia* 147:236–239.

Cobb, C.R., deVries, H.A., Urban, R.T., Luekens, C.A., and Bagg, R.J. (1975). Electrical activity in muscle pain. *American Journal of Physical Medicine* 54:80–87.

Conway, H. and Svenson, J. (1998). Occupational injury and illness rates, 1992–1996: Why they fell. *Monthly Labor Review* November:36–58.

Cornefjord, M., Sato, K., Olmarker, K., Rydevik, B., and Nordborg, C. (1997). A model for chronic nerve root compression studies. Presentation of a porcine model for controlled, slow-onset compression with analyses of anatomic aspects, compression onset rate, and morphologic and neurophysiologic effect. *Spine* 22:946–57.

deKrom, M.C.T., Kester, A.D.M., Knipschild, P.G., and Spaans, F. (1990). Risk factors for carpal tunnel syndrome. *American Journal of Epidemiology* 132:1102–1110.

Dellon, A.L. (1983). The vibrometer. *Plastic and Reconstructive Surgery* 71:427–431.

Dellon, A.L. and Kallman, C.H. (1983). Evaluation of functional sensation in the hand. *Journal of Hand Surgery (Am)* 8:865–870.

Dempsey, P.G. (2007). Effectiveness of ergonomics interventions to prevent musculoskeletal disorders: Beware of what you ask. *International Journal of Industrial Ergonomics* 37:169–173.

Dunham, W., Haines, G., and Spring, J.M. (1972). Bowler's thumb ulnovolar neuroma of the thumb. *Clinical Orthopaedics* 83:99–101.

Dyck, P.J., Lais, A.C., Giannini, C., and Engelstad, J.K. (1990). Structural alterations of nerve during cuff compression. *Proceedings of the National Academy of Sciences* 87:9828–9832.

Ekberg, K., Björkqvist, B., Malm, P., Bjerre-Kiely, B., Karlsson, M., and Axelson, O. (1994). Case-control study of risk factors for disease in the neck and shoulder area. *Occupational and Environmental Medicine* 51:262–266.

Ekberg, K., Karlsson, M., and Axelson, O. (1995). Cross-sectional study of risk factors for symptoms in the neck and shoulder area. *Ergonomics* 38:971–980.

Elliott, B.G. (1992). Finkelstein's test: A descriptive error than can produce a false positive. *Journal of Hand Surgery (Br)* 17B:481–482.

English, C.J., Maclaren, W.M., Court-Brown, C., Hughes, S.P.F., Porter, R.W., and Wallace, W.A. (1995). Relations between upper limb soft tissue disorders and repetitive movements at work. *American Journal of Industrial Medicine* 27:75–90.

Faulkner, J.A. and Brooks, S.V. (1995). Muscle fatigue in old animals. Unique aspects of fatigue in elderly humans. *Advances in Experimental Medicine and Biology* 384:471–480.

Faulkner, J.A., Brooks, S.V., and Zerba, E. (1990). Skeletal muscle weakness and fatigue in old age: Underlying mechanisms. *Annual Review of Gerontology and Geriatrics* 10:147–166.

Feldman, R.G., Travers, P.H., Chirico-Post, J., and Keyserling, W.M. (1987). Risk assessment in electronic assembly workers: Carpal tunnel syndrome. *Journal of Hand Surgery* 12A:849–855.

Ferguson, D. (1971a). Repetition injuries in process workers. *Medical Journal of Australia* 2:408–412.

Ferguson, D. (1971b). An Australian study of telegraphists' cramp. *British Journal of Industrial Medicine* 28:280–285.

Ferguson, D. (1973). A study of neurosis and occupation. *British Journal of Industrial Medicine* 30:187–198.

Ferguson, D.A. (1987). "RSI": Putting the epidemic to rest. *Medical Journal of Australia* 147:213–214.

Finkelstein, J. (1939). Stenosing tendovaginitis at the radial styloid process. *Journal of Bone and Joint Surgery* 12:509–540.

Fleiss, J.L. (1981). *Statistical Methods for Rates and Proportions*. New York: John Wiley & Sons.

Frank, J.W., Pulcins, I.R., Mickey, S.K., Shannon, H.S., and Stansfeld, S.A. (1995). Occupational back pain—An unhelpful polemic. *Scandinavian Journal of Work, Environment & Health* 21:3–14.

Freivalds, A. (2009). *Niebel's Methods, Standard and Work Design*, 12th edn, New York: McGraw-Hill, pp. 387–389.

Friis, R.H. and Sellers, T.A. (1996). *Epidemiology for Public Health Practice*. Gaithersburg, MD: Aspen Publishers.

Gellman, H., Gelberman, R.H., Tan, A.M., and Botte, M.J. (1986). Carpal tunnel syndrome: An evaluation of the provocative diagnostic tests. *Journal of Bone and Joint Surgery* 68A:735–737.

Ghavnini, M.R. and Haghighat, M. (1998). Carpal tunnel syndrome: Reappraisal of five clinical tests. *Electromyography and Clinical Neurophysiology* 38:437–441.

Greenberg, R.S. (1986). Prospective studies. In: S. Kotz and N.L. Johnson (eds), *Encyclopedia of Statistical Sciences*, Vol. 7. New York: John Wiley & Sons, pp. 315–319.

Greenberg, R.S., Daniels, S.R., and Flanders, D.W. (1996). *Medical Epidemiology*, 3rd edn, New York: McGraw-Hill.

Hadler, N. (1986). Industrial rheumatology—The Australian and New Zealand experiences with arm pain and backache in the workplace. *Medical Journal of Australia* 144:191–195.

Hadler, N. (1990). Cumulative trauma disorders, an iatrogenic concept. *Journal of Occupational Medicine* 32:38–41.

Hadler, N. (1993). *Occupational Musculoskeletal Disorders*. New York: Raven Press.

Hagberg, M. and Wegman, D.H. (1987). Prevalence rates and odds ratios of shoulder-neck diseases in different occupational groups. *British Journal of Industrial Medicine* 44:602–610.

Hales, T.R. and Fine, L. (1989). Hazard evaluation and technical assistance report: Cargill Poultry Division, Buena Vista, CA. NIOSH Report No. HHE 89-251-1997. Cincinnati, OH: U.S. Department of Health and Human Services, National Institute for Occupational Health and Safety.

Hales, T.R., Sauter, S.L., Petersen, M.R., Fine, L.J., Putz-Anderson, V., Schleifer, L.R., Ochs, T.T., and Bernard, B.P. (1994). Musculoskeletal disorders among visual display terminal users in a telecommunications company. *Ergonomics* 37:1603–1621.

Hammer, W. (1993). *Product Safety Management and Engineering*. Englewood Cliffs, NJ: Prentice-Hall.

Hart, D.A., Frank, C.B., and Bray, R.C. (1995). Inflammatory processes in repetitive motion and overuse syndromes: Potential role of neurogenic mechanisms in tendons and ligaments. In: S.L. Gordon, S.J. Blair, and L.J. Fine (eds), *Repetitive Motion Disorders of the Upper Extremity*. Rosemont, IL: American Academy of Orthopaedic Surgeons. pp. 247–262.

Hedlund, U. (1989). Raynaud's phenomenon of fingers and toes of miners exposed to local and whole-body vibration and cold. *International Archives of Occupational & Environmental Health* 61:457–461.

Herberts, P., Kadefors, R., Andersson, G., and Petersen, I. (1981). Shoulder pain in industry: An epidemiological study on welders. *Acta Orthopaedica Scandinavica* 52:299–306.

Herberts, P., Kadefors, R., Högfors, C., and Sigholm, G. (1984). Shoulder pain and heavy manual labor. *Clinical Orthopaedics* 191:166–178.

Hoekstra, E.J., Hurrell, J.J., and Swanson, N.G. (1994). Hazard evaluation and technical assistance report: Social Security Administration Teleservice Centers, Boston, MA, Fort Lauderdale, FL. NIOSH Report No. HHE 92-382-2450. Cincinnati, OH: U.S. Department of Health and Human Services, National Institute for Occupational Health and Safety.

Holmström, E.B., Lindell, J., and Moritz, U. (1992). Low back and neck/shoulder pain in construction workers: Occupational workload and psychosocial risk factors. *Spine* 17:663–671.

Hosmer, D.W. and Lemeshow, S. (1989). *Applied Logistic Regression*. New York: John Wiley & Sons.

Houtman, I.L.D., Bongers, P.M., Smulders, P.G.W., and Kompier, M.A.J. (1994). Psychosocial stressors at work and musculoskeletal problems. *Scandinavian Journal of Work, Environment & Health* 20:139–145.

Howell, E. and Leach, R.E. (1970). Bowler's thumb. *Journal of Bone and Joint Surgery* 52A:379–381.

Hughes, R.E., Silverstein, B.A., and Evanoff, B.A. (1997). Risk factors for work-related musculoskeletal disorders in an aluminum smelter. *American Journal of Industrial Medicine* 32:66–75.

Hünting, W., Läubli, T.H., and Grandjean, E. (1981). Postural and visual loads at VDT workplaces, I. Constrained postures. *Ergonomics* 24:917–931.

Hurrell, J.J. and Murphy, L.R. (1992). Psychological job stress. In: W.N. Rom (ed.), *Environmental and Occupational Medicine*, 2nd edn, New York: Little, Brown and Co., pp. 675–684.

Jennings, D.E. (1986). Judging inferences adequacy in logistic regression. *Journal of the American Statistical Association* 81:471–476.

Jensen, R. (1996). Mechanisms of spontaneous tension-type headaches: An analysis of tenderness, pain thresholds and EMG. *Pain* 64:251–256.

Jensen, R. and Olesen, J. (1996). Initiating mechanisms of experimentally induced tension-type headache. *Cephalalgia* 16:175–182.

Johnson, E.W. (1989). The myth of skeletal muscle spasm. *American Journal of Physical Medicine and Rehabilitation* 68:1.

Kaji, R. (2000). Facts and fancies on writer's cramp. *Muscle Nerve* 23:1313–1315.

Kamwendo, K., Linton, S.J., and Moritz, U. (1991). Neck and shoulder disorders in medical secretaries. Part I. Pain prevalence and risk factors. *Scandinavian Journal of Rehabilitation Medicine* 23:127–133.

Karasek, R.A., Gardell, B., and Lindell, J. (1987). Work and non-work correlates of illness and behaviour in male and female Swedish white collar workers. *Journal of Occupational Behavior* 8:187–207.

Kiken, S., Stringer, W., and Fine, L.J. (1990). Hazard evaluation and technical assistance report: Perdue Farms, Lewistown, N.C.; Robersonville, N.C. NIOSH Report No. HHE 89-307-2009. Cincinnati, OH: U.S. Department of Health and Human Services, National Institute for Occupational Health and Safety.

Kivekäs, J., Riihimäki, H., Husman, K., Hänninen, K., Härkönen, H., Kuusela, T., Pekkarinen, M., Tola, S., and Zitting, A.J. (1994). Seven-year follow-up of white-finger symptoms and radiographic wrist findings in lumberjacks and referents. *Scandinavian Journal of Work, Environment & Health* 20, 101–106.

Kuan, T.B. (2009). Current studies on myofascial pain syndrome. *Current Pain and Headache Reports* 13:365–369.

Kukkonen, R., Luopajärvi, T., and Riihimäki, V. (1983). Prevention of fatigue among data entry operators. In: T.O. Kvalseth (ed.), *Ergonomics of Workstation Design*. London, UK: Buttersworth, pp. 28–34.

Kumar, S. (2001). Theories of musculoskeletal injury causation. *Ergonomics* 44:17–47.

Kuorinka, I. and Forcier, L. (1995). *Work Related Musculoskeletal Disorders (WMSDs): A Reference Book for Prevention*. London: Taylor & Francis.

Kuorinka, I. and Koskinen, P. (1979). Occupational rheumatic diseases and upper limb strain in manual jobs in a light mechanical industry. *Scandinavian Journal of Rehabilitation Medicine* 5 (Suppl 3): 39–47.

Kurppa, K., Viikari-Juntura, E., Kuosma, E., Huuskonen, M., and Kivi, P. (1991). Incidence of tenosynovitis or peritendinitis and epicondylitis in a meat-processing factory. *Scandinavian Journal of Work, Environment & Health* 17:32–37.

Kvarnström, S. (1983). Occurrence of musculoskeletal disorders in a manufacturing industry with special attention to occupational shoulder disorders. *Scandinavian Journal of Rehabilitation Medicine* 15 (Suppl 8):1–114.

Lagerström, M., Wenemark, M., Hagberg, M., and Hjelm, E.W. (1995). Occupational and individual factors related to musculoskeletal symptoms in five body regions among Swedish nursing personnel. *International Archives of Occupational & Environmental Health* 68:27–35.

Larsson, S.E., Bodegard, L., Henriksen, K.G., and Öberg, P.A. (1990). Chronic trapezius myalgia: Morphology and blood flow studied in 17 patients. *Acta Orthopaedica Scandinavica* 61:394–398.

Lawrence, R.C., Helmick, C.G., Arnett, F.C., Deyo, R.A., Felson, D.T., Giannini, E.H., Heyse, S.P., Hirsch, R., Hochberg, M.C., Hunder, G.G., Lian, M.H., Pillemer, S.R., Steen, V.D., and Wolfe, F. (1998). Estimates of the prevalence of arthritis and selected musculoskeletal disorders in the United States. *Arthritis and Rheumatism* 41:778–799.

Leclerc, A., Franchi, P., Cristofari, M.F., Delemotte, B., Mereau, P., Teyssier-Cotte, C., and Touranchet, A. (1998). Carpal tunnel syndrome and work organisation in repetitive work: A cross sectional study in France. Study Group on Repetitive Work. *Occupational & Environmental Medicine* 55:180–187.

Lemasters, G.K., Atterbury, M.R., Booth-Jones, A.D., Bhattacharya, A., Ollila-Glenn, N., Forrester, C., and Forst, L. (1998). Prevalence of work related musculoskeletal disorders in active union carpenters. *Occupational & Environmental Medicine* 55:421–427.

Letz, R., Cherniack, M.G., Gerr, F., Hershman, D., and Pace, P. (1992). A cross-sectional epidemiological survey of shipyard workers exposed to hand-arm vibration. *British Journal of Industrial Medicine* 49:53–62.

Linton, S.J. and Kamwendo, K. (1989). Risk factors in the psychosocial work environment for neck and shoulder pain in secretaries. *Journal of Occupational Medicine* 31:609–613.

Lowe, B.D. and Freivalds, A. (1999). Effect of carpal tunnel syndrome on grip force coordination on hand tools. *Ergonomics* 42:550–564.

Lundborg, G. (1988). *Nerve Injury and Repair*. Edinburgh, U.K.: Churchill Livingstone.

Lundborg, G., Lie-Stenström, A.K., Sollerman, C., Strömberg, T., and Pyykko, I. (1986). Digital vibrogram: A new diagnostic tool for sensory testing in compression neuropathy. *Journal of Hand Surgery* 11A:693–699.

Luopajärvi, T., Kuorinka, I., Virolainen, M., and Holmberg, M. (1979). Prevalence of tenosynovitis and other injuries of the upper extremities in repetitive work. *Scandinavian Journal of Rehabilitation Medicine* 5 (Suppl 3):48–55.

Magnavita, N., Bevilacqua, L., Mirk, P., Fileni, A., and Castellino, N. (1999). Work-related musculoskeletal complaints in sonologists. *Journal of Occupational and Environmental Medicine* 41:981–988.

Malaviya, P., Butler, D.L., Boivin, G.P., Smith, F.N., Barry, F.P., Murphy, J.M., and Vogel, K.G. (2000). An in vivo model for load-modulated remodeling in the rabbit flexor tendon. *Journal of Orthopaedic Research* 18:116–125.

Mantel, N. and Haenszel, W. (1959). Statistical aspects of the analysis of data from retrospective studies of disease. *Journal of National Cancer Institute* 22:719–748.

Marcus, M. and Gerr, F. (1996). Upper extremity musculoskeletal symptoms among female office workers: Associations with video display terminal use and occupational psychosocial stressors. *American Journal of Industrial Medicine* 29:161–170.

Mathiowetz, V., Kashman, N., Volland, G., Weber, K., Dowe, M., and Rogers, S. (1985). Grip and pinch strength: Normative data for adults. *Archives for Physical Medicine and Rehabilitation* 66:69–72.

McComas, A. (1996). *Skeletal Muscle Form and Function*. Champaign, IL: Human Kinetics.

McCully, K.K. and Faulkner, J.A. (1985). Injury to skeletal muscle fibres of mice following lengthening contractions. *Journal of Applied Physiology* 59:119–126.

McKenna, K., McGrann, S., Blann, A., and Allen, J. (1993). An investigation into the acute vascular effects of riveting. *British Journal of Industrial Medicine* 50:160–166.

Mense, S. and Simons, D.G. (2000). *Muscle Pain, Understanding Its Nature, Diagnosis, and Treatment*. Philadelphia, PA: Lippincott Williams & Wilkins.

Mense, S., Simons, D.G., Hoheisel, U., and Quenzer, B. (2003). Lesions of rat skeletal muscle after local block of acetylcholinesterase and neuromuscular stimulation. *Journal of Applied Physiology* 94:2494–2501.

Milerad, E. and Ekenvall, L. (1990). Symptoms of the neck and upper extremities in dentists. *Scandinavian Journal of Work, Environment & Health* 16:129–134.

Mirbod, S.M., Yoshida, H., Komura, Y., Fujita, S., Nagata, C., Miyashita, K., Inaba, R., and Iwata, H. (1994). Prevalence of Raynaud's phenomenon in different groups of workers operating hand-held vibrating tools. *International Archives of Occupational and Environmental Health* 66:13–22.

Moore, J.S. and Garg, A. (1994). Upper extremity disorders in a pork processing plant: Relationship between job risk factors and morbidity. *American Industrial Hygiene Association Journal* 55:703–715.

Morgenstern, H., Kelsh, M., Kraus, J., and Margolis, W. (1991). A cross-sectional study of hand/wrist symptoms in female grocery checkers. *American Journal of Industrial Medicine* 20:209–218.

Mosconi, T. and Kruger, L. (1996). Fixed-diameter polyethylene cuffs applied to the rat sciatic nerve induce a painful neuropathy: Ultrasound morphometric analysis of axonal alterations. *Pain* 64:37–57.

Nagata, C., Yoshida, H., Mirbod, S., Komura, Y., Fujita, S., Inaba, R., Iwata, H., Maeda, M., Shikano, Y., and Ichiki, Y. (1993). Cutaneous signs (Raynaud's phenomenon, sclerodactylia, and edema of the hands) and hand-arm vibration exposure. *International Archives of Occupational and Environmental Health* 64:587–591.

Nathan, P.A., Meadows, K.D., and Doyle, L.S. (1988). Occupation as a risk factor for impaired sensory conduction of the median nerve at the carpal tunnel. *Journal of Hand Surgery* 13B:167–170.

Nathan, P.A., Keniston, R.C., Myers, L.D., and Meadows, K.D. (1992). Longitudinal study of median nerve sensory conduction in industry: Relationship to age, gender, hand dominance, occupational hand use, and clinical diagnosis. *Journal of Hand Surgery* 17A:850–857.

National Research Council. (2001). *Musculoskeletal Disorders and the Workplace*. Washington DC: National Academy of Press.

Necking, L.E., Lundstrom, R., Dahlin, L.B., Lundborg, G., Thornell, L.E., and Friden, J. (1966). Tissue displacement is a causative factor in vibration-induced muscle injury. *Journal of Hand Surgery (Br)* 21:753–757.

Nicholas, J.A. (1990). Clinical observations on sports-induced soft-tissue injuries. In: W.B. Leadbetter, J.A. Buckwalter, and S.L. Gordon (eds), *Sports-Induced Inflammation: Clinical and Basic Science Concepts*. Rosemont, IL: American Academy of Orthopedic Surgeons, p. 143.

Nilsson, T., Burström, L., and Hagberg, M. (1989). Risk assessment of vibration exposure and white fingers among platers. *International Archives of Occupational and Environmental Health* 61:473–481.

NIOSH. (1989). *Carpal Tunnel Syndrome: Selected References*. Cincinnati, OH: National Institute for Occupational Safety and Health.

NIOSH. (1995). Cumulative trauma disorders in the workplace: Bibliography. Report No. 95-119. Cincinnati, OH: National Institute for Occupational Safety and Health.

NIOSH. (1997). Musculoskeletal disorders and workplace factors. Report No. 97-141. Cincinnati, OH: National Institute for Occupational Safety and Health.

Noonan, T.J., Best, T.M., Seaber, A.V., and Garrett, W.E. (1994). Identification of a threshold for skeletal muscle injury. *American Journal of Sports Medicine* 22:257–261.

Ohlsson, K., Hansson, G.A., Balogh, I., Strömberg, U., Pålsson, B., Nordander, C., Rylander, L., and Skerfving, S. (1994). Disorders of the neck and upper limbs in women in fish processing industry. *Occupational and Environmental Medicine* 51:826–832.

Ohlsson, K., Attewell, R., Pålsson, B., Karlsson, B., Balogh, I., Johnsson, B., Ahlm, A., and Skerfving, S. (1995). Repetitive industrial work and neck and upper limb disorders in females. *American Journal of Industrial Medicine* 27:731–747.

Okutsu, I., Ninomiya, S., Hamanaka, I., Kuroshima, N., and Inanami, H. (1989). Measurement of pressure in the carpal canal before and after endoscopic management of carpal tunnel syndrome. *Journal of Bone and Joint Surgery* 71A:679–683.

Olsen, N. and Nielsen, S.L. (1988). Vasoconstrictor response to cold in forestry workers: A prospective study. *British Journal of Industrial Medicine* 45:39–42.

Osorio, A.M., Ames, R.G., Jones, J., Castorina, J., Rempel, D., Estrin, W., and Thompson, D. (1994). Carpal tunnel syndrome among grocery store workers. *American Industrial Hygiene Association Journal* 25:229–245.

Owen, R.D. (1994). Carpal tunnel syndrome: A products liability prospective. *Ergonomics* 37:449–476.

Parker, K.G. and Imbus, H.R. (1992). *Cumulative Trauma Disorders*. Chelsea, MI: Lewis Publishers.

Phalen, G.S. (1966). The carpal-tunnel syndrome. *The Journal of Bone and Joint Surgery* 48A:211–228.

Pocekay, D., McCurdy, S.A., Samuales, S.J., Hammond, K., and Schenker, M.B. (1995). A cross-sectional study of musculoskeletal symptoms and risk factors in semiconductor workers. *American Journal of Industrial Medicine* 28:861–871.

Praemer, A., Furner, S., and Rice, D.P. (1999). *Musculoskeletal Conditions in the United States*. Rosemont, IL: American Academy of Orthopaedic Surgeons.

Punnett, L., Robins, J.M., Wegman, D.H., and Keyserling, W.M. (1985). Soft-tissue disorders in the upper limbs of female garment workers. *Scandinavian Journal of Work, Environment & Health* 11:417–425.

Punnett, L., Fine, L.J., Keyserling, W.M., Herrin, G.D., and Chaffin, D.B. (1991). Back disorders and nonneutral trunk postures of automobile assembly workers. *Scandinavian Journal of Work, Environment & Health* 17:337–346.

Putz-Anderson, V. (1994). *Cumulative Trauma Disorders: A Manual for Musculoskeletal Diseases of the Upper Limbs*. London: Taylor & Francis.

Reinstein, L. (1983). DeQuervain's stenosing tenosynovitis in a video game player. *Archives of Physical Medicine and Rehabilitation* 64:434–435.

Rempel, D. (1995). Musculoskeletal loading and carpal tunnel pressure. In: S.L. Gordon, S.J. Blair, and L.J. Fine (eds), *Repetitive Motion Disorders of the Upper Extremity*. Rosemont, IL: American Academy of Orthopaedic Surgeons, pp. 123–133.

Ritz, B.R. (1995). Humeral epicondylitis among gas and waterworks employees. *Scandinavian Journal of Work, Environment & Health* 21:478–486.

Robert, A.W., Cynthia, B., and Thomas, J.A. (1994). Reverse Phalen's maneuver as an aid in diagnosing carpal tunnel syndrome. *Archives of Physical Medicine and Rehabilitation* 75:783–786.

Roland, M.O. (1986). A critical review of the evidence for a pain-spasm-pain cycle in spinal disorders. *Clinical Biomechanics* 1:102–109.

Roquelaure, Y., Mechali, S., Dano, C., Fanello, S., Benetti, F., Bureau, D., Mariel, J., Martin, Y.H., Derriennic, F., and Penneau-Fontbonne, D. (1997), Occupational and personal risk factors for carpal tunnel syndrome in industrial workers. *Scandinavian Journal of Work, Environment & Health*. 23:364–369.

Rossignol, A.M., Morse, E.P., Summers, V.M., and Pagnotto, L.D. (1987). Video display terminal use and reported health symptoms among Massachusetts clerical workers. *Journal of Occupational Medicine* 29:112–118.

Roto, P. and Kivi, P. (1984). Prevalence of epicondylitis and tenosynovitis among meatcutters. *Scandinavian Journal of Work, Environment & Health* 10:203–205.

Rydevik, B., Lundborg, G., and Nordborg, C. (1976). Intraneural tissue reactions induced by internal neurolysis. *Scandinavian Journal of Plastic and Reconstructive Surgery* 10:3–8.

Sackett, D.L. (1979). Bias in analytic research. *Journal of Chronic Diseases* 32:51–63.

Sahai, H. and Khurshid, K. (1996). *Statistics in Epidemiology*. New York: CRC Press.

Sakakibara, H., Miyao, M., Kondo, T., and Yamada, S. (1995). Overhead work and shoulder-neck pain in orchard farmers harvesting pears and apples. *Ergonomics* 38:700–706.

Sauter, S.L. and Swanson, N.G. (1996). Model of musculoskeletal disorders in office work. In: S. Moon and S. Sauter (eds), *Beyond Biomechanics Psychosocial Factors and Musculoskeletal Disorders*. Office work London: Taylor & Francis, pp. 2–18.

Schibye, B., Skov, T., Ekner, D., Christiansen, J., and Sjögaard, G. (1995). Musculoskeletal symptoms among sewing machine operators. *Scandinavian Journal of Work, Environment & Health* 21:427–434.

Schottland, J.R., Kirschberg, G.J., Fillingim, R., Davis, V.P., and Hogg, F. (1991). Median nerve latencies in poultry processing workers: An approach to resolving the role of industrial "cumulative trauma" in the development of carpal tunnel syndrome. *Journal of Occupational Medicine* 33:627–631.

Sheehy, M.P. and Marsden, C.D. (1982). Writer's cramp—A focal dystonia. *Brain* 105:461–480.

Shurr, D.G., Blair, W.F., and Bassett, G. (1986). Electromyographic changes after carpal tunnel release. *Journal of Hand Surgery (Am)* 11:876–880.

Silverstein, B.A., Fine, L.J., and Armstrong, T.J. (1987). Occupational factors and the carpal tunnel syndrome. *American Journal of Industrial Medicine* 11:343–358.

Simons, D.G. and Travell, J.G. (1983). Myofascial origins of low back pain. *Postgraduate Medicine* 73:66–73.

Simonsen, E.B., Klitgaard, H., and Bojsen-Moller, F. (1995), The influence of strength training, swim training and ageing on the Achilles tendon and m. soleus of the rat. *Journal of Sports Sciences* 13:291–295.

Sjøgaard, G. and Jensen, B.R. (1997). Muscle pathology with overuse. In: Ranney, D. (ed), *Chronic Musculoskeletal Injuries in the Workplace*. Philadelphia, PA: W.B. Saunders Co., pp. 17–40.

Sjøgaard, G. and Søgaard, K. (1998). Muscle injury in repetitive motion disorders. *Clinical Orthopaedics and Related Research* 351:21–31.

Skie, M., Zeiss, J., Ebraheim, N.A., and Jackson, W.T. (1990). Carpal tunnel changes and median nerve compression during wrist flexion and extension seen by magnetic resonance imaging. *Journal of Hand Surgery* 15A:934–939.

Sommer, C., Gailbraith, J.A., Heckman, H.M., and Myers, R.R. (1993). Pathology of experimental compression neuropathy producing hyperesthesia. *Journal of Neuropathology and Experimental Neurology* 52:223–233.

Sorock, G.S. and Courtney, T.K. (1996). Epidemiologic concerns for ergonomists: Illustrations from the musculoskeletal disorder literature. *Ergonomics* 39:562–578.

Stenlund, B., Goldie, I., Hagberg, M., Hogstedt, C., and Marions, O. (1992). Radiographic osteoarthrosis in the acromioclavicular joint resulting from manual work or exposure to vibration. *British Journal of Industrial Medicine* 49:588–593.

Stewart, J.D. and Eisen, A. (1978). Tinel's sign and the carpal tunnel syndrome. *British Medical Journal* 2(6145):1125–1126.

Strömberg, T., Dahlin, L.B., Brun, A., and Lundborg, G. (1997). Structural nerve damage at wrist level in workers exposed to vibration. *Occupational and Environmental Medicine* 54:307–311.

Takeuchi, T., Futatsuka, M., Imanishi, H., and Yamada, S. (1986). Pathological changes observed in the finger biopsy of patients with vibration-induced white finger. *Scandinavian Journal of Work, Environment & Health* 12:280–283.

Tanaka, S., Wild, D.K., Cameron, L., and Freund, E. (1997). Association of occupational and non-occupational risk factors with the prevalence of self-reported carpal tunnel syndrome in a national survey of the working population. *American Journal of Industrial Medicine* 32:550–556.

Tanaka, S., Wild, D.K., Seligman, P.J., Haperin, W.E., Behrens, V.J., and Putz-Anderson, V. (1995). Prevalence and work-relatedness of self-reported carpal tunnel syndrome among U.S. workers' analysis of the Occupational Health Supplement data of the 1988 National Health Interview Survey. *American Journal of Industrial Medicine* 27:451–470.

Taylor, W. (1982). Vibration white finger in the workplace. *Journal of the Society of Occupational Medicine* 32:159–166.

Taylor, W., Wasserman, D., Behrens, V., Reynolds, D., and Samueloff, S. (1984). Effect of the air hammer on the hands of stonecutters. The limestone quarries of Bedford, Indiana, revisited. *British Journal of Industrial Medicine* 41:289–295.

Thun, M., Tanaka, S., Smith, A.B., Halperin, W.E., Lee, S.T., Luggen, M.E., and Hess, E.V. (1987). Morbidity from repetitive knee trauma in carpet and floor layers. *British Journal of Industrial Medicine* 44:611–620.

Tine, J. (1915). Le signe du "fourmillement" dans les lésions des nerfs périphériques ('Pins and needles' signs of peripheral nerve lesions). *Presse Médicale* 23:388–389.

Tola, S., Riihimäki, H., Videman, T., Viikari-Juntura, E., and Hänninen, K. (1988). Neck and shoulder symptoms among men in machine operating, dynamic physical work and sedentary work. *Scandinavian Journal of Work, Environment & Health* 14:299–305.

Toomingas, A., Theorell, T., Michelsen, H., and Nordemar, R. (1997). Associations between self-rated psychosocial work conditions and musculoskeletal symptoms and signs. Stockholm MUSIC I Study Group. *Scandinavian Journal of Work, Environment & Health* 23:130–139.

Travell, J.G. and Simons, D.G. (1983). *Myofascial Pain and Dysfunction—The Trigger Point Manual.* Baltimore, MD: Williams & Wilkins.

Travell, J., Rinzler, S., and Herman, M. (1942). Pain and disability of the shoulder and arm. *Journal of the American Medical Association* 120:417–422.

Veiersted, K.B. and Westgaard, R.H. (1994). Subjectively assessed occupational and individual parameters as risk factors for trapezius myalgia. *International Journal of Industrial Ergonomics* 13:235–245.

Viegas, S.F. and Torres, F.G. (1989). Cherry pitter's thumb. Case report and review of the literature. *Orthopaedic Review* 18:336–338.

Viikari-Juntura, E.J., Kurppa, K., Kuosma, E., Huuskonen, M., Kuorinka, I., Ketola, R., and Kanni, U. (1991a). Prevalence of epicondylitis and elbow pain in the meat processing industry. *Scandinavian Journal of Work, Environment & Health* 17:38–45.

Viikari-Juntura, E.J., Vuori, J., Silverstein, B., Kalimo, R., Kuosma, E., and Videman, T. (1991b) A life-long prospective study on the role of psychosocial factors in neck-shoulder and low back pain. *Spine*, 16, 1056–1061.

Viikari-Juntura, E.J., Riihimäki, H., Tola, S., Videman, T., and Mutanen, P. (1994). Neck trouble in machine operating, dynamic physical work and sedentary work: A prospective study on occupational and individual risk factors. *Journal of Clinical Epidemiology* 47:1411–1422.

Warren, G.L., Hayes, D.A., Lowe, D.A., Prior, B.M., and Armstrong, R.B. (1993). Material fatigue initiates eccentric contraction-induced injury in rat soleus muscle. *Journal of Applied Physiology* 464:477–489.

Welch, L.S., Hunting, K.L, and Kellogg, J. (1995). Work-related musculoskeletal symptoms among sheet metal workers. *American Journal of Industrial Medicine* 27:783–791.

Wells, J.A., Zipp, J.F., Shuette, P.T., and McEleney, J. (1983). Musculoskeletal disorders among letter carriers. *Journal of Occupational Medicine* 25:814–820.

Wieslander, G., Norback, D., Gothe, C.J., and Juhlin, L. (1989). Carpal tunnel syndrome (CTS) and exposure to vibration, repetitive wrist movements, and heavy manual work: A case-referent study. *British Journal of Industrial Medicine* 46:43–47.

Wilks, S. (1878). *Lectures on Diseases of the Nervous System*. London: Churchill, pp. 452–460.

Woo, S.L., Ritter, M.A., Amiel, D., Sanders, T.M., Gomez, M.A., Kuei, S.C., Garfin, S.R., and Akeson, W.H. (1980). The biomechanical and biochemical properties of swine tendons—Long term effects of exercise on digital extensors. *Connective Tissue Research* 7:177–183.

Woodward, M. (1999). *Epidemiology, Study Design and Data Analysis*. New York: Chapman & Hall.

You, H. (1999). The development of a risk assessment model for carpal tunnel syndrome. Unpublished PhD thesis. University Park, PA: Penn State University.

You, H., Simmons, Z., Freivalds, A., Kothari, M.J., Naidu, S.H., and Young, R. (2004). The development of risk assessment models for carpal tunnel syndrome: A case-reference study. *Ergonomics* 47:668–709.

Yu, I.T.S. and Wong, T.W. (1995). Musculoskeletal problems among VDU workers in a Hong Kong bank. *Occupational Medicine* 46:275–280.

Yu, Z.S., Chao, H., Qiao, L., Qian, D.S., and Ye, Y.H. (1986). Epidemiologic survey of vibration syndrome among riveters, chippers and grinder in the railroad system of the People's Republic of China. *Scandinavian Journal of Work, Environment & Health* 12:289–292.

7

Instrumentation

7.1 Introduction

Any biomechanics instrumentation or measurement technique, whether for research or industrial or in-the-field evaluations, needs to meet certain criteria for usefulness (Brand and Crowninshield, 1981; Chaffin et al., 1999). These include the following:

1. The measured parameter should correlate accurately with the human function of interest, i.e., the instrument should be valid.
2. The measurement should be both accurate and repeatable, i.e., the instrument should be reliable.
3. The measurement should distinguish between normal and abnormal results, i.e., the instrument should be specific and sensitive.
4. The measurement should not significantly alter the function of interest.
5. The instrument or technique should be safe to use.
6. The instrument should be simple to use, relatively portable, relatively inexpensive, and insensitive to external noise.

The quantitative aspects of validity, reliability, sensitivity, and specificity are discussed in greater detail in Chapter 8. This chapter describes the different equipment and tools needed to evaluate human capability and capacities of the upper limbs, especially as related to the likelihood of developing musculoskeletal disorders. The practicalities of these measurements with respect to the above criteria are also discussed.

7.2 Wrist- and Finger-Motion Measurements

7.2.1 Types of Measurement Devices

Various technologies for measuring wrist motions have been developed, but none has received universal acceptance. One such approach is based on videotape analysis of wrist motion. Developed by Armstrong et al. (1982), it utilizes a frame-by-frame analysis of videotape that records wrist flexion/extension in one of five categories and radial/ulnar deviation in one of three categories. This method requires considerable time and effort because each individual frame has to be analyzed manually, and yields absolute resolutions of only 30° for flexion/extension and 20° for radial/ulnar deviation. In addition, dynamic variables of the wrist, such as angular velocity and acceleration, are not easily obtainable with this type of analysis.

Another such method of wrist-motion measurement was developed by Logan and Groszewski (1989) and utilizes an electromagnetic three space-digitizer sensor system to obtain real-time six degrees of freedom position information. Sensors determine specific x, y, z coordinates and θ, φ, ψ orientation angles with respects to a coordinate system based on a low-frequency magnetic field. Further analysis of this data provides flexion/extension, radial/ulnar deviation, and pronation/supination angles. Although this system provided useful information for a number of work tasks in the food processing industry, the system appeared to require excessive amount of time for data acquisition and reduction and had limitations due to its instrumentation and magnetic noise.

Another very common approach is the simple goniometer with its output assessed electrically or mechanically. Typically, goniometers are relatively small and lightweight offering quick and objective measurements of wrist joint motions (Nicole, 1987; Ojima et al., 1991; Hansson et al., 1996; Buchholz and Wellman, 1997). Numerous studies have already been performed using electrogoniometers (goniometers with electrical output) in laboratory, factory, and clinical fields. For example, Smutz et al. (1994) employed an electrogoniometer for measuring wrist posture in their ergonomic assessment of keyboard design. Moore et al. (1991) used the electrogoniometer to quantify wrist motion of ergonomic risk factors, and Ojima et al. (1991) performed a dynamic analysis of wrist circumduction using the electrogoniometer in clinical field. However, in all these studies extensive calibration techniques were required.

Schoenmarklin and Marras (1993) developed an electromechanical goniometer to collect online data of wrist movements of flexion/extension, radial/ulnar deviation, and pronation/supination planes simultaneously. Further analyses of the data yielded angular velocity and acceleration. This wrist monitor was composed of two thin metal strips, placed on two adjacent segments with a rotary potentiometer placed at the center of the joint. This system produced relatively accurate and repeatable results. However, it was relatively uncomfortable and obtrusive for hand motion.

There are several commercial goniometers (Biometrics Ltd, Gwent, United Kingdom, and BIOPAC Systems Inc., Santa Barbara, California; http://www.biopac.com/) currently available for measuring both wrist flexion/extension and radial/ulnar deviation, and forearm rotation of pronation/supination. These devices consist of two plastic end blocks that are separated by a flexible spring protecting a strain wire (see Figure 7.1). The goniometers incorporate gauge elements that measure bending strain along or around a particular axis. Biaxial goniometers measure orthogonal rotational axes simultaneously (e.g., wrist flexion/extension and radial/ulnar deviations), while torsiometers are used to measure angular twisting (e.g., forearm pronation/supination) as opposed to bending. Hansson et al. (1996), Rawes et al. (1996), Buchholz and Wellman (1997), Spielholz (1998), and Marshall et al. (1999) have used biaxial goniometers and torsiometers to continuously measure wrist motions and forearm rotations.

One common problem of such biaxial devices is various types of measurement errors. When the forearm rotates, the distal and proximal end blocks do not rotate together, causing a twist in the goniometer wire. The twist is primarily the result of the kinesiology of forearm rotation, in which the proximal end block of the goniometer is attached toward the middle of the forearm so that it rotates less than does the distal end block. The resulting twist leads to *crosstalk* and *zero drift* errors, which are fairly common due to complexity of human joints and should be continually corrected. Correction formulas for the Biometrics or BIOPAC Systems flexible goniometers were developed by Buchholz and Wellman (1997). A summary of the motion measurement devices, with their respective advantages and disadvantages is given in Table 7.1.

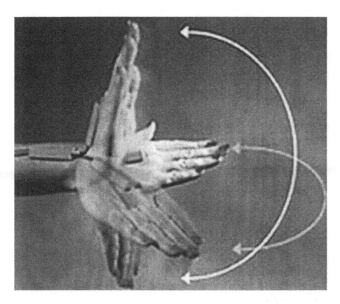

FIGURE 7.1
Flexible biaxial electrogoniometers. (Courtesy of BIOPAC Systems Inc., Santa Barbara, CA, http://www.biopac.com)

TABLE 7.1

Common Wrist-Motion Measurement Devices

Measurement Device	Accuracy	Reliability	Cost	Advantages	Disadvantages
Videotape analysis	Low	Low	Low	Hard copy	Time intensive
3D digitizer	High	High	High	Computer control	Problems with noise
Electromechanical goniometer	High	High	Low	Simple, direct measurement	Uncomfortable, intrusive
Flexible goniometers	High	High	Medium	Small, light, relatively unobtrusive	Noise, crosstalk
				Measure two planes simultaneously	

7.2.2 Calibration Methods

Calibration errors can occur at several levels: the accuracy of the instrument in the measurement of a known fixed angle, the procedural errors, the repeatability of measurements, and the correction procedures for any errors. Buchholz and Wellman (1997) constructed a calibration fixture to allow accurate measurement of true angles in one wrist plane for various forearm rotations. The fixture consisted of a protractor element for measuring true wrist angles and a rotary element for controlling forearm rotation. They also developed correction procedures that included a slope transformation and zero drift transformation to adjust for errors due to crosstalk and zero drift. The equations of the slope-transformed values of flexion/extension (F/E_S) and radial/ulnar deviation (R/U_S) from goniometer measurements of flexion/extension (F/E_M) and radial/ulnar deviation (R/U_M) were

$$\frac{F}{E_S} = \left(\frac{F}{E_M^2} + \frac{R}{U_M^2}\right)^{1/2}\left[\sin\left(\tan^{-1}\left\{\frac{F/E_M}{R/U_M}\right\} + \phi\right)\right] \tag{7.1}$$

$$\frac{R}{U_S} = \left(\frac{F}{E_M^2} + \frac{R}{U_M^2}\right)^{1/2}\left[\cos\left(\tan^{-1}\left\{\frac{F/E_M}{R/U_M}\right\} + \phi\right)\right] \tag{7.2}$$

The angle ϕ is the twist in goniometer wire due to forearm rotation.

The second transformation of zero drift was made for corrected flexion/extension (F/E_C) and radial/ulnar deviation (R/U_C) angles from slope-transformed zero point averages of flexion/extension (F/E_0) and radial/ulnar deviation (R/U_0) angles as follows:

$$\frac{F}{E_C} = \frac{F}{E_S} + \frac{F}{E_0} \tag{7.3}$$

$$\frac{R}{U_C} = \frac{R}{U_S} + \frac{R}{U_0} \tag{7.4}$$

Based on the slope transformation and zero-drift equations, they performed a nonlinear optimization minimizing the error (as seen below) and calculated true flexion/extension (F/E_T) and radial/ulnar deviation (R/U_T) angles.

$$\min\sum\left(\left|\frac{F}{E_T} - \frac{F}{E_C}\right| + \left|\frac{R}{U_T} - \frac{R}{U_C}\right|\right) \tag{7.5}$$

Hansson et al. (1996) introduced a test jig allowing independent setting of three planes of wrist angles, thus simulating the biomechanics of the wrist and forearm, and developed correction equations to induce actual wrist angles from recorded wrist angles as follows:

$$\frac{F}{E'} = S \times \cos(\phi - C \times R) \tag{7.6}$$

$$\frac{R}{U'} = S \times \sin(\phi - C \times R) \tag{7.7}$$

$$S = \left(\frac{F}{E^2} + \frac{R}{U^2}\right)^{0.5} \quad \phi = \sin\left(\frac{R}{U}\right) \times \arctan\left(\frac{F/E}{R/U}\right) \tag{7.8}$$

where
  F/E' is the recorded flexion/extension angle
  R/U' is the recorded radial/ulnar deviation angle
  F/E is the actual flexion/extension angle
  R/U is the actual radial/ulnar deviation angle
  R is the forearm rotation angle
  C is the a transducer-dependent constant

Ojima et al. (1991) measured the output of the electrogoniometer during wrist circumduction using a specially developed calibration apparatus. It consisted of a horizontal flat board and table, a universal joint at the end of the board, a metal straight bar joined to universal joint, and a vertical board with round hole and sliding side bar. The results showed that the measurement errors for flexion/extension and radial/ulnar deviation were within

FIGURE 7.2
Calibration mockup for electrogoniometer testing. (Reproduced from Jang, H., The effects of dynamic wrist workloads on risks of carpal tunnel syndrome, PhD dissertation, The Pennsylvania State University, University Park, PA, 2002. With permission.)

$4°$ and $1°$, respectively, and that *hysteresis* was barely measurable, especially when subjects' forearms were fixed to eliminate forearm rotation.

Jang (2002) developed a calibration device (see Figure 7.2) similar to Ojima et al. (1991) but used a simulated flexible ball joint rather than a human wrist. Static calibration of the Biometrics biaxial goniometer at nine different wrist flexion/extension angles and seven different radial/ulnar deviation angles produced an essentially linear ($r^2 = 0.999$, $p < .001$) relationship between true and measured angle. Nonrepeatabilities for flexion/extension and radial/ulnar deviation planes were 4.0% and 3.3%, respectively, while nonlinearities were 1.6% and 0.93%, respectively (see Figure 7.3).

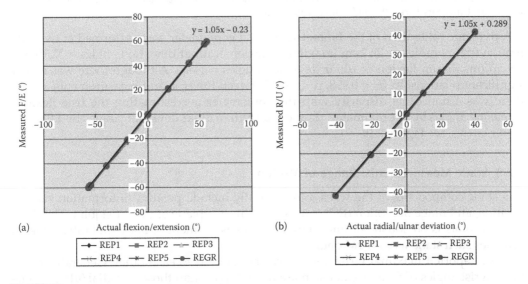

FIGURE 7.3
True and goniometer-measured angles during static calibration: (a) flexion/extension plane and (b) radial/ulnar deviation plane. (Reproduced from Jang, H., The effects of dynamic wrist workloads on risks of carpal tunnel syndrome, PhD dissertation, The Pennsylvania State University, University Park, PA, 2002. With permission.)

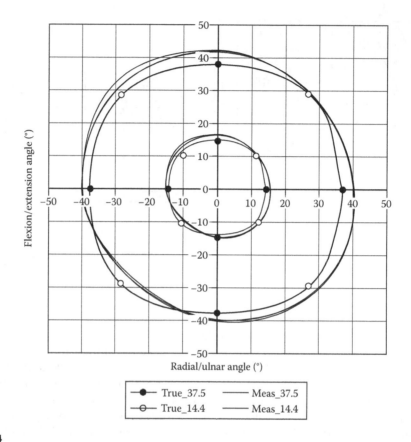

FIGURE 7.4
True and goniometer-measured angles during dynamic calibration. (Reproduced from Jang, H., The effects of dynamic wrist workloads on risks of carpal tunnel syndrome, PhD dissertation, The Pennsylvania State University, University Park, PA, 2002. With permission.)

A dynamic calibration of the Biometrics biaxial goniometer was performed at two calibration fixture radiuses: 26.2 cm (maximum flexion or ulnar deviation angles = 37.5°) and 8.8 cm (maximum flexion or ulnar deviation angles = 14.4°). Although there was a very significant relationship (r^2 = 0.998, p < .001) between the true and measurements angles, there was a noticeable disparity with the goniometer overestimating the true flexion/extension angles by approximately 2° and true radial/ulnar deviation angles by 1.08° (i.e., wider circles, see Figure 7.4).

7.2.3 Static Measurements: Range of Motion

The static components of the wrist joint typically include postural information such as position, and range of motion (ROM) measured in each plane of the wrist joint. The ROM of body joints is obviously an important factor in assessment of body mobility. Table 7.2 provides such static wrist ROM data.

These reported maximal wrist angles are very similar to each other. Generally, maximum wrist angles of flexion/extension are much larger than those of radial/ulnar deviation, and maximum ulnar deviation and supination angles are much larger than maximum radial deviation and pronation angles, respectively. Wrist angles under static conditions are much larger than those found under dynamic conditions, when measured from the

TABLE 7.2

Maximum ROM Data of the Wrist Joint

Previous Studies	Maximum Wrist Angle (°)					
	Flexion	Extension	Radial Deviation	Ulnar Deviation	Pronation	Supination
Boone and Azen (1979)	76	75	19	33	—	—
Bonebrake et al. (1990)	86	62	34	68	105	120
Schoenmarklin and Marras (1993)	62	57	21	28	81	101
Marshall et al. (1999)	67	73	21	47	—	—

beginning to the end of maximal dynamic movement. Schoenmarklin and Marras (1993) rationalized that the subjects might have focused more on the exertion and less on the maximal ROM in dynamic movements.

Another consideration of static wrist joint measurements is forearm posture. Maximum wrist angles increase as the arm and shoulder muscles are used to rotate the forearm and hand. Therefore, when measuring the maximum ROM in the wrist joint, the location and fixation of the arm and shoulder must be carefully constrained and documented.

7.2.4 Dynamic Measurements: Angular Velocity and Acceleration

Dynamic components of wrist typically include angular velocity and angular acceleration. Unfortunately, until fairly recently these have not be studied in detail. Schoenmarklin and Marras (1993) first established an important database on maximum dynamic capability in the three planes of wrist joint. Table 7.3 shows the maximum angular velocities and accelerations as a function of direction of movement.

The Table 7.3 reveals that maximum angular velocity and acceleration of pronation/ supination plane are much higher than those for flexion/extension, and maximum angular velocity and acceleration of flexion/extension movements are much greater than those for radial/ulnar deviation movements. The magnitude of dynamic wrist capability depends on the movement direction in each plane as shown in Table 7.3. Flexion movement (from extreme extension angle to flexion, E → F), ulnar movement (R → U), and supination movement (P → S) generate greater maximum angular velocities and accelerations than opposing movements. Schoenmarklin and Marras (1993) indicated that high dynamic

TABLE 7.3

Maximum Angular Velocity and Acceleration as a Function of Movement Direction

Variables		Flexion/Extension		Radial/Ulnar Deviation		Pronation/ Supination	
		F → E	E → F	R → U	U → R	P → S	S → P
Velocity (°/s)	Dominant hand	−914	1,049	−436	356	−2,202	1,898
	Nondominant hand	−926	1,069	−447	378	−2,072	1,784
Acceleration (°/s²)	Dominant hand	−12,007	16,092	−7,640	5,055	−45,034	36,336
	Nondominant hand	−12,051	16,020	−7,473	5,393	−39,367	33,217

Source: Adapted from Schoenmarklin, R.W. and Marras, W.S., *Int. J. Ind. Ergonom.*, 11, 207, 1993.

TABLE 7.4

Mean and Peak Wrist Positions and Angular Velocity and Acceleration in the Three Planes

Previous Studies	Variable	Task	F/E		R/U		P/S	
			Mean	Peak	Mean	Peak	Mean	Peak
Marras and	Position	High risk	−12.0[b]	6.6	−6.7	4.7	8.3	47.4
Schoenmarklin		Low risk	−10.1	4.4	−7.6	10.1	2.5	37.4
(1993)	Angular velocity	High risk	42	174	26	116	91	449
		Low risk	29	120	17	77	68	300
	Angular acceleration	High risk	824	4,471	494	3,077	1,824	11,291
		Low risk	494	2,588	301	1,759	1,222	7,169
Hansson et al. (1996)	Position	Fish processing	−1	n.a.	12	n.a.	n.a.	n.a.
	Angular velocity	Fish processing	61	142	36	84	n.a.	n.a.
Marklin and Monroe[a] (1998)	Angular velocity	Bone trimming	45	239	30	156	100	540
	Angular acceleration	Bone trimming	844	4,895	578	3,593	1,872	12,522
Serina et al. (1999)	Position	Typing	−21.7	n.a.	−16.7	n.a.	86.8	n.a.
	Angular velocity	Typing	24	n.a.	12	n.a.	13	n.a.
	Angular acceleration	Typing	306	n.a.	134	n.a.	168	n.a.

[a] Data are maximum values among three intervals.
[b] "_" denotes extension and ulnar deviation.

capabilities of the flexion and supination movements were probably due to the greater biomechanical potentials of flexor and supinator muscles rather than of the extensor and pronator muscles, respectively. Also, the greater peak velocity and acceleration of ulnar movement were probably attributable to the effect of gravity.

Several studies have attempted to use the angular velocity and acceleration variable as potential risk factors in their epidemiological research (Marras and Schoenmarklin, 1993; Hansson et al., 1996; Marklin and Monroe, 1998; Serina et al., 1999). These values are summarized in Table 7.4.

Marras and Schoenmarklin (1993) performed a quantitative surveillance study on the factory floor. Based on a total of 40 subjects from 8 industrial plants, wrist deviation, angular velocity, and acceleration variables were measured in three planes of wrist movements using dichotomous WRMSD risk levels (low and high risk). Table 7.4 indicates that the mean and maximum position, angular velocity, and acceleration values of high-risk tasks are generally much higher than these of low-risk tasks in all three planes of wrist movements. Besides, angular velocity and acceleration appear to separate WRMSD risk levels more reliably than wrist deviation. The angular velocity and acceleration measures in high-risk tasks showed increases of 46.2% and 67.1%, respectively, over the same measures in low-risk tasks. These results show the importance of dynamic components on assessing WRMSD risk.

Hansson et al. (1996) investigated the position and angular velocity variables for tasks in the fish-processing industry as means for characterizing static and dynamic properties of wrist movements. The results indicated that wrist deviations in fish-processing tasks are much smaller than these in the low-risk tasks reported by Marras and Schoenmarklin (1993). However, the angular velocities for F/E and R/U planes were 45% and 39%, respectively, higher than those for high-risk tasks. Serina et al. (1999) found that mean angular velocities and accelerations of typing task were similar to those of industrial tasks reported by Marras and Schoenmarklin (1993). In a clinical application, Ojima et al. (1991) found that angular-velocity/wrist-angle loci for healthy men were larger than for carpal tunnel syndrome (CTS) patients.

Most of the previous studies simply differentiated angular data collected from goniometers. However, differentiation of angle data, especially data with spikes and not mathematically smoothed (which produces a different sort of problems), can very easily create larger spikes with increasing errors. As an alternative, small, lightweight, and relatively inexpensive accelerometers can be used to collect acceleration data directly. The sensors utilize piezoelectric crystals, which upon deformation from accelerations produce a voltage signal proportional to that acceleration. Traditionally, by proper placement of six linear accelerometers in orthogonal orientations, both linear and angular accelerations of a body segments can be found (Morris, 1973). However, with low-cost tri-axial accelerometers (some under $100, www.gcdataconcepts. com), the amount of sensors for a given segment is reduced or conversely, more body segments can be measured. The calculation of segment velocities and displacements requires integration of the original data and can also result in erroneous values unless very careful calibration and integration procedures are not followed. In addition, sensor signal drift and even small noise levels can create large integration errors (Mayagoitia et al., 2002). In general, the use of accelerometers is a tradeoff between a relatively inexpensive, direct measurement technique not requiring a direct line of sight (as needed for cameras or other optical systems) and the relatively complicated coordination of multiple sensors, calibration of initial conditions, and careful signal processing (Chao, 1978). However, for relatively simple workplace studies of one segment (rather than complex complete whole motion analysis), accelerometers are quite useful. For example, Estill et al. (2000) used accelerometers in the form of activity monitors to assess risk factors for WRMSDs in an industrial setting. The activity monitors showed statistically significant differences between three different occupational groups and correlated significantly with observational ratings. Note, that with increasing concern for adult obesity, such tri-axial accelerometer based activity monitors have become very easily commercially obtainable, with data logging and software processing included. Two common ones are the Actitrac (www.theactigraph.com/) and RTC (www.stayhealthy.com) activity monitors for under $300.

Accelerometer measurements are much more important for understanding the effects of worker exposure to vibration from power tools, such as grinders, sanders, and polishers, with respect to hand–arm vibration syndrome. These measurements will require the traditional accelerometers and also more sophisticated data-processing hardware (A/D converters) and software (Fourier processing) so as to create power spectra and identify the critical frequencies.

These studies demonstrate the need for measuring dynamic aspects (i.e., angular velocity and acceleration) of wrist motions as potential contributing risk factors for WRMSDs. Also, it is important to measure all three planes of wrist motions (flexion/extension, radial/ulnar deviation, and pronation/supination) simultaneously for best results.

7.3 Pressure- and Force-Distribution Measurements

7.3.1 Early Pressure Devices

In one of the earliest, simplest, nonquantitative approaches Swearingen et al. (1962) seated a subject on absorbent paper placed over an inked cloth. The density of ink transferred indicated a crude measure of pressure intensity. A similar approach was used by Fellows and Freivalds (1991) to identify critical areas on a tool handle for a more specific placement of pressure sensors. Subjects dipped their hands in finger paint and grasped the tool handle. Areas of highest pressure maintained the least amounts of paint which spread to the areas of lowest pressure. Similarly, Dillon (1981) used strips of wax placed on top of the seat cushion. Lighter, ectomorphic individuals produced narrower and deeper indentations than heavy, endomorphic individuals. Lindan et al. (1965) used a bed of mechanical springs with over 1000 sensors at 1.4 cm intervals to measure the whole body pressure distribution. In a slightly different approach, thermography, with greater weight on a given area allowing less body heat to escape, was used to establish relatively nonquantitative pressure distributions (Trandel et al., 1975). However, reactive hyperemic thermal flare ups distorted the results. Also, all of these approaches are relatively crude, with problems in repeatability, resolution, and accuracy.

For quantitative data, a large matrix of numerous sensors that can individually measure pressure is needed. The earliest such systems used mechanical valves with compressed air (Houle, 1969) or in a cruder approach without valves, plunger-activated liquid-filled manometers (Jürgens, 1969). Unfortunately, the major disadvantage with these systems is the need for a large apparatus with numerous relatively large pressure-gage elements and a relatively large, mechanical control system. Later use of smaller sensors (Mooney et al., 1971), electronic controls and switches (Garber et al., 1978), and air as the pressure sensing medium (Bader et al., 1984) reduced some of the bulk in this approach. Based on the further work of Bader and Hawken (1986), the commercially available Talley Pressure Monitor (Talley Medical, Romsey, Hampshire, United Kingdom; http://www.talleymedical.co.uk/) was developed. Further testing (Ferguson-Pell and Cardi, 1991; Gyi et al., 1998) indicated high accuracy and repeatability as compared to force-sensing resistor systems but also several limitations: large (20 mm) sensor sizes, static measurements requiring at least 1 min of scanning, and relatively few sensors yielding poor resolution of the pressure distribution. The main advantage of pressure bladders is the ability to measure peak forces regardless of the orientation of the force.

Optical systems based on the prototype developed by Elftman (1934) have been used for both foot pressure (Betts et al., 1980; Franks et al., 1983) and seated pressure measurements (Mayo-Smith and Cochran, 1981; Kadaba et al., 1984; Treaster and Marras, 1987; Shields and Cook, 1988). This approach uses an acrylic sheet covered with a beaded silicone rubber baromat (Biomechanics, LeMesa, California) incorporated into the seat pad or seat back. The working principle is based on differences in the optical properties of the acrylic–air and acrylic–rubber interfaces. A fluorescent light is attached along one edge of the acrylic sheet. The light enters the sheet but cannot be reflected out unless baromat contacts the sheet. The greater the pressure on the rubber baromat, the more the beads deform and the more light is refracted from the acrylic sheet. The refracted light is photographed with a camera located either below the seat pan or reflected out with a mirror to a stationary camera. Processing of the refracted light is crucial for resolution, which has ranged from 9 levels using color (Shields and Cook, 1988) to 256 levels (Treaster and Marras, 1987) using direct digitization of the video signal and the available levels of gray scales on the video system. One problem with this system is creep that occurs in all viscoelastic materials. If pressure is applied for a significant length of time (on the order of a half minute depending on the type of rubber used), then due to the continuous deformation of the rubber in contact with the acrylic, increased light output will occur for the same applied pressure (Betts et al., 1980). This will especially be a problem for dynamic measurements, such as measuring restlessness during long-term sitting.

Hertzberg (1972) developed a "pressure-measuring blanket" that consisted of an array of closely spaced thin flexible capacitors, each 1 cm^2 in area. Increased pressure was measured by a change in capacitance. This approach was improved by Drummond et al. (1982) by incorporating microprocessor control with a matrix of 64 strain-gage resistive transducers instead of capacitors. Although quantitative specifications were not provided, the resistive transducers appeared to provide better sensitivity than the capacitors. However, the resistive transducers were fabricated onto an aluminum plate and then attached to a second aluminum base plate. Such a device is only useful for pressure measurements on a hard, uncountoured surface.

7.3.2 Force-Sensing Electronic Components

The development of a new, lighter, and more flexible type of sensor provided more opportunities for pressure-measurement applications. This force-sensing resistor (FSR), (Interlink Electronics, Camarillo, California; http://www.interlinkelectronics.com; or in Europe, Electrade GmbH, Gräfelfing, Germany; http://www.electrade.com/html/FSRtm. htm) consists of two sheets of polymer film, with conductive interdigitating fingers and the other with a conductive film overlying the fingers, separated by a spacer. Applying a force to the resulting sandwich causes the resistance between the two contact surfaces to decrease, which can be measured through a voltage divider (Fellows and Freivalds, 1989). The force–resistance relationship is quite nonlinear (see Figure 7.5, note the log–log scale) and, therefore, the sensors need to be calibrated carefully (Park, 1999). Since FSRs are quite flexible, one of the first applications involved measuring grip pressure distributions for different types of tool-handle surfaces (Fellows and Freivalds, 1991) as well as seat pressure distributions with a matrix of 32 FSRs placed between two thin sheets of plastic and placed on the seat pans of two different automobile seats (see Figure 7.6; Yun et al., 1992). A similar but larger mat of 225 sensors was used to model seating comfort in a car seat (Gross et al., 1994) and also to measure seated postural shifts (Fenety et al., 1994, 2000).

Although convenient and inexpensive, FSRs do have several problems. Although termed "force sensing," they, in fact, measure pressure or force per unit area. Localized or directed applications of a force to a relatively large sensor will not yield a correct value. Also, directionality of the forces, including shear loading, as well as bending the sensor can produce errors. To create a sensor that responds to force rather than pressure, Jensen et al. (1991) developed

FIGURE 7.5
Force sensor calibration curves. (Reproduced from Park, S.K., The development of an exposure measurement system for assessing risk of work-related musculoskeletal disorders, Unpublished PhD thesis, The Pennsylvania State University, University Park, PA, 1999. With permission.)

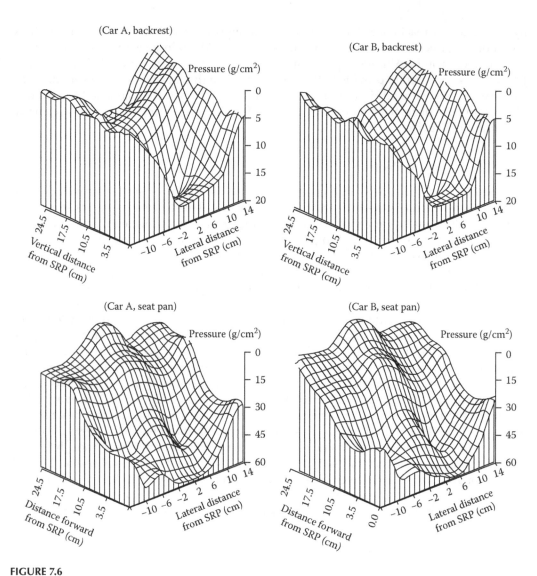

FIGURE 7.6
Pressure distribution curves for automobile seat pans and seat backs. (Reproduced from Yun, M.H., et al., Using force sensitive resistors to evaluate driver seating comfort, in S. Kumar (ed.), *Advances in Industrial Ergonomics and Safety IV*, Taylor & Francis, London, U.K., 1992.)

the method of forming an epoxy dome over the sensing area to better direct the applied forces to the sensor. This also helped stiffen the sensor area and keep it rigid during loading.

Park (1999) performed detailed calibration studies on UniForce FSRs (see Figure 7.7, now available as Flexiforce sensors from Tekscan Inc., South Boston, Massachusetts; http://www.tekscan.com/flexiforce.html), finding repeatability ranging from 87% to 94% for domed and 75% to 91% for undomed sensors, considerably worse than the 95% claimed by the manufacturer. Repeatability was worst for lowest forces. Also, there was a tendency for the sensor to flatten their logarithmic relationship by approximately 6% per day of usage (see Figure 7.8). Once sensor performance drops below a given threshold and fails to provide good calibration, the sensor can be considered to have failed. Park (1999) estimated failure to occur in 19 days for undomed sensors and 34 days for domed sensors.

FIGURE 7.7
FlexiForce force-sensing resistor. (Courtesy of Tekscan Inc., http://www. tekscan.com/flexiforce.html)

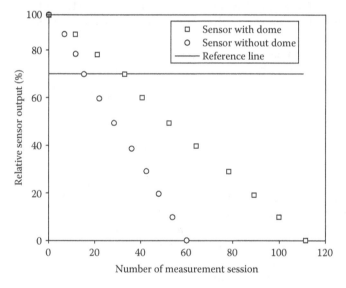

FIGURE 7.8
Force-sensing resistor decay. (Reproduced from Park, S.K., The development of an exposure measurement system for assessing risk of work-related musculoskeletal disorders, Unpublished PhD thesis, The Pennsylvania State University, University Park, PA, 1999. With permission.)

The concept of the domed force sensor was further expanded by Carvalho and Radwin (1996). By sandwiching the traditional FSR between two layers of spring steel, placing the sandwich on an annular ring support and covering it with a Torlon polymer dome, the usable force range was expanded by almost 100% and the resulting error was decreased by almost 50%. In another approach, Beebe et al. (1998) developed a completely new silicon-based force sensor with lower hysteresis and higher repeatability than the original sensor.

Another type of pressure sensor can be formed from piezoelectric film, which produces an electric current during displacement. Sorab et al. (1988) used piezoelectric sensor attached directly to a surgeon's hands to measure finger forces during delivery of newborns. However, the material is very fragile and, due to the transient nature of the electric signal, would serve poorly in static pressure measurements.

More recently, the force-sensing technology has been expanded to ready-made pressure sensing mats (Tekscan Inc., South Boston, Massachusetts; http://www.tekscan.com/flexiforce.html). Two thin, flexible polyester sheets, with electrically conductive electrodes deposited in perpendicular directions (i.e., rows for one and columns for the other), sandwich an intermediate layer with semi-conductive ink. A grid pattern is formed, creating a sensing location at each intersection. With an applied force, there is electrical resistance change at each of the intersecting points of the grid pattern, which can be mapped to create a pressure-distribution pattern. Since the grid lines can be as close as 0.5 mm, there can be over 170 sensors per square centimeter, establishing a very high resolution matrix, albeit at a considerable cost. Primary applications have been for in-the-shoe pressure measuring systems (Woodburn and Helliwell, 1997), pressure measurements under burn garments (Mann et al., 1997) and also for seat pan pressure distributions for wheel-chair users (Ferguson-Pell and Cardi, 1993). However, the system showed considerable hysteresis (±20%), creep (19%), and poor repeatability, but was liked by clinicians for its real-time display capabilities (Ferguson-Pell and Cardi, 1993).

A variation of the above resistive matrix approach is a conductive rubber sheet which has the unique property in that it conducts electric current when compressed but acts as insulator when the pressure is released (Yokohama Image System Co. Ltd, Technical Development Center, Kanagawa, Japan; http://www.y-i-s.co.jp/CSAEnglish.html). Thus, in a gross sense it acts as a switching function, but when used carefully, its electrical resistance varies according to the applied pressure and has been used to measure pressure distributions within the wrist (Hara et al., 1992) and to evaluate comfort while lying on different types of bedding (http://www.hql.or.jp/gpd/eng/www/nwl/n14/ergo.html).

Another recent product that provides a highly detailed pressure distribution is the Fuji pressure film (Fuji Medical Systems, Stamford, Connecticut; http://www.prescale.com/E/E_index.htm). Pressure-sensitive film is constructed of a color-developing layer and a microcapsule layer sandwiched between polyethylene terephthaylate (PET) bases. The film comes in several pressure ranges. Once exposed to pressure, the film changes color and the resultant color pressure density is established with a specially designed densitometer, reading areas down to 1 mm. Typical applications so far have been for measuring occlusal forces in dental surgery (Harada et al., 2000), joint forces (Konrath et al., 1999), but not seating distributions. Although, this approach appears to be quite sensitive for distribution, there has been some concern over errors of 10%–15% in the pressure readings due to the contact pressure exceeding the film threshold or due to the rate of pressure loading (Hale and Brown, 1992). Using multiple ranges of film simultaneously showed considerable variations in readings due to the stacking order and interactions of the microcapsule layers and may not completely solve the first problem (Atkinson et al., 1998). Calibrating the film with the same rate of loading as anticipated experimentally, may alleviate the second problem (Haut, 1989).

The most recent pressure-sensing mat is a highly flexible capacitive matrix with up to 1024 sensors developed by Novel GmbH (http://novel.de/). Each sensor can measure pressures in the range 20–600 kPa with 5% accuracy and can be scanned up to 400 times per second. Lemerle et al. (2008) found these sensor mats to be very useful in detecting significant decreases in grip forces with antivibration handles on vibratory breakers (jack hammers).

A comparison of various pressure- and force-distribution measurement systems, in terms of cost, accuracy, advantages, and disadvantages, is given in Table 7.5. Resolution has not been addressed, since the systems provide either continuous or discrete distributions. For the discrete systems, the resolution depends on how many sensors have been used. Only qualitative assessments have been made, since very few studies have provided quantitative data on reliability, validity, etc.

TABLE 7.5

Comparison of Pressure and Force Distribution Measurement Systems

Type of Measurement	Distribution	Accuracy	Cost	Advantages	Disadvantages
Paint, wax, heat	Continuous	Low	Low	Simple and inexpensive	Not easily quantified
Baromat, optical scan	Continuous	Medium	Medium	Quantification of continuous data	Rubber creep, data conversion
Pneumatic, hydraulic	Discrete	High	Medium	Directionality unimportant	Cumbersome equipment
Force sensing resistors	Discrete	Medium	Low	Simple, inexpensive, easy to apply	Directionality, daily calibration
Pressure mats	Discrete	High	High	High resolution, many shapes	Cost, repeatability, hysteresis
Pressure film	Continuous	Medium	Medium	Nonintrusive	Sensitive to rate of loading

7.3.3 Integrated-Touch Glove System

Yun et al. (1997) developed an integrated system, termed the "touch glove," to coordinate and facilitate real-time hand motion and grip force measurements in the field. The main component is the Cyberglove by Virtual Technologies of Palo Alto, California (http://www.immersion.com/products/3d/interaction/overview.shtml). The Cyberglove uses 22 strain gauge sensors: three bend sensors and one abduction sensor per finger, to measure finger flexion/extension and abduction/adduction angles. In conjunction with a Polhemus magnetic sensor, the position of the hand with respect to a reference is also established. Analog signals for the strain gauges are digitized via an analog-to-digital (A/D) converter on the host computer. For a typical application, an 8 bit A/D converter (0–255 point) provides sufficient accuracy to map the appropriate ROM in degrees ($< 140°$) for the fingers. For greater accuracy, 12 bit A/D converters will be more than sufficient. A device similar to that described in Section 7.2.2 but for the fingers would be needed to calibrate the glove.

The second component for the touch-glove system is a force sensor matrix, consisting of 12 force-sensing resistors (FSRs) described in Section 7.3.2, overlaying the Cyberglove. Although the number of sensors and their locations are freely changeable, the current system utilized sensors on the distal and metacarpal phalanges of each finger, except for the thumb, where only one sensor was attached to the distal phalanx. Three other sensors were placed on the thenar and hypothenar eminences as shown in Figure 7.9. The location for the sensors was determined by the rough contact area hand produced by gripping a cylindrical handle sprayed with paint following the procedures of Fellows and Freivalds (1991). The fully integrated touch glove holding a hand tool is also shown in Figure 7.9.

The touch glove was the utilized in a set of laboratory calibration experiments to measure joint angles and finger forces as a function of handle diameter (Yun, 1994; Yun et al., 1997). The results indicated, as could be hypothesized, that finger flexion angles decreased as grip diameter increased (see Figure 7.10). Force distribution results (see Figure 7.11) indicated that the fingertip forces were greater than metacarpal forces, thumb fingertip forces increased with increasing grip diameter, little fingertip forces decreased with increasing grip diameter, while the finger tip forces for middle fingers remained roughly constant. These results and the touch glove system were the basis for further research on optimal handle diameter (see Section 9.3.2) and handle shapes (see Section 9.3.3). It has also been

FIGURE 7.9
Sensor distribution on touch glove system. (Reproduced from Yun, M.H., A hand posture measurement systems for the analysis of manual tool handling tasks, PhD dissertation, The Pennsylvania State University, University Park, PA, 1994. With permission.)

FIGURE 7.10
Index finger joint angles as a function of grip diameter. (Reproduced from Yun, M.H. et al., *IEEE Trans. Syst. Man Cybernet. B*, 27, 835, 1997. With permission.)

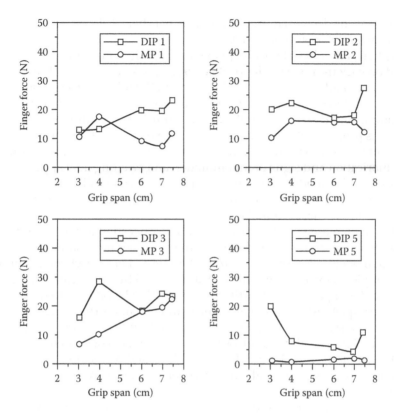

FIGURE 7.11
Finger forces as a function of grip diameter. (Reproduced from Yun, M.H. et al., *IEEE Trans. Syst. Man Cybernet. B*, 27, 835, 1997. With permission.)

used successfully in the field measuring pinch forces during warehouse handling of glass windshields (Lowe and Freivalds, 1997).

7.4 Nerve-Conduction Measurements

7.4.1 Basic Concepts

Currently, the most reliable technique for diagnosing and assessing the severity of CTS is nerve-conduction assessment (Kembel, 1968; Melvin et al., 1973; Jackson and Clifford, 1987; Stevens, 1987; Kimura, 1989; Ghavanini and Haghighat, 1998). Electromyographic (EMG) instrumentation (see Section 7.5) is used to measure and quantify nerve conduction parameters such as latency, amplitude, duration, and conduction velocity, by measuring the time required for an electrical impulse to travel from a stimulus site to the measurement site, typically on the median nerve. The results are then compared against reference values, which have been established for both healthy and symptomatic populations. CTS patients show prolonged median motor nerve latency and/or decreased median motor nerve amplitude as compared to normal subjects (Simpson, 1956; Thomas, 1960; Kimura, 1979, 1989). Similarly, CTS patients also demonstrate a prolonged median sensory nerve latency and/or decreased amplitude (Kembel, 1968; Felsenthal and Spindler, 1979; Kimura and Ayyar, 1985; Stevens, 1987).

The conceptual pathophysiological explanation for such changes in median nerve conduction is based on various models (Moore et al., 1991; Tanaka and McGlothlin, 1993; Hagberg et al., 1995; Werner and Armstrong, 1997) leading to the following scenario. Occupational risk factors such as forceful exertion, repetitive motions, and awkward postures may cause muscular fatigue and discomfort to the carpal tunnel at wrist during work. If sufficient recovery time is provided after such, the fatigue and discomfort is short lived. However, if work is continued despite fatigue and discomfort, the tendons may become strained due to inadequate lubrication and signs of inflammation and swelling may appear within carpal tunnel (Sissons, 1979). Tendon structures are especially susceptible, since tendon sheaths appear to require a much longer time recovery time than muscles. This swelling causes a further increase in the carpal tunnel pressure.

With sufficient increase in pressure, local venous congestion occurs within the vascular structure of the nerve, as well as ischemia in the arterioles nourishing the nerve, leading to endoneurinal edema (Sunderland, 1976). The role of neural ischemia is supported by the relatively rapid recovery from acute CTS after carpal tunnel release surgery and or the development of CTS symptoms by artificially restricting blood flow to the nerve with the pneumatic tourniquet test (Moore, 1992). The neural edema further increases the effect of the original compression, thus creating a vicious circle. If this condition persists for a prolonged period of time, it leads to progressive long-term axonal deterioration resulting in the characteristic symptoms for CTS, numbness, tingling, and pain in the areas corresponding to distribution of the nerves (Tanaka and McGlothlin, 1993). Mechanical pressure to the nerve, on the other hand, causes direct histologic changes to the nerve, including thinning or shearing of the myelin under the area of compression (Armstrong, 1994).

7.4.2 Nerve Stimulation and Recording

Since Simpson (1956) first measured median nerve latency in CTS patients, the technique has been continually improved to improve its sensitivity and specificity for CTS diagnosis. However, the technique basically still consists of two components: sensory nerve conduction with stimulating and recording electrodes on the median nerve (or other nerve of interest) and motor nerve conduction with stimulating electrodes on the nerve and recording electrodes in the muscles innervated by that nerve.

Either surface or needle electrodes may be used to stimulate the nerve. Stimulating electrodes consist of a *cathode* (negative pole) and an *anode* (positive pole). As the current flows between them, negative charges that accumulate under the cathode depolarize the nerve and forms an action potential (see Section 3.3). Most commercially available stimulators provide a probe that mounts the cathode and the anode at a fixed distance, usually 2–3 cm apart. The anode must be placed proximal to cathode while stimulating (see Figure 7.12).

The pulses of moderate intensity are used to adjust the positions of the cathode until further relocation causes no change in the size of the muscle action potential. With the cathode at the best stimulating site, one then defines the maximal intensity that just elicits a maximal potential. Increasing the stimulus another 20%–30% supramaximal, then, guarantees the activation of all the nerve axons innervating the recorded muscle (but does not further increase the muscle potential).

Surface stimulations of 0.1 ms duration, and 100–300 V or 5–40 mA intensities are usually sufficient to fully activate a healthy nerve but cause no particular risk to an ordinary patient. Special care to safeguard the patient includes proper grounding and the placement

(a)   (b)

FIGURE 7.12
Set up for median nerve conduction studies: (a) sensory nerve (antidromic) and (b) motor nerve (orthodromic). (Reproduced from Jang, H., The effects of dynamic wrist workloads on risks of carpal tunnel syndrome, PhD dissertation, The Pennsylvania State University, University Park, PA, 2002. With permission.)

of the stimulator with a sufficient distance from a pacemaker or other implanted electronic devices (AAEE, 1984). Stimulation by a needle electrode inserted subcutaneously close to the nerve requires much less current than surface stimulation to elicit the same response. The anode may be a surface electrode located on the skin or a second needle electrode inserted in the vicinity of cathode.

Recording the response potentials again requires a pair of surface electrodes or needle electrodes, the cathode and the anode. With this arrangement, the propagating action potential, originating under the cathode, gives rise to a simple biphasic waveform with initial negativity. Surface electrodes, in general, are better than needle electrodes for recording compound motor nerve action potentials in assessing contributions from all discharging units, because its onset latency indicates the conduction time of the fastest fibers, whereas its amplitude is approximately proportional to the number of available axons. The use of a needle electrode improves the recording from small atrophic muscles because the needle electrode registers only a small portion of the muscle action potential with less interference from neighboring discharges.

Routine recording of the sensory nerve action potential, in general is performed with surface ring electrodes which provide adequate and reproducible information noninvasively. (Tashjian et al., 1987; Jackson and Clifford, 1989; Kimura, 1989; Burnham and Steadward, 1994). Some, however, prefer needle electrodes placed perpendicular to the nerve to improve the resolution, and to improve the signal-to-noise ratio (Rosenfalck, 1978). Sensory studies are usually performed with filters set at 20 Hz–2 kHz while motor studies are usually performed with filter set at 2 Hz–10 kHz.

The nerve can be either be stimulated in the normal conduction direction, termed *orthodromic*, or in the reverse direction, termed *antidromic*. For example, in a sensory nerve fiber, stimulation at a distal point and recording proximal to the point of stimulation is orthodromic nerve conduction. If the process is reversed by stimulating the sensory nerve fibers proximal to the recording points, then the technique is antidromic nerve conduction (see Figure 7.13a). This is also sometimes termed distal nerve conduction.

The major advantage of an orthodromic technique is that only sensory fibers are stimulated and recorded. It has also been suggested that orthodromic nerve conduction

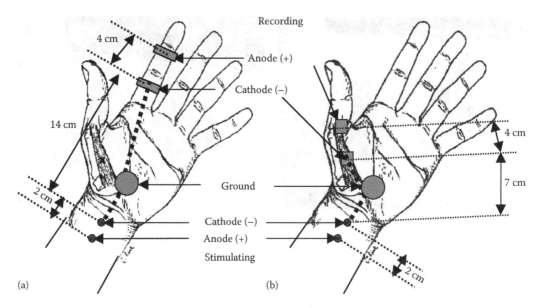

FIGURE 7.13
Electrode placements for median nerve conduction studies: (a) sensory nerve (antidromic) and (b) motor nerve (orthodromic). (Reproduced from Jang, H., The effects of dynamic wrist workloads on risks of carpal tunnel syndrome, PhD dissertation, The Pennsylvania State University, University Park, PA, 2002. With permission.)

parameters are less affected by change of temperature (Chodoroff et al., 1985). The primary advantage of the antidromic technique is larger response amplitude compared to the orthodromic technique because the digital nerves lie nearer to the surface. The amplitude of sensory nerve action potential is essential to establish the severity of CTS and its progress. MacDonnel et al. (1990) reported the antidromic technique is a more sensitive method for assessing mild CTS.

The conventional site for stimulation of both sensory and motor nerves is the wrist (see Figure 7.13b). At the wrist, the cathode may be placed 3 cm proximal crease of the wrist (Kimura, 1989). Alternative techniques use a fixed distance from the recording electrode, most commonly 12–14 cm (DiBenedetto et al., 1986; Carroll, 1987; Jackson and Clifford, 1989). Sensory potentials can be recorded from the first, second, or third digits with surface ring electrodes usually placed around the proximal (cathode) and distal interphalangeal joints (anode), at fixed distance of 4 cm between cathode and anode (Dumitru and Walsh, 1988) (see Figure 7.13a). Motor potentials are recorded at the abductor pollicus brevis muscle at the base of the thumb (see Figure 7.13b). Table 7.6 describes the common sites of electrode placement for the median, ulnar, and radial nerves.

7.4.3 Response Measures

Typical nerve conduction measures are identified in the sample response waveform shown in Figure 7.14. *Onset latency* (SO, in ms) is the time between nerve stimulation and the initial response detected at the active recording electrode. *Peak latency* (SP in ms) is time between nerve stimulation and peak response detected at the active recording electrode. The amplitude of the waveform (in mV for motor NCS, μV for sensory NCS) can be measured between the baseline and negative peak (OP) or between the negative peak and the positive peak (PT). The duration of the waveform (in ms) is the time between the initial

TABLE 7.6

Common Electrode Placements for Nerve Conduction Studies

Nerve	Fibers	Stimulation Site			Recording Site		
		Cathode	Anode	Distance	Cathode	Anode	Ground Site
Median	Motor	Fixed distance from recording electrode mostly 7–8 cm, or 3 cm proximal to the distal crease at wrist	2–3 cm proximal to cathode	7–8 cm	The belly of the abductor pollicis brevis (APB) at thumb	The tendon of abductor pollicis brevis (APB) at thumb	Palm (metacarpal phalanges of third digit)
	Sensory	Fixed distance from recording electrode mostly 12–14 cm, or 3 cm proximal to the distal crease at wrist	2–3 cm proximal to cathode	12–14 cm	Proximal interphalangeal joints (PIP) of second or third digits	Distal interphalangeal (DIP) joints or 4 cm distal to cathode	Palm (metacarpal phalanges of third digit)
Ulnar	Motor	Fixed distance from recording electrode mostly 7–8 cm, or 3 cm proximal to the distal crease at wrist	2 cm proximal to cathode	7–8 cm	Belly of the abductor digiti minimi (ADM)	Tendon of the abductor digiti minimi (ADM), 3 cm distally	Palm (metacarpal phalanges of third digit)
					Belly of the first dorsal interosseous muscle	Tendon of the first dorsal interosseous muscle	Dorsum side of palm
	Sensory	Fixed distance from recording electrode mostly 12–14 cm, or 3 cm proximal to the distal crease at wrist	2–3 cm proximal to cathode	12–14 cm	Proximal interphalangeal (PIP) joints of the fifth or fourth digits	Distal interphalangeal (PIP) joints of the fifth or fourth digits	Palm (metacarpal phalanges of third digit)
Radial	Motor	Forearm at lateral edge of the extensor carpi ulnaris (ECU) muscle 8–10 cm proximal to the styloid process	2 cm proximal to cathode	—	Monopolar needle electrode in the extensor indicis	Dorsum of hand laterally	Posterior forearm, 4–5 cm proximal to distal crease at wrist
	Sensory	Lateral edge of the radius in the distal forearm	2–3 cm proximal to cathode	—	Metacarpal phalangeal (MP) joint of first digit	Intercarpal (IP) joints of first digit	Posterior forearm, 4–5 cm proximal to distal crease at wrist

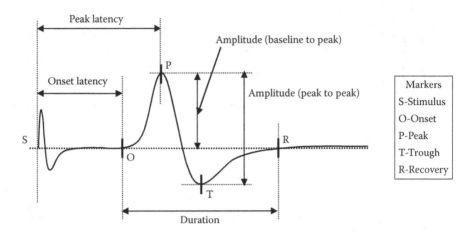

FIGURE 7.14
Typical median nerve conduction waveform. (Reproduced from Jang, H., The effects of dynamic wrist workloads on risks of carpal tunnel syndrome, PhD dissertation, The Pennsylvania State University, University Park, PA, 2002. With permission.)

deviation from the baseline and the ultimate return to the baseline (OR). The conduction velocity (in m/s) is calculated by dividing stimulated nerve length by the peak latency.

For motor nerve conduction studies, latency consists of two components: (1) nerve conduction time from the stimulus point to the nerve terminal and (2) neuromuscular transmission time from the axonal terminal to the motor end plate, including the time required for generation of muscle action potentials. Thus, onset latency is a measure of the fastest conducting motor fibers (Kimura, 1989). To calculate the pure motor nerve conduction velocity, one must eliminate the time for neuromuscular transmission and generation of muscle action potentials. The difference between the two latency responses elicited at two separate points excludes the two components common to both stimuli. Thus, it represents the time necessary for the nerve impulse to travel between the two stimulus points. The motor nerve conduction velocity is derived as the ratio between the distance from one point of stimulation (Site A) to the next (Site B) and the corresponding latency difference between them.

The reliability of results depends on accuracy in determining the length of the nerve segment, estimated with the surface distance along the course of the nerve. Unlike motor latency, which includes neuromuscular transmission, sensory latency consists only of the nerve conduction time from the stimulus point to the recording electrode. Therefore, stimulation of the nerve at a single site is enough for calculation of sensory nerve conduction velocity, which is calculated by dividing stimulated nerve length by onset latency.

CTS patients, compared to normals, have been shown to have prolonged median motor nerve latencies, decreased median motor nerve amplitudes (Simpson, 1956; Thomas, 1960; Kimura, 1979, 1989) and decreased median motor nerve conduction velocities in the presence of CTS (Thomas, 1960; Kimura, 1979; Kimura and Ayyar, 1985). However, even normal values (see Table 7.7) show considerable variability, with distal onset latency usually ranging between 3.2 and 3.7 ms, motor nerve amplitude ranging between 12.6 and 13.2 mV, and conduction velocity ranging between 48.8 and 59.6 m/s. The upper limits for normals and lower limit for CTS diagnosis is usually defined as mean plus two standard deviations, yielding values of 4.5 ms for latency, 3.0 mV for amplitude, and 32.4 m/s for conduction velocity. However, it is important to note that there was a considerable variability in distal median motor nerve conduction parameters reported by these

TABLE 7.7

Normal Values for Median Motor Nerve Conduction

Authors	Onset Latency (ms)		Amplitude (mV)		Conduction Velocity (m/s)	
	Normal	Abnormal (>2 SD)	Normal	Abnormal (<2 SD)	Normal	Abnormal (<2 SD)
Burnham and Steadward (1994)	3.63 ± 0.28	4.2	12.8 ± 4.0	4.6	59.6 ± 3.7	52.0
Jackson and Clifford (1989)	3.2 ± 0.27	3.8	12.6 ± 3.22	6.1	—	—
Kimura (1989)	3.49 ± 0.34	4.2	—	—	48.8 ± 5.3	38.0
Kimura (1979)	3.6 ± 0.36	4.3	—	—	49.0 ± 5.7	37.4
Melvin et al. (1973)	3.7 ± 0.3	4.5	13.2 ± 5.0	3.0	56.7 ± 3.8	48.9
Thomas et al. (1967)	3.4 ± 0.48	4.4	—	—	59.1 ± 5.2	48.5
Johnson and Olsen (1960)	—	—	—	—	53.0 ± 6.4	40.0
Average	3.5	4.2	12.9	4.6	54.7	44.7

Note: All data are antidromic.

investigators, with various experimental settings, different room and skin temperatures, and a variety of conduction distances.

Similar to median motor nerve studies, the results of median sensory nerve conduction studies indicated that between 49% and 66% of patients with CTS demonstrate a prolonged median sensory peak latency, a reduced median sensory nerve amplitude or even a complete absence of sensory nerve action potential between the wrist and a specific digit (Kembel, 1968; Felsenthal and Spindler, 1979; Kimura and Ayyar, 1985; Stevens, 1987). Most researchers used the index finger for stimulation or recording, but some used the middle finger. Normal values (see Table 7.8) indicate that distal onset latency ranges between 2.5 and 2.8 ms, peak latency ranges between 3.0 and 3.2 ms, sensory nerve amplitude ranges between 32.9 and 44.9 mV, and conduction velocity ranges between 56.2 and 58.3 m/s. The upper limits for normals and lower limit for CTS diagnosis is again defined as mean plus two standard deviations, yielding values of 3.5 ms for onset latency, 4.0 ms for peak latency, 0 mV for amplitude. and 44.4 m/s for conduction velocity.

7.4.4 Limitations

There are a variety of factors that influence nerve conduction parameters and that need to be carefully controlled or noted so as to avoid false-positive CTS diagnoses based on erroneous interpretation of nerve conduction measurement. These factors include skin temperature and age and, perhaps, gender and body mass index.

Skin temperature has a profound effect on nerve conduction parameters (Baysal et al., 1993; Letz and Gerr, 1994). As the skin temperature decreases, the nerve conduction action potential recorded from a nerve demonstrates an increased amplitude and prolonged latency. Tashjian et al. (1987) reported that the antidromic median sensory nerve latency was delayed by 0.06 ms/deg., with cooling, and median sensory nerve amplitude was found to increase with upper extremity cooling with the antidromic technique by 3.5 µV/deg. Lee et al. (1993) claim that this temperature effect on latency may be as large as 0.1 ms/deg. Conversely, nerve impulses conduct faster at higher body temperature. The conduction velocity increases almost linearly, by 2.4 m/s/deg., as the temperature measured near the nerve increases from 29°C to 38°C (Johnson and Olsen, 1960).

TABLE 7.8

Normal Values for Median Sensory Nerve Conduction

Authors	Onset Latency (ms)		Peak Latency (ms)		Amplitude (μV)		Conduction Velocity (m/s)	
	Normal	Abnormal (>2 SD)	Normal	Abnormal (>2 SD)	Normal	Abnormal (<2 SD)	Normal	Abnormal (<2 SD)
Burnham and Steadward (1994)	—	—	—	—	44.9 ± 14.8	15.1	58.3 ± 5.7	46.7
Jackson and Clifford (1989)	2.47 ± 1.2	2.7	3.16 ± 0.16	3.5	32.9 ± 10.4	11.9	—	—
Kimura (1989)	2.84 ± 3.4	3.5	—	—	38.5 ± 15.6	7.1	56.2 ± 5.8	44.4
Kimura (1979)	2.82 ± 2.8	3.4	—	—	41.3 ± 19.3	2.5	57.3 ± 6.9	45.1
Melvin et al. (1973)	—	—	3.2 ± 0.2	3.8	41.6 ± 25.0	0.0	56.9 ± 4.0	48.7
Johnson and Melvin (1967)	—	—	3.0 ± 0.4	4.0	—	—	—	—
Average	2.7	3.2	3.1	3.8	39.8	7.3	57.2	46.2

Note: All data are antidromic.

Correction factors for skin temperature are typically only employed when wrist temperature exceed normal ranges, defined as 29.6°C–33.4°C (Halar et al., 1983). However, to improve the sensitivity of nerve conduction studies, Jackson and Clifford (1989) suggested applying correction factors when the skin temperature measured at the wrist midline exceeded 31.0°C.

Slowing of median nerve function occurs naturally with increasing age though not necessarily leading to the development of CTS (Nathan et al., 1988, 1992). Specifically, median sensory nerve conduction velocity decreases by as much as 1.3 m/s per decade of age (Stetson et al., 1992; Letz and Gerr, 1994). Similarly, sensory nerve conduction velocity has been shown to decline by 1 m/s per decade (Chodoroff et al., 1985).

Effects of the body mass index on median nerve conduction are conflicting. Nathan et al. (1992) reported a strong positive correlation, while Letz and Gerr (1994) reported a small negative association between measures. If other variables are carefully accounted for, then gender differences in median nerve conduction parameters have been minimal (Nathan et al., 1988, 1992; Stetson et al., 1992; Robinson et al., 1993).

To improve the sensitivity of nerve conduction tests and to clarify the confounding effects of a generalized peripheral neuropathy, clinicians have suggested comparing median nerve conduction to ulnar or radial nerve conduction. Felsenthal and Spindler (1979) performed a 14 cm antidromic sensory nerve action potential technique to index finger and little finger for comparison of median and ulnar nerve. They concluded that a difference greater than 0.46 ms between median and ulnar sensory nerve peak latencies in the same hand was suggestive of CTS. Similarly, Johnson et al. (1981) and Jackson and Clifford (1989) recommended differences of median and ulnar peak latency of 0.3 and 0.35 ms, respectively, suggestive of CTS.

Johnson et al. (1987) established a comparison study of median-to-radial sensory nerve in thumb with a 10 cm antidromic sensory nerve action potential technique. They concluded that a peak latency disparity of greater than 0.4 ms between median and radial is suggestive of CTS because 93% of normal subjects demonstrated a difference of 0.4 ms or less. Carroll (1987) and Jackson and Clifford (1989) also reported differences of 0.3–0.4 ms as suggestive of CTS. Normal ulnar and radial sensory conduction values to be used in comparison with median nerve values are summarized in Table 7.9. Note, that the amplitude and conduction velocity of little finger are slightly larger and faster than for the ring finger.

TABLE 7.9

Normal and Abnormal Values for Ulnar and Radial Sensory Nerve

Nerve	Authors	Latency (ms)		Amplitude (µV)		Conduction Velocity (m/s)	
		Normal	Abnormal (>2 SD)	Normal	Abnormal (<2 SD)	Normal	Abnormal (<2 SD)
Ulnar nerve	Burnham and Steadward (1994)	—	—	26.7 ± 9.8 (Digit 4) 42.7 ± 18.0 (Digit 5)	7.1 6.7	55.7 ± 4.7 (Digit 4) 58.1 ± 5.7 (Digit 5)	46.3 46.7
	Kimura (1989)	2.54 ± 0.29 (Digit 5)	3.12	35.0 ± 14.7 (Digit 5)	5.6	54.8 ± 53 (Digit 5)	44.2
Radial nerve	Burnham and Steadward (1994)	—	—	—	—	59.4 ± 5.6 (Digit 1)	48.2
	Kimura (1989)	2.37 ± 0.22 (Digit 1)	2.81	13.0 ± 7.5 (Digit 1)	0.0	58.0 ± 6.0 (Digit 1)	46.0

7.5 Electromyography

As discussed in Chapter 3, the neuromuscular system consists of many muscles, each containing many motor units, each of which consists of a nerve innervating a collection of muscle fibers. For the muscle to produce force, these motor units need to be recruited according to the size principle, from the smallest to the largest, and from lower to higher thresholds. To recruit a given motor unit, nerve action potentials proceed from the cell body (which has received similar action potentials, either from higher centers in the central nervous system, or from other neurons in the peripheral nervous system), along the axon, across the synapse to each of the corresponding muscle fibers. There, through depolarization of the cell membrane, a similar muscle action potential is generated, which passes along the muscle fiber, depolarizing the membranes of sarcoplasmic reticulum, releasing calcium ions to promote the crossbridging of thick and thin filaments, and, ultimately, causing force production in the muscle. For a muscle twitch, a few small motor units may be involved at relatively low firing frequencies with a small amount of muscle action potentials. For maximum muscle contraction, all of the motor units need to be recruited at tetanic frequencies, resulting in a high level of muscle action potentials or electrical activity in the muscle. This muscle electrical activity, termed *electromyography* (EMG) for short, can be measured by placing electrodes either on the surface of the skin or placed within the muscle and suitably amplifying and processing the signal. Since, the electrical activity varies with the amount of motor unit recruited and thus the force produced by the muscle, EMG is a good measure of muscle force production, especially in occupational activities, where the force cannot be measured directly without interfering with the task on hand. However, over time as the muscle fatigues, force production drops, but motor unit recruitment and corresponding electrical activity increases. Therefore, EMG is also very useful in quantifying localized muscle fatigue.

7.5.1 EMG Instrumentation

The most crucial step in measuring a noise-free electrical signal is the proper attachment of electrodes to the individual. This can be either *invasive*, within the muscle, by using needle electrodes, or *noninvasive*, on the surface of the skin over the belly of the muscle of interest, by using surface electrodes. Needle electrodes yield a more sensitive signal, to the point of even isolating individual motor units. However, since they are invasive, they typically require the supervision of a medically trained expert and, thus, are better suited for a clinical setting rather than an industrial setting. Surface electrodes, being, noninvasive, do not require such medical supervision, and, being slightly less sensitive to electrical noise, are better suited to an industrial environment. They should be high-quality silver/silver-chloride electrodes used in conjunction with specialized electrode paste to improve the electrical conductance. However, to achieve as low an *electrical impedance* as possible (and reduce the effect of electrical noise) is also important to prepare the subject, by shaving the individual's hair, abrading the skin to remove the dry, scaling surface layer, rubbing electrode paste into the skin to further reduce skin resistance, and letting the electrode paste "soak" into the skin for 10–20 min. before the start of experimentation. By such means it is often possible to decrease skin resistance from values as high as 200,000 Ω to as low as 5,000 Ω.

The electrodes can be attached either in a *unipolar* or *bipolar* mode. In the unipolar mode, one active electrode is attached over the belly of the muscle to obtain the largest signal possible from the greatest number of motor units. The reference and ground electrodes are placed on nearby bony parts with minimal electrical activity. In the bipolar mode, the two active electrodes are placed over different areas of the muscle in order to obtain a differential reading, with the ground again placed on a bony part. The unipolar mode is best suited for industrial applications, in which overall muscle force is being estimated, while the bipolar modes is used for muscular dysfunction in clinical applications.

Next, the electrodes should be inserted into a small portable preamplifier worn on the subject as close as possible to the measuring site. By reducing the length of the electrode leads it is possible to minimize noise received from the *antenna effect* and to minimize motion artifacts. Amplification of the desired signal close to the origin also reduces the effects of any electrical noise added later in the circuitry. The preamplifier should have a high input impedance, up to 100 MΩ or at least 100 times the electrode impedance. The preamplifier should also contain a fuse or some other circuitry to limit faulty circuits.

The preamplified signal is next sent to an amplifier for further amplification (preferably variably controlled) and preprocessing. The amplifier should have a high *common-mode signal-to-noise rejection ratio* of at least 80–90 dB. This serves to reduce input lead capacitance differences and electrical noise from 60 Hz line current or other electrical instruments or machines in the vicinity. The amplifier should have wide preferably adjustable, *bandwidth*, on the order of 10–1000 Hz and an adjustable notch filter (or two) to reduce noise at critical frequencies, such as 60 Hz. The amplifier output levels should be in the range of ±5 V expected for analog-to-digital converters on computers.

Foulke et al. (1981) developed one such EMG measuring system for industrial use that met the above criteria. It used a commercially available but slightly modified AC voltmeter to provide both instantaneous raw outputs compatible with computer input as well as an RMS (root-mean-square) signal processor (discussed in Section 7.5.2). The system was successfully used in several industrial studies of hand-intensive work potentially leading to WRMSDs (Armstrong et al., 1982; Freivalds, 1990; Park et al., 1991). Further details on surface electromyography and EMG instrumentation can be found in Basmajian and De Luca (1985), Cram et al. (1988), NIOSH (1990), DeLuca (1997), and Chaffin et al. (1999).

7.5.2 EMG Analysis

The raw EMG signal can be analyzed in one of four different approaches based on the variables analyzed and the complexity of the analysis: EMG amplitude, EMG frequency, EMG-force relationships, and amplitude probability distributions. The simplest and most straightforward analysis is to process the raw signal through an EMG system similar to that described in Section 7.5.1 and obtain an *RMS signal* defined as extracting the square root of the mean of the function squared:

$$\text{RMS} = \left\{ \frac{1}{T} \int_0^T v^2(t)dt \right\}^{\frac{1}{2}} \tag{7.9}$$

where
  v(t) is the raw voltage signal
  T is the time period for the periodic signal

In practice, many amplifiers or processors may not produce an exact RMS value, but will produce a *smoothed-rectified signal* close in value. Note that rectification, or creating positive values from negative values, is comparable to squaring the function and then taking the square root. Smoothing, through a resistor–capacitor (RC) circuit with a time constant of

$$\tau = \frac{1}{RC} \tag{7.10}$$

is comparable to integration. Note also, that term *integrated EMG* applies to EMG values obtained by charging a capacitor (Bigland and Lippold, 1954). It does not correspond to the smooth-rectified or RMS EMG, which rises or falls, depending on the raw signal, as opposed to the integrated EMG, which would continually keep on rising until the capacitor is discharged.

As would be expected from the general description of EMG at the beginning of Section 7.5, the relationship of EMG_{RMS} to muscle force is monotonically increasing and provides the basis for estimating muscle tension during an activity. This relationship was first observed by Lippold (1952) and characterized as a direct linear relationship (Bigland and Lippold, 1954). Later, more detailed analyses, led to observations of a nonlinear upward trend (Nightingale, 1960; Zuniga and Simons, 1969), while others claimed a nonlinear downward trend (Milner-Brown et al., 1973; Kosarov and Gydikov, 1976).

Figure 7.15 may explain the controversy. There are two simultaneous events occurring during force production. Initially as a motor unit is recruited, successive twitches increase the force rapidly as the firing rate also increases rapidly. With more action potential, the contribution to the amplitude of the EMG signal increases, yielding an upward slope (Slope 1 in Figure 7.15). Near tetanic frequency, the force is leveling off at the maximum tension level for the motor unit, and the firing frequency, although still increasing, has become cyclical, at which point, the RMS value changes little and the contribution to the EMG amplitude decreases with a shallower slope (Slope 2 in Figure 7.15). This process is

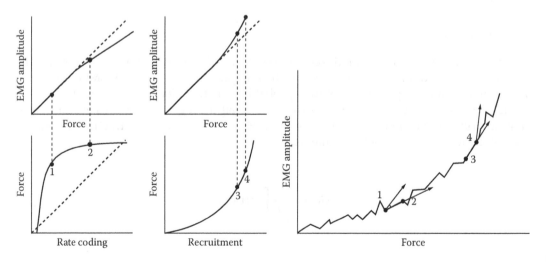

FIGURE 7.15
Theoretical basis for EMG amplitude–force relationship (see text for explanation).

termed *rate coding* (Milner-Brown et al., 1973). Simultaneously, additional motor units are also recruited. However, based on the size principle, each additional motor unit is larger, producing more force, but is also recruited at a higher threshold, with higher frequency and larger muscle action potentials and adding more contribution to EMG amplitude (Slopes 3 and 4 in Figure 7.15).

Complicating matters further is that electrode position on the muscle can also affect EMG (Zuniga et al., 1970) while, from Chapter 3, muscle size, length, and velocity affect force development. Therefore, most force prediction models (Cholewicki and McGill, 1994; Granata and Marras, 1995) take the general form of

$$F = g \times f_l \times f_v \times EMG_{RMS} \tag{7.11}$$

where
  F is the predicted muscle force
  g is the gain factor for a given muscle, individual, etc.
  f_l is the scaling factor for muscle length
  f_v is the scaling factor for velocity of muscle contraction

The *gain* factor g is very critical and methods for determining it, especially for multiple-muscle systems, have been formulated (Cholewicki and McGill, 1994). Thus, in most cases, it is important to standardize the shape of the EMG amplitude–force relationship for a given individual, a given muscle, or a specific activity. Then this curve can be used to reasonably estimate the forces required to perform other more complex activities by that same person.

To compare across individuals or tasks, a frequently used practice is to normalize the EMG signal for each muscle or subject as follows:

$$EMG_{Norm} = \frac{EMG_i - EMG_{Min}}{EMG_{Max} - EMG_{Min}} \tag{7.12}$$

where
  EMG_i is the EMG signal at time i
  EMG_{Min} is the minimum EMG signal, typically taken at rest
  EMG_{Max} is the maximum EMG signal obtained from that muscle

Normalization allows EMG values to be compared across a variety of conditions. For example, electrode placement could vary from muscle to muscle, day to day, or individual to individual. Normalization then allows data to be compared as a relative value across muscles, days, individuals, or other factors of interest. However, one needs to be careful in using this technique on dynamic exertions, which could lead to large errors, if the normalization is performed at an arbitrary muscle or joint position. Instead, any normalization of an EMG signal taken at a given joint angle must be normalized with minimum and maximum EMG signals taken at the same joint angle (Mirka, 1991).

Note that as a muscle fatigues, individual motor units may reduce the level of force production or even completely drop out, even though the motoneuron is still firing and muscle action potentials are still being created. As the result, for a given level of force production, EMG amplitude increases (Lippold et al., 1961) and the EMG amplitude–force relationship shown in Figure 7.15 shifts upward. If EMG amplitude is found to increase over the course of a working shift for the same activity, then one could surmise that muscle fatigue is occurring. From Chapter 3, it would be expected that muscle fatigue would occur once static muscle forces exceeded 15% of maximum voluntary contraction (MVC), i.e., the point at which the blood flow to the muscle starts being occluded, reducing the amount of oxygen being supplied to the working muscle.

In addition during fatigue, as motor units drop out, the frequency characteristics of the EMG signal will also change, leading to the second type of EMG analysis. As discussed in Chapter 3, the larger motor units are higher frequency, faster twitch, and more fatigable, while the smaller motor units are lower frequency, slower twitch, and more fatigue resistant. Thus, there is tendency for the fast fatigable motor units to drop out first, leaving behind the slower, and more fatigue-resistant motor units in the active pool. Consequently, there is a drop in the frequency characteristics of the EMG signal or a downward shift in the mean power of the signal and serves as a clear measure of the occurrence of muscle fatigue (see Figure 7.16) (Chaffin, 1969, 1973). Again, the frequency characteristics vary with many of the same factors that affect EMG amplitude but, with careful control, *frequency analysis* can be a useful tool for biomechanical studies (Herberts et al., 1980; Hagberg, 1981; Hansson et al., 1992). Typically, the raw EMG is filtered appropriately, digitally sampled (twice as fast as the highest frequency of interest), and processed with a fast Fourier transform to produce a *power spectrum* (IEEE, 1967; Bergland, 1969). As an alternative to software analysis, there are also a variety of commercially available spectrum analyzers.

The shape of the EMG amplitude–force curve is the basis for the third type of EMG analysis. deVries (1968) postulated that the functional state of muscle may be better assessed by examining the slope of the EMG amplitude–force curve, termed the *efficiency of electrical activity*, rather than assessing muscle strength alone, which may be influenced by psychological factors such as motivation. de Vries (1968) found that the slope decreased with improved muscle function for athletes and increased with disuse atrophy. Whereas de Vries (1968) only considered linear slopes, Chaffin et al. (1980) expanded the concept to the more common nonlinear formulation and used a two-part piecewise linear regression

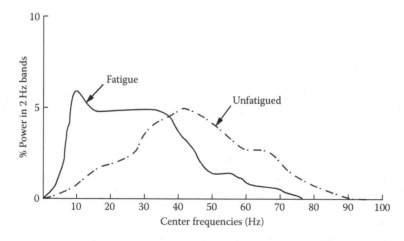

FIGURE 7.16
Average EMG power spectrum with reference to fatigue. (Adapted from Chaffin, D.B., *J. Occup. Med.*, 15, 346, 1973. With permission.)

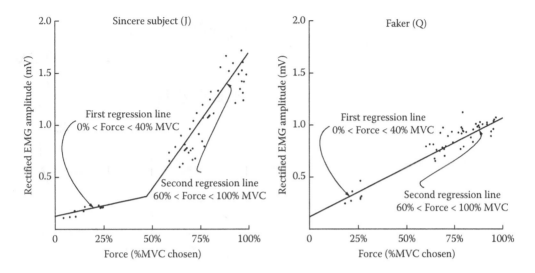

FIGURE 7.17
Piecewise regression analysis of EMG amplitude–force relationship. (Reproduced from Chaffin, D.B. et al., *Med. Sci. Sports Exerc.*, 12, 205, 1980. With permission.)

to model the Type I and Type II motor units (see Figure 7.17). This type of EMG analysis was then found to be successful in correctly identifying 21 of 22 individuals who were either "faking" or providing sincere muscular exertions and in significantly ($r^2 = 0.6$, $p < .001$) predicting their true MVC.

The fourth type of EMG analysis, developed by Jonsson (1978), is the most involved in that it combines several of the above techniques into one measure. The smooth-rectified EMG signal from a manual task over a given time period (see Figure 7.18, Steps A, B, D) is compared to a previously developed individual-specific EMG amplitude–force curve (Step C) to produce a force over time curve (Step E). The resulting force data is then sorted by amplitude in ascending order to produce a cumulative probability distribution termed the amplitude distribution function (Step F). Jonsson (1978) suggested load limits for continuous work: (1) the 90th percentile (peak) should not exceed 50%–70% MVC, (2) the 50th percentile (mean) should not exceed 1%–14% MVC, and (3) the 10th percentile (static) should not exceed 2%–5% MVC. Figure 7.19 depicts the resulting amplitude distribution function when applied to a variety of manual tasks in comparison to recommended exertion levels (shaded arc). Task A depicts an acceptably low muscular load on the trapezius muscle when using a light tool. Tasks B, C, and D all place excessively high muscular loading, Task C at the static loading level (at 8%–10% MVC exceeding the static level), Task D at the peak level, while Task B exceeds all three levels throughout the full range of exertion.

This technique has since been used by several other researchers (Hagberg, 1979; Linderhed, 1993) but, perhaps, has been less popular because of its complexity and extreme limits. The Jonsson (1978) recommended static loading of 2%–5% MVC is much lower than the Rohmert (1960) 15% MVC level discussed in Chapter 3 and could be difficult to achieve in many industries. Furthermore, one needs to be careful not confuse Jonsson's 10th percentile static load level with the more generic term static task and mean %MVC measured for that task. In that case, it would be better to compare mean %MVC values with Jonsson's (1978) 10%–14% (Ankrum, 2000). Further details on EMG analyses can be obtained from Desmedt (1973), NIOSH (1990), and Kumar and Mital (1996).

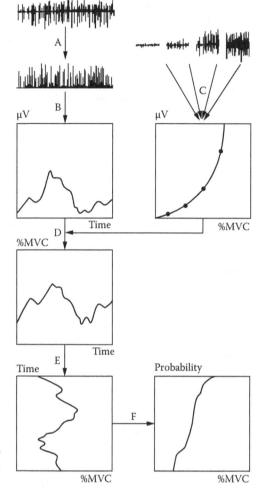

FIGURE 7.18
Formation of the amplitude distribution function (see text for details). (Reproduced from Jonsson, B., *Scand. J. Rehabil. Med.*, 10, 69, 1978. With permission.)

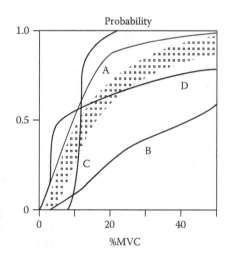

FIGURE 7.19
Application of the amplitude distribution function to manual tasks (see text for details). (Reproduced from Jonsson, B., *Scand. J. Rehabil. Med*, 10, 69, 1978. With permission.)

Questions

1. What are the characteristics needed for a "good" measurement system?
2. Compare and contrast common motion measurement systems.
3. What are crosstalk, zero drift, and hysteresis?
4. Compare and contrast force distribution measurement systems.
5. Discuss the problem of force versus pressure measurements found in many force distribution measurement systems. How may a force-sensitive sensor be improved in this regard?
6. What is the conceptual explanation for changes in nerve conduction found in many WRMSDs?
7. Describe the equipment and procedures used in nerve conduction velocity measurement.
8. What is the difference between orthodromic and antidromic stimulation? When would each be used?
9. What is the difference between onset and peak latency? Which would be preferred and why?
10. What are some of the factors that may limit the validity and reliability of nerve conduction velocity measurements?
11. Describe the equipment and procedures used to record EMG.
12. How do common-mode rejection ratios, bandwidth, and filtering affect the EMG signal?
13. How may EMGs be used to estimate muscle force?
14. Compare and contrast RMS, smooth-rectified, and integrated EMG signals.
15. Why are EMG signals sometimes normalized?
16. What information does frequency analysis of an EMG signal provide?
17. What is efficiency of electrical activity? Why is the curve nonlinear?
18. Explain the usefulness of distribution analysis for EMG signals.

Problems

1. Calculate the RMS value for a sinusoid with a peak-to-peak amplitude of 1 mV.
2. Calculate the normalized value for a 0.1 mV response in the signal of Problem 7.1.

References

AAEE—American Association of Electromyography and Electrodiagnosis. (1984). *Guidelines in Electrodiagnostic Medicine*. Rochester, MN: Professional Standard Committee, AAEE.

Ankrum, D.R. (2000). On the confusion between static load level and static task. *Applied Ergonomics* 31:545–546.

Armstrong, T.J. (1994). *Cumulative Trauma Disorders of the Hand and Wrist: Ergonomic Guides*. Akron, OH: American Industrial Hygiene Association.

Armstrong, T.J., Foulke, J.A., Joseph, B.S., and Goldstein, S.A. (1982). Investigation of cumulative trauma disorders in a poultry processing plant. *American Industrial Hygiene Association Journal* 43:103–116.

Atkinson, P.J., Newberry, W.N., Atkinson, T.S., and Haut, R.C. (1998). A method to increase the sensitive range of pressure sensitive film. *Journal of Biomechanics* 31:855–859.

Bader, D.L. and Hawken, M.B. (1986). Pressure distribution under the ischium of normal subjects. *Journal of Biomedical Engineering* 8:353–357.

Bader, D.L., Gwilliam, J., Newson, T., and Harris, J.D. (1984). Pressure mapping at the interface. *Care: Science and Practice* 8:67–69.

Basmajian, J.V. and De Luca, C.J. (1985). *Muscles Alive: Their Functions Revealed by Electromyography*, 5th edn, Baltimore, MD: Williams & Wilkins.

Baysal, A.I., Chang, C.W., and OH, S.J. (1993). Temperature effects on nerve conduction studies in patients with carpal tunnel syndrome. *Acta Neurologica Scandinavica* 88:213–216.

Beebe, D.J., Denton, D.D., Radwin, R.G., and Webster, J.G. (1998). Silicon-based tactile sensor for finger-mounted applications. *IEEE Transactions on Biomedical Engineering* 45:151–159.

Bergland, G.D. (1969). A guided tour of the fast Fourier transform. *IEEE Spectrum* 7:41–52.

Betts, R.P., Duckworth, T., Austin, I.G., Crocker, S.P., and Moore, S. (1980). Critical light reflection at a plastic/glass interface and its application to foot pressure measurements. *Journal of Medical Engineering and Technology* 4:136–142.

Bigland, B. and Lippold, O.C.J. (1954). The relation between force, velocity, and integrated electrical activity in human muscles. *Journal of Physiology* 123:214–224.

Bonebrake, A.R., Fernandex, J.E., Marley, R.J, Dahalan, J.B., and Kilmer, K.J. (1990). A treatment for carpal tunnel syndrome: Evaluation of objective and subjective measures. *Journal of Manipulative and Physiological Therapeutics* 13:507–520.

Boone, D.C. and Azen, S.P. (1979). Normal range of motion in joints of male subjects. *Journal of Bone and Joint Surgery* 61:756–759.

Brand, R.A. and Crowninshield, R.D. (1981). Comment on criteria for patient evaluation tools. *Journal of Biomechanics* 14:655.

Buchholz, B. and Wellman, H. (1997). Practical operation of a biaxial goniometer at the wrist joint. *Human Factors* 39:119–129.

Burnham, R.S. and Steadward, R.D. (1994). Upper extremity peripheral nerve entrapments among wheelchair athletes. *Archives of Physical Medicine and Rehabilitation* 75:519–524.

Carroll, G. (1987). Comparison of median and radial nerve sensory latencies in the electrophysiological diagnosis of carpal tunnel syndrome. *Electroencephalography and Clinical Neurophysiology* 68:101–106.

Carvalho, A.A. and Radwin, R.G. (1996). New method for extending the range of conductive polymer sensors for contact force. *International Journal of Industrial Ergonomics* 17:285–290.

Chaffin, D.B. (1969). Surface EMG frequency analysis as a diagnostic tool. *Journal of Occupational Medicine* 11(3):109–115.

Chaffin, D.B. (1973). Localized muscle fatigue—Definition and measurement. *Journal of Occupational Medicine* 15(4):346–354.

Chaffin, D.B., Lee, M.W., and Freivalds, A. (1980). Muscle strength assessment from EMG analysis. *Medicine and Science in Sports and Exercise* 12:205–211.

Chaffin, D.B., Andersson, G.B.J., and Martin, B.J. (1999). *Occupational Biomechanics*, 3rd edn, New York: John Wiley & Sons.

Chao, E.Y. (1978). Experimental methods for biomechanical measurement of joint kinematics. In: B.N. Feinberg and D.G. Fleming (eds), *CRC Handbook for Engineering in Medicine and Biology*, Vol. 1. Boca Raton, FL: CRC Press, pp. 385–411.

Chodoroff, G., Tashjian, E., and Ellenberg, M. (1985). Orthodromic vs antidromic sensory nerve latencies in healthy persons. *Archives of Physical Medicine and Rehabilitation* 66:589–591.

Cholewicki, J. and McGill, S.M. (1994). EMG assisted optimization: A hybrid approach for estimating muscle forces in an indeterminate biomechanical model. *Journal of Biomechanics* 27:1287–1289.

Cram, J.R., Kasman, G.S., and Holtz, J. (1988). *Introduction to Surface Electromyography*. Gaithersburg, MD: Aspen Publishers.

DeLuca, C.J. (1997). The use of surface electromyography in biomechanics. *Journal of Applied Biomechanics* 13:135–163.

Desmedt, J.E., ed. (1973). *New Development in Electromyography and Clinical Neurophysiology*. Basel, Switzerland: Karger.

deVries, H.A. (1968). "Efficiency of electrical activity" as a physiological measure of the functional state of muscle tissue. *American Journal of Physical Medicine* 47:10–22.

DiBenedetto, M., Mitz, M., Klingbeil, G., and Davidoff, D.D. (1986). New criteria for sensory nerve conduction especially useful in diagnosing carpal tunnel syndrome. *Archives of Physical Medicine and Rehabilitation* 67:586–589.

Dillon, J. (1981). The role of ergonomics in the development of performance tests for furniture. *Applied Ergonomics* 12:169–175.

Drummond, D.S., Narechania, R.G., Rosenthal, A.N., Breed, A.L., Lange, T.A., and Drummond, D.K. (1982). A study of pressure distributions measured during balanced and unbalanced sitting. *The Journal of Bone and Joint Surgery* 64A:1034–1039.

Dumitru, D. and Walsh, N. (1988). Practical instrumentation and common sources of error. *American Journal of Physical Medicine and Rehabilitation* 67:55–65.

Elftman, H. (1934). A cinematic study of the distribution of pressure in the human foot. *Anatomical Record* 59:481–487.

Estill, C.F., MacDonald, L.A., Wenzl, T.B., and Petersen, M.R. (2000). Use of accelerometers as an ergonomic assessment method for arm acceleration—A large-scale field trial. *Ergonomics* 43:1430–1445.

Fellows, G.L. and Freivalds, A. (1989). The use of force sensing resistors in ergonomic tool design. *Proceedings of the Human Factors Society* 33:713–717.

Fellows, G.L. and Freivalds, A. (1991). Ergonomic evaluation of a foam rubber grip for tool handles. *Applied Ergonomics* 22:225–230.

Felsenthal, G. and Spindler, H. (1979). Palmer conduction time of median and ulnar nerves of normal subjects and patients with carpal tunnel syndrome. *American Journal of Physical Medicine and Rehabilitation* 58:131–138.

Fenety, A., MacLeod, D., and Crouse, J. (1994). Use of a pressure mat to continuously measure seated postural shifts. *Proceedings of the 12th Triennial Congress of the International Ergonomics Association*, Vol. 2. Mississauga, Ontario, Canada: Human Factors Association of Canada, pp. 92–94.

Fenety, P.A., Putnam, C., and Walker, J.M. (2000). In-chair movement: Validity, reliability and implications for measuring sitting discomfort. *Applied Ergonomics* 31:383–393.

Ferguson-Pell, M. and Cardi, M.D. (1991). Evaluation of three advanced pressure mapping systems for clinical applications in seating and positioning. *Annals of Biomedical Engineering* 19:643.

Ferguson-Pell, M. and Cardi, M.D. (1993). Prototype development and comparative evaluation of wheelchair mapping system. *Assistive Technology* 5:788–791.

Foulke, J.A., Goldstein, S.A., and Armstrong, T.J. (1981). An EMG preamplifier system for biomechanical studies. *Journal of Biomechanics* 14:437–438.

Franks, C.I., Betts, R.P., and Duckworth, T. (1983). Microprocessor-based image processing system for dynamic foot pressure studies. *Medical & Biological Engineering & Computing* 21:566–572.

Freivalds, A. (1990). Pinching forces sustained during lens polishing operations. *International Journal of Industrial Ergonomics* 6:261–266.

Garber, S.L., Krouskop, T.A., and Carter, R.E. (1978). A system for clinically evaluating wheelchair pressure-relief cushions. *The American Journal of Occupational Therapy* 32:565–570.

Ghavanini, M.R. and Haghighat, M. (1998). Carpal tunnel syndrome: Reappraisal of five clinical tests. *Electromyography and Clinical Neurophysiology* 38:437–441.

Granata, K.P. and Marras, W.S. (1995). An EMG-assisted model of trunk loading during free-dynamic lifting. *Journal of Biomechanics* 28:1309–1317.

Gross, C.M., Goonetilleke, R.S., Menon, K.K., Banaag, J.C.N., and Nair, C.N. (1994). The biomechanical assessment and prediction of seat comfort. In: R. Lueder and K. Noro (eds), *Hard Facts about Soft Machines: The Ergonomics of Seating*. London, U.K.: Taylor & Francis, pp. 231–253.

Gyi, D.E., Porter, M., and Robertson, N.K.B. (1998). Seat pressure measurement technologies: Considerations for their evaluation. *Applied Ergonomics* 27:85–91.

Hagberg, M. (1979). The amplitude distribution of surface EMG in static and intermittent static muscular performance. *European Journal of Applied Physiology* 40:265–272.

Hagberg, M. (1981). Work load and fatigue in repetitive arm elevation. *Ergonomics* 24:543–555.

Hagberg, M., Silverstein, B., Wells, R., Smith, M.J., Hendrick, H.W., Carayon, P., and Perusse, M. (1995). *Work-Related Musculoskeletal Disorders (WMSDs): A Reference Book for Prevention*. London, U.K.: Taylor & Francis.

Halar, E.M., DeLisa, J.A., and Soine, T.L. (1983). Nerve conduction studies in upper extremities: Skin temperature corrections. *Archives of Physical Medicine and Rehabilitation* 64:412–416.

Hale, J.E. and Brown, T.D. (1992). Contact stress gradient detection limits of pressensor film. *Journal of Biomechanical Engineering (Transactions of the ASME)* 114:352–357.

Hansson, G.A., Strömberg, U., Larsson, B., Ohlsson, K., Balogh, I., and Moritz, U. (1992). Electromyographic fatigue in neck/shoulder muscles and endurance in women with repetitive work. *Ergonomics* 35:1341–1352.

Hansson, G.A., Balogh, I., Ohlsson, K., Rylander, L., and Skerfving, S. (1996). Goniometer measurement and computer analysis of wrist angles and movements applied to occupational repetitive work. *Journal of Electromyography and Kinesiology* 6:23–35.

Hara, T., Horii, E., An, K.N., Cooney, W.P., Linscheid, R.L., and Chao, E.Y. (1992). Force distribution across wrist joint: Application of pressure sensitive conductive rubber. *Journal of Hand Surgery* 17:339–347.

Harada, K., Watanabe, M., Ohkura, K., and Enomoto, S. (2000). Measure of bite force and occlusal contact area before and after bilateral split ramus osteotomy of the mandible using a new pressure-sensitive device: A preliminary report. *Journal of Oral Maxillofacial Surgery* 58:370–373.

Haut, R. (1989). Contact pressures in the patello-femoral joint during impact loading on the human flexed knee. *Journal of Orthopaedic Research* 7:272–280.

Herberts, P., Kadefors, R., and Broman, H. (1980). Arm positioning in manual tasks: A electromyographic study of localized muscle fatigue. *Ergonomics* 23:655–665.

Hertzberg, H.T.E. (1972). *The Human Buttocks in Sitting: Pressures, Patterns, and Palliatives*, SAE Technical Paper No. 720005. Warrendale, PA: Society of Automotive Engineers.

Houle, R.J. (1969). Evaluation of seat devices designed to prevent ischemic ulcers in paraplegic patients. *Archives of Physical Medicine and Rehabilitation* 50:587–594.

IEEE. (1967). Special issue on fast Fourier transform and its application to digital filtering and spectral analysis. *IEEE Transactions on Audio and Electroacoustics* AU-15:1–117.

Jackson, D.A. and Clifford, J.C. (1989). Electrodiagnosis of mild carpal tunnel syndrome. *Archives of Physical Medicine and Rehabilitation* 70:199–204.

Jang, H. (2002). The effects of dynamic wrist workloads on risks of carpal tunnel syndrome. PhD dissertation. University Park, PA: The Pennsylvania State University.

Jensen, T.R., Radwin, R.G., and Webster, J.G. (1991). A conductive polymer sensor for measuring external finger forces. *Journal of Biomechanics* 24:851–858.

Johnson, E.W. and Melvin, J.L. (1967). Sensory conduction studies of median and ulnar nerves. *Archives of Physical Medicine and Rehabilitation* 48:25–30.

Johnson, E.W. and Olsen, K.J. (1960). Clinical value of motor nerve conduction velocity determination. *Journal of the American Medical Association* 172:2030–2035.

Johnson, E.W., Kukla, R., and Wongsam, P. (1981). Sensory latencies to the ring finger: Normal values and relation to carpal tunnel syndrome. *Archives of Physical Medicine and Rehabilitation* 62:206–208.

Johnson, E.W., Sipski, M., and Lammertse, T. (1987). Median and radial sensory latencies to digit I: Normal values and usefulness in carpal tunnel syndrome. *Archives of Physical Medicine and Rehabilitation* 68:140–141.

Jonsson, B. (1978). Quantitative electromyographic evaluation of muscular load during work. *Scandinavian Journal of Rehabilitation Medicine* 10(Suppl. 6):69–74.

Jürgens, H.W. (1969). Die Verteilung des Körperdrucks auf Siztfläche und Rückenlehne als Problem der Industrieanthropologie (Distribution of body weight on the seat pan and seat back as an ergonomics problem). *Ergonomics* 12:198–205.

Kadaba, M.P., Ferguson-Pell, M.W., Palmieri, V.R., and Cochran, G.V.B. (1984). Ultrasound mapping of the buttock-cushion interface contour. *Archives of Physical Medicine and Rehabilitation* 65:467–469.

Kembel, F. (1968). Electrodiagnosis of the carpal tunnel syndrome. *Journal of Neurology, Neurosurgery and Psychiatry* 31:23–27.

Kimura, J. (1979). The carpal tunnel syndrome—Localization of conduction abnormalities within the distal segment of the median nerve. *Brain* 102:619–635.

Kimura, J. (1989). *Electrodiagnosis in Diseases of Nerve and Muscle: Principles and Practice*, 2nd edn, Philadelphia, PA: Davis Company.

Kimura, J. and Ayyar, D.R. (1985). The carpal tunnel syndrome: Electrophysiological aspects of 639 symptomatic extremities. *Electroencephalography and Clinical Neurophysiology* 25:151–164.

Konrath, G.A., Hamel, A.J., Guerin, J., Olson, S.A., Bay, B., and Sharkey, N.A. (1999). Biomechanical evaluation of impaction fractures of the femoral head. *Journal of Orthopaedic Trauma* 13:407–413.

Kosarov, D. and Gydikov, A. (1976). Dependence of the discharge frequency of motor units in different human muscles upon the level of the isometric muscle tension. *EMG Clinical Neurophysiology* 16:293–306.

Kumar, S. and Mital, A. (1996). *Electromyography in Ergonomics*. London, U.K.: Taylor & Francis.

Lee, H.J., DeLisa, J.A., and Bach, J.R. (1993). The effect of temperature on antidromic median sensory conduction. *Electromyography and Clinical Neurophysiology*. 33:125–128.

Lemerle, P., Klinger, A., Cristalli, A., and Geuder, M. (2008). Application of pressure mapping techniques to measure push and gripping forces with precision. *Ergonomics* 51:168–191.

Letz, R. and Gerr, F. (1994). Covariates of human peripheral nerve function: Nerve conduction velocity and amplitude. *Neurotoxicology and Teratology* 16:95–104.

Lindan, O., Greenway, R.M., and Piazza, J.M. (1965). Pressure distribution on the surface of the human body: I. Evaluation in lying and sitting positions using a "bed of springs and nails." *Archives of Physical Medicine* 46:378–385.

Linderhed, H. (1993). A new dimension to amplitude analysis of EMG. *International Journal of Ergonomics* 11:243–247.

Lippold, O.C.J. (1952). The relation between integrated action potentials in a human muscle and its isometric contraction. *Journal of Physiology* 117:492–499.

Lippold, O.C.J., Redfearn, J.W.T., and Vučo, J. (1961). The electromyography of fatigue. *Ergonomics* 4:121–131.

Logan, S.E. and Groszewski, P. (1989). Dynamic wrist motion analysis using six degree of freedom sensors. *Biomedical Sciences Instrumentation* 25:213–220.

Lowe, B.D. and Freivalds, A. (1997). Analyses of glove types and pinch forces in windshield glass handling. In: B. Das (ed.), *Advances in Occupational Ergonomics and Safety*. Amsterdam, the Netherlands: IOS Press, pp. 477–480.

MacDonnel, R.A., Schwartz, M.S., and Swash, M. (1990). Carpal tunnel syndrome—Which finger should be tested? An analysis of sensory conduction in digital branches of the median nerve. *Muscle and Nerve* 13:601–606.

Mann, R., Yeong, E.K., Moore, M.L., and Engrav, LH. (1997). A new tool to measure pressure under burn garments. *Journal of Burn Care & Rehabilitation* 18:160–163.

Marklin, R.W. and Monroe, J.F. (1998). Quantitative biomechanical analysis of wrist motion in bone trimming jobs in the meat packing industry. *Ergonomics* 41:227–237.

Marras, W.S. and Schoenmarklin, R.W. (1993). Wrist motions in industry. *Ergonomics* 36:341–351.

Marshall, M.M., Mozrall, J.R., and Shealy, J.E. (1999). The effects of complex wrist and forearm posture on wrist range of motion. *Human Factors* 41:205–213.

Mayagoitia, R.E., Nene, A.V., and Veltlink, R.H. (2002). Accelerometer and rate gyroscope measurement of kinematics: An inexpensive alternative to optical motion analysis systems. *Journal of Biomechanics* 35:537–542.

Mayo-Smith, W. and Cochran, G.V.B. (1981). Wheelchair cushion modification: Device for locating high-pressure regions. *Archives of Physical Medicine and Rehabilitation* 62:135–136.

Melvin, J.L., Schuchmann, J.A., and Lanese, R.R. (1973). Diagnostic specificity of motor and sensory nerve conduction variables in the carpal tunnel syndrome. *Archives of Physical Medicine and Rehabilitation* 54:69–74.

Milner-Brown, H.S., Stein, R.B., and Yemm, R. (1973). Changes in firing rate of human motor units during linearly changing voluntary contractions. *Journal of Physiology* 230:371–390.

Mirka, G. (1991). The quantification of EMG normalization error. *Ergonomics* 34:343–352.

Mooney, V., Einbund, M.J., Rogers, J.E., and Stauffer, E.S. (1971). Comparison of pressure distribution qualities in seat cushions. *Bulletin of Prosthetic Research* 10–15:129–143.

Moore, J.S. (1992). Carpal tunnel syndrome. *Occupational Medicine: State of the Art Reviews* 7:741–763.

Moore, A., Wells, R., and Ranney, D. (1991). Quantifying exposure in occupational manual tasks with cumulative trauma disorder potential. *Ergonomics* 34:1433–1453.

Morris, J.R.W. (1973). Accelerometry—A technique for the measurement of human body movement. *Journal of Biomechanics* 6:729–736.

Nathan, P.A., Meadows, K.D., and Doyle, L.S. (1988). Relationship of age and sex to sensory conduction of the median nerve at the carpal tunnel and association of slowed conduction with symptoms. *Muscle and Nerve* 11:1149–1153.

Nathan, P.A., Keniston, R.C., Myers, L.D., and Meadows, K.D. (1992). Longitudinal study of median nerve sensory conduction in industry—Relationship to age, gender, hand dominance, occupational hand use and clinical diagnosis. *Journal of Hand Surgery* 17A:850–857.

Nicole, A.C. (1987). A flexible electrogoniometer with wide spread applications. In: B. Jonsson (ed.), *International Series on Biomechanics: Biomechanics XB*. Champaign, IL: Human Kinematics, pp. 1029–1033.

Nightingale, A. (1960). Relationship between muscle force and EMG in stand-at-ease position. *Annals of Physical Medicine* 5:187–191.

NIOSH. (1990). *Surface Electromyography Procedures Manual for Use in the Industrial Setting*. Morgantown, WV: National Institute for Occupational Safety and Health.

Ojima, H., Miyake, S., Kumashiro, M., Togami, H., and Suzeki, K. (1991). Dynamic analysis of wrist circumduction: A new application of the biaxial flexible electrogoniometer. *Clinical Biomechanics* 6:221–229.

Park, D., Yun, M.H., and Freivalds, A. (1991). Knife replacement studies at an automobile carpet manufacturing plant. *Proceedings of the Human Factors Society, 35th Annual Meeting*. Santa Monica, CA: The Human Factors and Ergonomics Society, pp. 848–852.

Park, S.K. (1999). The development of an exposure measurement system for assessing risk of work-related musculoskeletal disorders. Unpublished PhD thesis. University Park, PA: The Pennsylvania State University.

Rawes, M.L., Richardson, J.B., and Dias, J.J. (1996). A new technique for the assessment of wrist movement using a biaxial flexible electrogoniometer. *Journal of Hand Surgery* 21:600–603.

Robinson, L.R., Rubner, D.E., Wahl, P.W., Fujimoto, W.Y. (1993). Influences of height and gender on normal nerve conduction studies. *Archives of Physical Medicine and Rehabilitation* 74:1134–1138.

Rohmert, W. (1960). Ermittlung von Erholungspausen für Statische Arbeit des Menschen (Determination of recovery times for human static work). *Internationale Zeitschrift für angewandte Physiologie einschliesslich Arbeitsphysiologie* 18:123–164.

Rosenfalck, A. (1978). Early recognition of nerve disorders by near-nerve recording of sensory action potentials. *Muscle and Nerve* 1:360–367.

Schoenmarklin, R.W. and Marras, W.S. (1993). Dynamic capabilities of the wrist joint in industrial workers. *International Journal of Industrial Ergonomics* 11:207–224.

Serina, E.R., Tal, R., and Rempel, D. (1999). Wrist and forearm postures and motions during typing. *Ergonomics* 42:938–951.

Shields, R.K. and Cook, T.M. (1988). Effect of seat angle and lumbar support on seat buttock pressure. *Physical Therapy* 68:1682–1686.

Simpson, J.A. (1956). Electrical signs in the diagnosis of carpal tunnel and related syndromes. *Journal of Neurology, Neurosurgery and Psychiatry* 19:275–280.

Sissons, H.A. (1979). Diseases of joints, tendon sheaths, bursae and other soft tissues. In: W.S. Symmers (ed.), *Systemic Pathology*, 2nd edn, Vol. 5. New York: Churchill Livingston, pp. 2492–2493.

Smutz, P., Serina, E., and Rempel, D. (1994). A system for evaluating the effects of keyboard design on force, posture, comfort and productivity. *Ergonomics* 37:1649–1660.

Sorab, J., Allen, R.H., and Gonik, B. (1988). Tactile sensory monitoring of clinician-applied forces during delivery of newborns. *IEEE Transactions of Biomedical Engineering* 35:1090–1093.

Spielholz, P. (1998). Development of an electrogoniometer calibration procedure for measurement of wrist angle and forearm rotation. In: S. Kumar (ed.), *Advances in Occupational Ergonomics and Safety*, Amsterdam: IOS Press, pp. 499–502.

Stetson, D.S., Albers, J.W., Silverstein, B.A., and Wolfe, R.A. (1992). Effects of age sex and anthropometric factors on nerve conduction measures. *Muscle and Nerve* 15:1095–1104.

Stevens, J.C. (1987). The electrodiagnosis of carpal tunnel syndrome. *Muscle and Nerve* 10:99–113.

Sunderland, S. (1976). The nerve lesion in the carpal tunnel syndrome. *Journal of Neural Neurosurgery and Psychiatry* 39:615–626.

Swearingen, J.J., Wheelwright, C.D., and Garner, J.D. (1962). *An Analysis of Sitting Areas and Pressures of Man*, Rep. No. 62-1. Oklahoma City, OK: U.S. Civil Aero-Medical Research Institute.

Tanaka, S. and McGlothlin, J.D. (1993). A conceptual quantitative model for prevention of work-related CTS. *International Journal of Industrial Ergonomics* 11:181–193.

Tashjian, E.A., Ellenberg, M.R., Gross, N., Chodoroff, G., and Honet, J.C. (1987). Temperature effect on antidromic and orthodromic sensory nerve action potential latency and amplitude. *Archives of Physical Medicine and Rehabilitation* 68:549–552.

Thomas, P.K. (1960). Motor nerve conduction in the carpal tunnel syndrome. *Neurology* 10:1045–1050.

Trandel, R.S., Lewis, D.W., and Verhonick, P.J. (1975). Thermographical investigation of decubitus ulcers. *Bulletin of Prosthetic Research* 10–24:137–155.

Treaster, D.E. and Marras, W.S. (1987). Measurement of seat pressure distributions. *Human Factors* 29:563–575.

Werner, R.A. and Armstrong, T.J. (1997). Carpal tunnel syndrome: Ergonomic risk factors and intra-carpal canal pressures. In: E.W. Johnson (ed.), *Carpal Tunnel Syndrome*. Philadelphia, PA: WB Saunders Company.

Woodburn, J. and Helliwell, P. (1997). Observations on the F-scan in-shoe pressure measuring system. *Clinical Biomechanics* 12:S16.

Yun, M.H. (1994). A hand posture measurement systems for the analysis of manual tool handling tasks. PhD dissertation. University Park, PA: The Pennsylvania State University.

Yun, M.H., Donges, L., and Freivalds, A. (1992). Using force sensitive resistors to evaluate driver seating comfort. In: S. Kumar (ed.), *Advances in Industrial Ergonomics and Safety IV*. London, U.K.: Taylor & Francis, pp. 403–410.

Yun, M.H., Cannon, D., Freivalds, A., and Thomas, G. (1997). An instrumented glove for grasp specification in virtual-reality based point-and-direct telerobotics. *IEEE Transactions on Systems, Man, and Cybernetics, Part B: Cybernetics*, 27:835–846.

Zuniga, E.N. and Simons, E.G. (1969). Nonlinear relationship between averaged EMG potential and muscle tension in normal subjects. *Archives of Physical Medicine and Rehabilitation* 50:613–620.

Zuniga, E.N., Truong, X.T., and Simons, E.G. (1970). Effects of skin electrode position of averaged electromyographic potentials. *Archives of Physical Medicine and Rehabilitation* 51:264–272.

8

Job and Worksite Analysis

8.1 The Need for Job Analysis

Chapter 6 presented data from epidemiological studies that identified WRMSD risk factors such as force, posture, repetition. These risk factors were primarily identified through statistical analysis of musculoskeletal injury records, tracking of injuries back to specific jobs, and detailed surveys of workers. Such approaches collectively form a system of *passive surveillance* but may not provide necessary information in sufficient detail.

A more active *surveillance* approach utilizes job and worksite analysis by trained ergonomists and provides more detailed information on worker postures, forces produced during work, the number of repetitions performed during a shift, etc. that will assist the analyst in identifying specific occupational risk factors. Such an active approach may identify potential problems or stressful conditions before workers develop symptoms severe enough to require medical treatment, potentially saving the company medical costs and lost time and wages.

Such a job or worksite analysis involves a systematic evaluation of the tasks, the duties, the workplace, the tools, and the working conditions necessary to perform the job in satisfactory manner and may include many of the measurements, techniques, and instruments described in Chapter 7. The results of such a structured approach should be a quantitative or semiquantitative evaluation of the risks involved with the particular job, with perhaps even a final risk score. This approach then lends itself to job redesign by providing a seminumerical guide for the reduction of the overall risk score. A consequent reduction of WRMSD risk and potential decrease in injuries and medical costs is the anticipated final goal for such a job and worksite analysis.

8.2 Reliability and Validity of Assessment Tools

8.2.1 Basic Concepts

Before any of posture or task analyses and WRMSD risk-assessment tools are to be used in either screening jobs or assigning workers to appropriate jobs, there arise concerns regarding the accuracy and precision of the observations, measurements, or analyses associated with these techniques and tools. An ergonomist would hope that these tools have characteristics of both *validity* and *reliability*.

Validity refers to the appropriateness, meaningfulness, and usefulness of a tool or survey to measure what it is supposed to measure. For example, a given WRMSD risk-assessment tool is supposed to measure and quantify the actual risk that is incurred for a given individual while performing a given task in a given work environment. A valid assessment tool will allow the ergonomist to make useful inferences about an individual working on a given job. There can be different types of validity, with the simplest being *face* or *content validity*. This refers to the content or format of the tool, which, on its face level, should measure what it is intended to measure. Thus, the content of any risk-assessment survey or checklist should include basic questions on the amount of time worked, the number and types of motions involved, the forces levels exerted, the types of tools or equipment handled, etc. Such content validity is typically determined opinion or judgment such as by a panel of experts.

A second type of validity is *criterion* or *predictive validity* and refers to the relationship of scores obtained using the tool and actual WRMSD injuries incurred which is the true criterion for considering a particular job risky. However, the whole purpose of these tools is to be able to predict or identify the risky jobs ahead of time before the actual injuries are incurred. Predictive validity can be determined by correlating model risk predictions with actual job injury rates. The third type of validity is *construct validity* and refers to physiological or psychological construct or characteristic being measured by the tool. It is most important in a basic theoretical research sense and perhaps less so to a practicing ergonomist in an industrial setting. Whereas the research might be interested in identifying all of the factors, force, frequency, posture, etc., that lead to potential injuries, the industrial ergonomist may be only interested in identifying the risky jobs. Construct validity is more difficult to quantify, and researchers may spend many years adjusting and fine tuning a prediction model.

Reliability refers to the consistency or stability of a measure, i.e., how consistent are the scores or values obtained by two different analysts on the same job, or how the scores vary over time, i.e., is there learning occurring. The importance of a reliable tool is obvious; an ergonomist could not use a tool or questionnaire that gives an unreliable measure of job risk, because, then, any job redesigns or worker reassignments would be meaningless as they were not based on the variables expected.

8.2.2 Reliability of Assessments

One can consider that any assessment consists of a true value superimposed with a random variable due to measurement errors. Since measurement errors are always present to some degree in research, it is important to be able to quantify the amount of variation or errors to be expected. The simplest measure of such variability is the *coefficient of variability* (CV) for a series of repeated measurements:

$$CV = \frac{s}{\bar{x}} \tag{8.1}$$

where
s is the standard deviation of the measurements
$\bar{x}$ is the mean of the measurements

Typically, the CV should be less than 10%, with 5% being even better.

More formal estimates of measurement errors are expressed as a *correlation* or *reliability coefficient*. For example, one common error component to be quantified is the consistency over time, referred to as *test–retest reliability*. To assess this type of reliability, the same analysis is performed on the same jobs with a certain amount of intervening time. The two sets of scores are correlated using the standard *Pearson product moment correlation coefficient* (Currier, 1984):

$$r = \frac{\sum x_i y_i - \sum x_i \sum y_i / n}{\left[\sum x_i^2 - \left(\sum x_i\right)^2 / n\right]^{\frac{1}{2}} \left[\sum y_i^2 - \left(\sum y_i\right)^2 / n\right]^{\frac{1}{2}}} \qquad (8.2)$$

where
 x_i is the scores from the first analysis
 y_i is the scores from the second analysis
 n is the number of jobs analyzed

The resulting correlation coefficient will range from 0 to ±1. A correlation coefficient of zero indicates no relationship between the two applications of the analysis and a very poor tool to be used for job analysis. A correlation coefficient of +1 indicates a perfect relationship and a very reliable analysis tool (very unlikely in real life). A score of –1 indicates a perfect inverse relationship. This would be very unlikely in these testing or analysis scenarios but could happen in a theoretical statistical sense between two unknown variables. Typically, for a tool to be reliable, the correlation coefficient should be roughly around 0.9.

Typically, the longer the time interval between measurements, the lower the correlation coefficient and the lower the reliability will be. This would indicate that something has changed over time; perhaps the analyst has forgotten key aspects of using the tool, or perhaps more training is required, or perhaps the job or person being analyzed has changed. On the other hand, reliability is typically increased, if there are several similar questions examining a particular variable of interest, especially for those with psychosocial aspects and more subjective evaluations. Although, no universally acceptable levels of reliability have been established, one appropriate scheme was suggested by Currier (1984). Values greater than 0.9 can be considered high reliability, values between 0.8 and 0.9 good reliability, values between 0.7 and 0.8 fair reliability and values below 0.7 poor reliability.

For situations where it is impractical to administer the same test to the same individuals (e.g., when workers may become sensitized to questions regarding pain or psychosocial aspects), an alternate approach to test–retest reliability is the *split-half procedure*. Two halves of a survey are scored separately for each person and correlation coefficient is calculated for the two sets of scores. The level of the correlation indicates the degree to which the two halves provide the same results and, thus, describes the internal consistency of the survey. The reliability coefficient for the full survey is computed using the *Spearman–Brown prophecy formula* (Fraenkel and Wallen, 1996), which for an exact split formulation is

$$r_{tot} = \frac{2r_{\frac{1}{2}}}{1 + r_{\frac{1}{2}}} \qquad (8.3)$$

where
 r_{tot} is the reliability for the full survey
 $r_{\frac{1}{2}}$ is the correlation coefficient for one-half the survey

A relatively low correlation coefficient of 0.8 for one-half the survey would result in an overall reliability coefficient of 0.889 for the full survey.

This demonstrates an important principle of reliability. The reliability of a survey can be increased by increasing its length with additional items similar to the original ones.

Three other statistical approaches can be used for internal-consistency checks. Two are not, strictly speaking, statistical tests, but computational formulas for a test's reliability from Kuder and Richardson (1937), specifically their formulas 20 and 21:

$$r = \frac{n}{n-1} \times \left\{ 1 - \frac{\sum p(1-p)}{s^2} \right\} \tag{8.4}$$

$$r = \frac{n}{n-1} \times \left\{ 1 - \frac{\bar{x}(1-\bar{x}/n)}{s^2} \right\} \tag{8.5}$$

where
   n is the number of items on test
   r is the estimate of test's reliability
   p is the proportion passing a given item
   s^2 is the variance of test
   $\bar{x}$ is the mean score of test

Equation 8.4 (Kuder–Richardson formula 20) is the most robust estimate of a test's reliability but requires more complex summations of test takers' proportion of passing items. Equation 8.5 (Kuder–Richardson formula 21) is considerably simpler to calculate but uses a more conservative assumption that all test items have the same difficulty. Note that for surveys or WRMSD risk assessments, "passing" would constitute exceeding a certain critical threshold value for risk for a given item. For example, if the mean score on a WRMSD screening survey with 40 items is 30, with a variance of 10, the reliability would be

$$r = \frac{40}{39} \times \left\{ 1 - \frac{30(1-30/40)}{10} \right\} = 0.256 \tag{8.6}$$

This reliability score of 0.256 is quite low considering that a value of 0 indicates no relationship and a value of 1 indicates perfect correlation. Many commercially available achievement tests in education (not for predicting WRMSD) have reliability coefficients exceeding 0.9 on the Kuder–Richardson formulas. Even classroom tests may have reliability coefficients exceeding 0.7 (Fraenkel and Wallen, 1996). The overall conclusion for this sample WRMSD screening test is that it would be quite unreliable and provide little use in identifying critical jobs or individuals who might be susceptible to WRMSD.

A variation of Kuder–Richardson formula 20 (Equation 8.4) was developed by Cronbach (1951) and termed *Cronbach's alpha*. Its primarily application is for tests or screening surveys where scoring is not simply right or wrong and more than one answer may be possible. It is formulated as

$$\alpha = \frac{n}{n-1} \times \left\{ 1 - \frac{\sum s_i^2}{s_t^2} \right\} \tag{8.7}$$

where
   s_i^2 is the variance of item scores
   s_t^2 is the variance of test scores
   α is the estimate of test's reliability

8.2.3 Reliability of Analysts

Another measure of the reliability and validity of an assessment is the amount of agreement between analysts. If the agreement between analysts is high, then there is a possibility, but not a guarantee, that the scoring reflects the measure or factor that it is meant to score. If their agreement is low, the usefulness of that assessment is very limited, because even the experts cannot even agree to what is being measured or scored. The simplest index of agreement is the overall proportion of agreement:

$$p_o = a + d \tag{8.8}$$

where
  p_o is the proportion of observations agreeing
  a is the proportion of observations in desired category agreeing
  d is the proportion of observations in opposite category agreeing

There may be several complicating factors in using proportions of observers agreeing. First, one of the categories may be quite rare, so either a or d, will be very likely quite large and thus inflate the value of p_o. Second, some degree of agreement is to be expected by chance alone. With pure random guessing, with $a = b = c = d = 0.25$ (Table 8.1), Equation 8.8 yields a p_o of 0.5. Therefore, there needs to be a way of correcting for chance. This was accomplished by Cohen (1960) with the *kappa statistic* (κ) defined as

$$\kappa = \frac{p_o - p_e}{1 - p_e} \tag{8.9}$$

where
  p_o is the proportion of agreement observed
  p_e is the proportion of agreement expected by chance

For most purposes, values of kappa greater than 0.8 may be considered excellent agreement beyond chance, values between 0.6 and 0.8, substantial agreement, values between 0.4 and 0.6 moderate agreement and values below 0.4 (even including possible negative values), poor agreement (Landis and Koch, 1977). Note, that, although kappa is an improvement over simple proportionality of agreement, it works best with dichotomous data. Grouping of continuous data into categories for the convenience of the analyst is not valid. The principal weakness of kappa is that it measures the frequency of exact agreement rather than the degree of approximate agreement.

A weighted kappa (Cohen, 1968) was developed to address this problem. However, the weighted kappa has its own set of problems, in that it allows the weights to be of arbitrary magnitude, distorting the resulting statistic (Maclure and Willett, 1987). Standardizing the

TABLE 8.1

Wrist Posture Counts

Analyst A	Analyst B	
	Ulnar Deviation	**Neutral Position**
Ulnar deviation	34 (a = 34/50)	5 (b = 5/50)
Neutral position	1 (c = 1/50)	10 (d = 10/50)

weights alleviates this problem and results in the weighted kappa becoming equivalent to Cronbach's alpha (Equation 8.7). Further information on interrater agreement can be found in Fleiss (1981). Note that the above discussion applies only to ordinal data or ranking. For continuous data measurements, as might be expected in a thorough exposure-assessment tool, standard statistical approaches, such as analysis of variance, are more appropriate. Even when continuous data is group into ordinal categories, serious errors can arise with the kappa statistic. Only time sample data should be used with the kappa statistic (Maclure and Willett, 1987).

Example 8.1: Measurement of the Amount of Agreement between Analysts

Consider a simple example of two analysts counting body postures, specifically whether the right wrist is in ulnar deviation (see Table 8.1). The analysts examine videos of 50 workers on an electronic assembly job. Their evaluation of the 50 workers yields the following data, with a, b, c, and d being proportions of the various combinations of interrater agreement.

The overall proportion of agreement is

$$p_o = \frac{34}{50} + \frac{10}{50} = 0.88 \tag{8.10}$$

The proportion agreement by chance is calculated from the revised contingency table where the expected values are the products of the intersection of the respective column and row totals divided by the grand total, similar to Equation 6.10. The resultant expected values for agreement, by row, are 27.3, 11.7, 7.7, and 3.3. The overall proportion agreement expected by chance is then

$$p_e = \frac{27.3}{50} + \frac{3.3}{50} = 0.612 \tag{8.11}$$

Correcting for chance agreement, the Kappa statistic, yields:

$$\kappa = \frac{p_o - p_e}{1 - p_e} = \frac{0.88 - 0.612}{1 - 0.612} = 0.691 \tag{8.12}$$

In either case, there is substantial agreement between analysts.

For continuous data, in which analysts give specific values of angle, force, or frequency, as opposed to categorical data, other methodologies need to be used. For two analysts, the two sets of scores can be simply correlated using the Pearson product moment correlation of Equation 8.2. For more than two analysts, *intraclass correlations* based on analysis of variance (ANOVA) of the data are utilized (Shrout and Fleiss, 1979). In a typical scenario, a analysts evaluate b jobs. In Case 1, each job is evaluated by a different set of a analysts, randomly selected from a larger population of analysts. In Case 2, a random sample of a analysts is randomly selected from a larger population of analysts. Each analyst then evaluates the same jobs. A very specific Case 3 could also be considered, in which the a analysts are the only analysts of interest. However, typically the results of any job analysis instrument would need to be generalized over a larger population of analysts and, therefore, Case 3 will not be considered.

Case 1 is analyzed as a one-way ANOVA yielding the intraclass correlation coefficient:

$$\text{ICC}_1 = \frac{\text{MS}_{\text{job}} - \text{MSE}}{\text{MS}_{\text{job}} + (a-1)\text{MSE}} \tag{8.13}$$

where
  ICC_1 is the intraclass correlation coefficient for Case 1
  MS_{job} is the between-jobs mean square
  MSE is the within-jobs mean square or mean square error
  a is the number of analysts

Case 2 is analyzed as a two-way ANOVA, yielding the intraclass correlation coefficient:

$$ICC_2 = \frac{MS_{job} - MSE}{MS_{job} + (a-1)MSE + a(MS_{analyst} - MSE)/b} \qquad (8.14)$$

where
  ICC_2 is the intraclass correlation coefficient for Case 2
  $MS_{analyst}$ is the between-analyst mean square
  b is the number of jobs

ICC_2 will typically be smaller than ICC_3 because of the added random effects of analysts and generalizability to a larger population of analysts. Similarly, ICC_1 will typically be smaller than ICC_2 because of the added variability due to a larger pool of analysts. Example 8.2 may help clarify the ICCs between Cases 1 and 2. More details on intraclass correlation coefficients and Case 3 can be obtained from (Shrout and Fleiss, 1979).

Example 8.2: Calculation of Intraclass Correlation Coefficients

Consider the frequency of wrist deviations for eight different jobs as observed by three different analysts shown in Table 8.2.
  For Case 1, a one-way ANOVA on wrist deviation frequencies yields:

Source	Degrees of Freedom	Sum of Squares	Mean Squares	F-Value	p-Value
Job	7	91.96	13.14	2.22	0.088
Error	16	94.67	5.92		
Total	23	186.63			

TABLE 8.2

Frequency of Wrist Deviations

Job No.	Analyst	Analyst	Analyst
1	2	5	8
2	1	3	2
3	4	6	8
4	1	2	6
5	5	6	9
6	2	4	7
7	6	8	12
8	3	5	8

The intraclass correlation coefficient for Case 1 from Equation 8.13 is

$$ICC_1 = \frac{MS_{job} - MSE}{MS_{job} + (a-1)MSE} = \frac{13.14 - 5.92}{13.14 + (2)5.92} = \frac{7.22}{24.98} = 0.29 \qquad (8.15)$$

For Case 2, a two-way ANOVA on wrist deviations yields:

Source	Degrees of Freedom	Sum of Squares	Mean Squares	F-Value	p-Value
Job	7	91.96	13.14	14.24	0.001
Analyst	2	81.75	40.88	44.30	0.001
Error	14	12.92	0.92		
Total	23	186.63			

The intraclass correlation coefficient for Case 2 from Equation 8.14 is

$$ICC_2 = \frac{MS_{job} - MSE}{MS_{job} + (a-1)MSE + a(MS_{analyst} - MSE)/b}$$

$$= \frac{13.14 - 0.92}{13.14 + (2)0.923 + 3(40.88 - 0.92)/8} = \frac{12.22}{29.97} = 0.41 \qquad (8.16)$$

8.2.4 Accuracy and Precision

Another way of examining validity and reliability is in the engineering context of *accuracy* and *precision* or *resolution*. An instrument is considered accurate if measurements are made with small errors or small deviations from the "true value." This can be considered in the context of target shooting. A rifle is considered accurate if it hits the bull's-eye or has a very small deviation from the center (Figure 8.1a). Similarly, an instrument may be considered as precise or having a high resolution, if it can detect very small quantities. In terms of target shooting, if the rifle produces a very small scatter, it is considered precise. However, it might not be scattered around the bull's-eye, in which case, it is not very accurate and needs to be resighted (Figure 8.1b). The opposite case, although it may be hard to interpret, is in which the rifle may be accurate, hitting the target, but with a large scatter. It may be

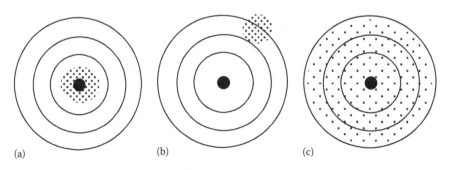

(a)   (b)   (c)

FIGURE 8.1
Comparison of accuracy and precision using the bull's-eye analogy: (a) good accuracy and good precision, (b) good precision but not accurate, (c) poor precision, maybe accurate (hard to judge).

TABLE 8.3

Sources of Variation and Procedures for Estimating the Reliability of an Assessment Instrument

Sources of Variation		Procedure	Specific Test
Instrument itself	Test–retest reliability (confounded with variation within testees)	Basic—give identical instrument twice within short time span	Pearson correlation coefficient r (Equation 8.2).
	Internal consistency (still confounded with variation between testees)	Better—divide instrument into equal halves and give both to testees	Split-half procedure, Pearson r (Equation 8.2) and Spearman–Brown prophecy r (Equation 8.3)
	Internal consistency (still confounded with variation between testees)	Better—give full instrument to testees	Kuder–Richardson r (Equations 8.4 and 8.5) or Cronbach α (Equation 8.7), ICC_1 (Equation 8.12).
Variation over time (effect of learning or sensitization of testees)		Give identical instrument two or more times over time period of interest	Pearson correlation coefficient r (Equation 8.2)
Variation in analysts, interrater agreement		Compare scores obtained by two or more analysts	Kappa (Equation 8.9), ICC_2 (Equation 8.13)

accurate, but the lack of precision makes it difficult to judge the accuracy (Figure 8.1c). Obviously, the best scenario is for the rifle to be both accurate and precise, i.e., hitting the bull's-eye with a small scatter (Figure 8.1a). Thus, accuracy is similar to validity and precision is similar to reliability. Note that, it is possible to have reliability without validity, but not validity without reliability. Further information on developing valid and reliable tests can be found in a variety of research methodology texts in both psychology and education (Thorndike and Hagen, 1977; Fraenkel and Wallen, 1996; Kerlinger and Lee, 2000). Also, Table 8.3 may be useful in identifying appropriate procedures for determining the reliability of a screening tool.

There are several other measures that indicate the usefulness of an assessment tool. *Sensitivity* refers to the assessment tool's ability to identify injurious jobs, i.e., jobs that will result in injuries in the future. It can be expressed as the fraction of injurious jobs that are correctly identified as being injurious from Table 8.2 or from the *signal-detection theory* analogy shown in Figure 8.2:

$$\text{Sensitivity} = \frac{\text{True positives}}{\text{True positives} + \text{False negatives}} \times 100\% = \frac{a}{a+c} \times 100\% \qquad (8.17)$$

In this analogy, safe jobs would score low on an assessment tool's risk rating and injurious jobs would have a high rating. Obviously, there would be a distribution of scores within safe jobs as well as for injurious jobs, with considerable overlap between the two distributions. The central vertical line represents the criterion level, at which point, based on the risk score, a job is classified as either being safe or injurious. Thus, some jobs, even though they may score low on a risk-assessment tool's rating, could still cause injuries. Being scored low, they would not be classified as injurious and would result in false negatives. Similarly, some safe jobs having no injuries may still be scored with a high value and would result in false positives. Correctly identified injurious jobs would be true positives and correctly identified safe jobs would be true negatives (Table 8.4).

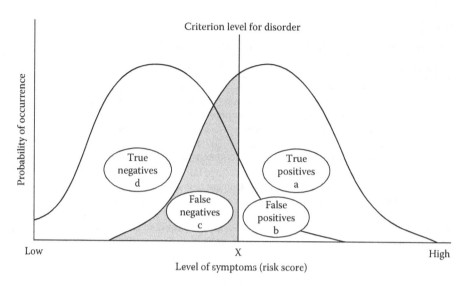

FIGURE 8.2
Signal-detection analogy for an assessment tool risk score.

TABLE 8.4

Classification Table for Test Results and the "True" Status of a Disorder

| Test Result | The "Truth" | | Total | |
	Disorder	No Disorder		
Positive	a = true positives	b = false positives	a + b	$\dfrac{a}{a+b}$ = positive predictive value
Negative	c = false negatives	d = true negatives	c + d	$\dfrac{d}{c+d}$ = negative predictive value
Total	a + c	b + d	n = a + b + c + d	
	$\dfrac{a}{a+c}$ = sensitivity	$\dfrac{d}{b+d}$ = specificity		$\dfrac{a+d}{a+b+c+d}$ = accuracy

Specificity refers to the assessment tool's ability to correctly identify safe jobs and would be expressed as

$$\text{Specificity} = \frac{\text{True negatives}}{\text{True negatives} + \text{False negatives}} \times 100\% = \frac{d}{d+b} \times 100\% \qquad (8.18)$$

Note that changing the criterion level to increase the sensitivity of the test will result in a tradeoff with a decrease in the specificity.

The *positive predictive value* of an assessment tool is the ability to predict which jobs will result in future musculoskeletal injuries, or

$$\text{Predictive value} = \frac{\text{True positives}}{\text{True positives} + \text{False positives}} \times 100\% = \frac{a}{a+b} \times 100\% \qquad (8.19)$$

Another less commonly used measure is accuracy. It measures the degree of agreement between an assessment tool and the *gold standard* (the best tool):

$$\text{Accuracy} = \frac{\text{True positives} + \text{True negatives}}{\text{Grand total}} = \frac{a+d}{a+b+c+d} \times 100\% \qquad (8.20)$$

Unfortunately, there are little data on the sensitivity, specificity, or predictive value for many of the assessment tools. These tools are simply not accurate enough to categorize all of the contributing risk factors. Or from another perspective, there is simply too much variability in the jobs and the individuals working on these jobs, which, at this point in time, are not understood well enough with the existing models to be accurately assessed.

8.2.5 Applications

The above issues of validity and reliability are very important in developing an exposure assessment instrument. The reliability will depend very much on the type of information sought and how it is collected. Self-reported information on work history, job titles and job duration can typically be considered reliable and valid with kappa values between 60% and 70% (Rona and Mosbech, 1989; Östlin et al., 1990). Questions on general physical activity, perhaps even gross postures, have reliability coefficients of 0.70–0.87 and can be considered sufficiently reproducible (Wiktorin et al., 1996). For more detailed information regarding level of activities and more detailed postures, the reliability becomes worse, with intraclass correlation coefficients ranging between 0.24 and 0.69 (Spielholz et al., 1999). Correlation coefficients between such questionnaire data and validation criteria (typically analysis of job videotapes or direct instrumented measurements) becomes much worse, between 0.1 and 0.3 (Lamb and Brodie, 1990; Ainsworth et al., 1993; Wiktorin et al., 1996; Spielholz et al., 2001). Even basic working postures or their durations as reported on questionnaires, can vary by as much as 34% from direct observation data (Baty et al., 1986) and have kappa values as low as 45% (Rossignol and Baetz, 1987).

In terms of WRMSD symptom severity, self-administered questionnaires have shown high test–retest reliabilities (Pearson correlation coefficient of $r = 0.91$) and internal consistencies (Cronbach alpha of $\alpha = 0.89$) (Levine et al., 1993). However, when such self-reported information is correlated to direct clinical evaluations, the correlations drop considerably. For two-point discrimination tests and monofilament tests the Spearman–Brown correlation coefficient ranged from $r = 0.12$ to $r = 0.42$ (Levine et al., 1993), while for direct nerve conduction latencies the Pearson correlation coefficient ranged from $r = 0.46$ to $r = 0.53$ (You et al., 1999). The highest correlations were obtained with primary symptoms of numbness, tingling, and nocturnal sensations as opposed to secondary symptoms of pain, weakness, and clumsiness.

In general, there is a tendency for the self-reported data to overestimate exposure (i.e., duration, force, postural angles) as compared to direct measurements, which Spielholz et al. (2001) attribute to a lack of adjustment of psychophysical rating scale on the part of the workers. Also, the rank ordering of self-reported data was similar to the rank ordering of direct measurements Although, both of these observations may allow the potential readjustment of self-reported data to yield more reliable and valid occupational risk assessments, the easiest approach may still be to use the simplest and most basic questions that will be understood by the general working population.

One would suspect that trained observers or analysts would provide more reliable data. Keyserling and Witting (1988) were the first to examine the agreement of expert ratings.

Five experts rated 10 jobs at 3 levels. Perfect agreement was found in only 30% of the cases, which, assuming perfect agreement by chance to be less than 1%, yields a kappa of 0.29. This is only fair agreement according to the Landis and Koch (1977) scale. If consensus agreement (i.e., three of five scores are identical) is considered, then 87.5% of the cases were in "agreement."

Genaidy et al. (1993) and Baluyutt et al. (1995) examined the reliability of visually estimating postural angles from videotapes. In general, the absolute error was almost 10°, with flexion/extension angles and lower back and neck postures easiest to estimate and wrist and elbow postures most difficult to estimate. Also, interestingly, estimates of angles exhibited a range effect; smaller angles were overestimated while larger angles were underestimated. Rather than estimating the angles directly, one can simply place the estimate into one of several postural angle categories. But then there is the problem of determining the optimal size for (or number of) postural angle categories used. There is a definite tradeoff between the accuracy of joint posture (size of the posture angle category) and the misclassification error (too many angle categories). Based on empirical data collection, van Wyk et al. (2009) found optimal posture category sizes of 30° for trunk, shoulder, and elbow flexion/extension, 30° for shoulder abduction/adduction and 15° for trunk lateral bending, very comparable to those used in previously published ergonomic assessments.

Burt and Punnett (1999) had two analysts evaluate postures for 70 jobs. Exact agreement between analysts ranged from a low of 26% for shoulder elevation to a high of 99% for wrist flexion. However, once chance agreement was introduced through kappa statistic, the proportion of agreement was much lower from 0.0 (with even a couple of slightly negative values) to a high of 0.55. Of the 18 posture assessments, only two exceeded the 0.4 threshold for moderate agreement, with the rest being fair or poor agreement. The reason for the relatively high percentage of basic agreement but low kappa was explained by the fact that some of the postures were observed rarely, therefore, artificially increasing the probability that the two analysts would indicate the same posture. On the other hand, the Burt and Punnett (1999) reasoned that a low value of kappa may be useful in deterring analysts from using an exposure assessment tool that has not be properly evaluated over a wide range of conditions.

In terms of force estimation, van der Beek et al. (1992) had two observers rate truck driver postures and force exertions at three levels. Interobserver reliability of force was 0.95 with a kappa of 0.81. Similarly deLooze et al. (1994) examined two analysts rating loads in nine different manual materials handling tasks. Interobserver reliability after 1 week practice was 0.76 with a kappa of 0.68. However, reliability with directly recorded values for load was lower at 0.63 with a kappa of 0.50. Their conclusion was that observations of the task may not be valid.

A better approach may be for the subject to estimate the task force through a simulated contraction on a measurement instrument (Kotani, 1995). Twenty subjects exerted various levels of a required task force on an instrumented tool. After each exertion, the subjects attempted to replicate the exact force level on a grip dynamometer. The relationships between the task force on the tool and the perceived for the grip dynamometer were significantly linear (mean $r^2 = 0.84$, $p < .001$) with a slight overestimation for low forces and a larger underestimation for high forces (see Figure 8.3). Interestingly, tool grip texture and wrist deviation significantly affected perceived force.

Such force matching was studied in more detail by Bao and Silverstein (2005) on several simulated industrial tasks. Both pinch and power grips only slightly overestimated actual forces, which tended to be on the low side. Similarly, Koppelaar and Wells (2005) examined, force estimation on five tasks. Correlations coefficients expressed as r^2 were significant for each method with values, 0.34 for force matching, 0.19 and 0.24 for two different EMG measurements, 0.34 for observation, and 0.27 for self-reported VAS. The accuracy of such estimation can be improved by using benchmarks to calibrate the subject prior to

FIGURE 8.3
Relationship between task force on tool (%T) and perceived force on a grip dynamometer (%P) for different textures. (Reproduced from Kotani, K., Modeling perception and production of force as a means of estimating force requirements in industrial tasks, PhD dissertation, The Pennsylvania State University, University Park, PA, 1995. With permission.)

force estimation. Marshall et al. (2004) had subjects estimate submaximal exertions on 12 simulated tasks. Using one benchmark (100% MVC) significantly decreased the error (estimated minus actual) from an average of 14% to 4% MVC, while using three benchmarks (25%, 75%, and 100% MVC) decreased the error to −3% MVC.

A recent study by Lowe and Krieg (2009) has perhaps the best summary of the relationships between various rater estimates and physical measurements of upper limb activity. Estimation of various upper limb force exertion levels gave ICC_2 values ranging from 0.43 to 0.78 for %MVC, from 0.05 to 0.6 for Borg ratings, and −0.04 to 0.54 for VAS scales (Section 8.3.2.3). Correlations of estimated to actual counts of wrist motion were significant but rather low at $r^2 = 0.21$. Correlations of ratings of hand activity level (Section 8.5.4) with measured joint velocities were again significant but modest with r^2 ranging from 0.28 to 0.50.

In general, interobserver reliability can be influenced by a variety of factors. The sequence of postures and activities can be memorized from one analysis session to another, resulting in a learning effect. This problem can be minimized if sufficient time is given between sessions or a variety of jobs are analyzed in a random order. Obviously, the reverse effect must also be taken into account. The analysts should be trained sufficiently well that any learning effects with regard to the assessment tool have leveled off. Interobserver reliability will also tend to decrease as the complexity of the assessment tool increases. The larger the number of simultaneously observed categories increases, the greater the variance in the responses that can be expected. A good review of the types of information that can be obtained and the various problems than can be expected to occur in observational analysis and exposure assessment is found in Kilbom (1994).

8.3 Initial Identification of Musculoskeletal Injury Problems

8.3.1 Initial Steps

The first step in evaluating the scope of WRMSDs in the workplace is a thorough review of existing medical, safety, and insurance records. In the United States, regulations issued by Occupational Safety and Health Administration (OSHA) require that most employers

FIGURE 8.4
Pareto distribution of injuries; 20% of jobs account for 80% of the injuries.

maintain records work-related injuries and disorders. These are maintained on the standard OSHA 300 log and are subject to review by OSHA inspectors as well are open to employees and union representatives. In addition, the company will most likely keep more detailed records for each injury or disorders, both for medical and workers compensation purposes. Therefore, there will be a variety data sources available for an initial attempt at identifying the problem.

One tool that may be useful in identifying problem areas is *Pareto analysis* (named after the Italian economist Vilfredo Pareto, 1848–1923). Items of interest (e.g., injuries in Figure 8.3) are identified and measured on a common scale and are then ordered in ascending order, creating a cumulative probability distribution. Typically 80% or more of the total activity is accounted by 20% of the ranked items; consequently, the technique is sometimes called the 80–20 rule. For example, in Figure 8.4, 81% of total injuries occur on three job titles, or less than 20% of all job titles. (In Vilfredo Pareto's original application, more than 80% of wealth was concentrated in less 20% of individuals.) Theoretically, the ergonomist concentrates the greatest effort on those few jobs that produce most of the problems and return the greatest benefit for the amount of effort or money invested. In many cases, the Pareto distribution can be transformed to a straight line using a log–normal transformation, from which further quantitative analyses can be performed (Herron, 1976).

8.3.2 Surveys and Subjective Ratings

In many cases, the medical records are incomplete or may not reflect the true nature of the problem. Many workers may be hesitant to report relatively minor arm pain at the workplace, thinking that it is not work related, and have it treated by their family physician. However, these may be the first signs of an oncoming epidemic that should be caught early on. Therefore, the next step should be to survey the workers. Questionnaires and surveys have been developed for this purpose. Note, however, that these surveys rely on the worker's recognition of the problem and willingness to respond. Therefore, unless special steps are taken, such as anonymity of responses and lack of retribution on the part of management, the response may be biased.

8.3.2.1 Symptom Surveys

A typical questionnaire, developed by OSHA (1990), is shown in Figure 8.5. The questions are designed to disclose the nature, location, and severity of the symptoms. Questions are also needed to determine whether the workers have received treatment for any previous musculoskeletal injuries and whether they have other conditions that may exhibit similar

---

Symptoms Survey

Date_____

Department_____ Job title_____

Number of years on this job_____ Previous job _____

1) Have you had any pain and discomfort during the last year?   Yes   No

   If yes, check area: Neck_____Shoulder_____Elbow/forearm_____Hand/wrist_____Fingers_____
   Upper back_____Low back_____Thigh/knee_____Lower leg_____Ankle/feet_____

2) Please put a check by the word(s) that best describe your problem:

_____Aching	_____Numbness	_____Tingling
_____Burning	_____Pain	_____Weakness
_____Cramping	_____Swelling	_____Loss of color
_____Stiffness	_____Other	

3) When did you first notice the problem?_____
4) How long does each episode last? (Mark an X along the line)

   1 hour   1 day   1 week   1 month   6 months

5) What do you think caused the problem?_____
6) Have you had this problem in the last 7 days?
7) How would you rate this problem now? (Mark an X along the line)   Yes   No

   None_____ Unbearable

8) How would you rate this problem at its worst? (Mark an X along the line)

   None_____ Unbearable

9) Have you had medical treatment for this problem?   Yes   No

   If no, why not?_____
   If yes, where and when did you receive treatment?_____
   If yes, did the treatment help?   Yes   No

10) How much time have you lost in the last year because of this problem?
11) How many days in the last year were you on restricted or light duty because of this problem?_____

Please comment on what you think would improve your symptoms.

_____
_____
_____

FIGURE 8.5

Typical symptoms survey questionnaire. (From OSHA [Occupational Safety and Health Administration], *Ergonomics Program Management Guidelines for Meatpacking Plants*, Bureau of National Affairs, Inc., Washington, DC, 1990.)

symptoms, such as arthritis, diabetes, thyroid disorders, gout, kidney disease, menstrual problems, pregnancy, and use of oral contraceptives. Thus, such a questionnaire is typically termed a *symptom survey*.

8.3.2.2 Body Discomfort Maps

Another common tool for surveying workers is the *body discomfort map* developed by Corlett and Bishop (1976) (see Figure 8.6). The worker marks each body part where pain or discomfort is experienced and then rates the level of that pain on a *visual analogue scale* (VAS). The VAS is typically a 10 cm line drawn on a piece of paper with endpoints of 0 (nothing at all) to 10 (almost maximum), on which the subject is asked to indicate the degree of perceived pain by putting a mark on the line (Neely et al., 1992). The use of such a subjective rating for pain has been found to be both valid and reliable (Reading, 1980; Price et al., 1983).

8.3.2.3 Subjective Ratings

An alternate but comparable rating scale is the Borg (1982) *category ratio scale* (CR-10) with several verbal anchors, originally designed for muscular exertion (see Figure 8.6), which may provide a higher level of precision than the VAS (Cameron, 1996). However, the VAS may be preferred by workers who do not have the time to read and to consider the anchor points individually (Ulin et al., 1990). Also, the VAS may not impose the need to exceed a threshold of sensation intensity at each level before proceeding to the next level as do the category ratio scales such as the CR-10 (Wilson and Jones, 1989). This type of approach has been successfully by a number of researchers

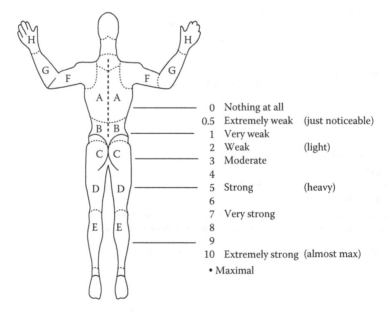

FIGURE 8.6
Body discomfort map with ratings of perceived pain. (Adapted from Corlett, E.N. and Bishop, R.P., *Ergonomics*, 19, 175, 1976; Borg, G.A.V., *Med. Sci. Sports Exerc*, 14, 377, 1982.)

to assess postural discomfort (Boussenna et al., 1982; Kuorinka, 1983; Bhatnagar et al., 1985; Harms-Ringdahl, 1986; Saldana et al., 1994) or the identification of WRMSDs in the workforce (Buckle et al., 1984).

Borg ratings are also widely used as estimates of hand force exertions used in task analyses and risk assessments (Sections 8.4 and 8.5). From a practical standpoint, such psychophysical ratings are much less costly, both in time and money, as compared with instrumented techniques or electromyography. However, the accuracy of these estimates are inherently subjective and are suspect in terms of validity. The estimates can be improved considerably by using guided calibration methods prior to the actual task exertion. Spielholz (2006) showed that mean estimation error for a 44.5 N power grip task was significantly reduced from 142.8 to 62.3 N.

Overall, such a visual map with rating scales is an especially tool useful for situations in which the working population may not be native born or do not have the sufficient English skills to read lengthy instructions or questions. This approach can also provide crude quantitative measures. By counting the number of times each body part was marked and dividing the by the number of total responses, a rough measure of the incidence of the problem is obtained. Furthermore, the mean level of the perceived pain ratings provides a rough measure of the severity of the problem.

8.3.2.4 Nordic Questionnaire

One comprehensive questionnaire that utilizes both body discomfort maps and detailed questions to elicit further information is the Nordic Questionnaire (Kuorinka et al., 1987). It consists of a general survey with specific sections for various body parts (see Figure 8.7). Test–retest reliabilities for samples of 20 workers showed identical responses from 77% to 100% of the questions and validity tests between a physiotherapist and 82 workers showed identical responses from 87% to 100% of the questions. The Nordic Questionnaire has been used quite successfully in identifying potentially injurious situations in a many studies (Dickinson et al., 1992; Bru et al., 1994; Deakin et al., 1994; Hagen et al., 1998).

An interesting alternative to the Nordic Questionnaire is the disabilities of the arm, shoulder, and head (DASH) questionnaire (Hudak et al., 1996). Although it was developed to assess the quality of life for patients before and after surgery (Gummesson et al., 2003), it does focus exclusively on the upper limbs and has been used successfully to analyze WRMSDs in the textile industry with high (0.92) test–retest reliability (Kitis et al., 2009).

8.3.3 Limitations of Surveys

Note that the results of any such questionnaires or surveys must be interpreted with caution. Workers may be hesitant in providing true and accurate responses. Pain tolerance varies considerably between individuals. Also, there are many technical factors that enter into the proper design, validation, and analyses of surveys. Some were discussed in Section 8.2.1, but others include the reading level of the respondents, the length and wording of the surveys, written or oral response, etc. Further details on survey design can be obtained from Warwick and Lininger (1975) and Berdie et al. (1986). Note also that is the only the starting point in identifying the problem. More in-depth worksite analyses will be necessary to identify the source of these WRMSDs.

SHOULDER

How to answer the questionnaire: By shoulder trouble is meant ache, pain or discomfort in the shaded area. Please concentrate on this area, ignoring any trouble you may have in adjacent parts of the body. There is a separate questionnaire for other areas of discomfort.

Please answer by putting a cross in the appropriate box—one cross for each question. You may be in doubt as to how to answer, but please do your best anyway.

9. Have you ever had shoulder trouble (ache, pain or discomfort)?

   1. No   2. Yes   □

If you answered No to Question 9, do not answer Questions 10 –17.

10. Have you ever hurt your shoulder in an accident?

    1. No   2. Yes, my right shoulder
            3. Yes, my left shoulder
            4. Yes, both shoulders   □

11. Have you ever had to change jobs or duties because of shoulder trouble?

    1. No   2. Yes   □

12. Have you had shoulder trouble during the last 12 months?

    1. No   2. Yes, in my right shoulder
            3. Yes, in my left shoulder
            4. Yes, in both shoulders   □

If you answered No to Question 12, do not answer Questions 13 –17.

13. What is the total length of time that you have had shoulder trouble during the last 12 months?

    1. 1–7 days
    2. 8–30 days
    3. More than 30 days, but not every day   □
    4. Every day

14. Has shoulder trouble caused you to reduce your activity during the last 12 months?

    a. Work activity (at home or away from home)?

       1. No   2. Yes   □

    b. Leisure activity?

       1. No   2. Yes   □

15. What is the total length of time that should trouble has prevented you from doing your normal work (at home or away from home) during the last 12 months?

    1. 0 days
    2. 1–7 days
    3. 8–30 days
    4. More than 30 days   □

16. Have you been seen by a doctor, physiotherapist, chiropractor or other such person because of shoulder trouble during the last 12 months?

    1. No   2. Yes   □

17. Have you had shoulder trouble at any time during the last 7 days?

    1. No   2. Yes, in my right shoulder
            3. Yes, in my left shoulder
            4. Yes, in both shoulders   □

FIGURE 8.7
The shoulder section of the Nordic Questionnaire for analysis of musculoskeletal symptoms. (Reprinted from Kuorinka, I. et al., *Appl. Ergon.*, 18, 233, 1987. With permission.)

8.4 Gross Posture and Task Analyses

8.4.1 Early Recording of Postures

Poor postures, as mentioned in Chapter 6, can be a major factor in the cause of musculoskeletal injuries. However, the accurate recording of postures is not an easy matter. Systems for recording postures were developed as early as the seventeenth century for choreography. Current variations of such systems, the Labanotation and Benesh notation, require several months of diligent training to achieve suitable skill and speed. These, obviously, would not be suitable for widespread use in industry or even more-detailed laboratory use.

A simpler system for defining a posture numerically was developed by Priel (1974). It noted the position and angle of each joint with respect to a reference level and independent of other joint positions. The angles were estimated in orthogonal planes in roughly 15° increments. The system is simple and can be learned quickly but requires considerable amount of data entries on the forms to obtain the final *posturegram*.

8.4.2 Owaco Working Posture Analysis System

Another readily learnt procedure is the Owaco Working Posture Analysis System (OWAS) developed at the Finnish Institute of Occupational Health for use in the steel industry (Karhu et al., 1977, 1981). The system uses a two-step procedure, the first of which collects data at regular intervals using a three-digit code based on the posture categories given in Figure 8.8. For example, the code 215 would represent a worker with a bent back, with both arms below shoulder level, and kneeling. A later version incorporates three levels of loading (<10, <20, and >20 kg).

The second step analyzes the data to provide frequency distributions of the postures, and rates the work phases into four levels of "action" categories, with category 4 being the worst. Although, somewhat simplistic, OWAS does provide a means of recording and categorizing working postures rather quickly. Also, test–retest correlations are very high, r = 0.97–1.0 (Mattila et al., 1993). Unfortunately, little detail is given to the upper limbs. An interesting extension of OWAS to the construction industry, termed posture, activity, tools, handling (PATH) was formulated by Buchholz et al. (1996). It has since been expanded to include upper extremity limb postures and Latko et al. (1997) hand activity levels and yielded interrater agreement kappa values of 0.4 or higher (Park et al., 2009).

8.4.3 Posture Targeting

A slightly more detailed approach for recording postures at random times during the workday was developed by Corlett et al. (1979). Termed *posture targeting*, the analyst records the body part angle on the body diagram shown in Figure 8.9 by blackening in the appropriate area on a target-like concentric circle arrangement. The first concentric circle represents 45° angular displacement from the standard anatomical position, while each succeeding circle is another 45° increment in displacement. The "target" itself represents azimuth angles in the coronal plane. For example, point 1 in Figure 8.9 indicates the arm is at 90° flexion (pointing horizontally) at 45° from the mid-sagittal plane. Point 2 indicates the wrist is in 45° extension. Note, that repeated observations over time could create a series of points or even a blackened area, indicating a range of movement or static postures. The procedure can be learned in less than an hour and provides test–retest correlations as high as r = 0.67–0.88. The approach allows the analyst to identify the most frequent and potential most stressful postures for more detailed biomechanical analysis and can be combined with worker reports of musculoskeletal pain to provide a comprehensive workplace evaluation (Corlett and Manenica, 1980).

8.4.4 Rapid Upper Limb Assessment

The above posture-targeting system of Corlett et al. (1979) was later refined by McAtamney and Corlett (1993) and Corlett (1995) into *RULA* (rapid upper limb assessment). Upper limb

FIGURE 8.8
The OWAS posture assessment tool. (Reprinted from Karhu, O. et al., *Appl. Ergon.*, 8, 199, 1977. With permission.)

postures (Group A) from Figure 8.10, for the left or right side are combined per Table 8.5 to yield an upper limb score. This score is adjusted upward by one point, if the posture is mainly static or repetitive, and by one, two, or three points, if a 2–10 kg intermittent load, 2–10 kg static load, and more than 10 kg load is handled, respectively. The same procedure is repeated for trunk and leg postures (Group B) from Figure 8.10 and combined per Table 8.6 to yield a trunk score. This score is similarly corrected and then combined with the upper limb score per Table 8.7 to yield a final grand score as a rudimentary musculoskeletal injury risk level, with values above 5 requiring changes (Table 8.7). RULA has shown good correlation with self-reported musculoskeletal discomfort (Hedge et al., 1995; Kilroy and Dockrell, 2000) and since been expanded to the whole body, the Rapid Entire Body Assessment—REBA (Hignett and McAtamney, 2000).

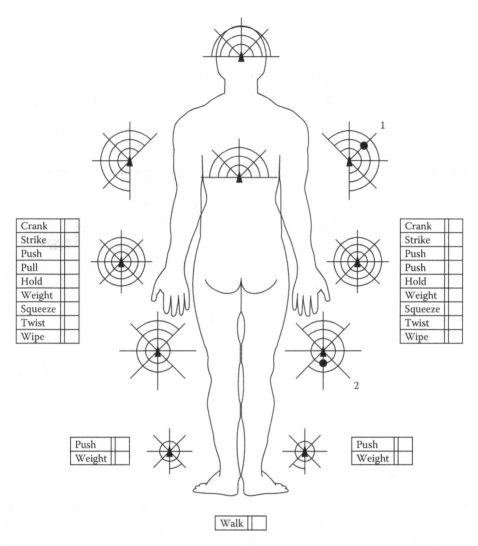

FIGURE 8.9
The posture targeting tool. (Reproduced from Corlett, E.N. et al., *Ergonomics*, 22, 357, 1979. With permission.)

8.4.5 Video Posture Analyses

These early systems were primarily relatively simple pencil-and-paper posture recording systems relying on visual observations. For more detailed analyses, both a permanent record and a finer breakdown or categorization is required. Armstrong et al. (1979, 1982) developed one such system for the upper extremities. First, the job was recorded either on film (as done by the authors) or on videotape (current approach). Next, the analyst selected frames at frequent, regular intervals and recorded shoulder, elbow, and wrist angles and hand posture according to one of six grasp specifications as shown in Figure 8.11. Also, some measure of hand forces were obtained indirectly from observation of forearm muscle EMG. The method was quite successful in identifying stressful tasks in poultry processing and later in the garment industry (Punnett and Keyserling, 1987), but at a relatively high cost of effort, several minutes per frame or several hours per minute of videotape.

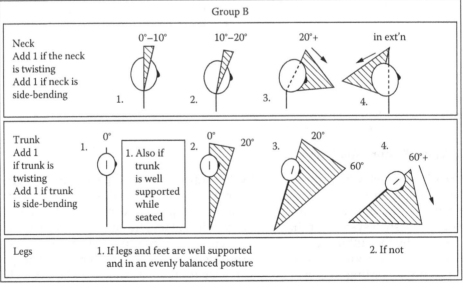

FIGURE 8.10
The RULA posture assessment tool. (Reproduced from Corlett, E.N., The evaluation of posture and its effects, in J. Wilson and E.N. Corlett (eds.,), *The Evaluation of Human Work*, 2nd edn., Taylor & Francis, London, U.K., 1995. With permission.)

TABLE 8.5

Upper Limb Posture Score (Group A) from the RULA Posture Assessment Tool

| | | Wrist Posture Score | | | | | | | |
| | | 1 | | 2 | | 3 | | 4 | |
Upper Arm	Lower Arm	Wrist 1	Twist 2	Wrist 1	Twist 2	Wrist 1	Twist 2	Wrist 1	Twist 2
1	1	1	2	2	2	2	3	3	3
	2	2	2	2	2	3	3	3	3
	3	2	3	3	3	3	3	4	4
2	1	2	3	3	3	3	4	4	4
	2	3	3	3	3	3	4	4	4
	3	3	4	4	4	4	4	5	5
3	1	3	3	4	4	4	4	5	5
	2	3	4	4	4	4	4	5	5
	3	4	4	4	4	4	5	5	5
4	1	4	4	4	4	4	5	5	5
	2	4	4	4	4	4	5	5	5
	3	4	4	4	5	5	5	6	6
5	1	5	5	5	5	5	6	6	7
	2	5	6	6	6	6	7	7	7
	3	6	6	6	7	7	7	7	8
6	1	7	7	7	7	7	8	8	9
	2	8	8	8	8	8	9	9	9
	3	9	9	9	9	9	9	9	9

Source: Corlett, E.N., The evaluation of posture and its effects. In: J. Wilson and E.N. Corlett (eds.), *The Evaluation of Human Work*, 2nd edn., Taylor & Francis, London, U.K., 1995, pp. 663–699. With permission.

TABLE 8.6

Trunk/Neck/Leg Posture Score (Group B) from the RULA Posture Assessment Tool

| | Trunk Posture Score | | | | | | | | | | | |
| Neck Posture Score | 1 Legs | | 2 Legs | | 3 Legs | | 4 Legs | | 5 Legs | | 6 Legs | |
	1	2	1	2	1	2	1	2	1	2	1	2
1	1	3	2	3	3	4	5	5	6	6	7	7
2	2	3	2	3	4	5	5	5	6	7	7	7
3	3	3	3	4	4	5	5	6	6	7	7	7
4	5	5	5	6	6	7	7	7	7	7	8	8
5	7	7	7	7	7	8	8	8	8	8	8	8
6	8	8	8	8	8	8	8	9	9	9	9	9

Source: Corlett, E.N., The evaluation of posture and its effects. In: J. Wilson and E.N. Corlett (eds.), *The Evaluation of Human Work*, 2nd edn., Taylor & Francis, London, U.K., 1995, pp. 663–699. With permission.

Other similar videotape approaches include: (1) the VIRA (Persson and Kilbom, 1983; Kilbom et al., 1986), which utilized two perpendicular cameras, a four part categorization scheme for the shoulder and neck and computer assistance to record time spent in the posture and (2) the Keyserling (1986) one-camera approach for trunk and shoulder angles with computer tabulation. The advantage of the latter approach is that the film can be run a real

TABLE 8.7

Grand Score Table

Upper Limb Score (A)	Trunk/Neck/Leg Score (B)						
	1	**2**	**3**	**4**	**5**	**6**	**8+**
1	1	2	3	3	4	5	5
2	2	2	3	4	4	5	5
3	3	3	3	4	4	5	6
4	3	3	3	4	5	6	6
5	4	4	4	5	6	7	7
6	4	4	5	6	6	7	7
7	5	5	6	6	7	7	7
8+	5	5	6	7	7	7	7

Source: McAtamney, L. and Corlett, E.N., *Appl. Ergon.*, 24, 91, 1993. With permission.

time, saving considerable time over frame-by-frame analysis. Also inexperienced analysts could be trained in 2 h and show very good consistency between observations.

Further automation of upper limb posture analysis was implemented by Yen and Radwin (2002) using the Armstrong et al. (1982) classification scheme and a computer-controlled VCR. (Further information on the multi-media video task analysis [MVTA] computer system is available at http://mvta.engr.wisc.edu/mvta.htm.) The average difference among analysts for average joint angle was 11.4°. MVTA has been used successfully assessing limb postures in manufacturing workers with interreliability coefficients ranging from 0.80 to 0.99 for neck and should postures and from 0.56 to 0.92 for wrist postures and considerably higher intrarater reliability coefficients (Dartt et al., 2009). An alternate approach using spectral analysis of goniometric data (previously presented in Radwin and Lin, 1993; Yen and Radwin, 1999) was much more consistent (average joint deviation angle was only 0.9°) and took only 16% of the time to perform than manual ratings by analysts. Even considering the additional time needed for setting up the instrumentation, total spectral analysis time was 77% of manual analysis time. However, no overall risk assessment was provided.

8.4.6 Task Analyses

Several other posture classification systems were developed based as a part of a general job or task analysis system. The first of these is the AET job analysis method of Rohmert and Landau (1983) and a later variation in the form of PLIBEL (Kemmlert, 1995). Later approaches to continuously record and classify postural changes have utilized the capabilities of personal computers (PCs). The first was a relatively crude classification of gross postures without specifying exact angles by Foreman, Davies, and Troup (1988). Later ones became more detailed by either specifying more accurately joint angles, the Portable Ergonomic Observation (PEO) method by Fransson-Hall et al. (1995), or by categorizing the loads involved, the Task Recording and Analysis on Computer (TRAC) method by van der Beek et al. (1992). Although, quite detailed, some, such as ARBAN (Holzmann, 1982; Wangenheim et al., 1986) are essentially computerized versions of the previously mentioned body discomfort map with a rating for perceived effort using the CR-10 scale at each of the body locations used to identify ergonomic hazards on a job. However, by providing a mean value of the summated ratings, ARBAN is also a coarse overall WRMSD risk-assessment instrument.

ANALYST: _____
DATE: _____

JOB: _____
HAND: RIGHT/LEFT

UPPER EXTREMITY POSTURES AND WORK ELEMENT RECORDING SHEET

FIGURE 8.11

Upper extremity postures and work element recording sheet. (Reproduced from Armstrong, T.J., *Am. Ind. Hyg. Assoc. J.*, 43, 103, 1982. With permission.)

Note, that all of the above systems focus primarily on gross posture and/or general task analysis and typically neglect the upper limbs and the key factors leading to WRMSDs in the upper limbs. One exception to this is the cube model for classifying hand-tool work of Sperling et al. (1993). It categorizes three factors, force, precision, and time, at three levels, during hand-tool usage and then defines acceptable limits. Although, it does not strictly define a risk level for developing WRMSDs in the upper limbs, the cube model is a step in the right direction. More detailed reviews of different postural assessment techniques are provided by Genaidy et al. (1994), Juul-Kristensen et al. (1997), and Kilbom (1994). For convenience purposes, the main posture assessment instruments are summarized and categorized by characteristics in Table 8.8.

8.5 Quantitative Upper Limb WRMSD Risk-Assessment Tools

8.5.1 Checklists

One of first risk-assessment tools developed specifically for identifying upper limb WRMSD was an Upper Extremity Checklist (see Figure 8.12) with questions grouped into five sections relating to repetitiveness, mechanical contact stresses, forceful exertions, awkward postures, and hand-tool usage (Stetson et al., 1991; Keyserling et al., 1993). Some questions required a simple binary response, corresponding to no/zero and yes, while others required categorization into a three-level scale, corresponding to zero/insignificant, moderate, and substantial ergonomic exposures. Once the checklist was completed, the total number of nonzero responses was summed to produce an overall stress score. The authors, however, emphasized that due to the qualitative nature of the responses and user interpretation of stressors, the checklist was designed primarily as a screening tool to identify critical jobs for later analyses and to view the overall risk score with caution.

The checklist was utilized by plant personnel on four work sites to evaluate 335 jobs and was considered to be a quick but effective screening tool (Keyserling et al., 1993). However, when the checklist was compared to results of expert (defined as "university personnel with extensive experience") analyses, the percent of analysts agreeing on the various categories ranged from a low 39% to a high of 90%, or in terms of the kappa statistic (Equation 8.9), from a low of −22% to a high of 80%. Only two of seven categories score a kappa in the range of substantial agreement. The poor agreement was attributed to exposure variability due to the fact that the checklist and expert analyses were often spaced months apart with different workers observed, perhaps using different methods.

8.5.2 Strain Index

Moore and Garg (1995) proposed a more quantitative job analysis methodology based on physiological considerations and job risk factors, which yielded a final risk score, Termed the Strain Index (SI), six task variables, intensity of exertion, duration of exertion, efforts per minute, wrist posture, speed of exertion, and duration of task were rated on an ordinal five-point exposure scale (see Table 8.9). The ratings were converted to six multipliers from

TABLE 8.8

Categorization of Posture Assessment and Gross Task Analysis Instruments (in Order of Complexity)

Type of Instrument (Key Ref.)	Equipment Used	Posture Levels of Categorization	Force	Frequency	Learning Time	Analysis Time	Test-Retest Reliability	Validity (With Standard)
Posture recording via sampling	*Paper/pencil*	*Gross postures*						
Posturegram (Priel, 1974)	Paper/pencil	Sh 6-Ro, Sh 8-A/A, Sh 8-F/E, El 4-Ro, El 6-F/E, Wr 3-F/E	—	—	Long	Medium	—	—
OWAS (Karhu et al., 1977)	Paper/pencil	Sh 3-F/E and trunk angles	Three levels	%Time	5 days	Short	$0.74 < r < 0.99$[a]	—
Posture targeting (Corlett et al., 1979)	Paper/pencil	Nominally 4 × 8 categories, but, in practice, infinite combinations	—	—	1h	Medium	$0.67 < r < 0.88$[a]	Upper arm $r = 0.32$[a], lower arm $r = 0.08$NS
RULA (McAtamney and Corlett, 1993)	Paper/pencil	Sh 5-F/E, Sh A/A, El 3-F/E, Wr 3-F/E, Wr 3-R/U	Four levels	Two levels	Medium	Short	—	—
Continuous posture recording	*Video*	*Micro postures*						
Armstrong (1979, 1982)	One camera, PC	Sh 5-F/E, Sh 4-A/A, Sh 4-Ro, El 4-F/E, El 2-Ro, Wr 5-F/E, Wr 3-R/U, 6 grasps	From EMG	Cycle time # grasp	Medium	Very long	—	—
VIRA (Persson and Kilbom 1983)	Two cameras, PC	Sh 5-F/E, Sh 4-A/A	—	Cycle time	0.5h	Medium	6% error[a]	—
Keyserling (1986)	One camera, PC	Sh 3-F/E and trunk angles	—	Cycle time	20h	Medium	Time, $r = 0.98$[a] Posture $r = 0.95$[a]	Time, $r = 0.99$[a]
Wrigley et al. (1991)	One camera, PC	Infinite, true motion analysis	—	—	Medium	Medium	$r = 0.99$[a]	Difference = 1.4°
MVTA (Yen and Radwin, 2002)	One camera, PC	Either Armstrong (1982) or infinite	—	Cycle time	Medium	Long or short	—	Difference = 11.4° or 0.9°

(continued)

TABLE 8.8 (continued)

Categorization of Posture Assessment and Gross Task Analysis Instruments (in Order of Complexity)

Type of Instrument (Key Ref.)	Equipment Used	Posture Levels of Categorization	Force	Frequency	Learning Time	Analysis Time	Test–Retest Reliability	Validity (With Standard)
Task (risk) analysis								
		Gross postures						
AET (Rohmert and Landau, 1983)	Paper/pencil	Arm, hand/finger, trunk	Five levels	Five levels	Long	Long	Good if trained	—
ARBAN (Holzmann, 1982)	Video, PC	El 3-Ro × 4-F/E, similar for other joints	Borg-CR10	Cycle time	Long	Long	Good if trained	—
TRAC (van der Beek et al., 1992)	Pocket PC	Four for arms and trunk, legs	Three levels	—	Short	Medium	$0.24 < r < 0.89$	$r = 0.98$[a], posture
PEO (Fransson-Hall et al., 1995)	Pocket PC video helps	Sh 2-F/E, wrist, neck, trunk,	Loads lifted	Cycle time # events	10h	Medium	Time, r[a] frequency, r NS	$r = 0.5$[a], for posture

Abbreviations: Sh, shoulder; El, elbow; Wr, wrist; A/A, abduction/adduction; F/E, flexion/extension; R/U, radian/ulnar deviation; Ro, rotation. —, unknown or not applicable; NS, not significant at p > .05.
[a] Significant at p < .05.

UPPER EXTREMITY CHECKLIST

Worker Information
Which hand is the operator's dominant hand? (circle one)
Left Hand   Right Hand   Both Hands
Circle a *, √ or to answer each question below.

Repetitiveness			No	Yes
1. Does the job involve repetitive use of the hands and wrists?			o	*

Answer "yes" if either of the following is true:
a. The work cycle is less than 30 s long, or
b. The hands repeat the same motions/exertions for more than ½ of the work cycle

Mechanical Stress		**Left Hand**		**Right Hand**		
		No	Yes	No	Yes	Element(s)
2. Do hard or sharp objects, tools, or parts of the workstation put localized pressure on the:						
a. Back or side of the fingers?		o	√	o	√	_____
b. Palm or base of the hand?		o	√	o	√	_____
c. Forearm or elbow?		o	√	o	√	_____
d. Armpit?		o	√	o	√	_____
3. Is the pain or base of the hand used as a striking tool (like a hammer)?		o	√	o	√	_____

Force						
4. Does the worker lift, carry, push or pull objects weighing more than 4.5 kg (10 lb)?		o	√	o	√	_____
5. Does operator grip an object or a tool that has a smooth, slippery (no texture or hand holds to reduce slipping)?		o	√	o	√	_____
6. Is the tip of a finger or thumb used as a pressing or pushing tool?		o	√	o	√	_____
7. Check box if no gloves are worn and skip this question. ☐						
If the operator wears gloves, do the gloves hinder gripping?		o	√	o	√	_____

FIGURE 8.12
Upper extremity checklist. (Reproduced from Keyserling, W.M., *Ergonomics*, 36, 807, 1993. With permission.)

TABLE 8.9

Strain Index Rating Criteria

Rating	Intensity of Exertion (%MVC)	Duration of Exertion (% of Cycle)	Efforts per min	Wrist Posture (Worst Case)			Speed of Work (% Speed Rating)	Duration per Day (h)
				Extension	Flexion	Ulnar Deviation		
1	<15	<10	<4	0°–10°	0°–5°	0°–10°	<80	<1
2	16–30	10–29	4–8	11°–25°	6°–15°	11°–15°	81–90	1–2
3	31–52	30–49	9–14	26°–40°	16°–30°	16°–20°	91–100	2–4
4	51–75	50–79	15–19	41°–55°	31°–50°	21°–25°	101–115	4–8
5	>75	≥80	≥20	>55°	>50°	>25°	>115	>8

Source: Moore, J. S. and Garg, A., *Am. Ind. Hyg. Assoc. J.*, 56, 443, 1994.

TABLE 8.10

Strain Index Multiplier Table (for Table 8.9)

Rating	Intensity of Exertion	Duration of Exertion	Efforts per min	Wrist Posture	Speed of Work	Duration per Day
1	1	0.5	0.5	1.0	1.0	0.25
2	3	1.0	1.0	1.0	1.0	0.50
3	6	1.5	1.5	1.5	1.0	0.75
4	9	2.0	2.0	2.0	1.5	1.00
5	13	3.0	3.0	3.0	2.0	1.50

Source: Moore, J. S. and Garg, A., *Am. Ind. Hyg. Assoc. J.*, 56, 443, 1994. With permission.

Table 8.10, which when multiplied together yield the final SI score. For example, a task with 20% MVC exertions over 60% of one cycle, with 12 efforts per minute, with 18° ulnar deviations, at 95% of normal pace for a full 8 h shift would yield ratings of 2, 4, 3, 3, 3, and 4 from Table 8.9, respectively. These ratings convert to multipliers of 3.0, 2.0, 1.5, 1.5, 1.0, and 1.0 from Table 8.10, respectively, and, when multiplied together, yield a final SI score of 13.5. SI scores above 5.0 were considered to be potentially hazardous.

The authors tested the SI methodology on data from an earlier study in a pork-processing plant (Moore and Garg, 1994). The SI correctly identified 11 of 12 jobs associated with WRMSD morbidity and all 13 jobs not associated with WRMSDs. The relative risk was 11.7 greater for the hazardous jobs (as defined by the SI) as opposed to the jobs deemed safe. A later studies established sensitivity, specificity, and positive predictive values for the SI of 0.86, 0.79, and 0.92, respectively, on 28 poultry processing jobs (Knox and Moore, 2001) and ICC_2 scores of 0.81 for individuals and 0.88 for teams on 61 job-video files over 5 month period (Stephens et al., 2006).

Note that the SI was originally designed for single-force exertion jobs and that it would not apply for jobs in which a worker may exert a variety of forces or, worse, a variety of different tasks. Bao et al. (2009) attempted to correct this problem with six different combined computational methods, which however resulted in different SI scores and thus different risk level classifications. The Spearman rank-order correlation coefficients between the different methods ranged from 0.61 to 0.97. In general, simpler methods generated more comparable SI scores and any method gave good correlations, such that a relative ranking of jobs was still valid.

8.5.3 OCRA

A more detailed exposure assessment tool for upper limbs, termed the OCRA exposure index, was proposed by Occhipinti (1998). The final exposure index is a ratio of the number of motions (termed technical actions) performed in repetitive tasks during a shift to the number of recommended or allowed motions for that shift. The categorization of motions follows a procedure developed by Colombini (1998) and shown in Figure 8.13. The calculation of the number of allowed motions is a fairly involved procedure involving multipliers for various risk factors (see tables in Figure 8.14) that is somewhat analogous to those in the SI of Moore and Garg (1995).

TASK INVOLVEMENT: *OPERATING A LEVER*

UPPER LIMB: ☑ RIGHT ☐ LEFT

	CYCLE	POSTURAL SCORE IN CYCLE/TASK (A + B = MAX 16)
SHOULDER POSITIONS AND MOVEMENT	|_0_|_0_|_0_|A2 CYCLE |_4_|B1	|_0_|_4_| SHOULDER
ELBOW MOVEMENTS	|_0_|_0_|_0_|A2 CYCLE |_4_|B2	|_0_|_4_| ELBOW

SHOULDER POSITIONS AND MOVEMENT

0°, 60°, 20°, 0°, 60°, 20°

- MOVEMENTS IN EXTREME ARTICULAR RANGE: THEY LAST: ☐ 1/3, ☐ 2/3, ☐ 3/3 of cycle/task time
- STEREOTYPE MOVEMENTS (SCORE 4):
  ☑ Performs work gestures of the same type involving the shoulder for more than 50% of the cycle task time.
- STATIC POSTURES (score 4):
  ☐ Keeps the arm raised (unsupported) at an angle more than 60° or in extension, for at least 10 sec conecutively once every cycle (short cycle: inf. 30 sec). For longer cycle time increase proportionally the time of the static constraction.
  ☐ Keeps the arm raised (unsupported) at an angle of:
    ☐ 60° for more than 1 min
    ☐ 40° for more than 2 min
    ☐ 20° for more than 3 min

ELBOW MOVEMENTS

0°, RANGE, Score 2, 0°, SUPINATION PRONATION

- MOVEMENTS IN EXTREME ARTICULAR RANGE: THEY STAND: ☐ 1/3, ☐ 2/3, ☐ 3/3 of cycle/task time
- LACK OF VARIATION (score 4): ☑ Performs work gestures of the same type involving the elbow for at least 50% of the cycle.

(continued)

FIGURE 8.13
Upper limb postures for the OCRA index of exposure. (Reproduced from Colombini, D., *Ergonomics*, 41, 1261, 1998. With permission.)

WRIST POSITION AND MOVEMENTS	|_0_|_0_|_0_|A3 CYCLE

EXTENSION   FLEXION   0°
 	
RADIAL   ULNAR
DEVIATION DEVIATION   0°
 	
– MOVEMENTS IN EXTREME ARTICULAR RANGE: THEY LAST: ☐ 1/3, ☐ 2/3, ☐ 3/3 of cycle/task time
– LACK OF VARIATION (SCORE 4):
  ☑ Performs work gestures of the same type involving the wrist for at least 50% of the cycle,
  ☐ Keeps the wrist flexed or extended (at an angle of over 45°) or deviated laterally (ulna or radius) for at least 50% of cycle/task time.
	|_4_|B3
	
	|_0_|_4_|
	WRIST/HAND

TYPE OF GRIP AND FINGER MOVEMENTS	|_1_|_1_|_1_|A4 SCORE
TIME OF THE GRIP AND FINGER POSITION SCORE TIGHT GRIP (1.5 cm) [ ] 1/3, ☐ 2/3, ☐ 3/3 2 PINCH [ ] 1/3, ☐ 2/3, ☐ 3/3 3 PALMAR GRIP [ ] 1/3, ☐ 2/3, ☐ 3/3 4 HOOK GRIP [ ] 1/3, ☐ 2/3, ☐ 3/3 4 KEYING [ ] 1/3, ☐ 2/3, ☐ 3/3 4 WIDE GRIP (4–5 cm) [ ] 1/3, ☐ 2/3, ☑ 3/3 1 .... [ ] 1/3, ☐ 2/3, ☐ 3/3 .... [ ] 1/3, ☐ 2/3, ☐ 3/3 .... LACK OF VARIATION (score 4): [1] Performs work gestures of the same type involving the same finger(s) for at least 50% of the cycle. [2] Holds an object in a pinch or palmar (or hook) grip for at least 50% of the cycle.	|_0_|B4 |_0_|_4_| GRIP/HAND

FIGURE 8.13 (continued)

Part A. Summary of data for calculating index of exposure to repetitive movements of the upper limbs.

Department or line...............	Station or task.................	Shift.....................

Characterization of repetitive tasks performed during shift

	A	B	C	D
• Duration of task in shift (min)				
• Mean cycle duration (s)				
• Action frequency (no. of action / min)				
• Total actions in task				

• Total actions in shift (sum of A, B, C, D) $\boxed{}$ A^e

Characterization of non-repetitive tasks performed during shift

	X	Y	X
• Duration (min)			
• Comparable to recovery			
• Not comparable to recovery			min

Total no. of minutes of non-repetitive task comparable to recovery

$\boxed{}$

Characterization of breaks during shift

• Duration of meal break (min)
• Other breaks
• Total duration of other breaks (min)

Time-wise distribution of tasks and breaks in shift
(describe exact sequence of tasks and breaks, and their relative duration in minutes)

1h

No. of hours in shift featuring lack of recovery times, N = _____

	A	B	C	D	
• Minutes spent with previous adequate recovery periods					D_{re}
• Minutes spent without previous adequate recovery periods					D_{so}

FIGURE 8.14
Worksheet for the calculation of the OCRA index of exposure. (Reproduced from Occhipinti, E., *Ergonomics*, 41, 1290, 1998. With permission.)

$$A_r = F_r \sum_1^n CF \times F_f \times F_p \times F_a \times D \tag{8.21}$$

where

A_r is the total number of motions recommended during shift
F_r is the multiplier for the lack of recovery period during the shift
CF is the reference number of motions per minute (typically 30)
F_f is the multiplier for the force risk factor
F_p is the multiplier for the posture risk factor
F_a is the multiplier for additional elements of risk
D is the duration of each repetitive task in minutes

The final index of exposure (IE) is then:

$$IE = \frac{A_e}{A_r} \tag{8.22}$$

where A_e is the total number of motions observed during the repetitive tasks.

Theoretically, when IE scores are below one, the exposures can be considered acceptable. As the index increases above one, the exposure becomes increasingly hazardous. However, Occhipinti (1998) adopted a three-level classification scheme analogous to the green/amber/red colors of a traffic light. For IE scores below 0.75 (green region), the exposure is acceptable. IE scores ranging between 0.75 and 4.00 (amber region) are borderline significant and need to be monitored more closely. IE scores above 4.00 (red area) are considered significant with corrections to the workplace required.

OCRA was validated over the course of eight studies involving 462 exposed and 749 nonexposed workers (Grieco, 1998). Linear regression by job category of the OCRA IE score with a normalized damage index, total number of WRMSDs divided by the total number of limbs at risk (because some workers had multiple disorders or even multiple disorders for a given limb), yielded a significant correlation ($r^2 = 0.72$, $p = .004$). A log transformation yielded an even better relationship ($r^2 = 0.88$, $p = .0002$). A more recent study (Occhipinti and Colombini, 2007) updated reference values and predictive models and established a database for 23 groups of workers. Although fairly complicated, the OCRA model seems to show promise.

8.5.4 Recent Developments

There has also been ongoing standards activity by a committee of the American National Standards Institute (ANSI Z-365) to standardize methodology for assessing upper limb WRMSD risks through the use of checklists. Although several working drafts have been released, no definitive methods or tools have been recommended so far. On the other hand, the American Conference on Government Industrial Hygienists just released a new threshold level value (TLV) to be used in the reduction of work-related musculoskeletal disorders (see Figure 8.15, ACGIH, 2003). Peak force is estimated by the Borg (1982) CR-10 scale or as fraction of %MVC, while hand activity level is estimated from a 10-point linear

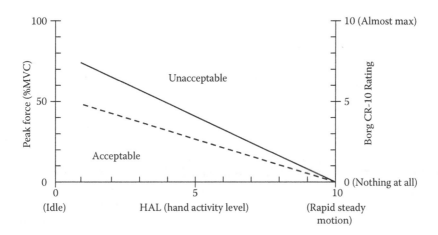

FIGURE 8.15
The TLV for reduction of WRMSDs based on hand activity level. The solid top line is the TLV, the dashed bottom line is an action level. (From ACGIH, *2002 TLVs and BEIs*, American Conference of Governmental Industrial Hygienists, Cincinnati, OH, 2002. With permission.)

scale with verbal anchors ranging from 0, hands idle most of the time, to 10, rapid steady motion based on Latko et al. (1997). The top line is the TLV, while the bottom line is an action limit for implementing corrective measures. As this is a new measure, no data is currently available on its reliability or validity.

8.6 Data-Driven Upper Limb WRMSD Risk Index

Another upper limb WRMSD risk-assessment index, similar to OCRA, was developed by Seth et al. (1999). However, two main differences separated this tool, termed the CTD Risk Index (available at http://www.ie.psu.edu/courses/ie327/CTDriskindex.htm), from the others previously discussed. First, wrist-posture data collected with the Yun et al. (1997) integrated touch glove system (see Section 7.3.3) was fed directly into the model. Second, WRMSD data from industry was used to develop the regression coefficients of the final model to yield a predicted incidence rate. The risk-assessment model is presented here in a step-by-step approach.

Wrist deviation and arm rotation cause a significant grip strength decrement as compared to a neutral wrist posture. These effects, from the data of Terrell and Purswell (1976), Imrahn (1991), and Hallbeck et al. (1992), were expressed as equations for maximum voluntary contraction (MVC) for power grip and various pinches produced in five wrist positions (neutral, flexion, extension, radial, and ulnar deviation) and in three arm rotations (pronation, mid-position, and supination) (see Table 8.11). Inputting the appropriate parameters yields the variable *Force Capacity Wrist*. Similarly, force decrements occur for both power and pinch grip depending on the grip span utilized. This effect again can be quantified from the data of Greenberg and Chaffin (1976) and Petrofsky et al. (1980) to yield average grip span strength decrements for spans ranging from 0 to 11 cm as shown in Table 8.12. Inputting the appropriate parameters yields the variable *Grip Span Force*.

TABLE 8.11

Force Capacity Wrist Equations

Grip Type	Wrist Position	%MVC as a Function of Wrist Angle A (Degrees)
Power	Flexion/extension/pronation	$-0.0113A^2 + 0.1826A + 88$
Power	Flexion/extension/midposition	$-0.0114A^2 + 0.1308A + 99$
Power	Flexion/extension/supination	$-0.0112A^2 + 0.0979A + 100$
Power	Radial/ulnar deviation/pronation	$-0.0337A^2 + 0.025A + 99$
Power	Radial/ulnar deviation/midposition	$-0.0538A^2 + 0.275A + 88$
Power	Radial/ulnar deviation/supination	$-0.0338A^2 + 0.075A + 100$
Lateral pinch	Flexion/extension/supination	$-0.0124A^2 + 0.1905A + 100$
Lateral pinch	Radial/ulnar deviation/pronation	$-0.0409A^2 + 0.1525A + 100$
Chuck pinch	Flexion/extension/supination	$-0.0158A^2 + 0.2191A + 98$
Chuck pinch	Radial/ulnar deviation/pronation	$-0.0626A^2 + 0.1275A + 98$
2-Point pinch	Flexion/extension/supination	$-0.0114A^2 + 0.1423A + 72.4$
2-Point pinch	Radial/ulnar deviation/pronation	$-0.00535A^2 + 72.4$

TABLE 8.12

Grip Span Force Equations

Grip Type	%MVC as a Function of Grip Span Width (G in cm)
Power	$-0.3624G^3 + 4.6865G^2 - 3.6186G + 14.4$
Lateral pinch	$-0.8308G^2 + 3.0288G + 97.59$
Chuck pinch	$-0.2363G^2 - 0.7093G + 100.22$
2-Point pulp pinch	$-0.3931G^2 + 1.6383G + 99.22$

Repeated exertions will result in muscle fatigue and reduced capacity for further exertions. This effect can be quantified from the data of Schutz (1972) as the maximum %MVC Allowed for a particular wrist motion based on the exertion time for the motion and the time between exertions or motions. If the %MVC Required for the motion is greater than that allowed as calculated below (%MVC Allowed), then a penalty is assessed to that motion.

$$\%\text{MVC Allowed} = [0.9503\,\text{TW}^{-0.394} \times \text{TR}^{0.2246} \times \text{MW}^{0.258} \times 0.475] \times 100 \qquad (8.23)$$

where
 TW is the work time of grip or motion (min)
 TR is the rest time between grips or motions (min)
 MW is the time worked during one shift (min)

For each motion a Force Capacity is calculated as the product of Force Capacity Wrist and Grip Span Force:

$$\text{Force Capacity} = \frac{\text{Force Capacity Wrist} \times \text{Grip Span Force}}{100} \qquad (8.24)$$

%MVC Required$_{Adj}$ is calculated based on %MVC Required for the motion and the previously calculated Force Capacity. %MVC Required is typically found by dividing the subjective job force requirement to the operator's MVC.

$$\%MVC\ Required_{Adj} = \frac{\%MVC\ Required}{Force\ Capacity} \times 100 \qquad (8.25)$$

The %MVC Required$_{Adj}$ is then compared to the %MVC Allowed for Equation 8.23. If the %MVC Allowed is less than the %MVC Required$_{Adj}$, then no penalty is assessed to that hand motion and that motion will have a Force Frequency Score (FFS) of one. If the %MVC Allowed is greater than the %MVC Required$_{Adj}$, then the FFS$_i$ for that individual motion is calculated as follows:

$$FFS_i = \frac{\%MVC\ Required_{Adj}}{\%MVC\ Allowed} \times n \qquad (8.26)$$

where n is the number of hand motions per job cycle.

The FFS$_i$ values for each individual hand motion are then summed to obtain an overall force frequency score:

$$FFS = \sum \frac{FES_i \times N}{10,000} \qquad (8.27)$$

where N is the number of job cycles per shift.

The scaling factor of 10,000 is the NIOSH (Hales et al., 1989) maximum recommended number of damaging wrist motions that can be performed in an 8h shift. The model then assesses which hand has a higher overall FFS and uses that value for further calculations.

Gross torso posture of a worker while performing a job is important because awkward postures can lead to fatigue. The resulting fatigue, defined as %Endurance Capacity, can be quantified in a manner similar to Equation 8.23:

$$\%Endurance\ Capacity = \left\{ 1 - \left[1.0996 \times F_{MVC}^{1.863} \times TW^{0.734} \times TR^{-0.413} \times MW^{0.481} \right] \right\} \times 100 \qquad (8.28)$$

where
  TW is the work time posture held (min)
  TR is the rest time between postures (min)
  MW is the minutes worked during one shift (min)
  F$_{MVC}$ is the relative weight, weight held divided by 51 lb (from the NIOSH Lifting Equation, Waters et al., 1993)

Five postures are considered: neck and back flexion, elbow and shoulder flexion, and shoulder abduction. For simplicity sake (and difficulty interpreting angles from job videotapes), *Points* are assigned to various angles as follows: for back flexion 0°–10° = 0, 10°–20° = 1, 20°–45° = 2, and >45° = 3 points; for neck flexion 0°–30° = 0, 30°–45° = 1, 45°–60° = 2, and >60° = 3 points; for elbow flexion/extension (with a 90° bent elbow being considered the neutral posture) 10° flexion to 30° extension = 0, everything else is 1 point; for shoulder flexion 0°–20° = 0, 20°–45° = 1, 45°–90° = 2 and >90° = 3 points; and for shoulder abduction 0°–30° = 0, 30°–60° = 1, 60°–90° = 2, >90° = 3 points.

The Posture Score for each body part is obtained by multiplying the point value by the %Endurance Capacity (Equation 8.28) and dividing the product into 50, which is considered as the limit for acceptable fatigue or endurance:

$$\text{Posture Score} = \frac{50}{(\%\text{Endurance Capacity} \times \text{Points})} \tag{8.29}$$

The Overall Posture Score (OPS) is the maximum of individual Posture Scores for each joint.

The final risk score is a weighted average (coefficients obtained from regression of a subset of jobs) of the FFS (Equation 8.27) and the OPS in the form of a predicted incidence rate (IR) normalized to 200,000 exposure hours:

$$\text{IR} = 3.41\,\text{FFS} + 1.87\,\text{OPS} \tag{8.30}$$

Regression of predicted incidence rates against the actual incidence rates experienced on 24 industrial jobs in the garment and the printing industry (involving a total of 288 worker) yielded a significant (p < .001) linear regression with $r^2 = 0.52$. As a comparison, Moore and Garg's (1995) SI yielded a nonsignificant (p = .2) regression with $r^2 = 0.17$ as did also the proposed ANSI Z-365 checklist ($r^2 = 0.22$). The only limitations found were for very short cycle jobs (typically under four second cycle times), in which any error in miscounting motions could be amplified into a large error for the final predicted incidence rate.

Novice ergonomists (university graduate students) required at least several trials in becoming proficient with the risk-assessment model. However, by the fifth trial, average time required for job analysis had decreased to 12 min, and test–retest reliability was up to $r^2 = 0.99$. A simplified version of this risk index has been developed into a paper-and-pencil checklist for use in industry (see Figure 8.16), with values greater than 1.0 indicating risk for injury. However, it has not been validated or checked for reliability.

Note that the roughly 48% of the variance unaccounted for, was thought to be due individual differences such as gender, age, physical fitness, etc. and the psychosocial risk factors discussed in Section 6.6. This leads to the need of further modeling efforts utilizing the multivariate tools discussed in Section 6.4.3 (You, 1999).

For convenience purposes, the main upper limb WRMSD risk-assessment instruments are summarized in Table 8.13. Also, many of these risk-assessment instruments are available as part of an Upper Extremity Assessment tools package from NexGen Ergonomics Inc. (Quebec, Canada; http://www.nexgenergo.com/)

CTD Risk Index					
Job Title:	VCT Counter No.:				Date:
Job Description:	Department:				Analyst:
Cycle Time (i minutes; obtain from videotape)					❶
#Cycle/Day = $\dfrac{(480 - \text{Lunch} - \text{Breaks})}{\text{CycleTime}}$ =			❷ a		❸ Larger of ❷ a or ❷ b:
# Parts/Day (if known)			❷ b		
# Handmotions/Cycle					❹
# Handmotions/Day (❸ × ❹)					❺
Frequency Factor (Divide ❺ by 10,000) =					

(Circle appropriate condition)	Points			
	0	1	2	3
Working Posture	Sit	Stand		
Hand Posture 1: Pulp Pinch	No	Yes		
Hand Posture 2: Lateral Pinch	No	Yes		
Hand Posture 3: Palm Pinch	No	Yes		
Hand Posture 4: Finger Press	No	Yes		
Hand Posture 5: Power Grip	Yes	No		
Type of Reach	Horizontal	Up/Down		
Hand Deviation 1: Flexion	No	Yes		
Hand Deviation 2: Extension	No	Yes		
Hand Deviation 3: Radial Dev.	No	Yes		
Hand Deviation 4: Ulnar Dev.	No	Yes		
Forearm Rotation	Neutral	In/Out		
Elbow Angle	=90°	≠90°		
Shoulder Abduction	0	<45°	<90°	>90°
Shoulder Flexion	0	<90°	<180°	>180°
Back/Neck Angle	0	<45°	<90°	>90°
Balance	Yes	No		
Total the Points for the Circled Conditions				❻
Posture Factor (Divide by ❻ by 10) =				
Grip or Pinch Force Used on Task	❼ lbs.		❾ Divide ❼ by ❽:	
Max Grip or Pinch Force	❽ lbs.			
Force Factor (Divide ❾ by 0.15) =				

(Circle appropriate condition)	Points			
	0	1	2	3
Sharp Edge	No	Yes		
Glove	No	Yes		
Vibration	No	Yes		
Type of Action	Dynamic	Intermittent	Static	
Temperature	Warm	Cold		
Total the Points for the Circle Conditions				❿
Miscellaneous Factor (Divide 10 by 3) =				
CTD Risk Index = 0.3 × (Frequency + Posture + Force Factors) + 0.1 × (Miscellaneous Factor)				
CTD Risk Index = 3 × (+ +) + 0.1 × ( ) =				

FIGURE 8.16

A simple CTD risk index. (Reproduced from Freivalds, A., *Niebel's Methods, Standards, and Work Design*, The McGraw-Hill Companies, New York, 2009. With permission.)

TABLE 8.13

Categorization of Upper Extremity WRMSD Risk-Assessment Instruments (in Order of Complexity)

Type of Instrument (Key Ref.)	Equipment Used	Posture (No. of Levels)	Force (No. of Levels)	Frequency (No. of Levels)	Duration per Cycle	Overall Duration	Learning Time	Analysis Time	Test–Retest Reliability	Validity (with Standard)
TLV (ACGIH, 2002)	Paper, pencil	—	Ten levels	Ten levels	—	One	Very short	Very short	—	—
Upper extremity checklist (Keyserling et al., 1993)	Paper, pencil	Three levels	Two levels	Two or four levels (two variations)	Two levels	None	Short	Short	—	$\kappa > 0.7$, 2 of 7 $\kappa > 0.4$, 5 of 7
Strain index (Moore and Garg, 1995)	Paper, pencil	Five levels	Five levels	Five levels	Five levels	Five levels	Short	Medium	—	86% sensitivity 79% specificity
OCRA (Grieco, 1998; Occhipinti, 1998)	Paper, pencil	Two or three levels	Ten levels	Count number of motions	Five levels	Eight levels	Medium	Medium	—	$r^2 = 0.88$, $p = .0002$
CTD risk index (Seth et al., 1999)	Touch glove, videotape PC	Torso, arms = four levels, wrist = continuous	Continuous	Count number of motions	Continuous	Continuous	Medium	Medium	$r = 0.72$	$r^2 = 0.52$, $p = .001$

Abbreviations: Sh, shoulder; El, elbow; Wr, wrist; A/A, abduction/adduction; F/E, flexion/extension; R/U, radian/ulnar deviation; Ro, rotation; —, unknown or not applicable.

Questions

1. What is the difference between passive and active surveillance? What implications does that have for a research study?

2. What is validity and how can it be further defined?

3. What is reliability and how can it be measured?

4. What does a correlation coefficient of –1 mean? Does that mean that assessment tool under evaluation is worthless?

5. What is a split-half procedure and why is it needed?

6. How can the reliability over time of an assessment tool be established?

7. How can the reliability of an assessment tool between analysts be established?

8. What is the purpose of the kappa statistic? That is, what benefits does it have?

9. What procedures can be used to establish the agreement between items or analysts given continuous data?

10. Compare and contrast the two classes of interclass correlation coefficients.

11. Compare and contrast accuracy and precision.

12. How does accuracy and precision of a test relate to the validity and reliability of a test?

13. What is the difference between the sensitivity and specificity of a test?

14. How does signal detection theory relate to the effectiveness of an assessment tool?

15. Discuss the tradeoffs of self-reports as compared to direct measurements of occupational risk factors.

16. How does the predictive value of a risk-assessment tool vary according to the prevalence of the WRMSD?

17. How may one initially identify the scope of WRMSDs in a workplace?

18. What is the purpose of symptom surveys? Describe some typical approaches.

19. Describe some of the different posture analysis tools. What are the advantages and disadvantages of each?

20. What are the tradeoffs in using a paper-and-pencil posture analysis tool such as RULA as opposed to a video-based tool such as VIRA or MVTA?

21. Discuss the tradeoffs between using a simple risk-assessment instruments such as the ACGIH (2002) TLV and the more complex OCRA.

Problems

1. On a 40 question test, the mean passing score is 35 and the variance is 5. What is Kuder–Richardson measure of reliability for this test?

2. A new risk-assessment tool is being developed to identify the risk for WRMSDs. Three hundred workers are screened by physicians for WRMSDs, yielding 100 confirmed cases. The risk-assessment tool yields 200 positives, of which 50 are true positives. Calculate the sensitivity, specificity, and predictive value of this tool.

3. A new test is being compared with the gold standard measurement with the following results:

	Gold Standard	
New Test	**+**	**−**
+	22	2
−	8	73

What is the sensitivity and specificity?

4. Two analysts are comparing their results on a posture assessment tool.

	Analyst B	
Analyst A	**+**	**−**
+	82	9
−	8	2

a. What is the percentage agreement?

b. What is kappa?

c. Is this a reliable tool? That is, is there reasonable agreement between analysts?

5. The prevalence of CTS in the general industry is approximately 1.5%. A large NIOSH study will screen approximately 10,000 workers. The sensitivity and specificity associated with this test is thought to be 22.9% and 99.8%, respectively.

a. What is the positive predictive value of this test?

b. What is the negative predictive value of this test?

6. An analyst counts the number of deviated wrist motions for eight jobs on April 2 and then repeats the analysis for the same eight jobs on April 19.

a. What is the test–retest reliability for this analysis?

b. What is a potential problem with this approach?

c. How could it be corrected?

Job Number	April 2	April 19
1	2	3
2	1	2
3	4	6
4	1	2
5	5	6
6	2	4
7	6	8
8	3	5

7. Two analysts separately estimated the forces required to perform ten different jobs.

a. What is the Pearson product moment correlation coefficient?

b. What is the intraclass correlation coefficient (Case 2)?

c. Is there good agreement between the analysts?

Job Number	Analyst A	Analyst B
1	20	50
2	10	30
3	40	60
4	10	20
5	50	60
6	20	40
7	60	80
8	40	30
9	60	30
10	30	50

8. The ratings of perceived exertion for six different jobs are given below.

   a. Given that four analysts were picked randomly for each job, find a measure of agreement for their ratings.

   b. Given that the same four analysts rated each job, find a measure of agreement for their ratings.

   c. Which approach gives better reliability? Why? Discuss the implications of the results.

	Analysts			
Jobs	A	B	C	D
1	9	2	5	8
2	6	1	3	2
3	8	4	6	8
4	7	1	2	6
5	10	5	6	9
6	6	2	4	7

9. Evaluate the following eight jobs, focusing on the right hand and assuming a grip force as stated (videoclips available at http://www2.ie.psu.edu/freivalds/courses/ie327new/design.htm):

   i. Stamping extrusions—30% MVC

   ii. Stamping end coupling—15% MVC

   iii. Flashlight assembly—15% MVC

   iv. Union assembly—15% MVC

   v. Hospital bed rail assembly—30% MVC

   vi. Stitching garments—30% MVC

   vii. Labeling garments—15% MVC

   viii. Cut and tack (garments)—30% MVC

      a. Use RULA to evaluate upper limb posture.

      b. Use the ACGIH (2002) TLV limits to evaluate WRMSD risk.

      c. Use the SI to evaluate WRMSD risk.

      d. Use the CTD Risk Index to evaluate WRMSD risk.

      e. Use the simplified CTD Risk Index (Figure 8.16) to evaluate WRMSD risk.

      f. How do the SI, CTD Risk Index, and simplified CTD Risk Index scores compare?

10. Consider that a "finger sensitivity" test (from a low of 0 [complete nerve loss] to a high of 10 [full sensitivity]) was used to screen the workers as a cheaper alternative to electrodiagnostic testing by a physician.

Trigger Finger	Sensitivity—Low	Sensitivity—High
Yes	11	3
No	13	33

a. What is the *sensitivity and accuracy* of this test? Explain what each means and relate to the above scenario.

b. Is this a good test? Why or why not?

References

ACGIH. (2003). *2003 TLVs and BEIs*. Cincinnati, OH: American Conference of Governmental Industrial Hygienists.

Ainsworth, B.E., Jacobs, D.R., Leon, A.S., Richardson, M.T., and Montoye, H.J. (1993). Assessment of the accuracy of physical activity questionnaire occupational data. *Journal of Occupational Medicine* 35:1017–1027.

Armstrong, T.J., Chaffin, D.B., and Foulke, J.A. (1979). A methodology for documenting hand positions and forces during manual work. *Journal of Biomechanics* 12:131–133.

Armstrong, T.J., Foulke, J.A., Joseph, B.S., and Goldstein, S.A. (1982). Investigation of cumulative trauma disorders in a poultry processing plant. *American Industrial Hygiene Association Journal* 43:103–116.

Baluyutt, R., Genaidy, A.M., Davis, L.S., Shell, R.L., and Simmons, R.J. (1995). Use of visual perception in estimating static postural stresses: Magnitudes and sources of error. *Ergonomics* 38:1841–1850.

Bao, S. and Silverstein, B. (2005). Estimation of hand force in ergonomic job evaluations. *Ergonomics* 48:288–301.

Bao, S., Spielholz, P., Howard, N., and Silverstein, B. (2009). Application of the Strain Index in multiple task jobs. *Applied Ergonomics* 40:56–68.

Baty, D., Buckle, P.W., and Stubbs, D.A. (1986). Posture recording by direct observation, questionnaire assessment and instrumentation: A comparison based on a recent field study. In: E.N. Corlett, J. Wilson, and I. Manenica (eds), The *Ergonomics of Working Postures*. London, U.K.: Taylor & Francis, pp. 283–292.

Berdie, D.R., Anderson, J.F., and Niebuhr, M.A. (1986). *Questionnaires: Design and Use*, 2nd edn, Metuchen, NJ: Scarecrow Press.

Bhatnagar, V., Drury, C.G., and Schiro, S.G. (1985). Posture, postural discomfort, and performance. *Human Factors* 27:189–199.

Borg, G.A.V. (1982). Psychophysical bases of perceived exertion. *Medicine and Science in Sports and Exercise* 14:377–381.

Boussenna, M., Corlett, E.N., and Pheasant, S.T. (1982). The relation between discomfort and postural loading at the joints. *Ergonomics* 25:315–322.

Bru, E., Mykletun, R. J., and Svebak, S. (1994). Assessment of musculoskeletal and other health complaints in female hospital staff. *Applied Ergonomics* 25:101–105.

Buchholz, B., Paquet, V., Punnett, L., Lee, D., and Moir, S. (1996). PATH: A work sampling-based approach to ergonomic job analysis for construction and other non-repetitive work. *Applied Ergonomics* 27:177–187.

Buckle, P.W., Stubbs, D.A., and Baty, D. (1984). Musculoskeletal disorders (and discomfort) and associated work factors. In: E.N. Corlett, J. Wilson, and I. Manenica (eds), The *Ergonomics of Working Postures*. London, U.K.: Taylor & Francis, pp. 19–30.

Burt, S. and Punnett, L. (1999). Evaluation of interrater reliability for posture observations in a field study. *Applied Ergonomics* 30:121–135.

Cameron, J.A. (1996). Assessing work-related body-discomfort: Current strategies and a behaviorally oriented assessment tool. *International Journal of Industrial Ergonomics* 18:389–398.

Cohen, J. (1960). A coefficient of agreement for nominal scales. *Educational and Psychological Measurement* 20:37–46.

Cohen, J. (1968). Weighted kappa: Nominal scale agreement with provision for scaled disagreement or partial credit. *Psychological Bulletin* 70:213–220.

Colombini, D. (1998). An observational method for classifying exposure to repetitive movements of the upper limbs. *Ergonomics* 41:1261–1289.

Corlett, E.N. (1995). The evaluation of posture and its effects. In: J. Wilson and E.N. Corlett (eds), *The Evaluation of Human Work*, 2nd edn, London, U.K.: Taylor & Francis, pp. 663–699.

Corlett, E.N. and Bishop, R.P. (1976). A technique for assessing postural discomfort. *Ergonomics* 19:175–182.

Corlett, E.N. and Manenica, I. (1980). The effects and measurement of working postures. *Applied Ergonomics* 11:7–16.

Corlett, E.N., Madeley, S.J., and Manenica, I. (1979). Posture targetting: A technique for recording working postures. *Ergonomics* 22:357–366.

Cronbach, L.J. (1951). Coefficient alpha and the internal structure of tests. *Psychometrika* 16:297–334.

Currier, D.P. (1984). *Elements of Research in Physical Therapy*. Baltimore, MD: Williams & Wilkins.

Dartt, A., Rosecrance, J., Gerr, F., Chen, P., Anton, D., and Merlino, L. (2009). Reliability of assessing upper limb postures among workers performing manufacturing tasks. *Applied Ergonomics* 40:371–378.

Deakin, J.M., Stevenson, J.M., Vail, G.R., and Nelson, J.M. (1994). Use of the nordic questionnaire in an industrial setting: A case study. *Applied Ergonomics* 25:182–185.

deLooze, M.P., Toussaint, H.M., Ensink, J., and Mangnus, C. (1994). The validity of visual observations to assess posture in a laboratory-simulated, manual material-handling task. *Ergonomics* 37:1335–1343.

Dickinson, C.E., Campion, K., Foster, A.F., Newman, S.J., O'Rourke, A.M.T., and Thomas, P.G. (1992). Questionnaire development: An examination of the Nordic Musculoskeletal Questionnaire. *Applied Ergonomics* 23:197–201.

Fleiss, J.L. (1981). *Statistical Methods for Rates and Proportions*, 2nd edn, New York: John Wiley & Sons, pp. 212–236.

Foreman, T.K., Davies, J.C., and Troup, J.D.G. (1988). A posture and activity classification system using a microcomputer. *International Journal of Industrial Ergonomics* 2:285–289.

Fraenkel, J.R. and Wallen, N.E. (1996). *How to Design and Evaluate Research in Education*, 3rd edn, New York, McGraw-Hill, pp. 153–169.

Fransson-Hall, C., Gloria, R., Kilbom, Å., and Winkel, J. (1995). A portable ergonomic observation method (PEO) for computerized on-line recording of postures and manual handling. *Applied Ergonomics* 26:93–100.

Freivalds, A. (2009). *Niebel's Methods, Standards and Work Design*, 12th edn, New York: McGraw-Hill.

Genaidy, A.M., Al-Shedi, A.A., and Karwowski, W. (1994). Postural stress analysis in industry. *Applied Ergonomics* 25:77–87.

Genaidy, A.M., Simmons, R.J., Guo, L., and Hidalgo, J.A. (1993). Can visual perception be used to estimate body part angles? *Ergonomics* 36:323–329.

Greenberg, L. and Chaffin, D.B. (1976). *Workers and Their Tools: A Guide to the Ergonomics of Hand Tools and Small Presses*. Midland, MI: Pendell Pub.

Grieco, A. (1998). Application of the concise exposure index (OCRA) to tasks involving repetitive movements of the upper limbs in a variety of manufacturing industries: Preliminary validations. *Ergonomics* 41:1347–1356.

Gummesson, C., Atroshi, I., and Ekdahl, C. (2003). The disabilities of the arm, shoulder and had (DASH) outcome questionnaire: Longitudinal construct validity and measuring self-rated health change after surgery. *BMC Musculoskeletal Disorders* 4:11.

Hagen, K.B., Magnus, P., and Vetlesen, K. (1998). Neck/shoulder and low-back disorders in the forestry industry: Relationship to work tasks and perceived psychosocial job stress. *Ergonomics* 41:1510–1518.

Hales, T., Habes, D., Fine, L., Hornung, R., and Boiano, J. (1989). *Health Hazard Evaluation Report, Bennett Industries, Peotone, IL*, HETA 89-146-2049. Cincinnati, OH: National Institute of Occupational Safety and Health.

Hallbeck, M.S., Kamal, M.S., and Harmon, P.E. (1992). The effects of forearm posture, wrist posture and hand on three peak pinch force types. *Proceedings of the Human Factors and Ergonomics Society 36th Annual Conference*. Santa Monica, CA: Human Factors and Ergonomics Society, pp. 801–805.

Harms-Ringdahl, K. (1986). On assessment of shoulder exercise and load-elicited pain in the cervical spine. Biomechanical analysis of load-EMG-methodological studies of pain provoked by extreme position. *Scandinavian Journal of Rehabilitation Medicine Supplement* 14:1–40.

Hedge, A., McCrobie, D., Land, B., Morimoto, S., and Rodriguez, S. (1995). Healthy keyboarding: Effects of wrist rests, keyboard trays, and a present tiltdown system on wrist posture, seated posture, and musculoskeletal discomfort. *Proceedings of the Human Factors and Ergonomics Society 39th Annual Conference*. Santa Monica, CA: Human Factors and Ergonomics Society, pp. 630–634.

Herron, D. (1976). Industrial engineering applications of ABC curves. *Transactions of the American Institute of Industrial Engineers* 8:210–218.

Hignett, S. and McAtamney, L. (2000). Rapid entire body assessment (REBA). *Applied Ergonomics* 31:201–205.

Holzmann, P. (1982). ARBAN—A new method for analysis of ergonomic effort. *Applied Ergonomics* 13:82–86.

Hudak, P.L., Amadio, P.C., and Bombardier, C. (1996). Development of an upper extremity outcome measure: The DASH (Disabilities of the arm, shoulder and head). *American Journal of Industrial Medicine* 29:602–608.

Imrahn, S.N. (1991). The influence of wrist posture on different types of pinch strength. *Applied Ergonomics* 22:379–384.

Juul-Kristensen, B., Fallentin, N., and Ekdahl, C. (1997), Criteria for classification of posture in repetitive work by observation methods: A review. *International Journal of Industrial Ergonomics* 19:397–411.

Karhu, O., Kansi, P., and Kuorinka, I. (1977). Correcting working postures in industry: A practical method for analysis. *Applied Ergonomics* 8:199–201.

Karhu, O., Härkönen, R., Sorvali, R., and Vepsäläinen, P. (1981). Observing working postures in industry: Examples of OWAS application. *Applied Ergonomics* 12:13–17.

Kemmlert, K. (1995). A method assigned for the identification of ergonomic hazards—PLIBEL. *Applied Ergonomics* 26:199–211.

Kerlinger, F.N. and Lee, H.B. (2000). *Foundations of Behavioral Research*. New York: Harcourt College Publishers.

Keyserling, W.M. (1986). Postural analysis of the trunk and shoulders in simulated real time. *Ergonomics* 29:569–583.

Keyserling, W.M. and Witting, S.J. (1988). An analysis of experts' ratings of ergonomic stress. *International Journal of Industrial Ergonomics* 2:291–304.

Keyserling, W.M., Stetson, D.S., Silverstein, B.A., and Brouwer, M.L. (1993). A checklist for evaluating ergonomic risk factors associated with upper extremity cumulative trauma disorders. *Ergonomics* 36:807–831.

Kilbom, Å. (1994). Assessment of physical exposure in relation to work-related musculoskeletal disorders—What information can be obtained from systematic observations? *Scandinavian Journal of Work Environment and Health* 20:30–45.

Kilbom, Å., Persson, J., and Jonsson, B. (1986). Risk factors for work-related disorders of the neck and shoulder—With special emphasis on working postures and movements. In: E.N. Corlett, J. Wilson, and I. Manenica (eds), *The Ergonomics of Working Postures*. London, U.K.: Taylor & Francis, pp. 44–53.

Kilroy, N. and Dockrell, S. (2000). Ergonomic intervention: Its effect on working posture and musculo-skeletal symptoms in female biomedical scientists. *British Journal of Biomedical Sciences* 57:199–206.

Kitis, A., Celik, E., Aslan, U.B., and Zencir, M. (2009). DASH questionnaire for the analysis of mus-culoskeletal symptoms in industry workers: A validity and reliability study. *Applied Ergonomics* 40:251–255.

Knox, K. and Moore, J.S. (2001). Predictive validity of the Strain Index in turkey processing. *Journal of Occupational and Environmental Medicine* 43:451–462.

Koppelaar, E. and Wells, R. (2005). Comparison of measurement methods for quantifying hand force. *Ergonomics* 48:983–1007.

Kotani, K. (1995). Modeling perception and production of force as a means of estimating force requirements in industrial tasks. PhD dissertation. University Park, PA: The Pennsylvania State University.

Kuder, G. F. and Richardson, M.W. (1937). The theory of the estimation of test reliability. *Psychometrika* 2:151–160.

Kuorinka, I. (1983). Subjective discomfort in a simulated repetitive task. *Ergonomics* 26:1089–1101.

Kuorinka, I., Jonsson, B., Kilbom, Å., Vinterberg, H., Biering-Sørensen, F., Andersson, G., and Jørgensen, K. (1987). Standardised nordic questionnaires for the analysis of musculoskeletal symptoms. *Applied Ergonomics* 18:233–237.

Lamb, K.L. and Brodie, D.A. (1990). The assessment of physical activity by leisure-time physical activity questionnaire. *Sports Medicine* 10:159–180.

Landis, R. and Koch, G.G. (1977). The measurement of observer agreement for categorical data. *Biometrics* 33:159–174.

Latko, W.A., Armstrong, T.J., Foulke, J.A., Herrin, G.D., Rabourn, R.A., and Ulin, S.S. (1997). Development and evaluation of an observational method for assessing repetition in hand tasks. *American Industrial Hygiene Association Journal* 58:278–285.

Levine, D.W., Simmons, B.P., Koris, M.J., Daltroy, L.H., Hohl, G.G., Fossel, A.H., and Katz, J.N. (1993). A self-administered questionnaire for the assessment of severity of symptoms and functional status in carpal tunnel syndrome. *The Journal of Bone and Joint Surgery* 75A:1585–1592.

Lowe, B.D. and Krieg, E.F. (2009). Relationship between observational estimates and physical mea-surements of upper limb activity. *Ergonomics* 52:569–583.

Maclure, M. and Willett, W.C. (1987). Misinterpretation and misuse of the kappa statistic. *American Journal of Epidemiology* 126:161–169.

Marshall, M.M., Armstrong, T.J., and Ebersole, M.L. (2004). Verbal estimation of peak exertion inten-sity. *Human Factors* 46:697–710.

Mattila, M., Karwowski, W., and Vilkki, M. (1993). Analysis of working postures in hammering tasks on building construction sites using the computerized OWAS method. *Applied Ergonomics* 24:405–412.

McAtamney, L. and Corlett, E.N. (1993). RULA: A survey method for the investigation of work-related upper limb disorders. *Applied Ergonomics* 24:91–99.

Moore, J.S. and Garg, A. (1994). Upper extremity disorders in a pork processing plant: Relationships between job risk factors and morbidity. *American Industrial Hygiene Association Journal* 55:703–715.

Moore, J. S. and Garg, A. (1995). The strain index: A proposed method to analyze jobs for risk of distal upper extremity disorders. *American Industrial Hygiene Association Journal* 56:443–458.

Neely, G., Ljundggren, G., Sylvén, C., and Borg, G. (1992). Comparison between the visual analogue scale (VAS) and category ratio scale (CR-10) for the evaluation of leg exertion. *International Journal of Sports Medicine* 13:133–136.

Occhipinti, E. (1998). OCRA: A concise index for the assessment of exposure to repetitive movements of the upper limbs. *Ergonomics* 41:1290–1311.

Occhipinti, E. and Colombini, D. (2007). Updating reference values and predictive models of the OCRA method in the risk assessment of work-related musculoskeletal disorders of the upper limbs. *Ergonomics* 450:1727–1739.

OSHA (Occupational Safety and Health Administration). (1990). *Ergonomics Program Management Guidelines for Meatpacking Plants.* Washington, DC: Bureau of National Affairs, Inc.

Östlin, P., Wärneryd, B., and Thorslund, M. (1990). Should occupational codes be obtained from census data or from retrospective survey data in studies in occupational health? *Social Indicators Research* 23:231–246.

Park, J.K., Boyer, J., Tessler, J., Casey, J., Schemm, L., Gore, R., and Punnett, L. (2009). Inter-rater reliability of PATH observations for assessment of ergonomic risk factors in hospital work. *Ergonomics* 52:820–829.

Persson, J. and Kilbom, Å. (1983). VIRA—En enkel videofilmteknik för registering och analys av arbetsställningar och rörelser, Undersökningsrapport (VIRA—A simple video technique for recording and analyzing working postures and motions, Research Report). Solna, Sweden: Arbetsmiljöinstitutet.

Petrofsky, J.S., Williams, C., Kamen, G., and Lind, A.R. (1980). The effect of handgrip span on isometric exercise performance. *Ergonomics* 23:1129–1135.

Price, D.D., McGrath, P.A., Rafii, A., and Buckingham, B. (1983). The validation of visual analogue scales as ratio scale measures for chronic and experimental pain. *Pain* 17:45–56.

Priel, V.Z. (1974). A numerical definition of posture. *Human Factors* 16:576–584.

Punnett, L. and Keyserling, W.M. (1987). Exposure to ergonomic stressors in the garment industry: Application and critique of job-site work analysis methods. *Ergonomics* 30:1099–1166.

Radwin, R.G. and Lin, M.L. (1993). An analytical method for characterizing repetitive motion and postural stress using spectral analysis. *Ergonomics* 36:379–389.

Reading, A.E. (1980). A comparison of pain rating scales. *Journal of Psychosomatic Research* 24:119–124.

Rohmert, W. and Landau, K. (1983). *A New Technique of Job Analysis.* London, U.K.: Taylor & Francis.

Rona, R.J. and Mosbech, J. (1989). Validity and repeatability of self-reported occupational and industrial history from patients in EEC countries. *International Journal of Epidemiology* 18:674–679.

Rossignol, M. and Baetz, J. (1987). Task-related risk factors for spinal injury: Validation of a self-administered questionnaire on hospital employees. *Ergonomics* 30:1531–1540.

Saldana, N., Herrin, G.D., Armstrong, T.J., and Franzblau, A. (1994). A computerized method for assessment of musculoskeletal discomfort in the workforce: A tool for surveillance. *Ergonomics* 37:1097–1112.

Schutz, R.K. (1972). Cyclic work-rest exercise's effect on continuous hold endurance capability. PhD dissertation. Ann Arbor, MI: University of Michigan.

Seth, V., Weston, R.L., and Freivalds, A. (1999). Development of a cumulative trauma disorder risk assessment model for the upper extremities. *International Journal of Industrial Ergonomics* 23:281–291.

Shrout, P.E. and Fleiss, J.L. (1979). Intraclass correlations: Uses in assessing rater reliability. *Psychological Bulletin* 86:420–428.

Sperling, L., Dahlman, S., Wikström, L., Kilbom, Å., and Kadefors, R. (1993). A cube model for the classification of work with hand tools and the formulation of functional requirements. *Applied Ergonomics* 24:212–220.

Spielholz, P. (2006). Calibrating Borg scale ratings of hand force exertion. *Applied Ergonomics* 37:615–618.

Spielholz, P., Silverstein, B., and Stuart, M. (1999). Reproducibility of a self-report questionnaire for upper extremity musculoskeletal disorder risk factors. *Applied Ergonomics* 30:429–433.

Spielholz, P., Silverstein, B., Morgan, M., Checkoway, H., and Kaufman, J. (2001). Comparison of self-report, video observation and direct measurement methods for upper extremity musculoskeletal disorder physical risk factors. *Ergonomics* 44:588–613.

Stephens, J.P., Vos, G.A., Stevens, Jr., E.M., and Moore, J.S. (2006). Test-retest repeatability of the Strain Index. *Applied Ergonomics* 37:275–281.

Stetson, D., Keyserling, W.M., Silverstein, B.A., and Leonard, J.A. (1991). Observational analysis of the hand and wrist: A pilot study. *Applied Occupational and Environmental Hygiene* 6:927–937.

Terrell, R. and Purswell, J.L. (1976). The influence of forearm and wrist orientation on static grip strength as a design criterion for hand tools. *Proceedings of the Human Factors and Ergonomics Society 36th Annual Conference*. Santa Monica, CA: Human Factors and Ergonomics Society, pp. 28–32.

Thorndike, R.L. and Hagen, E.P. (1977). *Measurement and Evaluation in Psychology and Education*. New York: John Wiley & Sons.

Ulin, S.S., Ways, C.M., Armstrong, T.J., and Snook, S.H. (1990). Perceived exertion and discomfort versus work height with a pistol-shaped screwdriver. *American Industrial Hygiene Association Journal* 51:588–594.

van der Beek, A.J., van Gaalen, L.C., and Frings-Dresen, M.H.W. (1992). Working postures and activities of lorry drivers: A reliability study of on-site observation and recording on a pocket computer. *Applied Ergonomics* 23:331–336.

van Wyk, P.M., Weir, P.L., Andrews, D.M., Fiedler, K.M., and Callaghan, J.P. (2009). Determining the optimal size for posture categories used in video-based posture assessment methods. *Ergonomics* 52:921–930.

Wangenheim, M., Samuelson, B., and Wos, H. (1986). ARBAN—A force ergonomic analysis method. In: E.N. Corlett, J. Wilson, and I. Manenica (eds), *The Ergonomics of Working Postures*. London, U.K.: Taylor & Francis, pp. 243–255.

Warwick, D.P. and Lininger, C.A. (1975). *The Sample Survey: Theory and Practice*. New York: McGraw-Hill.

Waters, T.R., Putz-Anderson, V., Garg, A., and Fine, L. (1993). Revised NIOSH equation for the design and evaluation of manual lifting tasks. *Ergonomics* 36:749–776.

Wiktorin, C., Hjelm, E.W., Winkel, J., and Köster, M. (1996). Reproducibility of a questionnaire for assessment of physical load during work and leisure time. *Journal of Occupational and Environmental Medicine* 38:190–201.

Wilson, R.C. and Jones, P.W. (1989). A comparison of the visual analogue scale and modified Borg scale for the measurement of dyspnea during exercise. *Clinical Science* 76:277–282.

Wrigley, T.V., Green, R.A., and Briggs, C.A. (1991). Microcomputer video image processing technology in working posture analysis. *Applied Ergonomics* 22:2–8.

Yen, T.Y. and Radwin, R.G. (1999). Automated job analysis using upper extremity biomechanical data and template matching. *International Journal of Industrial Ergonomics* 25:19–28.

Yen, T.Y. and Radwin, R.G. (2002). A comparison between analysis time and inter-analyst reliability using spectral analysis of kinematic data and posture classification. *Applied Ergonomics* 33:85–93.

You, H. (1999). The development of a risk assessment model for carpal tunnel syndrome. Unpublished PhD thesis. University Park, PA: Penn State University.

You, H., Simmons, Z., Freivalds, A., Kothari, M.J., and Naidu, S.H. (1999). Relationships between clinical symptom severity scales and nerve conduction measures in carpal tunnel syndrome. *Muscle & Nerve* 22:497–501.

Yun, M.H., Cannon, D., Freivalds, A., and Thomas, G. (1997). An instrumented glove for grasp specification in virtual-reality based point-and-direct telerobotics. *IEEE Transactions on Systems, Man, and Cybernetics, Part B: Cybernetics* 27:835–846.

9

Hand Tools

9.1 Introduction

9.1.1 Historical Development of Tools

Tools are as old as the human race itself. The hands and feet could be considered as tools given to the human by nature. However, tools as we know them were developed as extensions of the hands and feet to reinforce the range, strength, and effectiveness of these limbs. Thus, the early man, by picking up a stone, could make the fist heavier and harder to produce a more effective blow. Similarly, by using a stick a longer and stronger arm was created.

The exact time when humans began to use and to make tools is not known. Leakey (1960), during his excavations in Africa, uncovered evidence that more than a million years ago the prehistoric human was already a toolmaker using stones for chipping bones and for leather work. Similarly, Napier (1962, 1963) indicated that with changing tasks, such as converting from the power to precision grip, there was a similar change in the anatomy of the hand as well as development of tools. An important milestone occurred when the stone tool was provided with a handle some 35,000 years ago. The addition of the handle increased the range and speed of action and increased the kinetic energy for striking tasks (Drillis, 1963). A still later change in tool development occurred with the change in tasks from food gathering to food production. New tools were required and developed accordingly. Surprisingly, many of these tools, with minor improvements and refinements, are still in use today. The reasons for such stagnation could be twofold: either the tool reached an optimal form very quickly with no room for improvement or there was not the impetus for further improvement. The latter is the resigned view that since a tool has been used by so many people for so many years, no further improvement is possible. The former view is obviously not true since Lehmann (1953) noted the existence of over 12,000 different styles of shovels in Germany in the 1930s, all essentially used for the same task. Indeed the last great change in tool development occurred with the start of the Industrial Revolution with a change in task from food production to manufacturing of goods.

9.1.2 Tools and Musculoskeletal Injuries

The parallel development of tools with changing technology has given rise to another problem. The current technology explosion has proceeded too quickly to permit the gradual development of tools appropriate for the new industrial tasks. The instant demand for new and specialized tools to match the needs of technology has, in many cases, bypassed the testing needed to fit these tools to the human users. This has resulted in a variety of hand-tool-generated work stressors, high force, high repetition, poor posture, leading to cumulative trauma and chronic problems, reducing productivity, disabling individuals, and increasing medical costs in the plant (Rothfleisch and Sherman, 1978; Cannon et al., 1981; Silverstein et al., 1987).

Approximately 6% of all compensable work injuries and 10% of all industrial injuries in the United States are caused by the use of hand tools (Mital and Sanghavi, 1986; Aghazadeh and Mital, 1987). This means over 73,000 injuries involving at least one work day lost amounting to over $10 billion annually in costs (Bureau of Labor Statistics, 1995). The most injured body parts by both non-powered and powered hand tools were the upper extremities (59.3% and 51.0%, respectively) followed by back, trunk, and lower extremities. Fingers accounted for 56% of upper extremity injuries or about 30% of all body parts (Aghazadeh and Mital, 1987).

9.1.3 General Tool Principles

An efficient tool has to fulfill some basic requirements (Drillis, 1963):

1. It must perform effectively the function for which it is intended. Thus, an axe should convert a maximum amount of its kinetic energy into useful chopping work, separate wood fibers cleanly, and be easily withdrawn.

2. It must be properly proportioned to the body dimensions of the operator to maximize efficiency of human involvement.

3. It must be designed to the strength and work capacity of the operator. Thus, allowances have to be made for the gender, training, and physical fitness of the operator.

4. It should not cause undue fatigue, i.e., it should not demand unusual postures or practices that will require more energy expenditure than necessary.

5. It must provide sensory feedback in the form pressure, some shock, texture, temperature, etc. to the user.

6. The capital and maintenance cost should be reasonable.

9.2 General Biomechanical Considerations of Tools

9.2.1 Anatomy and Types of Grip

As discussed in Chapter 1, the human hand is a complex structure of bones, arteries, nerves, ligaments, and tendons. The fingers are controlled by the extensor carpi and flexor carpi muscles in the forearm. The muscles are connected to the fingers by tendons which pass through a channel in the wrist, formed by the bones of the back of the hand on one side and the transverse carpal ligament on the other. Through this channel, called the carpal tunnel, pass also various arteries and nerves. The bones of the wrist connect to two long bones in the forearm, the ulna and the radius. The radius connects to the thumb side of the wrist and ulna connects to the little finger side of the wrist. The orientation of the wrist joint allows movement in only two planes, each at 90° to the other. The first gives rise to palmar flexion and dorsiflexion. The second movement plane gives ulnar and radial deviation. The ulna and radius of the forearm connect to the humerus of the upper arm. The biceps brachii, brachialis, and brachioradialis control elbow flexion and to some degree supination (outward rotation) of the wrist. The triceps, acts as an elbow extensor.

Probably, the most unique feature of the above upper extremity is the manual, dexterity produced by the hand. Napier (1956) defined the prehensile movements of the human hand in terms of a power grip and a precision grip. In a power *grip* the tool, whose axis is more or less perpendicular to the forearm, is held in a clamp formed by the partly flexed fingers and the palm, with opposing pressure being applied by the thumb (see Figure 9.1). There are three subcategories of the power grip, differentiated by the line of action of force: (1) force parallel to the forearm, as in sawing; (2) force at an angle to forearm, as in hammering; and (3) torque about the forearm, as when using a screwdriver. As the name implies, the power grip is used for power or for holding heavy objects (Bendz, 1974).

In a *precision grip*, the tool is pinched between the flexor aspects of the fingers and the opposing thumb. The relative position of the thumb and fingers determines how much force is to be applied and provides sensory surface for receiving feedback necessary to give the precision needed. There are two types of precision grip (see Figure 9.1): (1) internal, in which the shaft of the tool (e.g., knife) passes under the thumb and is thus internal to the hand; and (2) external, in which the shaft (e.g., pencil) passes over the thumb and is thus external to the hand (Konz and Johnson, 2000). The precision grip is used for control. There is also the hook grip, which used to support weight by the fingers only, as in holding a box, a lateral pinch, as in holding a key, a pulp or tip pinches, depending if the pulpy part or nails of the fingers touch. A finer gradation of grips

| Power grip | Two-point pinch | Internal precision |
| Hook grip | Lateral pinch | External precision |

FIGURE 9.1
Types of grip. (Reproduced from Freivalds, A., Ergonomics of hand tools, In: W. Karwowski and W.S. Marras (eds.), *Occupational Ergonomics Handbook*, CRC Press, Boca Raton, 1999. With permission.)

TABLE 9.1

Relative Forces for Different Types of Grips

Grip	Male (N)	Female (N)	% of Power Grip
Power grip	400	228	100
Tip pinch	65	45	18
Pulp pinch	61	43	17
Lateral pinch	109	76	30

Source: Adapted from An, K.N. et al., Biomechanics and functional assessment of upper extremities, In: W. Karwowski (ed.), *Trends in Ergonomics/Human Factors III*, Elsevier, Amsterdam, The Netherlands, 1986.

is also possible, as presented by Kroemer (1986). Note that all of these pinches have a significantly decreased strength capability as compared to the power grip (see Table 9.1) and, therefore, large forces should never be applied using pinch grips. Normative data for gender, age, and different types of pinches can be found in Mathiowetz et al. (1986) and Rice et al. (1998).

9.2.2 The Biomechanics of a Power Grip

One theory of gripping forces has been described by Pheasant and O'Neill (1975) and by Grieve and Pheasant (1982). The hand gripping a cylindrical handle forms a closed system of forces in which portions of the digits and palm are used, in opposition to each other, to exert compressive forces on the handle (Figure 9.2). The strength of the grip (G) may be defined as the sum of all components of forces exerted normal to the surface of the handle:

$$G = \sum g \tag{9.1}$$

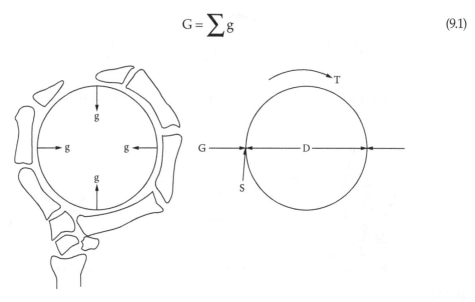

FIGURE 9.2
Mechanics of gripping. (Reproduced from Freivalds, A., *Int. Rev. Ergon.*, 1, 43, 1987. With permission.)

When exerting a turning action on the handle, the maximum torque, as given at the moment of hand slippage, is given by

$$T = S \cdot D \qquad (9.2)$$

where
  T is the torque
  S is the total frictional or shear force
  D is the handle diameter

where S can be defined by

$$S = \mu G \qquad (9.3)$$

where μ is the coefficient of friction.

Thus, torque is directly dependent upon handle diameter and indirectly upon diameter squared, since the gripping force also depends on the circumference of the handle gripped. This was confirmed experimentally by Pheasant and O'Neill (1975). For thrusting motions in the direction of the long axis of the handle, the diameter is not involved and determination of maximum force is more complicated. For handles larger than the grip span diameter, the gripped area no longer increases in proportion of the diameter. An analysis of such conditions was performed by Replogle (1983) who concluded that for handles up to twice the grip span diameter the relative ungripped area of the handle increases, reducing the effective gripped area. Torque is then dependent on handle diameter as follows:

$$T = \frac{3d^2(4-d)}{(d+2)^2} \qquad (9.4)$$

where d is the ratio of handle diameter to grip span diameter. For larger handle diameters the expression for torque becomes much more complicated (Replogle, 1983).

Torque is also dependent on the direction of movement. Clockwise torque was found to be 45% greater than counterclockwise torque (movement toward thumb) (Seo et al., 2008). The authors attributed this to measurements of normal contact forces (g's in Figure 9.2) that were 19% greater for clockwise motion as opposed to counterclockwise motion. This phenomenon has interesting implications for workers in that assembly operations (tightening screws) should be less fatiguing than disassembly operations (loosening tight screws).

The individual fingers do not contribute equally to force production in a power grip. The middle finger is the strongest at 28.7% of the grip force, followed by the index, ring, and little fingers, with percentage contributions of 26.5%, 24.6%, and 20.2%, respectively (see Figure 9.3, Kong, 2001; Kong and Freivalds, 2003). Similar values have been found by An et al. (1978), Amis (1987), Ejeskar and Örtengren (1981), Chen (1991), and Radhakrishnan and Nagaravindra (1993) while more recent studies found a slight reversal with the ring finger being stronger than the index finger, with the four

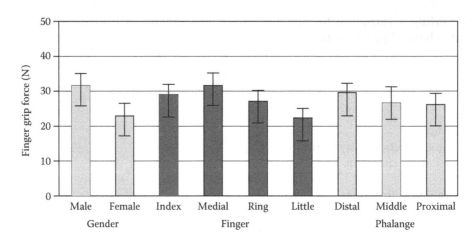

FIGURE 9.3
Finger forces by finger, phalange, and gender. (Adapted from Kong, Y.K. and Freivalds, A., *Int. J. Ind. Ergon.*, 32, 12, 2003. With permission.)

fingers contributing 22%, 36%, 38%, and 14% of the grip force, respectively (Kong and Lowe, 2005a,b; Lee et al., 2009).

These different finger force contributions may be explained by the mechanical characteristics of bone and muscle. From the bone point of view, the middle finger is at the center of the hand and longer than the others and, thus, may have the mechanical advantage over the other fingers. The index and the ring fingers are located about the same distance from the center of the hand and, consequently, exert a similar amount of force. The little finger is the farthest from the center of the hand, and, therefore, may have a mechanical disadvantage over the other fingers when gripping.

From the muscle point of view, each finger has different muscle characteristics such as mass, volume, and length of muscle fibers. Brand et al. (1981) reported that the mass or volume of muscle is proportional to the total work capacity and showed that the FDS of the middle finger has the largest mass fraction of total weight, followed by the FDP of the middle finger. The FDS of the little finger has the lowest mass fraction. Ketchum et al. (1978) also reported that the FDS of the middle finger was strongest and the combined force of both the superficialis and the profundus tendons was also the strongest in the middle finger, followed by the index, ring, and little finger.

Phalange force distributions are also non uniform. The force imposed by the distal phalange (35.9%) was significantly higher than that imposed by the middle (32.4%) and the proximal (31.7%) phalanges in the gripping task (see Figure 9.3, Kong, 2001; Kong and Freivalds, 2003). These findings are confirmed by An et al. (1978), Amis (1987), Chao et al. (1989), and Lee and Rim (1990). Note that these results only apply to a gripping task. For a pulling task utilizing a power grip, a greater amount of the force is applied by the proximal (37.6%) and middle (33.6%) phalanges and lesser amount by the distal phalange (28.8%) (Kong, 2001; Kong and Freivalds, 2003). Note also that female power grip force is roughly 70% of male power grip force (see Figure 9.3).

9.2.3 The Biomechanics of a Precision Grip

Precision or pinch grip can be modeled as follows (see Figure 9.4). The application force (F_A) is transmitted to the workpiece (in addition to the tool weight) through the axis of the

FIGURE 9.4
Forces of a precision grip. (Reproduced from Lowe, B.D. and Freivalds, A., *Ergonomics*, 42, 550, 1999. With permission.)

tool. In static equilibrium, a reactive force (F_R) is directionally opposite and equal in magnitude to the application force plus the weight of the tool (W):

$$F_R = F_A + W \tag{9.5}$$

When F_A is applied, the tendency for the reactive force, F_R, to push the tool upward through the grasp, is resisted by the frictional forces (F_{f1} and F_{f2}) between the fingertip surfaces and tool grip surface material. The sum of these frictional forces must be greater than the force applied with the tool (F_A) to resist the slip. In this paradigm, the frictional forces at each digit (F_f) are a result of the pinch forces normal to the tool surface (F_P) multiplied by the static coefficient of friction (μ) between the digital pulpar skin and the tool grip surface material. Further, the forces applied by the thumb and index finger (F_{P1} and F_{P2}) are equal in magnitude and opposite in direction (due to net zero horizontal translation of the tool) so that the total frictional force downward is equal to $2\mu F_P$:

$$F_{f1} + F_{f2} \geq F_R - W \tag{9.6}$$

$$2\mu F_P \geq F_R - W \tag{9.7}$$

Provided that the tool does not slip within the grip, $2F_{p(task)}$ must be greater than the minimum pinch force required to prevent slip, $2F_{p(slip)}$. At the instant of slip, $2F_{p(slip)}$ is directionally opposite and equal in magnitude to ($F_R - W$), so the coefficient of friction can be defined by

$$2F_{P(slip)}\,\mu = F_R - W \tag{9.8}$$

$$\mu = \frac{F_R - W}{2F_{P(slip)}} \tag{9.9}$$

Conversely, if μ is known, calculation of the minimum required pinch force (pinch force at slip) as a function of reactive force F_R is

$$F_{p(slip)} = \frac{F_R - W}{2\mu} \tag{9.10}$$

The pinch force *safety margin* (SM) is defined as the excessive pinch force (sum of thumb and index finger force) exceeding the minimum pinch force resisting slip, $2F_{p(slip)}$:

$$SM = 2F_{p(task)} - 2F_{p(slip)} \tag{9.11}$$

$$SM = \frac{2F_{p(task)} - F_R - W}{\mu} \tag{9.12}$$

Note that the safety margin increases with increasing push forces in a lateral pinch. A fourfold increase was observed in going from 7% to 65% MVC exertions (Seo, 2009). One possible explanation for such a large chance could simply be a fear factor, increased consequences with increased forces. A more physiological explanation could be that the larger motor units recruited for the increased exertions have much less force fine-tuning ability as compared to the smaller motor units. Note, also, that the safety margin can be an unreliable measure of excess grip force because it relies on the skin coefficient of friction, which can be difficult to measure and generally is estimated. One can also define a *force ratio* as the ratio of grip to application forces. The force ratio is not dependent on unreliable estimates of frictional coefficients, but, since it is a unitless ratio, it cannot provide any information on the absolute magnitude of excess grip force.

9.2.4 Measurement of Skin Coefficient of Friction

The *coefficient of friction* between the digital pulpar skin and the grip surface has been measured by determining peak shear force as a function of normal (pinch) force (Buchholz et al., 1988). The subjects pinched, between alcohol-cleansed (to remove oils) thumb and index fingertips, an instrumented "tool." Based on visual feedback of force displayed on an oscilloscope, the subjects attempted to maintain a constant normal (pinch) force while slowly pulling upward on the clamped tool, which also measured axial force. As the upward pull force increased, the fingertip shear forces were estimated from axial forces on the tool. Eventually, the fingertips slipped, with the ratio of the maximum axial force immediately preceding the slip to the sum of the two normal forces yielding the coefficient of friction. The coefficients ranged approximately from 0.25 to 0.55 for different materials, with large inter- and intrasubject variabilities. Cloth and suede material exhibited higher values as compared to aluminum. Also, the coefficient of friction was inversely related to the pinch force applied by the digits, decreasing approximately 0.1 per each 30 N of pinch force. The calculation of the coefficient of friction is further complicated by the difficulties subjects had in maintaining a constant pinch force and avoiding the reflexive pinch force increase or a *slip reflex* which occurs approximately 75 ms after the onset of slip between the fingertips and the object (Cole and Abbs, 1987; Johansson and Westling, 1987).

Later research found very similar results, but with significantly lower values of friction for older adults (Cole, 1991; Lowe and Freivalds, 1999). This could be attributed to the reduced eccrine sweat gland output (Cole, 1991), but with regular cleansing of the finger tip surfaces, this should not be a major factor. An alternative explanation may be related to skin deformation characteristics and changes in the viscoelasticity of the pulpar skin that may occur with age. Young skin viscoelastic properties deviate considerably from Amonton's laws (Comaish and Bottoms, 1971), aging would only exacerbate that. The deviations Amonton's laws were demonstrated quite dramatically by Bobjer et al. (1993) in measuring coefficients of friction for textured and non-textured surfaces contaminated with oil and lard. In many conditions, they found coefficients of friction well above the theoretical limit of 1.0.

The results also presented trade-off problems for designers of hand tools. Smooth, non-textured handles produced highest coefficients of friction for clean hands ($\mu = 1.4$), but lowest coefficients of friction ($\mu = 0.2$) when the hands were contaminated, as one would reasonably expect. By adding texture, the friction was increased for contaminated conditions, perhaps, by channeling them away. However, with normal (cleansed with alcohol) hands, any texture decreased the coefficient of friction, perhaps because of the decreased area of contact with the skin (Bobjer et al., 1993).

Very similar results were found by O'Meara and Smith (2002). Smooth, dry surfaces gave highest coefficients of friction ($\mu = 1.87$ for chrome, $\mu = 1.72$ for textured aluminum, and $\mu = 1.67$ for knurled steel). Wetting the surface decreased friction for chrome and aluminum by 34% and 6%, respectively, but increased it for knurled steel by 15%. However, a soapy solution decreased all the coefficients of friction, but least (to $\mu = 0.654$) for knurled steel. Perhaps the optimum situation with acceptable coefficients of friction for all conditions (approximately uniform at $\mu = 0.75$) can be achieved with a coarse texture of alternating 2 mm ridges and 2 mm grooves (Bobjer et al., 1993).

9.2.5 Grip Force Coordination

Coordination was defined by Athènes and Wing (1989) as "the way in which different motor acts are coupled with regard to their temporal and spatial characteristics to allow for a more efficient motor performance." Neurophysiological studies of grip force coordination in simple lift and hold maneuvers have revealed that individuals apply a higher grip force than demanded by mechanical conditions (mainly friction) of the external object (Johansson and Westling, 1984; Westling and Johansson, 1984). The higher grip force represents a safety margin (Johansson, 1991), or buffer, against unanticipated perturbing forces or slip of the tools from the grip. The minimum ratio of grip force to the load force (external force demand) is governed by mechanical conditions of the hand–object interface and the force which is transmitted through the grasped object to its external environment. The actual ratio of these forces is scaled above this minimum slip force to achieve an adequate margin of safety. The scaling of the ratio of these forces determines the efficiency of an individual's grip force coordination and represents a clear trade-off between maintaining a margin of safety and minimizing excess grip force on the object.

Under conditions in which there is impairment of the sensory nerves, such as anesthesia of the digital pulpy areas, subjects have experienced difficulties in modulating grip force in parallel with the load force (Johansson et al., 1992). Microneurographic recordings from the afferent tactile mechanoreceptors have shown that cutaneous feedback from these receptors is critical in transmitting information regarding the conditions preceding slip at the grip interface (Westling and Johansson, 1987). When, the mechanoreceptors are anesthetized, individuals lose this feedback. Similarly, Cole (1991) observed force coordination impairments in elderly individuals that were attributed to an age-related decrement in tactile sensibility.

FIGURE 9.5

Conceptual model of the relationship between the required force, safety margin, and risk threshold. (a) Employee B exerts only 29% higher grip force on the tool, but the grip force exceeding the risk threshold is 83% higher than that of employee A. (b) Employee B's grip force, which exceeds the risk threshold, is attributable exclusively to a higher safety margin while employee A's grip force is below the risk threshold. (Reproduced from Lowe, B.D. and Freivalds, A., *Ergonomics*, 42, 550, 1999. With permission.)

Compression neuropathies of the median nerve, such as carpal tunnel syndrome (CTS), result in decreased tactile sensitivity of the thumb and first digits (Jackson and Clifford, 1989) and could be hypothesized to consequently also degrade the ability to coordinate pinch grip, resulting in higher grip force levels. Reviews of epidemiological studies have suggested that force exertions exceeding 15%–20% of an individual's maximum voluntary contraction (MVC) maybe linked with musculoskeletal disorders (Kroemer, 1989, 1992). This suggestion appears to be based on previous findings that force exertions below 15% MVC are associated with an essentially infinite endurance time while recovery periods are need for larger exertions (Monod and Scherrer, 1965; Rohmert, 1973).

The effects of a deficit in grip force coordination efficiency relative to a 15% MVC threshold is illustrated conceptually in Figure 9.5 (Lowe and Freivalds, 1999). Two individuals (A and B) of equivalent maximum strength may actually exert very different grip forces when performing identical tasks. The model illustrates that the employee who exerts a higher grip force as a result of reduced grip force coordination efficiency (higher safety margin) has an amplified risk. When the force requirement is below the risk threshold, an individual with reduced grip force coordination efficiency may apply a grip force above the threshold purely as a result of the safety margin. For those individuals who already are slightly impaired with a median nerve entrapment disorder would exhibit even higher grasp forces and would have even greater risk.

Grip coordination was tested further by Lowe and Freivalds (1999) with an instrumented hand tool (shown in Figure 9.4) on seven patients diagnosed with CTS and seven matched controls. The subjects were required to track a sinusoidal target force (varying both in amplitude and frequency between conditions) presented on an oscilloscope display by applying a tool application force (F_A). The application force and pinch force ($2F_P$) were recorded (see Figure 9.6) and used to calculate two measures of grip coordination. The *modulation index* indicated the percentage of maximum pinch force as it modulated between the minimum and maximum tool application force:

$$\text{Modulation index} = \frac{F_{Pmax(t)} - F_{Pmin(t)}}{F_{Pmax(t)}} \tag{9.13}$$

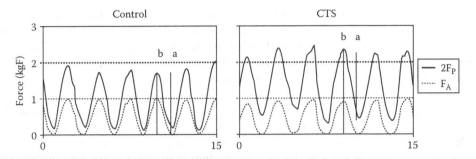

FIGURE 9.6

Grip force (2F$_P$) and application force (F$_A$) performance for a typical control group subject (left panel) and CTS group subject (right panel). The modulation index is the ratio of the lengths of line segments a (difference between maximum and minimum pinch forces) and b (peak pinch force). (Reproduced from Lowe, B.D. and Freivalds, A., *Ergonomics*, 42, 550, 1999. With permission.)

The modulation index ranged from 0 (no grip force modulation) to 1 (most efficient grip force modulation). The force ratio represented the ratio of total grip force to the applied force, integrated over one period of the application force cycle:

$$\text{Force ratio} = \int \frac{2F_{P(t)}}{F_{R(t)}} dt \qquad (9.14)$$

On average, the CTS group exerted significantly higher pinch forces at equivalent levels of application force (see Figure 9.7a) and modulated their grip force less (see Figure 9.6), indicating a lower efficiency of grip force coordination. More specifically, the mean value for the modulation index was 12.4% lower for the CTS group, while the force ratio was 54% higher for the CTS group (see Figure 9.7b). The link between median nerve compression and decreased grip coordination is hypothesized to be an adaptive, compensatory rescaling of the force ratio to a higher safety margin. The increased force ratio (and safety margin) serves a larger buffer against localized slips which may be "undetected" by a less sensitive afferent system. The higher grip forces indicate higher flexor tendon forces as they glide within the carpal tunnel, further aggravating the compression of the medium nerve through the tendon pulley model (see Chapter 5). For example, Chao et al. (1976) estimated that the flexor digitorum profundus tendon forces to be 4.32 times the

FIGURE 9.7

(a) Mean modulation indices and (b) mean force ratios. Each bar is the subject's mean for 24 trials. (Reproduced from Lowe, B.D. and Freivalds, A., *Ergonomics*, 42, 550, 1999. With permission.)

external force measured at the finger tip. A 54% average increase in the force ratio for CTS patients as compared to controls, would now yield tendon forces as 6.5 times the external force, further accelerating the risk for further injury. However, by increasing the friction characteristics of the tool surface (in this case, suede material), the force ratio for CTS patients was reduced significantly almost to the same level as found in controls (Lowe and Freivalds, 1999).

Note that grip force coordination is quite complex and that the measurement and prediction of multi-finger strength is relatively poor (r^2 between 0.45 and 0.64, DiDomenico and Nussbaum, 2003, 2008). This is because multi-finger prehension necessarily has to consider *motor redundancy* (more degrees of freedom than constraints, first formulated by the Russian neurophysiologist, Nikolai Berstein, [Berstein, 1967]) and the complex synergy between the fingers. Instead of complete independence between the finger muscles, there is considerable *enslaving*, i.e., the involuntary force production by fingers not explicitly recruited in the grasp (Zatsiorsky et al., 2000). For more information on motor control consider Zatsiorsky and Latash (2009) and Latash (2008).

9.2.6 Static Muscle Loading

When tools are used in situations in which the arms must be elevated or tools have to be held for extended periods, muscles of the shoulders, arms, and hands may be loaded statically, resulting in fatigue, reduced work capacity, and soreness. Abduction of the shoulder with corresponding elevation of the elbow will occur if work has to be done with a straight tool on a horizontal workplace. An angled tool reduces the need to raise the arm (Eastman Kodak Company, 1983). A good example of such a tool is the redesigned soldering iron described by Tichauer and Gage (1977).

Prolonged work with arms extended can produce soreness in the forearm for assembly tasks done with force. By rearranging the workplace so as to keep the elbows at 90° most of the problem can be eliminated (see Figure 9.8). Similarly, continuous holding of an activation switch can result in fatigue of the fingers and reduced flexibility. Thus tool activation forces should be kept low to reduce this loading, or a power grip bar instead of a single-finger trigger should be used. For a two-handled tool, a spring-loaded return saves the fingers from having to return the tool to its starting position (Eastman Kodak Company, 1983).

FIGURE 9.8
Optimum working posture with elbow bent at 90°.

9.2.7 Awkward Wrist Position

As the wrist is moved from its neutral position there is loss of grip strength (Terrell and Pursewell, 1976). Starting from a neutral wrist position, full pronation decreases grip strength by 12%, full flexion/extension by 25%, and full radial/ulnar deviation by 15% (see Figure 9.9). This degradation of maximum grip strength available can be quantified by

$$\%\text{Grip Strength} = 95.7 + 4.3\,\text{PS} + 3.8\,\text{FE} - 25.2\,\text{FE}^2 - 16.8\,\text{RU}^2 \qquad (9.15)$$

where
PS is 1 if the wrist is fully pronated or supinated and 0 if in a neutral position
FE is 1 if the wrist is fully flexed or extended and 0 if in a neutral position
RU is 1 if the wrist is fully in radial or ulnar deviate and 0 if in a neutral position

Furthermore, awkward hand positions may results in soreness of the wrist, loss of grip and, if sustained for extended periods of time, occurrence of WRMSDs. To reduce this problem, the workplace of the tools should be redesigned to allow for straight wrist, i.e., lowering work surfaces and edges of containers, tilting jigs toward the hand, etc., using a pistol grip on knives (Armstrong et al., 1982), using a pistol handle on powered tools for vertical surfaces and in-line handles for horizontal surfaces (Armstrong, 1983), and putting a bend in the tool handle to reflect the axis of grasp such as the Tichauer and Gage (1977) pliers.

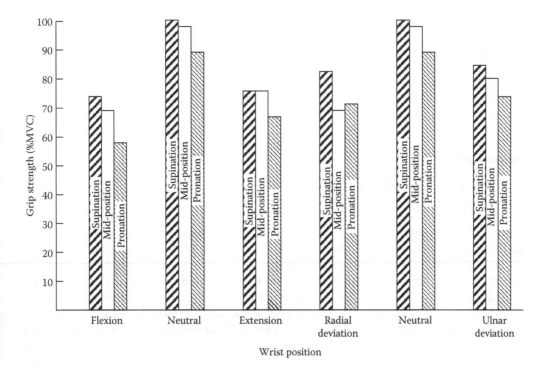

FIGURE 9.9
Grip strength as a function of wrist and forearm position. (Adapted from Terrell, R. and Purswell, J., *Proc. Hum. Fact. Soc.*, 20, 28, 1976. With permission.)

TABLE 9.2

Maximal Static Finger Flexion Forces

Digit	Maximum Force (N)	% of Force of Thumb
Thumb	73	100
Index	59	81
Middle	64	88
Ring	50	69
Little	32	44

Source: Adapted from Hertzberg, H.T.E., Engineering anthropometry, In: H. Van Cott and R. Kincaid (eds), *Human Engineering Guide*, Government Printing Office, Washington, DC, U.S., 1973.

9.2.8 Tissue Compression

Often in the operation of a hand tool considerable force is applied by the hand. Such actions can concentrate considerable compressive force on the palm of the hand or the fingers, resulting in ischemia, obstruction of blood flow to the tissues and eventual numbness and tingling of the fingers. Handles should be designed to have large contact surfaces to distribute the force over a larger area or to direct it to less sensitive areas such as the tissue between the thumb and index finger. Similarly, finger grooves or recesses in tool handles should be avoided. Since hands vary considerably in size, the grooves will accommodate a fraction of the population (McCormick and Sanders, 1982).

9.2.9 Repetitive Finger Action

If the index finger is used excessively for operating triggers, symptoms of trigger finger develop. Trigger forces should be kept low, preferably below 10 N (Eastman Kodak Company, 1983) to reduce the load on the index finger. Two- or three-finger-operated controls are preferable. Finger strip controls are even better, because they require the use of more and stronger fingers. Absolute finger flexion strengths are shown in Table 9.2.

9.3 Handles for Single-Handled Tools

9.3.1 Handle Length

A cut-out handle should be large enough to provide space for all four fingers. Hand breadth across the metacarpals ranges from 71 mm for a 5% female to 97 mm for a 95% male (Garrett, 1971). Thus, 100 mm may be a reasonable minimum, but 125 mm may be more comfortable (Konz and Johnson, 2000). Eastman Kodak Company (1983) recommended 120 mm. If the grip is enclosed or gloves are used, even larger openings are recommended. For an external precision grip, the tool shaft must be long enough to be supported at the base of the first finger or thumb. A minimum value of 100 mm is suggested (Konz and Johnson, 2000). For an internal precision grip, the tool should extend past the palm, but not so far as to hit the wrist (Konz and Johnson, 2000). It is interesting to note that screwdriver torque was experimentally found to be proportional to the handle grip length (Magill and Konz, 1986).

9.3.2 Handle Diameter

For a power grip on screwdrivers, Rubarth (1928) recommended a diameter of 40 mm. Basing their recommendation on empirical judgments of stair handrails, Hall and Bernett (1956) suggested 32 mm while Dusenberry et al. (2009) recommended 51 mm for round force-instrumented rails. Based on minimum EMG activity, Ayoub and LoPresti (1971) found a 51 mm handle diameter to be best. However, based on the maximum number of work cycles completed before fatigue and on the ratio of grip force to EMG activity, they suggested a 38 mm diameter. Pheasant and O'Neill (1975) found that muscle strength deteriorates when using handles greater than 50 mm in diameter. Rigby (1973), for full encirclement of the hand and heavy loads, recommended 38 mm. For handles on boxes, Drury (1980) found diameters of 31–38 mm to be best in terms of least reduction in grip strength. Eastman Kodak Company (1983), based on company experiences, recommended 30–40 mm with an optimum of 40 mm for power grips and 8–16 mm with an optimum of 12 mm for precision grips. More recently, a highly instrumented handle to measure various grip force components with adjustable caps still yielded an optimum grip size of 38.1 mm (Edgren et al., 2004). In a completely opposite approach but with the same results, female subjects rated 35 mm handle diameters and male subjects rated 40 mm handle diameters as the most comfortable sizes for maximum grip force exertions. These handle sizes corresponded to 19.7% of the user's hand length (Kong and Lowe, 2005a).

The above handle dimensions were derived from maximum grip forces. However, as the task changes, the handle diameter will also change. Replogle (1983), in validating his gripping model, found maximum torques at twice the grip span diameter. With average spans of about 25 mm, this yields a handle diameter of 50 mm. For maximum torque tasks, female subjects rated 37–44 mm diameter handles as the most comfortable, while male subjects rated 41–48 mm diameter handles as most comfortable. These handle sizes corresponded to 23.3% of user's hand length (Kong and Lower, 2005b). Using various handles of non-circular cross section, Cochran and Riley (1982, 1986b) found largest thrust forces in handles of 130 mm circumference (or 41.4 mm equivalent circular diameter) for both males and females. For manipulation, however, the smallest handles of 22 mm were found to be best (Cochran and Riley, 1983).

Based on the above data, one could summarize that handle diameters should be in the range of 31–50 mm with the upper end best for maximum torque and the lower end for dexterity and speed. However, it would also be best to size the handle to each individual's hand size. This was first succinctly observed by Fox (1957) in that a handle which allows some overlap between the thumb and index finger may be better than a larger handle that matches the individual's grip diameter. Similarly Yakou et al. (1997) found that maximum holding force was optimum at handle diameters around 35–40 mm, which also corresponding to the largest contact area of the hand to the handle. Grant et al. (1992) later confirmed that handles 1 cm smaller than the inside grip diameter maximized grip strength as compared to handles 1 cm larger or those matching the inside grip diameter.

Kong (2001) went further by defining normalized handle size (NHS) as the ratio of the handle circumference to hand length, as measured from the wrist crease to the tip of the middle finger. Thirty subjects, ranging from 5th percentile females to 95th percentile males, with hand lengths ranging from 160 to 205 mm, gripped a variety of handle sizes in several different tasks. This resulted in NHS ranging from 45% to 90%. Maximum grip forces and minimum subjective ratings of perceived exertion were obtained roughly in the range of 50%–55% NHS or absolute handle sizes in the range of 30.6–39.2 mm, depending on the individuals hand length. A more detailed analysis indicated that a better match yet is for the handle size to conform to individual finger lengths, with the ratio of the handle circumference to the length of finger ranging from 90% to 110%. This would result in a handle shape that is of an asymmetrical double frustum shape described further in the next section.

9.3.3 Handle Shape

As early as 1928, Rubarth investigated handle shape and concluded that, for a power grip, one should design for maximum surface contact so as to minimize unit pressure of the hand. Thus, a tool with a circular cross section was found to give largest torque. Pheasant and O'Neill (1975) concluded that the precise shape of handles was irrelevant and recommended simple knurled cylinders. Evaluation of handle shape on grip fatigue in manual lifting (which is a different action than for tool use) did not indicate any significant differences in shapes (Scheller, 1983). Maximum pull force, though, was obtained with a triangular cross section, apex down. For thrusting forces, the circular cross section was found to be worst and a triangular best (Cochran and Riley, 1982). However, for a rolling type of manipulation, the triangular shape was slowest (Cochran and Riley, 1983). A more comprehensive study indicated that no one shape may be perfect, and that shape may be more dependent on the type of task and motions involved than initially thought (Cochran and Riley, 1986b). A rectangular shape of width: height ratios, from 1:1.25 to 1:1.50 appeared to be a good compromise. A further advantage of a rectangular cross section is that the tool does not roll when placed on a table (Konz and Johnson, 2000). It should also be noted that handles should not have the shape of a true cylinder except for a hook grip. For screwdriver type tools, the handle end is rounded to prevent undue pressure at the palm and for hammer type tools the handle may have some flattening curving to indicate the end of the handle.

In a departure from the circular, cylindrically shaped handles, Bullinger and Solf (1979) proposed a more radical design using a hexagonal cross section, shaped as two truncated cones joined at the largest ends. Such a shape fits the contours of the palm and thumb best in both precision and power grips and yielded highest torques (9 Nm) in comparison with more conventional handles. A more detailed study by Kong (2001) identified four asymmetric double frustum cone handle sizes that would fit most of the adult population:

Small—corresponding to a 5th percentile female hand (160 mm)

Medium—corresponding to a 50th percentile female/5th percentile male hand (175 mm)

Large—corresponding to a 50th percentile male/95th percentile female hand (190 mm)

Extra large—corresponding to a 95th percentile male hand (205 mm)

The double frustum shape, with thick ends joined, allows one handle to fit all four fingers naturally. The index and middle fingers are larger, thus the slant of the top cone is less (6.9°) than for the bottom cone (15.4°). The total length of the handle is 130 mm, i.e., 65 mm for each cone. Specific diameters (mm) for each of the four handles are given in Table 9.3.

A final note on shape is that T-handles yield much better performance than straight screwdriver handles, Pheasant and O'Neill (1975) reported as much as 50% increase in torque. Optimum handle diameter was found to be 25 mm and optimum angle was 60°, i.e., a slanted T (Saran, 1973). The slant allows the wrist to remain straight and thus generate larger forces.

TABLE 9.3

Recommended Sizes for a Set of Four Double-Frustum Handles

Handle Feature	Small	Medium	Large	Extra Large
Large top end	22.7	25.5	28.5	31.3
Connecting middle part	30.6	33.4	36.4	39.2
Small bottom end	12.7	15.4	18.4	21.3

9.3.4 Texture and Materials

For centuries, wood was the material of choice for tool handles. Wood was readily available, and easily worked. It has good resistance to shock and to thermal and electrical conductivity and has good frictional qualities even when wet. Since wooden handles can break and stain with grease and oil, there has been a shift to plastic and even metal. Plastic handles are typically knurled or cross-hatched with grooves to improve the hand/tool frictional interface (Pheasant and O'Neill, 1975).

Such grooved fiberglass handles were evaluated with respect to traditional wooden handles by Chang et al. (1999). Although the focus was primarily on weight and efficiency of shoveling, with hollow handles requiring 12% less energy expenditure than solid handles, the subjects rated the grooved fiberglass handles more acceptable than wooden handles in terms of tactile feeling and slipperiness.

Metal should be covered with rubber or leather to reduce shock and electrical conductance and increase friction (Fraser, 1980). The latter effect can produce up to 52% greater torque for high-friction rubber handles ($\mu = 0.78$) than for low-friction ($\mu = 0.38$) aluminum handles (Seo et al., 2008). In addition, such a resilient covering may also aid in the reduction of hand discomfort. Fellows and Freivalds (1991) found that a 4 mm foam covering on wooden handled garden tools provided a significantly more uniform grip force distribution and lower ratings of perceived discomfort as compared to plain wooden handles. Unfortunately, in most cases, the total grip forces were higher for the foam-covered handles due to an excessive deformation of the foam and a "loss-of-control" feeling in the subjects. The authors hypothesized that a thinner layer of foam would have provided more control, but still maintained a better grip force distribution.

9.3.5 Angulation of Handle

As discussed in Section 9.2.7, deviations of the wrist from the neutral position under repetitive load can lead to a variety of cumulative trauma disorders as well as decreased grip strength (see Figure 9.9). Therefore, angulation of tool handles, e.g., power tools, may be necessary so as to maintain a straight wrist. The handle should reflect the axis of grasp, i.e., about 78° from the horizontal, and should be oriented so that the eventual tool axis is in line with the index finger (Fraser, 1980). This principle was first applied to pliers (see Figure 9.10) by Tichauer and Gage (1977) and then later to soldering irons, knives, and other tools.

An interesting extension of this concept has been promoted as Bennett's handle (Emanuel et al., 1980). Bennett developed this concept based on the angle formed by the index finger and the life line under the thumb. This angle of 19°, used for his handles, is claimed to maintain a straight wrist, generate increased strength and control and reduce stress, shock, and fatigue (Bennett Ergonomic Labs, 1983). Bennett's claims initially were supported by anecdotal evidence of improved performance by various individuals

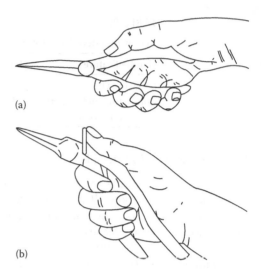

(a)

FIGURE 9.10
(a) Conventional pliers causing ulnar deviation.
(b) Ergonomically redesigned pliers allowing the hand
to work in line with the forearm. (Reproduced from
Freivalds, A., *Int. Rev. Ergon.*, 1, 43, 1987. With permission.)   (b)

(Emanuel et al., 1980). Since then Konz and his colleagues (Granada and Konz, 1981; Krohn and Konz, 1982; Konz and Streets, 1984; Konz, 1986) have conducted a variety of tests to evaluate the effectiveness of Bennett's handle on a hammer in comparison with a standard hammer. In the second study, a variety of angled handles were evaluated and subjects rated a 10° bend as being most preferred. In the third study, performance in driving nails was evaluated using various bent hammers. No performance difference was found. The 10° bend was again rated significantly higher. In the final study, using a semantic-differential questionnaire, Konz (1986) concluded that although no significant performance effects were found, subjects preferred a slight (5°–10°) bend rather than the 19° of Bennett's handle. An independent study by Knowlton and Gilbert (1983) used cinematography to evaluate a curved and conventional claw hammer. Bilateral grip strength was, measured before and after a task, nail driving. The curved hammer produced a smaller strength decrement and caused less ulnar deviation than the hammer. Thus, a bent handle does give some benefits but may be task dependent. The same effect was found for bent-handled pliers. Although they were 5.3% faster on one task, straight-handle pliers were 4.9% faster on another task. Furthermore, if the operators were allowed to use the pliers in a grip configuration of their own choosing, the postural benefits were considerably reduced (Duke et al., 2004). Therefore, operators should be trained in using tools properly.

9.4 Handles for Two-Handled Tools

9.4.1 Grip Span

Grip strength and the resulting stress on finger flexor tendons vary with the size of the object being grasped. Maximum grip strength is achieved at about 75–80 mm (Pheasant and Scriven, 1983; Chaffin et al., 1999). The smaller values of 75 mm were obtained on a dynamometer with parallel sides (Pheasant and Scriven, 1983), whereas the larger values of 75–80 mm were obtained on a dynamometer with handles angled inward (see Figure 9.9). This relationship can be modeled as

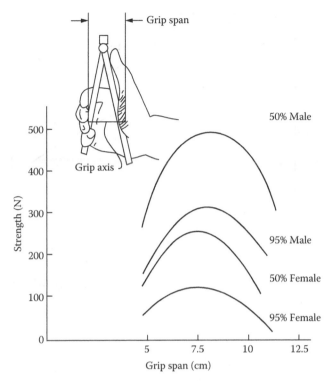

FIGURE 9.11
Grip strength capability for various grip spans. (Reproduced from Greenberg, L. and Chaffin, D.B., *Workers and Their Tools*, Pendell, Midland, MI, 1976. With permission.)

$$\%\text{Grip Strength} = 100 - 0.11 * S - 10.2 * S^2 \tag{9.16}$$

where S is the given grip span minus optimum grip span in cm.

Also, as is seen in Figure 9.11, there is quite a large variation in strength capacity over the population. To accommodate this population variability, maximal grip requirements should be limited to less than 90 N.

A similar effect is found for pinch strength (see Figure 9.12). However, the overall 4-point pulp pinch force is at a much more reduced force level (approximately 17% of power grip, see Table 9.1 for other types of pinches) and drops sharply beyond a 4–5 cm pinch span (Heffernan and Freivalds, 2000).

9.4.2 Gender

Female grip strength typically ranges from 50% to 67% of male grip strength (Pheasant and Scriven, 1983; Chaffin and Andersson, 1984; Konz and Johnson, 2000), i.e., the average male can be expected to exert approximately 500 N while the average female can be expected to exert approximately 250 N. An interesting survey by Ducharme (1975) examined how tools and equipment that were physically inadequate for female workers hampered their performance. The worst offenders were crimpers, wire strippers, and soldering irons. Females have a twofold disadvantage—an average lower strength and an average smaller grip span. Ducharme concluded that women could be integrated more quickly and safely into the work if tools were designed to accommodate smaller dimensions.

On the other hand, Pheasant and Scriven (1983) challenged Ducharme's assertions based on their findings that optimal performance for both males and females occurred at similar

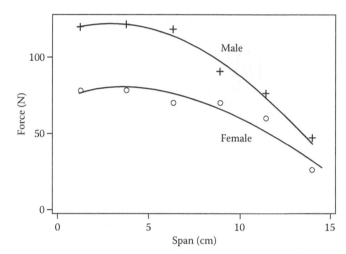

FIGURE 9.12
Pulp pinch strength capability for various grip spans. (Adapted from Heffernan, C. and Freivalds, A., *Appl. Ergon.*, 31, 409, 2000. With permission.)

conditions. Males had sufficient strength to overcome the deficiencies in tool design which posed much greater problems for females.

9.4.3 Handedness

Alternating hands permits reduction of local muscle fatigue. However, in many situations this is not possible as the tool use is one handed. Furthermore, if the tool is designated for the user's preferred hand, which for 90% of the population is the right hand, then 10% are left out (Konz, 1974). Laveson and Meyer (1976) gave several good examples of right-handed tools that cannot be used by a left-handed person, i.e., a power drill with side handle on the left side only, a circular saw, and a serrated knife leveled on one side only.

A few studies have compared task performance using dominant and nondominant hands. Shock (1962) indicated the non-preferred hand grip strength to be 80% of the preferred hand grip strength. Miller and Freivalds (1987) found right-handed males to show a 12% strength decrement in the left hand while right-handed females showed a 7% strength decrement. Surprisingly, both left-handed males and females had nearly equal strengths in both hands. They concluded that left-handed subjects were forced to adapt to a right-handed world. Using time study ratings, Konz and Warraich (1985) found decrements, ranging from 9% for an electric drill to 48% for manual scissors, for ratings using the non-preferred hand as opposed to the preferred hand.

9.5 Other Tool Considerations

9.5.1 Posture

A series of studies were performed by Mital and colleagues to examine various tool and operator factors on torque capability (Mital 1985, 1986; Mital et al., 1985; Mital and Sanghavi, 1986). In general, unless the posture is extreme, i.e., standing versus lying, torque exertion capability was not affected substantially. The height at which torque was applied had no influence on peak torque exertion capability. On the other hand, torque exertion capability decreased linearly with increasing reach distance. Another interesting requirement for proper tool usage is the volume or space envelope generated during operation of the tool. Comprehensive data on a variety of tools have been collected by Baker et al. (1960).

9.5.2 Weight

The weight of a hand tool will determine how long it can be held or used and how precisely it can be manipulated. For tools held in one hand with the elbow at 90° for extended periods of time, Greenberg and Chaffin (1976) recommend a load of no more that 2.3 kg. A similar value is suggested by Eastman Kodak Company (1983). For precision operations, tool weights greater than 0.4 kg are not recommended unless a counter-balanced system is used. Heavy tools, used to absorb impact or vibration, should be mounted on a truck to reduce effort for the operator (Eastman Kodak Company, 1983).

9.5.3 Gloves

Gloves are often used with hand tools for safety and comfort, but have adverse effects on task performance, tactility, dexterity, and strength (Bishu and Muralidhar, 1999). Safety gloves are seldom bulky, but gloves worn in subfreezing climates can be very heavy and interfere with grasping ability. The wearing of woolen or leather gloves may add 5 mm to the hand thickness and 8 mm to the hand breadth at the thumb, while heavy mittens add 25 and 40 mm, respectively (Damon et al., 1966). Gloves generally decrease grip strength by 5%–30%, depending on the type of glove as measured directly on grip strength (Hertzberg, 1973; Mital et al., 1994; Rock et al., 2001; Willms et al., 2009) or by a 15% increase in muscle activation to maintain a given force (or a corresponding decrease in endurance time) as measured by EMG (Larivière et al., 2004). In terms of performance, neoprene gloves slowed manual task times by 12.5% over barehanded performance, terry cloth by 36%, leather by 45%, and PVC by 64% (Weidman, 1970). On the other hand in certain cases, by protecting the hand, gloves could improve operational speed (Bradley, 1969a,b). Gloves consistently reduced torque production on small knobs (Swain et al., 1970), whereas Kevlar fiber gloves doubled torque production over bare-handed knife gripping (Claudon, 2006). The first effect was probably due to small size, while the second effect was due to increased friction, given that the knives had been coated with fat-simulating meat-packing conditions. Thus, typically, there is a trade-off to be considered between increased safety and reduced performance while using gloves.

9.5.4 Vibration

Vibration is a separate and very complex problem with powered hand tools. Vibration can induce white-finger syndrome, the primary symptom of which is a reduction in blood flow to the fingers and hand due to vasoconstriction of the blood vessels. As a result, there is loss of sensory feedback and decreased performance. The effect is dependent on the RMS level of the vibration, characteristic frequencies and individual susceptibility to the condition. It is a very complex and separate problem that is discussed in other sources (McCormick and Sanders, 1982).

The control of such vibration is probably best done in the design of the power tools itself. After market fixes will most likely be much less effective. For example, gloves, especially those with a label of "anti-vibration," are commonly recommended for workers using power tools and have been included as part of ergonomic intervention studies (Smith et al., 2000; Jetzer et al., 2003; Hull, 2007). However, the effectiveness of these gloves is difficult to interpret, especially since any reductions in WRMSDs are probably confounded with other interventions. Very few studies have shown clear reductions in vibration transmissibility for all frequencies (Goel and Rim, 1987; Reynolds and Jetzer, 1998). Most studies show that, typically, gloves will reduce transmissibility for higher frequencies (>200 Hz or so), but may actually increase transmissibility for lower frequencies (<200 Hz) (Rens et al., 1987; Jack, 2005). The latter effect may also vary due to the amount of push force that the operator applies to the power tool, with higher push forces associated with increased transmissibility (Paddan and Griffin, 1998). The only type of glove that may avoid the material compression due to push forces is one with air bladder technology (Reynolds and Jetzer, 1998). Therefore, as one South African mining study concluded, presently available commercial anti-vibration gloves are not a suitable intervention to prevent HAVS (Sampson and Van Niekerk, 2003). However, gloves will reduce the cooling of the hands (Suizu and Harada, 2005), which is a contributory factor in HAVS and also major factor in white-finger and Raynaud's syndromes.

9.5.5 Rhythm

The operation of hand tools involves repetition of a particular pattern of motion. A skilled operator acquires a basic motor pattern that will be most economical in terms of energy expenditure and is thus one attribute of skill. Once this pattern is established it is continued with very consistent velocity and acceleration through kinesthetic and aural feedback. Optimum rhythms have been observed by Drillis (1963) as follows: filing at 78 strokes/min, chiseling at 60 strokes/min, shoveling at 14–17 strokes/min, and cranking at 35 revolutions/min.

9.5.6 Miscellaneous

Tools should not have protruding sharp edges or corners. Two-handed tools should have stop limits to limit closure of the tools and prevent pinching of the fingers. Locking tools should not engage until the tool closes to the point where the fingers cannot be inserted. Tool surfaces should have matted surfaces to reduce glare (Fraser, 1980). Further details on efficient tool design can be found in Freivalds (1999).

9.6 Agricultural and Forestry Tools

9.6.1 Shovels and Spades

Spades are used to cut turf and lift and turn soil, while shovels are used to lift, move, and toss loose soil or grain. The blade is fastened to the shaft through a socket which, if stamped from a flat sheet, is generally rolled over to form a crimp known as a frog. This produces a compensating hollow in the back, yielding a hollow-back socket. The shaft may either taper to an end or have a handle. The handle traditionally has been of a T form, but more lately of a D form. Long spade shafts are generally 1.2–1.27 m long, while the short D handle is about 0.7 m long. The angle of the shaft with respect to the horizontal is called the lift and provides the tool with added leverage.

The task of shoveling was first examined scientifically by Taylor, at the Bethlehem Steel Works in 1898 (Taylor, 1913; Copley, 1923), who found that maximum performance was attained using a load of 9.7 kg. Since then many studies have examined various aspects of shoveling. The results of these studies are summarized by the particular feature investigated.

9.6.1.1 Shoveling Rate

Most of the studies (Lehmann, 1953; Dressel et al., 1954; Müller and Karrasch, 1956; Wyndham et al., 1966) consistently agreed on a high rate of shoveling in the range of 18–21 scoops/mill. Adjusted data from the two most complete studies (Lehmann, 1953; Müller and Karrasch, 1956) are plotted in Figure 9.13. Although quite different in other aspects, both data sets clearly show increasing efficiency with increasing shoveling rates. The effect levels out at higher rates, and, with other factors such as recovery pulse rate tending to limit shoveling, rates, values of 18–21 scoops/min are quite reasonable. This result can be explained primarily by the ergonomic principle of utilizing frequent and short work–rest cycles to gain maximum benefit from exponential recovery curves.

9.6.1.2 Shovel Load

The consensus on shovel load is not as clear as for shoveling rate. The range for an optimum load is 5–11 kg, depending on the decision criterion, the shoveling rate and the weight of the shovel used (which was not always specified). Thus, based on shoveling performance, Taylor (1913) recommended a 9.7 kg load. Wenzig (1928, 1932), using efficiency as the criterion, indicated 7–8 kg to be optimum for a rate of 8 scoops/min. Kommerell (1929) indicated 11 kg for low rates of 5–8 scoops/min. Spitzer (1950) and Dressel et al. (1954) recommended 8 kg for faster rates of 15–20 scoops/min. Müller and Karrasch (1956) indicated 5 kg, based on heart-rate recovery. For constrained mining conditions, Wyndham et al. (1969) specified 6.8 kg at 5–6 scoops/min.

FIGURE 9.13
Efficiency of shoveling as a function of shoveling rate and load. (Reproduced from Freivalds, A., *Ergonomics*, 29, 3, 1986. With permission.)

Adjusted data from the two most complete studies (Lehmann, 1953; Müller and Karrasch, 1956) are also plotted in Figure 9.13. The results are quite different. Lehmann's data indicate increasing efficiency with increasing loads. However, the concomitant increased static load gives rise to increased circulatory stress in the form of increased heart rate. Thus, Müller and Karrasch (1956) used recovery pulse rate as a second criterion. Maximizing efficiency given constrained recovery pulse rates yielded optimum loads between 5 and 7 kg. Thus, for high rates of shoveling (18–20 scoops/min), the lower end of the load range (5–7 kg) may be more appropriate (which follows the principles of reducing static loading on the circulatory system) while for lower rates (6–8 scoops/min), the higher end of the load range (8 kg) may be acceptable (which follows the principles of increasing efficiency with larger loads).

9.6.1.3 Throw Height

Two conflicting decision criteria are found in the literature. Increasing the throw height, especially above 1 m, increased the efficiency of the shoveling task (Wenzig, 1928, 1932; Spitzer, 1950), as shown in Figure 9.14. However, it also increased total energy expenditure rate ($\dot{E}$). Thus, if reasonably possible considering task constraints, the throw height should be reduced, e.g., a reduction in height from 2 to 0.5 m reduced $\dot{E}$ by 50% (Spitzer, 1950). On the other hand, since the shoveling performance was reasonably constant up to a height of 1.3 m (Stevenson and Brown, 1923), an acceptable throw height may be as high as 1–1.3 m.

9.6.1.4 Throw Distance

The same conflicting criteria that apply to throw height also apply to throw distance. Wenzig (1928, 1932) and Spitzer (1950) found minimum efficiency at a distance of 2 m with steadily increasing efficiencies thereafter, as shown in Figure 9.14. Again, however, energy expenditure increased correspondingly. Stevenson and Brown (1923) observed uniform shoveling performance up to a distance of 1.22 m. Since these lower distances have a lower $\dot{E}$ and a greater efficiency than at 2 m (due to the incomplete utilization of necessary body movements), then throw distances of up to 1.2 m may be optimum.

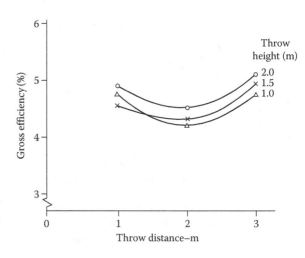

FIGURE 9.14
Efficiency of shoveling as a function of throw height and throw distance. (Reproduced from Freivalds, A., *Ergonomics*, 29, 3, 1986. With permission.)

9.6.1.5 Posture

Constraining the posture used in shoveling (typically by decreasing the height of the workspace, as in a low-seam mine) increases the energy expended as well as decreases the efficiency of the task. Thus, lowering the working height from 1.2 to 1.0 m increased $\dot{E}$ by 10% (Kommerell, 1929); lowering the height from 1.83 to 0.71 m reduced efficiency by 35% (Wyndham et al., 1969); and reducing the working height from erect to 60% of erect height increased $\dot{E}$ by 13% (Morrissey et al., 1983). The kneeling posture typically requires 6.5% less energy for the same task as a standing posture (Morrissey et al., 1983). A lying posture typically requires 1 kcal/min less than a standing posture (Humphreys et al., 1962).

9.6.1.6 Technique

The technique used in shoveling can also change the amount of energy expended. Thus, Wenzig (1932) recommended standing in front of the destination but facing away and shoveling over the shoulder, rather than standing and shoveling sideways, as the former was 18% more efficient. Dressel et al. (1954) found that scraping the material along the bottom of the pile to fill the shovel is 15% more efficient than digging directly into the pile.

9.6.1.7 Lift Angle

Lift angle was examined by Freivalds (1986b) using an experimental shovel with an adjustable lift of 16° intervals. The energy cost of shoveling sand at a constant rate of 18 scoops/min normalized to the amount of sand shoveled indicated a significantly lower normalized energy cost for lift angles of 16° and 32° as opposed to 0° and 48°. Predicted low-back compressive forces were significantly lower at 48° than at the other angles. This suggested that in order to reduce low-back stresses one should use the steepest lift angle. Unfortunately, such a steep angle caused much of the scooped material to slide out during the shoveling motion resulting in less productive work. Thus, a lift angle of 32° appeared to be the best compromise, which corresponded closely to the 37° angle found on most typical shovels.

9.6.1.8 Length of Handle

Wenzig (1932) observed the 0.64 m shovel to be slightly more efficient than a longer or shorter shovel. Kommerell (1929) found a 0.66 m shovel to be 10% more efficient than a 0.9 m shovel, which was very reasonable in his constrained (1.0 and 1.2 m heights) working environment. Lehmann (1953) agreed that short handles were more efficient in constrained environments but felt that there were insufficient data to justify a recommendation for unconstrained environments. Freivalds (1986b) found a significant improvement in efficiency for long-handled as compared to short-handled shovels in an unconstrained environment. Thus, the deciding criterion for shovel length is the amount of head room and posture used.

9.6.1.9 Handle Material

Traditionally, tool handles have been manufactured from wood, a surprisingly good material in that it is relatively light and resistant to transfer of heat, electricity, and even vibration. However, recently, probably due to cost of shaping the wood into the appropriate size and shape, there has been a trend to manufacture the handles from other materials

such as metal or fiberglass. Metal is a very poor material in that it is heavy and trans-
mits heat, electricity, and vibrations. On the other hand, fiberglass does not seem to have
such limitations. Chang et al. (1999) examined shoveling performance, grip force, forearm
flexor, and biceps brachii EMG, and Borg ratings of perceived exertion for three types of
gardening tools, shovel, rake, and hoe, with three different handles, wood, solid fiberglass,
and hollow fiberglass. The most effective measure for shovels was shoveling efficiency,
i.e., sand shoveled per minute divided by the increase in heart rate per minute. The hollow
fiberglass handle was 12% more efficient that either the wood or solid fiberglass handle,
probably due to the decreased load handled, as discussed in the next section. Subjective
ratings were also significantly lower for the hollow handle, part of which may have also
been attributed to the ribbed texture which provided the subjects with a better tactile feel.

9.6.1.10 Shovel Weight

Kirsch (1939) found that lighter shovels were 20% more efficient than heavier shovels.
Müller and Karrasch (1956) recommended a shovel weight of 1.5–1.8 kg based on an incomplete study in which shovel weight was dependent on shovel load. Freivalds (1986b) found
that subjects gave higher preference ratings to lighter shovels, although there were other
shovel parameters that could not be controlled and could have influenced their ratings.
Obviously, reducing shovel weight should greatly increase shoveling efficiency, especially
if one considers the unproductive weight to be one-third to one-half of the total shovel load
(e.g., Morrissey et al., 1983, used a 4 kg shovel with loads less than 8 kg).

9.6.1.11 Blade Size, Shape, and Thickness

Kirsch (1939) and Lehmann (1953) both agreed that blade size should depend on the density of the material being shoveled: the less dense the material the larger the blade size. The
optimum shape of the blade also depends on the material being shoveled (Kirsch, 1939): for
coarse-grained materials (e.g., rock, coal, and ore), a square point and flat blade with raised
edges; and for fine-grained materials (e.g., sand, soil), a round point and curved blade with
slightly raised edges. In terms of penetrating the material being shoveled, the coarser and
grainier the material being shoveled, the more energy will be expended. Thus, Dressel
et al. (1954) observed that shoveling coarse gravel required 37% more energy than sand.
Blade thickness (in the range 0.5–1.0 mm) was found to be unimportant as long as the blade
was properly sharpened (Vennewald, 1939).

Note that there should be a trade-off between blade size and shovel load handled (plus
the weight of the shovel itself). For small blades, a relatively small load is handled with
comparatively greater energy expenditure for moving the trunk and the shovel itself.
For large blades and large loads, excessively high energy expenditures will lead to quick
fatigue, for which the individual may compensate by using less than full scoops. This
trade-off was examined by Freivalds and Kim (1990) while shoveling sand with various
sized blades and shovel weights. The dependent variable, energy expenditure, was normalized to the individual's body weight and load shoveled (including shovel weight). The
blade size and shovel weight characteristics were combined into one independent variable, the ratio of blade size to shovel weight. The resulting quadratic functional relationship (shown in Figure 9.15) yielded a minimum energy cost at a blade/weight ratio of
$0.0676 \, m^2/kg$, which for an average-weight subject (77 kg) resulted in an energy expenditure of 5.16 kcal/min, just below the acceptable 8 h energy expenditure rate of 5.2 kcal/h as
recommended by Lehmann (1953). For larger blade sizes and theoretically larger loads and

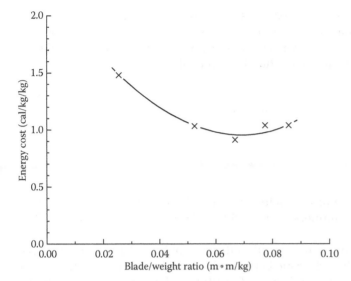

FIGURE 9.15
Energy cost as a function of blade-size/shove-weight ratio. (Reprinted from Freivalds, A. and Kim, Y.J., *Appl. Ergon.*, 21, 39, 1990. With permission.)

higher energy expenditures, the subjects compensated by taking less than full loads. More details on other shovel parameters may be found in Freivalds (1986a,b).

9.6.2 Axes and Hammers

9.6.2.1 Length and Striking Efficiency

Axes and hammers are striking tools designed to transmit a force to an object by direct contact and thereby change its shape or drive it forward. The tool's efficiency in doing this may be defined as the ratio of the energy utilized in striking to the energy available in the stroke. Using geometric methods, Drillis et al. (1963) showed that the tool's efficiency could be further defined by

$$\eta = 1 - \frac{S^2}{\rho_1^2} \qquad (9.17)$$

where
  η is the efficiency
  S is the distance from the mass center to the line of action (OB in Figure 9.3)
  ρ_1 is the radius of gyration with respect to the center of action

For the efficiency to be 100%, the center of mass should coincide with the line of action, which is impossible with a shafted tool. In the hand axe of stone-age man, the total energy of the stroke movement was converted into useful energy giving maximum efficiency, although the force was fairly weak. The opposite extreme is a uniform rod held at one end, which has an efficiency of only 25% but provides quite a bit more relative force.

Two comparable formulae for tool efficiency were developed by Gorjatschkin (1924, cited in Drillis et al., 1963).The first related tool efficiency to the ratio of S to the tool length, L:

$$\eta = 1 - 1.5 \frac{S}{L} \qquad (9.18)$$

Again, this indicates that the efficiency increases as the ratio of S to L increases. Physically, this is achieved by placing the mass center as close as possible to the center of action, i.e., increasing the mass of the tool head relative to the handle. A second way of expressing the above observation is to relate the mass of the handle to the total mass:

$$\eta = 1 - 0.75 \frac{m_1}{m_1 + m_2} \tag{9.19}$$

where
  m_1 is the mass of handle
  m_2 is the mass of tool head

Drillis et al. (1963) indicated that efficiencies for typical striking tools ranged from 0.8 to 0.95 for axes, from 0.7 to 0.9 for hammers, from 0.55 to 0.85 for scutches, and from 0.3 to 0.65 for hoes.

Regarding impacting tools such as hammers, the efficiency of impact and recoil are very important. When two bodies collide, the ratio between their relative velocities after impact to that before impact is defined as the coefficient of restitution. This can be used to derive the energy of recoil and eventually the efficiency of impact (Drillis et al., 1963).

In the case of forging this can be defined as

$$\eta = \frac{1}{1 + m_0/m} \tag{9.20}$$

where
  m_0 is the mass of hammer
  m is the mass of other object (e.g., forging and anvil)

The aim is to transform as much of the kinetic energy of the hammer into deforming the object's shape as possible. Thus the mass of the hammer should be small relative to the mass of the forging and anvil. On the other hand, in driving a nail the intent is to transform the kinetic energy of the hammer into the kinetic energy of the nail. Then the mass of the hammer should be great in relation to the mass of the nail and the efficiency becomes

$$\eta = \frac{1}{1 + m/m_0} \tag{9.21}$$

The overall efficiency of the system including the operator becomes the product of the efficiency of the tool, the efficiency of the stroke movement, the efficiency of impact and the physiological efficiency of the human operator. This latter factor can range from a low of 3%–4% for relatively static tasks such as shoveling (Freivalds, 1986b) to a high of 25%–30% for dynamic tasks such as cycling (Lehmann, 1953). Drillis et al. (1963) computed the overall efficiency of hammering a 6 in. (15 cm) nail into a wooden block as 57%, not counting the physiological efficiency. Using an average value of 15% for physiological efficiency, overall system efficiency reduces to 8.6%.

9.6.2.2 Weight and Striking Efficiency

The effect of the weight of the head on swing characteristics dynamics of striking tools, especially axes, was further investigated by Widule et al. (1978) and Corrigan et al. (1981).

Using cinematography, they analyzed the dropping motion of the subjects using four axes with head weights of 0.85, 1.6, 2.2, and 3.6 kg. Accelerations as well as kinetic energy for various points of interest were calculated frame by frame from the film.

The results supported the hypothesis that an increase in head weight led to an increase in kinetic energy. However, a noticeable drop-off in angular velocity and kinetic energy was found for the heaviest axe. Thus, there appeared to be a limit to the ability of an individual to achieve rotational inertia and adding additional mass may have been counterproductive in terms of physiological energy costs. The authors concluded that the heavy axes (heads ranging from 2.2 kg and above) used to clear the American forests in the late 1800s, although more taxing in terms of energy expenditure, were more efficient in clearing forests. Rapid bursts of energy were used to chop down a tree, and necessary rest periods could be obtained during preparation of the cut, sharpening the axe and chopping off branches. The authors also concluded that the American axe, distinguished from the European axe by its possession of a poll (a lump of metal at the rear of the head—see Figure 9.16a) was more efficient. The poll counterbalanced the protruding blade and gave the axe better handling characteristics.

Such observations were confirmed by Drillis et al. (1963) based on his survey of 521 axes used in Latvia. Average head weight was found to be 1.4 kg or about 2% of the user's weight. Average handle length was found to be 0.6 m or about 35% of the user's height. He concluded that these values compared very favorably to folk norms. Optimum swing height to achieve maximum kinetic energy for wood splitting was found to be approximately 1.1 m.

Some variations on these optimum values were noted by German work physiologists. In a study of sledgehammers, Meyer (1930) examined hammers ranging in weight from 4.4 to 10.6 kg. He concluded though that to get a more lively action (i.e., increased acceleration) one should use lighter hammers. Gläser (1933, cited in Lehmann, 1953) investigated axes with head weights under 2 kg for forestry use. He found the opposite and concluded that the "liveliest action" was to be achieved using axes weighing 3–4 kg. A mitigating

(a)

(b)

FIGURE 9.16

(a) Determination of striking tool efficiency (American axe); O = mass center, B = center of action, C = center of percussion (ideal point for holding), L = length of the tool, W = weight of the tool. (b) European axe. (Reproduced from Freivalds, A., *Int. Rev. Ergon.*, 1, 43, 1987. With permission.)

factor is that the Germans most likely measured the weight of the whole implement. Subtracting approximately 0.6–0.8 kg for the handle yields values more closely in line with the other studies.

9.6.2.3 Other Considerations

Further design principles for striking tools are given by Fraser (1980). The handles should not be cylindrical, but appropriately contoured for a power grip with an enlargement at the end to prevent slippage. Plastic handles are susceptible to fatigue and fracture. Metal handles are only useful if covered with leather or rubber to prevent slippage and reduce shock. Wooden handles, made from ash or hickory, are hard and dense with high shock resistance. The shaft is wedged into the hammerhead with iron wedges to insure additional security. Handle diameter is in the range of 25–40 mm. For more specialized carpentry hammers handle lengths will be shorter, around 0.3 m (Fraser, 1980).

9.6.3 Saws

9.6.3.1 General Considerations

The action of heavy sawing involves a power grip with repetitive flexion and extension at the elbow, while the action of light sawing requires a precision grip with manipulation of the wrist. A large two-man crosscut saw may require use of two hands, one superimposed upon the other, although at times one hand can be used. Typical American and European hand saws cut as they are pushed through the wood, while Oriental hand saws cut as they are pulled through the wood (Bleed et al., 1982). For most saws a "pistol grip" is typically used, except for the lightest saws in which a cylindrical screwdriver type handle serves best for a precision grip.

Several studies on sawing have indicated a variety of optimum features. Gläser (1933, cited in Lehmann, 1953) investigated a variety of postures and techniques to be used with two-man crosscut saws in forestry work. Using the one-handed stooped posture as the baseline for relative comparisons, Gläser found the following (Table 9.4).

A two-handed action provided more force and better performance, but at a higher energy cost. Most efficient was the kneeling position in which less torso support was needed and less energy was expended. Thus, posture plays an important part in tool usage.

9.6.3.2 Pulling versus Pushing

The effect of pulling versus pushing action in sawing, i.e., Oriental versus American saws, was tested by Bleed et al. (1982). Oxygen consumption was measured while sawing

TABLE 9.4

A Comparison of Sawing Postures and Techniques

	Normalized Cutting Performance (m²/min)	Normalized Energy Expenditure (kcal/min)	Normalized Energy Cost/Output (kcal/m²)
One-handed stooped	100	100	100
Two-handed stooped	130	141	108
Two-handed kneeling	130	120	92

Source: Adapted from Gläser, H. Beiträge zur Form der Waldsäge und zur Technik des Sägens (Contributions to the design of forestry saws and sawing techniques), Dissertation, Eberswalde, Germany, 1933.

identical beams using the two saws, plus a bow saw that could either be pushed or pulled. Sawing times were not significantly different while oxygen consumption for the Oriental saws was significantly lower than for the American saw (2.59 versus 3.4 L), and pushing the bow saw was significantly lower than for pulling it (3.28 versus 4.55 L). The authors indicated that a push stroke is superior to a pull stroke, except that for a Japanese saw a thinner blade and different handle style allowed for more efficient use. However, there is evidence that in a low posture (i.e., 50% of height), an unbraced pull can be stronger than an unbraced push (Ayoub and McDaniel, 1974; Materials Handling Research Unit, 1980), which could also explain the Japanese saw's superiority. The differences observed in the bow saw cannot be explained.

9.6.4 Other Agricultural Tools

9.6.4.1 Hoes

Although not really applicable in today's mechanized agriculture, an interesting study with evaluations of a variety of agricultural tools and techniques was performed by Barnstaet and Kogelschatz (1933). Some of the results illustrate general ergonomic concepts that can be applied in modern day tasks. First, an evaluation of hoes used in digging for potatoes was performed. The characteristics of the two opposite extreme hoes are given in Table 9.5.

Obvious differences in performance can be seen with hoe A being 58% more efficient than hoe D in retrieving potatoes and 72% more efficient in hoeing a given area. Decisive factors against hoe D were that the longer blade required greater force and more of a chopping action to penetrate the ground. The shallow blade of hoe A allowed it to be used more in a pulling action.

9.6.4.2 Wheelbarrows

Various techniques have been examined in beet and potato harvesting. Traditional methods use either a stoop posture or crawling on the knees. Barnstaet and Kogelschatz (1933) implemented a cart with wheels to support the torso with a 35% savings in energy expenditure. A similar effect was produced using a stool in potato harvesting. Thus, supporting the torso and eliminating a stooped posture provided large savings in energy expenditure and improved productivity significantly. A third factor of concern not examined in the study is that supporting the upper torso is also likely to alleviate stresses in the low back.

Lehman (1953) also examined the wheelbarrow and found that a typical wheelbarrow was not properly balanced, so either considerable weight was carried by the user or the center of gravity was so high that extra effort was needed to balance the wheelbarrow. Using a proper design and rubber tires a saving of 20% in energy expenditure was

TABLE 9.5

Characteristics and Performance of Two Hoes Used for Digging Potatoes

Hoe	Angle between Handle and Blade (°)	Weight (kg)	Handle Length (m)	Blade Area (m²)	Performance Number of Potatoes	Number of Strokes	Potatoes/ Stroke
A	72	0.75	1.42	153	179	651	0.275
D	85	1.50	1.28	89	184	1058	0.174

Source: Adapted from Barnstaet, K. and Kogelschatz, H., *Landwirtschaftliches Jahrbuch der Schweiz*, 76, 861, 1933.

obtained, although smoothness of the rolling surface was probably judged to be an even more significant factor, decreasing energy expenditure even more.

For other more obsolete agricultural tools such as the scythe, scutch, flail, etc. please refer to Drillis et al. (1963).

9.7 Industrial Tools

9.7.1 Pliers

Pliers and related tools—wire strippers, pincers, and nippers—are tools with a head in the form of jaws which can have a variety of configurations, a joint which may be simple or complex, and two handles. Although, sometimes, the handles are straight, more typically they are curved outwards to conform roughly to the position of grasp. The grasp, depending on use, can be of the precision or power type (Fraser, 1980).

In their simple form (see Figure 9.10), pliers are a very common tool and, if used casually for short periods of time, will give reasonable performance with little fatigue. However, the relationship of the handles to the head forces the wrist into ulnar deviation (see Figure 10a), a posture which cannot be held repeatedly or for prolonged periods of time without fatigue or occurrence of tenosynovitis. A further problem is that such a deviation reduces the range of wrist rotation by 50%, so reducing productivity (Tichauer, 1966). Certain industries, such as the electronics assembly industry, place just such demands on the workers. In the case of pliers, a radical ergonomic design has been instituted with remarkable success in reducing medical problems. By bending the handles of the pliers, the wrists of the user can be kept straight, reducing stress on the wrist (see Figure 9.10b). In the case of two groups of Western Electric Co. trainees, one using conventional straight pliers and the other the redesigned bent pliers, during a 12 week training program there was a sixfold increase in symptoms for the group using the straight pliers as opposed to the group using the bent pliers (Tichauer, 1976, 1978). A similar problem occurred at Eli Lilly and Co. involving diagonal cutting pliers used with considerable wrist extension. After numerous complaints, the pliers were redesigned with a similar bend and used successfully (Yoder et al., 1973).

Specifics on modern pliers design have been detailed by Lindstrom (1973, cited in Fraser, 1980). Four factors relating to the hand need to be considered in the design of pliers: size, strength, endurance, and working position. Lindstrom (1973) recommended a working hand width of 90 mm for men and 80 mm of women and a handle length of 110 mm for men and 100 mm for women. Longer handles would limit the opening of the tool head.

With regard to strength, Lindstrom (1973) cited a maximum grip strength of 588 N for the male dominant hand and 392 N for the female (or approximately 70% of male strength). By age 60–65, these values will have been reduced by 30%. For repeated or continuous operations, Lindstrom recommended a working strength of 33%–50% of the above values. Two-handed operation can increase the force produced by 60%–70%.

The working posture of the hand is extremely crucial since the finger flexor muscles cross the wrist and are located in the forearm. Thus, when the wrist is flexed, extended, or deviated the grip force may be reduced by as much as 30%. This phenomenon is another reason for the need to modify the tool to fit the requirements of the user as in the case of the Western Electric pliers.

Lindstrom (1973) also noted that application forces are not always limited by the lack of strength, but also by hand discomfort. For repeated operations, the pressure should not exceed 100 kPa for females, 200–400 kPa for males, and 700 kPa for an occasional maximum. To minimize the applied pressure, it is necessary to enlarge and flatten handles and avoid pressure producing ridges. Thus, indentation of the handles for the fingers is undesirable. Encasing the basic metal handles in a rubber or plastic sheath provides insulation and improves the tactile feel (Fraser, 1980).

9.7.2 Screwdrivers

The handles of screwdrivers (and similar tools: files, chisels, etc.) can either be used with a precision grip for stabilization or a power grip for torque. The handle must also be capable of being approached equally effectively from all directions. Crucial factors to be considered in screwdriver use are size, shape, and texture of the handle.

Rubarth (1928) examined maximum torque from a power grip on a screwdriver handle. The best shape was cylindrical with a rounded end. Within the range of diameters used, 18–40 mm, an increase in diameter allowed for a greater force production. Hunt (1934) studied speed of use as a function of handle diameter. The time taken to drive a screw with a 7.6 mm diameter handle was 1.9 s, while with a 16 mm handle it was 3.6 s. Thus, the smaller the diameter the less time was needed for rotation of the handle. Pheasant and O'Neill (1975) measured torque for various sized cylindrical handles as well as actual screwdriver handles. Again torque was found to increase with an increase in handle diameter size. Knurled cylinders allow for significantly greater torque production than smooth cylinders. Maximum torque was achieved with knurled cylinders 50 mm in diameter. Actual screwdriver handles compared favorably to knurled cylinder handles. Differences in the precise shape of handles were not significant, as long as the hand did not slip around the handle. Similarly, Habes and Grant (1997a) found increased torque capability and decreased EMG-torque ratios (i.e., improved muscle contraction efficiency) with larger diameter handles (3.7 versus 2.9 cm).

Further studies on the shape of the handle have shown some inconsistencies in results. Fraser (1980) indicated that a tool manufacturer in Germany had introduced a successful version of a screwdriver handle with a triangular cross section. The planes of the sections allowed better use of the fingers in torque application. Magill and Konz (1986) found that a similar screwdriver with three large shallow flutes also produced the largest torque. They confirmed that torque was proportional to grip volume and grip length and time on task was inversely related to grip volume and length. On the other hand, a new series of ergonomic screwdrivers produced by Ergo in Sweden and marketed by Bahco in the United States use essentially a cylindrical handle with a circular cross section (Bobjer, 1984). The presence of large flutes created pressure concentrations in the palm of the hand and were omitted. To give better frictional characteristics, the handle incorporated 40 axial grooves with cross grooves. A second innovation was that small screwdrivers for precision work were fitted with normal length handles. The lowest part of the handle assisted in finding directions during a precision task. The contradiction in handle shape is not easily explainable and is examined more closely in Section 9.3.3 on handles shapes.

A final study on screwdrivers and posture (Huston et al., 1984) indicated that greater torque could be produced standing rather than sitting and at the lowest of three body positions, elbow, rather than shoulder or eye height. Similarly, Habes and Grant (1997a) found increased torque capability and decreased EMG-torque ratios (i.e., improved muscle contraction efficiency) with a vertical (as opposed to horizontal) orientation of the screw-driver, decreased point-of-operation heights, and decreased reach distances.

9.7.3 Knives

Although a very old tool, the knife has recently reappeared in the literature as a possible cause for the increase in cumulative trauma disorders in the butchering industry. The first study investigated a rash of cumulative trauma disorders in a poultry processing plant (Armstrong et al., 1982). Detailed Methods, Time and Measurement (MTM) analyses as well as a frame-by-frame film analysis of the hand motions during cutting were performed. Certain modifications to the currently used boning knife were suggested. A pistol type grip would allow the operator to hold the blade and the forearm horizontal so as to eliminate ulnar deviation and wrist flexion. A circular or elliptical shaped handle with a larger circumference of 99 mm, as well as a strap, were recommended to allow the hand to relax between exertions without losing grip of the knife. Later research by Habes and Grant (1997b) also confirmed the use of pistol grip knives to promote the use of stab grip as opposed to holding the knife in-line with the forearm axis in a slice grip. The stab grip allowed a higher force capability and minimized EMG to force ratios in various muscles, indicating more efficient muscle contractions.

The fish canning industry in Sweden has also been plagued by cumulative trauma disorders (Karlqvist, 1984). The common straight knives, which during the cutting action caused large ulnar deviations, were identified as possible causes for the medical incidents. Of the four knives used in different operations, one was fitted with a pistol grip similar to Armstrong et al.'s (1982), while the others were fitted with larger diameter handles for better balance and movement.

Knife safety is also of concern during butchering operations. Long hours of static loading on the forearm flexors can result in accelerated fatigue. Due to body fluids causing slippery handles, there are frequent instances of the operator's hand, upon impact or abrupt stoppage of the knife penetration, sliding down the handle and over the blade, resulting in severe injury. Cochran and Riley (1986a) examined tangs (barriers to the blade projecting perpendicular from the handle) of various heights and found that guard heights of 1.52 cm were optimal for safety with lower heights being inadequate. Knife sharpness is also critical to safety (less potential slips) and also for lowering biomechanical stresses, with significantly lower EMGs for the FDS, biceps brachii, triceps, and deltoid muscles (Claudon and Marsot, 2006).

9.7.4 Meat Hooks

Meat hooks are used to control the accessibility of meat during meat-processing operations, typically placed in the nondominant hand (the dominant hand holds a knife or other cutting tool) and is suspected to be the cause of many incidences of tenosynovitis in the nondominant hand ring finger. The current model is a 5 mm thick piece of flat polyethylene with a hook inserted in the middle of the piece (Hook A, see Figure 9.17). The thin shape leads to high compressive forces while the location of the hook places high forces on the ring finger (which is only the third strongest finger). Another current model uses a polyethylene frustum with the hook inserted off-center at the smaller end (Hook B, see Figure 9.17). Potentially better new designs tested include Hook C, with the hook at the larger end of the frustum, Hook D, a double frustum with the hook offset (between the two strongest fingers) and Hook E, a double frustum with the hook centered (Kong and Freivalds, 2003).

FIGURE 9.17
Different types of meat hooks. Hook A is a traditional design, Hooks B and C have the hook off center, Hooks D and E have a double frustum handle, Hooks F and G have an oval cross section. (Reprinted from Kong, Y.K. and Freivalds, A., *Int. J. Ind. Ergon.*, 32, 12, 2003. With permission.)

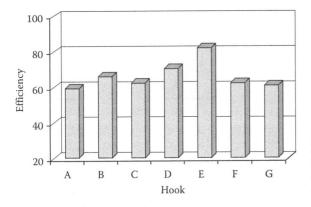

FIGURE 9.18
Efficiency (maximum force per normalized EMG) of meat hooks. (Reprinted from Kong, Y.K. and Freivalds, A., *Int. J. Ind. Ergon.*, 32, 12, 2003. With permission.)

Force-sensing resistors (FSRs) were used to measure finger forces during simulated meat-pulling tasks. The resulting finger force distributions were compared to the theoretically optimal finger contribution distributions mentioned in Section 9.2.2 with Hook E deviating least from the optimal finger force distribution. Incorporating the empirical FSR forces into the biomechanical hand model (discussed in Section 5.5), produced individual tendon forces which were normalized per unit external force. This latter measure can be considered as a form of grip efficiency and was best for Hook E (see Figure 9.18). The lowest Borg rating of perceived exertion was obtained with Hook D (see Figure 9.19). Therefore, a double frustum-shaped meat hook handle is most efficient for gripping and, producing least amount of tendon forces. The only uncertainty is the placement of the hook.

9.7.5 Power Tools

9.7.5.1 Power Drills

In a power drill, or other power tools, the major function of the operator is to hold, stabilize, and monitor the tool against a workpiece, while the tools perform the main effort of the job. Although the operator may at times need to shift or orient the tool, the main function for the operator is to effectively grasp and hold the tool. A drill is comprised of a head, body, and handle, with all three, ideally, being in line. The line of action is from

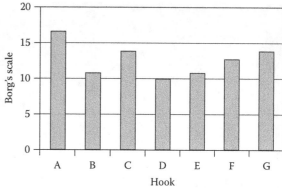

FIGURE 9.19
Borg's rating of perceived exertion for meat hooks. (Adapted from Kong, Y.K. and Freivalds, A., *Int. J. Ind. Ergon.*, 32, 12, 2003. With permission.)

FIGURE 9.20
Proper orientation of power tools in the workplace. (Reprinted from Freivalds, A. *Int. Rev. Ergon.*, 1, 43, 1987. With permission.)

the line of the extended index finger so that in the ideal drill, the head is off-center with respect to the central axis of the body. Handle configuration is important, with the choices being pistol-grip, in-line, or right-angle. As a rule of thumb, in-line and right-angle are best for tightening downward on a horizontal surface while pistol-grips are best for tightening on a vertical surface (Figure 9.20) with the aim being to obtain a standing posture with a straight back, upper arms hanging down, and a straight wrist (Figure 9.8). For the pistol grip, this results in the handle being at angle of approximately 78° with horizontal (Fraser, 1980).

Another factor of importance is the center of gravity. If it is too far forward in the body of the tool, a turning moment is created, which must be overcome by the muscle of the hand

and forearm, creating muscular effort additional to that required for holding, positioning and pushing the drill into the workpiece. They recommend placing the primary handle directly under the center of gravity, such that the body juts out behind the handle as well as in front. For heavy drills, a secondary supportive handle may be needed, either to the side or preferably below the tool, such that the supporting arm can be tucked in against the body rather than being abducted (Fraser, 1980).

9.7.5.2 Nutrunners

Nutrunners, especially common in the automobile industry, are used to tighten nuts, screws, and other fasteners. They come in a variety of handle configurations (in line, pistol grip, right angle), torque outputs, shut-off mechanisms, speeds, weights, and spindle diameters, and are commercially available from a variety of sources. Torque levels range from 1 to 5000 N m and, for pneumatic tools, are generally lumped into approximately 22 power levels (M1.6–M45) depending on motor size and gearing required to drive the tool. The torque is transferred from the motor to the spindle through a variety of mechanisms such that the power (often air) can be quickly shut-off once the nut or other fastener is tight. The simplest and cheapest mechanism is a direct-drive, which is under the operator's control but, because of the long time to release the trigger once the nut is tightened, transfers a very large *reaction torque* to the operator's arm. Mechanical friction clutches will allow the spindle to slip, reducing some of this reaction torque. A better mechanism for reducing the reaction torque is the air-flow shut-off which automatically senses when to cut off the air supply as the nut is tightened. A still faster mechanism is an automatic mechanical clutch shut-off. The most recent mechanisms include the hydraulic pulse system where the rotational energy from the motor is transferred over a pulse unit containing an oil cushion (filtering off the high frequency pulses as well as noise) and a similar electrical pulse system, both of which, to a large extent, reduce the reaction torque (Freivalds and Eklund, 1993).

Variation of torque delivered to the nut depends on a variety of conditions including properties of the tool, the operator of the tool, properties of the joint, i.e., the combination of the fastener and material being fastened (ranging from soft, with the materials having elastic properties such as body panels, to hard, when two stiff surfaces, such as pulleys on a crankshaft, are brought together), stability of the air supply, etc. The torque experienced by the user (the reaction torque) depends on the above factors (see Figure 9.21) plus the torque shut-off system and is believed to contribute to the development of cumulative

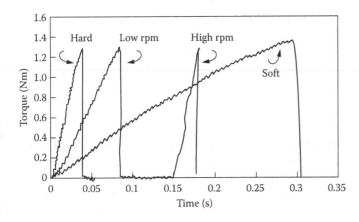

FIGURE 9.21
Nutrunner reaction torques as a function of soft or hard joints and low (100) or high (400) rpm levels. (Reprinted from Freivalds, A. and Eklund, J., *Appl. Ergon.*, 24, 158, 1993. With permission.)

FIGURE 9.22
Comparison of nutrunners torque impulse levels with subjective ratings. (Reprinted from Freivalds, A. and Eklund, J., *App. Ergon.*, 24, 158, 1993. With permission.)

trauma disorders. In general, using electrical tools at lower than normal rpm levels or under powering pneumatic tools resulted in larger reaction torques and more stressful ratings (see Figure 9.22). Pulse type tools produced the lowest reaction torques and were rated as less stressful. It was hypothesized that the short pulses "chop up" or allow the inertia of the tool to resist the reaction torque. A more recent study found that electrical tools produced significantly lower peak hand accelerations than pneumatic tools, due to the servo systems that are incorporated into electrical tools and assist in reducing the ergonomic impact of the reaction torques (Potvin et al. 2004). Another possibility is to provide reaction torque bars (Freivalds and Eklund, 1993).

9.7.5.3 Handle Sizes

The expectation would be that handle size requirements for powered tools should be no different than powered tools. Johnson (1988) examined the handle diameter for powered in-line screwdrivers (similar to nutrunners discussed above, except that they tend to have smaller torque levels and are typically either in line or pistol grip) by adding aluminum sleeves to the basic tool. Interestingly, larger diameters (5.0–6.35 cm) showed decreased EMG levels as compared to smaller diameters (2.86 cm). These numbers would appear to be larger than those recommended for manual circular tool handles (Section 9.3.2). However, there might be a confounding factor in that the additional aluminum sleeve may have absorbed some the vibration or reaction torques discussed above and required less force (i.e., EMG) to grip and control the tool. Oh and Radwin (1993) modified a pistol-grip tools to have an adjustable handle. Larger spans (5–6 cm) required least amount of grip force during the task requirements, which is comparable to the grip span for two-handled tools (Section 9.4.1). Also, as could be expected, extended triggers decreased finger forces and palmar forces during tool operation.

9.7.6 Railroad Tools

Use of large hand tools in the railroad industry has produced many injuries which are exceeded in number only by injuries from slips, falls, and material injuries. In addition, the injuries are not confined to the hand and wrist, but include a large number (up to 30%) of torso injuries. Striking and leverage tools are possible sources for these problems and thus were examined in a series of studies (Marras, 1986; Marras and Rockwell, 1986;

Rockwell and Marras, 1986). The first task involved swinging a 4.5 kg maul about the trunk and hitting a spike (Marras and Rockwell, 1986). This required both strength and skill as the spike surface area was only 3.9 cm^2 and the maul striking surface area was 5.3 cm^2. Six to 10 swings were required to drive the spike completely. Three tool weights, three tool striking surface areas and six spiking methods were utilized in the experimental design. Spiking force was measured by a load cell, and electromyograms (EMG) of the low back musculature were recorded.

The most obvious results were differences between professional railroad men and novice subjects. Force levels produced during spiking were greater for professionals and enlarging the striking surface area increased spiking force. The latter effect was due to the worker using a greater ballistic motion because less control was needed to strike the surface. However, too large an area would impede work close to the rails. Thus, the long narrow heads typically used are a compromise. Tool weights in the narrow range selected (3.6–5.5 kg) were not significant. The method of tool use significantly affected spiking force for novice subjects but not for professionals, probably because the professionals had already adapted to their preferred techniques. For the novice subjects methods involving less control, such as back motion alone without hand motion, produced greater ballistic motion and spiking force. The EMG data indicated that using the back alone produced lowest spinal stresses, especially in novice subjects. The overall conclusions were that professionals benefitted most from tool changes while novices benefitted most from technique changes (Marras and Rockwell, 1986).

In a second experiment, Rockwell and Marras (1986) examined the clawbar used to remove spikes from rails. It is a heavy (12.6–13.6 kg) tool leading to injuries when the tool suddenly releases and one operator falls. Two angles of leverage on the claw bar (44° or 66°) and various methods of performing the task were tested. Again the results indicated significant differences between professionals and novices with professionals producing 50% greater lifting forces. The best technique involved snapping or jerking the bar downward to create a peak force over a short time. The short impulse was more likely to free a spike and produced less bending in the bar, which could also be a cause for injuries. Tool design in terms of leverage angle was not a significant factor for tool performance. Bar weight and length have some effect, but were not studied (Rockwell and Marras, 1986).

9.7.7 Mining Tools

A significant proportion of underground mining accidents are attributed to the use of hand tools. The worst tools in coal mining in this respect are scaling bars, jacks, pry-bars, hammers, axes, and drills. For metal and non-metal mining, the worst tools are jacks, drills, and scaling bars, which account for 85% of the lost days in hand-tool accidents (Lavender et al., 1986). In almost all the above cases, the injuries are over-exertion injuries to the trunk or having the tool strike various body parts. Although the authors did not address specific tools, they suggested that "struck-by" accidents could be reduced by improved lighting, better work site preparation and improved training.

9.7.8 Miscellaneous Tools

9.7.8.1 Soldering Irons

A variety of other tools have been ergonomically redesigned to fit the human operator. The electronics assembly industry uses many bench-top assemblies that require the operator to abduct their arms so that they are nearly horizontal. This is often caused by tools and workspace designs requiring the forearm to angle down into the area of work, such as soldering wires to terminals on circuit boards lying flat on the workbench. Tichauer (1966) redesigned the soldering iron to include a bend between the tip and the handle, which eliminated the shoulder abduction and lowered the forearm.

9.7.8.2 Surgical Instruments

Surgical instruments such as the bayonet forceps have also been examined and redesigned (Miller et al., 1971). The problems with the original forceps included a tendency for it to roll in the fingers while in use, for fatigue to develop in the finger flexor muscles and for improper passing from nurse to surgeon. Using motion times and electromyographic recordings of the finger flexors, alternative designs were evaluated until one showed a reduction in grasp times of 25% and in muscle workload of 40%.

9.7.8.3 Dental Instruments

Hoping to improve efficiency in dentistry, dental instruments were evaluated and modified by Evans et al. (1973). Instead of the current dental syringe (providing air, water, and air–air–water spray with a separate suction device), the authors combined all four into one multi-function instrument. Field tests indicated a somewhat improved performance, reducing the number of hand movements required by dental assistants from 64 to 42 and reducing the dentist's cutting time from 91 to 84 s. Energy expenditure, however, did not change. The authors concluded that with more practice time and better control coding, larger improvements would have been obtained.

9.7.8.4 Food Scoops

The design of food scoops was examined by Konz (1975).The traditional food scoop used a thumb-activated clearing mechanism. The control required 17% of mean male thumb strength and could not be shifted to the other hand. Thus, fatigue would be a serious problem and left-handed operators could not use the tool. A second design used a power-grip activator. However, a large force, 10% of male grip strength, was still required. A third alternative design was especially suitable for ice-cream since it eliminated the need for a clearing bar. A liquid center transferred heat from the hand to the scoop melting residual ice cream.

9.7.8.5 Writing Instruments

The ergonomics of writing instruments were examined by Kao (1976, 1977, 1979). Evaluation of writing speed for ballpoint pens, felt-tip pens, fountain pens, and pencils indicated the ballpoint as being best and the fountain-pen worst. For least fatiguing writing, i.e., requiring least pressure, the felt-tip was best and the ballpoint was worst. Considering the trade-offs in speed and fatigue, the felt-tip was judged best overall (Kao, 1979). For any writing instrument, increasing the size of the grip area with a flared design up to a diameter of 13.6 mm should significantly reduce gripping force. This was found to be the case for ball point pens as measured by the EMG of the flexor pollicis brevis and pain scores for various hand regions during extended writing (Udo et al., 2000).

9.7.8.6 Scissors

Scissors were evaluated as a means of controlling upper extremity disorders in an automobile upholstery plant (Tannen et al., 1986). Traditional scissors were considered as well as various blades connected with a C-shaped handle and spring to produce a self-opening scissors. The commercial self-opening blade elicited fewest complaints. However, each instrument had a minority of unsatisfied users. The authors concluded that choice of hand tools appears to be a highly individualized decision, requiring the input of the users.

Scissors used by barbers were redesigned in a study by Bullinger and Solf (1979). Handles were bent 22° with respect to the blades in the plane of the scissors, while the planes of the cutting edges were twisted 30° from the plane of the handles. The redesigned scissors were 50% more efficient than conventional scissors and increased heart rate only 3% as opposed to 21% for the conventional scissors in an experimental shearing task.

9.7.8.7 Toothbrushes

Even the common toothbrush has been redesigned using ergonomic principles (Guilfoyle, 1977). Based on time and motion studies, expert opinions, and survey data, a smaller bristle to concentrate brushing action, an angle handle for easier manipulation, and a contoured thumb area for comfort were incorporated in the new design.

A variety of other interesting tool and handle redesigns are presented in Roubal and Kovar (1962).

Questions

1. Why might there still be need for ergonomic tool design when many of these tools have been in existence for hundreds if not thousands of years?

2. What are some of the basic considerations that all tools need to fulfill?

3. What are the differences between a precision and a power grip? What are the implications for work and resulting injuries?

4. What is a safety margin and what implications does it have for work and resulting injuries?

5. What is a slip reflex and what implications does it have?

6. What may explain the coefficient of friction for skin exceeding the theoretical limit of 1.0?

7. What biomechanical arguments may be used to justify the need to maintain a neutral wrist posture?

8. What biomechanical arguments may be used to justify an "optimum" handle shape?

9. What biomechanical factors are important in designing a two-handled tool such as pliers?

10. Discuss the trade-offs of using gloves with tools.

11. What are some of key factors in designing shovels and a shoveling task for optimum performance?

12. What determines the striking efficiency of a hammer or other striking tool?

13. What factors are important in screwdriver design?

14. What is reaction torque and what power tool and task characteristics will affect it?

Problems

1. Plot the relative torque produced as handle diameter increases from practically zero to double the grip span diameter.

2. What is the loss in grip strength for an average male using channel-lock pliers with a grip span of 10 cm held in full ulnar deviation (as would be the case for most work on a horizontal work surface)?

3. What is the loss of efficiency for a cheap hammer that is made completely of cast iron as compared to a hammer with a very light weight handle? (*Hint:* Assume the center of gravity for the first hammer is at the mid-position of the handle.)

4. Assume that a typical shovel has a blade size of 0.06 m² and weighs 2.2 kg. What effect does doubling the blade size for the same weight have? What effect would reducing the weight of the shovel by 50% have?

References

Aghazadeh, F. and Mital, A. (1987). Injuries due to hand tools. *Applied Ergonomics* 18:273–278.

Amis, A.A. (1987). Variation of finger forces in maximal isometric grasp tests on a range of cylindrical diameters. *Journal of Biomedical Engineering* 9:313–320.

An, K.N., Cooney, W.P., Chao, E.Y., and Linscheid, R.L. (1978). Functional strength measurement of normal fingers. *ASME Advances in Bioengineering*, New York, pp. 89–90.

An, K.N., Askew, L.J., and Chao, E.Y. (1986). Biomechanics and functional assessment of upper extremities. In: W. Karwowski (ed.) *Trends in Ergonomics/Human Factors III*. Amsterdam, The Netherlands: Elsevier, pp. 573–580.

Armstrong, T.J. (1983). *An Ergonomic Guide to Carpal Tunnel Syndrome*. Akron, OH: American Industrial Hygiene Association.

Armstrong, T.J., Foulke, J.A., Joseph, B.S., and Goldstein, S.A. (1982). Investigation of cumulative trauma disorders in a poultry processing plant. *American Industrial Hygiene Association Journal* 43:103–116.

Athènes, S. and Wing, A. (1989). Knowledge-directed coordination in reaching for objects in the environment. In: S.A. Wallace (ed.) *Perspectives on the Coordination in Movement*. Amsterdam, The Netherlands: North Holland, pp. 284–301.

Ayoub, M. and LoPresti, P. (1971). The determination of an optimum size cylindrical handle by use of electromyography. *Ergonomics* 14:509–518.

Ayoub, M.M. and McDaniel, J.W. (1974). Effects of operator stance on pushing and pulling tasks. *American Institute of Industrial Engineers Transactions* 6:185–195.

Baker, P.T., McKendry, J.M., and Grant, G. (1960). Volumetric requirements for hand tool usage. *Human Factors* 2:156–162.

Barnstaet, K. and Kogelschatz, H. (1933). Die Untersuchung verschiedener landwirtschaftlicher Arbeiten mit Hilfe des Respirationsapparatus (Investigation of agricultural work using a respirometer). *Landwirtschaftliches Jahrbuch der Schweiz* 76:861–888.

Bendz, P. (1974). Systematization of the grip of the hand in relation to finger motor, systems. *Scandinavian Journal of Rehabilitation Medicine* 6:158–165.

Bennett Ergonomic Labs. (1983). *Why Bennett's Biocurve?* Minneapolis, MN: Bennett's Bend, Inc.

Bernstein, N.A. (1967). *The Co-Ordination and Regulation of Movements.* New York: Pergamon Press.

Bishu, R. and Muralidhar, A. (1999). Gloves. In: W. Karwowski and W.S. Marras (eds), *The Occupational Ergonomics Handbook.* Boca Raton, FL: CRC Press, pp. 865–876.

Bleed, A.S., Bleed, P., Cochran, D.J., and Riley, M.W. (1982). A performance comparison of Japanese and American hand saws. *Proceedings of the Human Factors Society* 26:403–407.

Bobjer, O. (1984). Screwdriver handles design for power and precision. *Proceedings of the 1984 International Conference on Occupational Ergonomics.* Ontario, Canada: Human Factors Association of Canada, pp. 443–446.

Bobjer, O., Johansson, S.E., and Piguet, S. (1993). Friction between hand and handle. Effects of oil and lard on textured and non-textured surfaces; perception of discomfort. *Applied Ergonomics* 24:190–202.

Bradley, J.V. (1969a). Effects of gloves on control operation time. *Human Factors* 11:13–20.

Bradley, J.V. (1969b). Glove characteristics influencing control manipulability. *Human Factors* 11:21–35.

Brand, P.W., Beach, R.B., and Thompson, D.E. (1981). Relative tension and potential excursion of muscles in the forearm and hand. *Journal of Hand Surgery* 6:209–218.

Buchholz, B., Frederick, L.J., and Armstrong, T.J. (1988). An investigation of human palmar skin friction and the effects of materials, pinch force and moisture. *Ergonomics* 31:317–325.

Bullinger, H.J. and Solf, J.J. (1979). *Ergonomische Arbeitsmittel-gestaltung II—Handgeführte Werkzeuge—Fallstudien* (Ergonomic improvements to dangerous hand tools). Dortmund, Germany: Bundesanstalt fur Arbeitsschutz und Unfallforschung.

Bureau of Labor Statistics. (1995). *Reports on Survey of Occupational Injuries and Illnesses in 1977–1994.* Washington, DC: U.S. Department of Labor.

Cannon, L.J., Bernacki, E.J., and Walter, S.D. (1981). Personal and occupational factors associated with carpal tunnel syndrome. *Journal of Occupational Medicine* 23:255–258.

Chaffin, D.B., Andersson, G.B.J., and Martin, B.J. (1999). *Occupational Biomechanics,* 3rd edn, New York: John Wiley & Sons, pp. 355–368.

Chang, S.R., Park, S., and Freivalds, A. (1999). Ergonomic evaluation of the effects of handle types on garden tools. *International Journal of Industrial Ergonomics* 24:99–105.

Chao, E.Y., Opgrande, J.D., and Axmear, F.E. (1976). Three-dimensional force analysis of finger joints in selected isometric hand functions. *Journal of Biomechanics* 9:387–396.

Chao, E.Y.S., An, K.N., Cooney, W.P., and Linsheid, R.L. (1989). *Biomechanics of the Hand: A Basic Research Study.* Singapore: World Scientific.

Chen, Y. (1991). An evaluation of hand pressure distribution for a power grasp and forearm flexor muscle contribution for a power grasp on cylindrical handles. Unpublished PhD dissertation. Lincoln, NE: University of Nebraska.

Claudon, L. (2006). Influence on grip of knife handle surface characteristics and wearing protective gloves. *Applied Ergonomics* 37:729–735.

Claudon, L. and Marsot, J. (2006). Effect of knife sharpness on upper limb biomechanical stresses—A laboratory study. *International Journal of Industrial Ergonomics* 36:239–246.

Cochran, D.J. and Riley, M.W. (1982). An evaluation of handle shapes and sizes. *Proceedings of the Human Factors Society* 26:408–412.

Cochran, D.J. and Riley, M.W. (1983). An examination of the speed of manipulation of various sizes and shapes of handles. *Proceedings of the Human Factors Society* 27:432–436.

Cochran, D.J. and Riley, M.W. (1986a). An evaluation of knife handle guarding. *Human Factors* 27:253–265.

Cochran, D.J. and Riley, R.W. (1986b). The effects of handle shape and size on exerted forces. *Human Factors* 28:295–301.

Cole, K.J. (1991). Grasp force control in older adults. *Journal of Motor Behavior* 23:251–258.

Cole, K.J. and Abbs, J.H. (1987). Kinematic and electromyographic responses to perturbation of a rapid grasp. *Journal of Neurophysiology* 57:1498–1510.

Comaish, S. and Bottoms, E. (1971). The skin and friction: Deviations from Amonton's laws and the effects of hydration and lubrication. *British Journal of Dermatology* 84:37–43.

Copley, F.B. (1923). *Frederick W. Taylor*, Vol. II. New York: Harper, pp. 56–67.

Corrigan, D.L., Foley, V., and Widule, C.J. (1981). Axe use efficiency—A work theory explanation of an historical trend. *Ergonomics* 24:103–109.

Damon, A., Stoudt, H.W., and McFarland, R.A. (1966). *The Human Body in Equipment Design*. Cambridge, MA: Harvard University Press.

DiDomenico, A. and Nussbaum, M.A. (2003). Measurement and prediction of single and multi-digit finger strength. *Ergonomics* 46:1531–1548.

DiDomenico, A. and Nussbaum, M.A. (2008). Estimation of forces exerted by the fingers using standardised surface electromyography from the forearm. *Ergonomics* 51:1858–871.

Dressel, G., Karrasch, K., and Spitzer, H. (1954). Arbeitsphysiologische Untersuchungen beim Schaufeln, Steinetragen, und Schubkarreschieben (Work physiology studies of shoveling, stone carrying and wheelbarrow pushing). *Zentralblatt für Arbeitswissenschaft und soziale Betriebspraxis* 3:33–48.

Drillis, R.J. (1963). Folk norms and biomechanics. *Human Factors* 5:427–441.

Drillis, R., Schneck, D., and Gage, H. (1963). The theory of striking tools. *Human Factors* 5:467–478.

Drury, C.G. (1980). Handles for manual materials handling. *Applied Ergonomics* 11:35–42.

Ducharme, R.E. (1975). Problem tools for women. *Industrial Engineering* Sep:46–50.

Duke, K., Mirka, G.A., and Sommerich, C.M. (2004). Productivity and ergonomic investigation of bent-handle pliers. *Human Factors* 46:234–243.

Dusenberry, D.O., Simpson, H., and DelloRusso, S.J. (2009). Effect of handrail shape on graspability. *Applied Ergonomics* 40:657–669.

Eastman Kodak Company. (1983). *Ergonomic Design for People at Work*. Belmont, CA: Lifetime Learning Publications, pp. 140–159.

Edgren, C.S., Radwin, R.G., and Irwin, C.B. (2004). Grip force vectors for varying handle diameters and hand sizes. *Human Factors* 46:244–251.

Ejeskar, A. and Örtengren, R. (1981). Isolated finger flexion force—A methodological study. *British Society for Surgery of the Hand* 13:223–230.

Emanuel, J.T., Mills, S.J., and Bennett, J.F. (1980). In search of a better handle. *Proceedings of the Symposium of Human F actors and Industrial Design in Consumer Products*. Medford, MA: Tufts University, pp. 34–40.

Evans, T.E., Lucaccini, L.F., Hazell, J.W., and Lucas, R.J. (1973). Evaluation of dental hand instruments. *Human Factors* 15:401–406.

Fellows, G.L. and Freivalds, A. (1991). Ergonomics evaluation of a foam rubber grip for tool handles. *Applied Ergonomics* 22:225–230.

Fox, K. (1957). The effect of clothing on certain measures of strength of upper extremities (Report EP-47). Natick, MA: Environmental Protection Branch, U.S. Army Quartermaster Research and Development Center.

Fraser, T.M. (1980). *Ergonomic Principles in the Design of Hand Tools*. Occupational Safety and Health Series, No. 44. Geneva, Switzerland: International Labour Office.

Freivalds, A. (1986a). The ergonomics of shovelling and shovel design—A review of the literature. *Ergonomics* 29:3–18.

Freivalds, A. (1986b). The ergonomics of shovelling and shovel design—An experimental study. *Ergonomics* 29:19–30.

Freivalds, A. (1987). The ergonomics of tools. *International Reviews of Ergonomics* 1:43–75.

Freivalds, A. (1999). Ergonomics of hand tools. In: W. Karwowski and W.S. Marras (eds), *Occupational Ergonomics Handbook*. Boca Raton: CRC Press, pp. 461–478.

Freivalds, A. and Eklund, J. (1993). Reaction torques and operator stress while using powered nut-runners. *Applied Ergonomics* 24:158–164.

Freivalds, A. and Kim, Y.J. (1990). Blade size and weight effects in shovel design. *Applied Ergonomics* 21:39–42.

Garrett, J. (1971). The adult human hand: Some anthropometric and biomechanical considerations. *Human Factors* 13:117–131.

Gläser, H. (1933). *Beiträge zur Form der Waldsäge und zur Technik des Sägens* (Contributions to the design of forestry saws and sawing techniques). Dissertation. Eberswalde, Germany.

Goel, V.K. and Rim, K. (1987). Role of gloves in reducing vibration: An analysis for pneumatic chipping hammer. *American Industrial Hygiene Association Journal* 48:9–14.

Gorjatschkin, W. (1924). Theory of striking hand tools. *Herald of Metal Industry*, Moscow, No. 4 (in Russian).

Granada, M. and Konz, S. (1981). Evaluation of bent hammer handles. *Proceedings of the Human Factors Society* 25:322–324.

Grant, K.A., Habes, D.J., and Steward, L.L. (1992). An analysis of handle designs for reducing manual effort: The influence of grip diameter. *International Journal of Industrial Ergonomics* 10:199–206.

Greenberg, L. and Chaffin, D.B. (1976). *Workers and Their Tools*. Midland, MI: Pendell.

Grieve, D. and Pheasant, S. (1982). Biomechanics. In: W.T. Singleton (ed.), *The Body at Work*. Cambridge, UK: Cambridge University Press, pp. 142–150.

Guilfoyle, J. (1977). Look what design has done for the toothbrush. *Industrial Design* 24:24–38.

Habes, D.J. and Grant, K.A. (1997a). An electromyographic study of maximum torques and upper extremity muscle activity in simulated screw driving tasks. *International Journal of Industrial Ergonomics* 20:339–346.

Habes, D.J. and Grant, K.A. (1997b). An electromyographic study of strength and upper extremity muscle activity in simulated meat cutting tasks. *Applied Ergonomics* 28:129–137.

Hall, N.B. and Bernett, E.M. (1956). Empirical assessment of handrail diameters. *Journal of Applied Psychology* 40:381–382.

Heffernan, C. and Freivalds, A. (2000). Optimum pinch grips in the handling of dies. *Applied Ergonomics*. 31:409–414.

Hertzberg, H.T.E. (1973). Engineering anthropometry. In: H. Van Cott and R. Kincaid (eds), *Human Engineering Guide*. Washington, DC: U.S. Government Printing Office, pp. 467–584.

Hull, S.S. (2007) *Evaluation of Ergonomic Interventions for Bucking Bars in Aircraft Manufacturing*. PhD Thesis. Wichita State University, Wichita, KS.

Humphreys, P.W., Lind, A.R., and Sweetland, J.S. (1962). The energy expenditure of coal miners at work. *British Journal of Industrial Medicine* 19:264–275.

Hunt, L.I. (1934). A study of screwdrivers for small assembly work. *The Human Factor* 8:70–73.

Huston, T.R., Sanghavi, N., and Mital, A. (1984). Human torque exertion capabilities on a fastener device with wrenches and screwdrivers. In: A. Mital (ed.), *Trends in Ergonomics/ Human Factors*, Vol. I. Amsterdam, The Netherlands: Elsevier, pp. 51–58.

Jack, R.L. (2005). The effectiveness of using two different types of anti-vibration gloves compared to bare hand condition at dampening the frequencies associated with hand-arm vibration syndrome. *Work* 25:197–203.

Jackson, D.A. and Clifford, J.C. (1989). Electrodiagnosis of mild carpal tunnel syndrome. *Archives of Physical Medicine Rehabilitation* 70:199–204.

Jetzer, T., Haydon, P., and Reynolds, D. (2003). Effective intervention with ergonomics, anti-vibration gloves, and medical surveillance to minimize hand-arm vibration hazards in the workplace. *Journal of Occupational and Environmental Medicine* 45:1312–1317.

Johansson, R.S. (1991). How is grasping modified by somatosensory input? In: D.R. Humphrey and H.J. Freund (eds), *Motor Control: Concepts and Issues*. Chichester, U.K.: John Wiley, pp. 331–355.

Johansson, R.S. and Westling, G. (1984). Roles of glabrous skin receptors and sensorimotor memory in automatic control of precision grip when lifting rougher or more slippery objects. *Experimental Brain Research*. 56:550–564.

Johansson, R.S. and Westling, G. (1987). Signals in tactile afferents from the fingers eliciting adaptive motor responses during precision grip. *Experimental Brain Research* 66:141–154.

Johansson, R.S., Huger, C., and Bäckström, L. (1992). Somatosensory control of precision grip during unpredictable pulling loads, III. Impairments during digital anesthesia. *Experimental Brain Research* 89:204–213.

Johnson, S.L. (1988). Evaluation of powered screwdriver design characteristics. *Human Factors* 30:61–69.

Kao, H. (1976). An analysis of user preference toward handwriting instruments. *Perceptual and Motor Skills* 43:522.

Kao, H. (1977). Ergonomics in penpoint design. *Acta Psychologica Taiwanica* 18:49–52.

Kao, H. (1979). Differential effects of writing instruments on handwriting performance. *Acta Psychologica Taiwanica* 21:9–13.

Karlqvist, L. (1984). Cutting operation at canning bench—A case study of handtool design. *Proceedings of the 1984 International Conference on Occupational Ergonomics*. Ontario, Canada: Human Factors Association of Canada, pp. 452–456.

Ketchum, L.D., Thompson, D., Pocock, G., and Wallingford, D. (1978). A clinical study of forces generated by the intrinsic muscles of the index finger and the extrinsic flexor and extensor muscles of the hand. *Journal of Hand Surgery* 3:571–578.

Kirsch, G. (1939). *Untersuchungen über die zweckmässigste Gestalt der Schaufelns* (Research on an effective shovel shape). Dissertation. Berlin-Charlottenberg, Germany: Technische Hochschule.

Knowlton, R.G. and Gilbert, J.C. (1983). Ulnar deviation and short term strength reductions as affected by a curve handled ripping hammer and a conventional claw hammer. *Ergonomics* 26:173–179.

Kommerell, G. (1929). Die Schaufelarbeit in gebückter Haltung (Shoveling while in a bent posture). *Arbeitsphysiologie* 1:278–295.

Kong, Y.K. (2001). Optimum design of handle shape through biomechanical modeling of hand tendon forces. Unpublished PhD dissertation. University Park, PA: The Pennsylvania State University.

Kong, Y.K. and Freivalds, A. (2003). Evaluation of meat-hook handle shapes. *International Journal of Industrial Ergonomics* 32:12–23.

Kong, Y.K. and Lowe, B.D. (2005a). Optimal cylindrical handle diameter for grip force tasks. *International Journal of Industrial Engineering* 35:495–507.

Kong, Y.K. and Lowe, B.D. (2005b). Evaluation of handle diameters and orientation in a maximum torque task. *International Journal of Industrial Engineering* 35:1073–1084.

Konz, S. (1974). Design of handtools. *Proceedings of the Human Factors Society* 18:292–300.

Konz, S. (1975). Design of food scoops. *Applied Ergonomics* 6:32.

Konz, S. (1986). Bent hammer handles. *Human Factors* 27:317–323.

Konz, S. and Johnson, S. (2000). *Work Design*, 5th edn, Scottsdale, AZ: Holcomb Hathaway, Inc.

Konz, S. and Streets, B. (1984). Bent hammer handles performance and preference. *Proceedings of the Human Factors Society* 28:438–440.

Konz, S. and Warraich, M. (1985). Performance differences between the preferred and non-preferred hand when using various tools. In: I.D. Brown, R. Goldsmith, K. Coombes, and M.A. Sinclair (eds), *Ergonomics International'85*. London: Taylor & Francis, pp. 451–453.

Kroemer, K.H.E. (1986). Coupling the hand with the handle: An improved notation of touch grip and grasp. *Human Factors* 27:337–339.

Kroemer, K.H.E. (1989). Cumulative trauma disorders: Their recognition and ergonomics measures to avoid them. *Applied Ergonomics* 20:274–280.

Kroemer, K.H.E. (1992). Avoiding cumulative trauma disorders in shops and offices. *American Industrial Hygiene Association Journal* 53:596–604.

Krohn, R. and Konz, S. (1982). Bent hammer handles. *Proceedings of the Human Factors Society* 26:413–417.

Larivière, C., Plamondon, A., Lara, J., Tellier, C., Boutin, J., and Dagenais, A. (2004). Biomechanical assessment of gloves. A study of the sensitivity and reliability of electromyographic parameters used to measure activation and fatigue of different forearm muscles. *International Journal of Industrial Ergonomics* 34:101–116.

Latash, M.L. (2008). *Neurophysiological Basis of Movement*, 2nd edn, Champaign, IL: Human Kinetics.

Lavender, S.A., Marras, W.S., Lundquist, R.G., Rockwell, T.H., and Bobick, T.G. (1986). Analysis of hand tool accidents in the underground mining industry. *Proceedings of the Human Factors Society* 30:1419–1423.

Laveson, J.K. and Meyer, R.P. (1976). Left out "lefties" in design. *Proceedings of the Human Factors Society* 20:122–125.

Leakey, L.S.B. (1960). Finding the world's earliest man. *National Geographic* 118:420–435.

Lee, J.L., Kong, Y.K., Lowe, B.D., and Song, S. (2009). Handle grip span for optimising finger-specific force capability as a function of hand size. *Ergonomics* 52:601–608.

Lee, J.W. and Rim, K. (1990). Maximum finger force prediction using a planar simulation of the middle finger. *Proceedings of the Institute of Mechanical Engineers* 204:167–178.

Lehmann, G. (1953). *Praktische Arbeitsphysiologie* (Practical Work Physiology). Stuttgart, Germany: Thieme, pp. 182–197.

Lindstrom, F.E. (1973). *Modern Pliers*. Enköping, Sweden: Bahco Verktyg.

Lowe, B.D. and Freivalds, A. (1999). Effect of carpal tunnel syndrome on grip force coordination on hand tools. *Ergonomics* 42:550–554.

Magill, R. and Konz, S. (1986). An evaluation of seven industrial screwdrivers. In: W. Karwowski (ed.), *Trends in Ergonomics/Human Factors*, Vol. III. Amsterdam, The Netherlands: Elsevier, pp. 597–604.

Marras, W.S. (1986). Measurements of spine loading components during the usage of large hand tools. In: W. Karwowski (ed.), *Trends in Ergonomics/Human Factors*, Vol. III. Amsterdam, The Netherlands: Elsevier, pp. 693–699.

Marras, W.S. and Rockwell, T.H. (1986). An experimental evaluation of method and tool effects in spike maul use. *Human Factors* 27:267–281.

Materials Handling Research Unit. (1980). *Force Limits in Manual Work*. Guildford; UK: IPC Science and Technology Press.

Mathiowetz, V., Wiemer, D.M., and Federman, S.M. (1986). Grip and pinch strength: Norms for 6- to 19-year olds. *American Journal of Occupational Therapy* 40:705–711.

McCormick, F.J. and Sanders, M.S. (1982). *Human Factors in Engineering Design*, 5th edn, New York: McGraw-Hill, pp. 283–309.

Meyer, F. (1930). Arbeitsgrösse, Arbeitsaufwand und Arbeitsökonomie beim hantieren schwerer Hammer. (Power, expenditure, and efficiency for work using a heavy hammer.) *Arbeitsphysiologie* 3:529.

Miller, G. and Freivalds, A. (1987). Gender and handedness in grip strength. *Proceedings of the Human Factors Society, 31st Annual Meeting*, Santa Monica, CA, pp. 906–909.

Miller, M., Ransohoff, J., and Tichauer, E.R. (1971). Ergonomic evaluation of a redesigned surgical instrument. *Applied Ergonomics* 2:194–197.

Mital, A. (1985). Effects of tool and operator factors on volitional torque exertion capabilities of individuals. In: I.D. Brown, R. Goldsmith, K. Coombes, and M.A. Sinclair (eds), *Ergonomics International'85*. London, U.K.: Taylor & Francis, pp. 262–264.

Mital, A. (1986). Effect of body posture and common hand tools on peak torque exertion capabilities. *Applied Ergonomics* 17:87–96.

Mital, A. and Sanghavi, N. (1986). Comparison of maximum volitional torque exertion capabilities of males and females using common hand tools. *Human Factors* 27:283–294.

Mital, A., Sanghavi, N., and Huston, T. (1985). A study of factors defining the operator-hand tool system at the work place. *International Journal of Production Research* 23:297–314.

Mital, A., Kuo, T., and Faard, H.F. (1994). A quantitative evaluation of gloves used with non-powered hand tools in routine maintenance tasks. *Ergonomics* 37:333–343.

Monod, H. and Scherrer, J. (1965). The work capacity of a synergic muscular group. *Ergonomics* 8:329–338.

Morrissey, S., Bethea, N.J., and Ayoub, M.M. (1983). Task demands for shoveling in non-erect postures. *Ergonomics* 26:297–951.

Müller, E.A. and Karrasch, K. (1956). Die grösste Dauerleistung beim Schaufeln (The longest shoveling work period). *Internationale Zeeitchrift für angewandte Physiologie einschliesslich Arbeitsphysiologie* 16:318–324.

Napier, J. (1956). The prehensile movements of the human hand. *Journal of Bone and Joint Surgery* 38B:902–913.

Napier, J. (1962). The evolution of the hand. *Scientific American* 207(12):56–62.

Napier, J. (1963). Early man and his environment. *Discovery* 24(3):12–18.

Oh, S. and Radwin, R.L. (1993). Pistol grip power tool handle and trigger size effects on grip exertions and operator preference. *Human Factors* 35:551–569.

O'Meara, D.M. and Smith, R.M. (2002). Functional handgrip test to determine the coefficient of static friction at the hand/handle interface. *Ergonomics* 45:717–731.

Paddan, G.S. and Griffin, M.J. (1998). Effect of push force on the transmission of shear vibration through gloves. *Eighth International Conference on Hand-Arm Vibration*, Arbetslivsrapport ISSN 1401-2928. Stockholm, Sweden: Arbetslivsinstitutet.

Pheasant, S.T. and O'Neill, D. (1975). Performance in gripping and turning—A study in hand/handle effectiveness. *Applied Ergonomics* 6:205–208.

Pheasant, S.T. and Scriven, J.G. (1983). Sex differences in strength—Some implications for the design of handtools. In: K. Coombes (ed.), *Proceedings of the Ergonomics Society's Conference 1983*. London: Taylor & Francis, pp. 9–13.

Potvin, J.R., Agnew, M.J., and Ver Woert, C. (2004). An ergonomic comparison of pneumatic and electrical pistol grip hand tools. *International Journal of Industrial Ergonomics* 34:467–478.

Radhakrishnan, S. and Nagaravindra, M.C. (1993). Analysis of hand forces in health and disease during maximum isometric grasping of cylinders. *Medicine and Biological Engineering and Computing* 31:372–376.

Rens, G., Dubrulle, P., and Malchaire, J. (1987). Efficiency of conventional gloves against vibration. *Annals of Occupational Hygiene* 31:249–254.

Replogle, J.O. (1983). Hand torque strength with cylindrical handles. *Proceedings of the Human Factors Society* 27:412–416.

Reynolds, D. and Jetzer, T. (1998). Use of air bladder technology to solve hand tool vibration problems. *Eighth International Conference on Hand-Arm Vibration*, Arbetslivsrapport ISSN 1401-2928. Stockholm, Sweden: Arbetslivsinstitutet.

Rice, M.S., Leonard, C., and Carter, M. (1998). Grip strengths and required forces in accessing everyday containers in a normal population. *American Journal of Occupational Therapy* 52:621–626.

Rigby, L.V. (1973). Why do people drop things? *Quality Progress* 6:16–19.

Rock, K.M., Mikat, R.P., and Foster, C. (2001). 'The effects of gloves on grip strength and three-point pinch. *Journal of Hand Therapy* 14:286–290.

Rockwell, T.H. and Marras, W.S. (1986). An evaluation of tool design and method of use of railroad leverage tools on back stress and tool performance. *Human Factors* 27:303–315.

Rohmert, W. (1973). Problems in determining rest allowances. *Applied Ergonomics* 4:91–95.

Rothfleisch, S. and Sherman, D. (1978). Carpal tunnel syndrome: Biomechanical aspects of occupational occurrence and implications regarding surgical management. *Orthopaedic Review* 7:107–109.

Roubal, J. and Kovar, Z. (1962). Tool handles and control levers of machines. *Annals of Occupational Hygiene* 5:37–40.

Rubarth, B. (1928). Untersuchung zur Festgestaltung von Handheften für Schraubenzieher und ähnliche Werkzeuge (Research on handles for screwdrivers and similar tools). *Industrielle Psychotechnik* 5:129–142.

Sampson, E. and Van Niekerk, J.L. (2003). Literature survey on anti-vibration gloves. Safety in Mines Research Committee (http://hdl.handle.net/10204/1304).

Saran, C. (1973). Biomechanical evaluation of T-handles for a pronation supination task. *Journal of Occupational Medicine* 15:712–716.

Scheller, W.L. (1983). The effect of handle shape on grip fatigue in manual lifting. *Proceedings of the Human Factors Society* 27:417–421.

Seo, N.J. (2009). Dependence of safety margins in grip force on isometric push force in lateral pinch. *Ergonomics* 52:840–847.

Seo, N.J., Armstrong, T.J., Chaffin, D.B., and Ashton-Miller, J.A. (2008). Inward torque and high-friction handles can reduce required muscle efforts for torque generation. *Human Factors* 50:37–48.

Shock, N. (1962). The physiology of aging. *Scientific American* 206:100–110.

Silverstein, B.A., Fine, L.J., and Armstrong, T.J. (1987). Occupational factors and carpal tunnel syndrome. *American Journal of Industrial Medicine* 11:343–358.

Smith, C.A., Mirka, G.A., and Myers, K.A. (2000). Ergonomic hand toll interventions for the furniture manufacturing industry. *Proceedings of the Human Factors and Ergonomics Society 2000 Congress,* 44(5):99–102.

Spitzer, H. (1950). Die Rationelle Ausführung der Körperarbeit (Rational organization of physical work). *Stahl und Eisen* 70:509–515.

Stevenson, A.G. and Brown, R.L. (1923). An investigation on the motion study of digging and the energy expenditure involved, with the object of increasing efficiency of output and economising energy. *Journal of the Royal Army Medical Corps* 40:340–349, 423–434; 41:39–45, 99–111.

Suizu, K. and Harada, N. (2005). Effects of waterproof covering on hand immersion tests using water at 10°C, 12°C and 15°C for diagnosis of hand-arm vibration syndrome. *International Archives of Occupational and Environmental Health* 78:311–318.

Swain, A.D., Shelton, G.G., and Rigby, L.V. (1970). Maximum torque for small knobs operated with and without gloves. *Ergonomics* 13:201–208.

Tannen, K.J., Stetson, D.S., Silverstein, B.A., Fine, L.J., and Armstrong, T.J. (1986). An evaluation of scissors for control of upper extremity disorders in an automobile upholstery plant. In: W. Karwowski (ed.), *Trends in Ergonomics/Human Factors,* Vol. III. Amsterdam, The Netherlands: Elsevier, pp. 631–639.

Taylor, F.W. (1913). *The Principles of Scientific Management.* New York: Harper & Row.

Terrell, R. and Purswell, J. (1976). The influence of forearm and wrist orientation on static grip strength as a design criterion for hand tools. *Proceedings of the Human Factors Society* 20:28–32.

Tichauer, E.R. (1966). Some aspects of stress on forearm and hand in industry. *Journal of Occupational Medicine* 8:63–71.

Tichauer, E.R. (1976). Biomechanics sustains occupational safety and health. *Industrial Engineer* Feb:46–56.

Tichauer, E.R. (1978). *The Biomechanical Basis of Ergonomics.* New York: Wiley.

Tichauer, E.R. and Gage, H. (1977). Ergonomic principles basic to hand tool design. *Journal of the American Industrial Hygiene Association* 38:622–634.

Udo, H., Otani, T., Udo, A., and Yoshinaga, F. (2000). A electromyographic study of two different types of ball point pens. *Industrial Health* 38:47–50.

Vennewald, H. (1939). Über die Zweckmässigkeit der Grabwerkzeugen (On the efficiency of graveyard tools). *Arbeitsphysiologie* 10:647–667.

Weidman, B. (1970). *Effect of Safety Gloves on Simulated Work Tasks* (AD 738981). Springfield, VA: National Technical Information Service.

Wenzig, K. (1928). Arbeitsphysiologische Studien VII, Beiträge zur Physiologie des Schaufelns (Contributions to the physiology of shoveling). *Arbeitsphysiologie* 1:154–186.

Wenzig, K. (1932). Arbeitsphysiologische Studien X, Beiträge zur Physiologie des Schaufelns (Contributions to the physiology of shoveling). *Arbeitsphysiologie* 5:252–268.

Westling, G. and Johansson, R.S. (1984). Factors influencing the force control during precision grip. *Experimental Brain Research* 53:277–284.

Westling, G. and Johansson, R.S. (1987). Responses in glabrous skin mechanoreceptors. *Experimental Brain Research* 66:128–140.

Widule, C.J., Foley, V., and Demo, F. (1978). Dynamics of the axe swing. *Ergonomics* 21:925–930.

Willms, K., Wells, R., and Carnahan, H. (2009). Glove attributes and their contribution to force decrement and increased effort in power grip. *Human Factors* 51:797–812.

Wyndham, C.H., Morrison, J.F., Williams, C.G., Heyns, R., Margo, E., Brown, A.M., and Astrup, J. (1966). The relationship between energy expenditure and performance index in the task of shovelling sand. *Ergonomics* 9:371–378.

Wyndham, C.H., Morrison, J.F., Viljoen, J.H., Strydom, N.B., and Heynes, R. (1969). Factors affecting the mechanical efficiency of men shovelling rock in stopes. *Journal of the South African Institute of Mining and Metallurgy* 70:53–59.

Yakou, T., Yamamoto, K., Koyama, M., and Hyodo, K. (1997). Sensory evaluation of grip using cylindrical objects. *International Journal of the Japanese Society of Mechanical Engineers* 40:730–735.

Yoder, T.A., Lucas, R.L., and Botzum, C.D. (1973). The marriage of human factors and safety in industry. *Human Factors* 15:197–205.

Zatsiorsky, V.M. and Latash, M.L. (2009). Multi-finger prehension: An overview. *Journal of Motor Behavior*. 40:446–476.

Zatsiorsky, V.M., Li, Z.M., and Latash, M.L. (2000). Enslaving effects in multi-finger force production. *Experimental Brain Research* 131:187–195.

10

The Office Environment

10.1 General Musculoskeletal Problems

Musculoskeletal problems in an office environment have existed as long as writing has been known. The cramping of the writer's hand was a common complaint and became the subject of clinical interest and controversy in England as early as 1855, when it was termed scrivener's palsy or, more typically, *writer's cramp*. With the growth of commerce in the Victorian era, a large number of scriveners were responsible for copying all the contracts by hand using a quill, whose thin shaft had to be gripped firmly. The resulting spasms were first described in detail by Wilks (1878) and later by others (Sheehy and Marsden, 1982) as resulting from the repetitive forceful contractions of the hand with complications induced by co-contractions of the forearm flexors and extensors. This interaction of various aspects of the motor system as well as the sensory system, technically termed *focal dystonia*, has only recently been counteracted by the use of peripheral sensory stimulation, high-frequency vibrations, and blocking of selected pathways with lidocaine or botulism (Kaji, 2000). In terms of preventing the problem, increasing the size of a ballpoint pen grip area with a flared design up to a diameter of 13.6 mm significantly reduced EMG of the flexor pollicis brevis and pain scores for various hand regions as compared to a common ballpoint pen during extended writing (Udo et al., 2000).

The gradual reduction of writing implements for data entry in favor of faster means by mechanical typewriters, then electronic typewriters and, eventually, keyboards linked to the personal computer did not eliminate the musculoskeletal problems associated with clerical work. If anything, complaints increased, but for different reasons and in different parts of the body. Whereas over-gripping a quill or pen resulted in writer's cramp, the more constrained posture and high force required to operate the keys of mechanical typewriters resulted in tenosynovitis of the fingers (Çakir et al., 1980). Early electronic keyboards were not much better with a high rate of fatigue and musculoskel et al complaints in Japanese keypunch operators in the 1960s (Komoike and Horiguchi, 1971; Maeda et al., 1982) leading to neck and upper arm pain, termed the cervicobrachial disorder (Maeda, 1977). Similar problems were later observed in Europe (Çakir et al., 1978; Hünting et al., 1981), in Australia (ACTU-VHTC, 1982; Ferguson, 1984; Hocking, 1987), and in the United States leading to a large NIOSH study of journalists and other office workers (NIOSH, 1981). Much of the early concerns were primarily related to non-biomechanical outcomes, such as visual fatigue, near sightedness, color vision changes, various occulomotor changes, radiation leakages leading to skin rashes, cataracts, and even miscarriages, resulting primarily from relatively crude early model visual displays terminals (VDTs) with low pixel densities.

Since then, as the electronics of the VDT improved, the emphasis has been primarily on the musculoskeletal disorders related to the constrained postures, physical layout, keyboards designs, etc. Numerous studies have been performed in this area, too many to cite here. However, there are a number of good reviews that summarize these studies and the various occupational factors leading to these musculoskeletal disorders of the upper extremities including National Research Council (1984), NIOSH (1989), NIOSH (1995), NIOSH (1997), and National Research Council (2001). Among the most commonly observed biomechanical work-related risk factors are high forces, high repetition, vibration, cold exposure, short cycle times (<10 s), hand tool use, deviated postures, acceleration, and hours of keyboard use. The combination of the two major factors, force and repetition, can increase the risk for injury (odds ratio) up to 30 times greater (Silverstein et al., 1986). There are also numerous psychosocial risk factors than enter into the picture: job satisfaction, work speed, monotony, relations with colleagues and supervisors, work content, and control of work. However, being non-biomechanical, these will not be discussed any further.

10.2 Seated Workplace

10.2.1 Seated Posture

The most common overall posture found in an office environment is sitting at a computer workstation. That is not to say, there are not some specialized tasks that are performed in a standing posture, such as copying, working with large-sized drawings, using light tables, and handling photographic reproductions, or some individuals may prefer to work in a standing posture (Thomas Jefferson is the prime historical example—http://standupdesks. com/tj.html), or standing workstations may be used to increase customer throughput by minimizing the time spent dawdling at library or public computer laboratory workstations. However, the vast majority of the time will be spent sitting, which causes large alterations to the shape of the spine and increases in disk pressure, potentially resulting in increased incidences of low-back pain and injuries in subjects who predominantly work in a sitting posture.

10.2.1.1 Spine

The spine or vertebral column is divided into four sections: the *cervical spine* of the neck, the *thoracic spine* of the upper back, the *lumbar spine* of the lower back, and the *sacrum*, primarily fixed within the pelvis. In a standing posture, from the sagittal plane, the spine appear to have an extended-S shape, with several distinctive curves, *lordosis* in the cervical area, *kyphosis* in the thoracic area, and the more critical lumbar lordosis (Figure 10.1). Anatomically, this curve is necessary to maintain the head upright, since the sacrum is tilted considerably down from horizontal (Chaffin et al., 1999). Functionally, one could argue that such curvature provides dampening of impacts to the brain during locomotion and other physical activity.

More importantly, when one moves from a standing to a seated posture, there is a considerable change to the shape of the spine. Because the lumbar spine is joined to the sacrum, which is practically fixed in the pelvis, a rotational movement of the pelvis also directly affects the shape of the lumbar spine. In the process of sitting down, the pelvis rotates

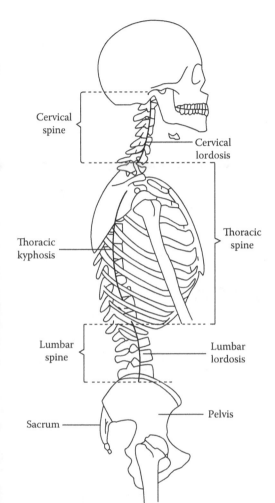

Cervical
spine

Cervical
lordosis

Thoracic
spine

Thoracic
kyphosis

Lumbar
spine

Lumbar
lordosis

Sacrum

Pelvis

FIGURE 10.1

Anatomy of the human spine. (Reproduced from Chaffin, D.B. et al., *Occupational Biomechanics*, 3rd edn., John Wiley & Sons, New York, 1999. With permission.)

backward, causing the lumbar spine to flatten and lose its lordotic shape (Figure 10.2b and c). Sometimes, as in slouching forward, even a pronounced kyphosis can develop (Figure 10.2d). This lumbar flattening has been verified from radiographic studies and can be prevented by the use of lumbar supports (Andersson et al., 1979) or a more posterior-leaning posture (Figure 10.2e; Chaffin et al., 1999).

As described in Chapter 1, the spine consists of the bony vertebrae separated by intervertebral disks, each with a gel-filled nucleus pulposus. Such a fluid-like center allowed for the insertion of a pressure transducer to directly the pressure changes within a disk during various postures (Nachemson and Morris, 1964). Later refinements with a strain-gauge transducer needle allowed more detailed experiments on various office and experimental chairs (Andersson and Örtengren, 1974a; Andersson et al., 1974a,b). These results are shown in Figure 10.3, with a resting sitting position with arms handing down normalized to 100% disk pressure. Disk pressures in a standing posture were found to be 35% lower, while, for reference purposes, a supine posture, with minimal effects of gravity on the disks, yielded a pressure of only 10%. When the arms were marginally supported during writing, disk pressures dropped slightly to 98%. Unsupported arms, as during typewriting, increased disk pressures to 116%. Holding a 1.2 kg with extended arms increased disk pressures to 135%.

FIGURE 10.2
Posture of the pelvis and the lumbar
spine: (a) standing, (b) sitting relaxed,
(c) sitting erect, (d) sitting forward,
and (e) sitting backward (note that
the head faces left). (Reproduced from
Andersson, G.B.J. et al., *Scand. J. Rehabil.
Med.*, 6, 104, 1974a. With permission.)

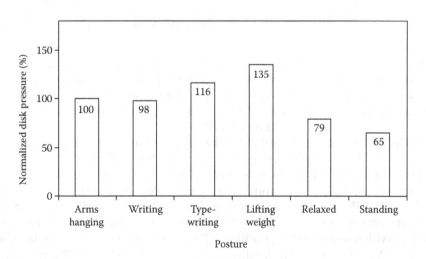

FIGURE 10.3
Mean normalized disk pressures measured in an office chair during simulated work activities (100% = 0.471
MPa or 47.1 N/cm^2). (Adapted from Andersson, G.B.J. and Örtengren, R., *Scand. J. Rehabil. Med.*, 6, 115, 1974a;
Andersson, G.B.J. et al., *Scand. J. Rehabil. Med.*, 6, 128, 1974b.)

10.2.1.2 Disk Compression Forces

In terms of the more commonly used *disk compression forces*, typically calculated from biomechanical modeling (Chaffin et al., 1999), normalized 100% disk pressure corresponds to an absolute pressure of $47.1\,N/cm^2$. Given an average lumbar disk area of $17\,cm^2$ (Pooni et al., 1986), the disk compression forces in a resting sitting posture with arms hanging down is $800\,N$. The criterion disk compression force used as the basis for the recommended weight limit in the NIOSH lifting equation (Waters et al., 1993) is only four times larger at $3400\,N$.

Overall, one can conclude that disk pressures increase considerably as the body goes from a standing to a sitting postures, and as additional loading is put on the shoulders, i.e., arms not supported. This change is pressure is thought to be due to an increase trunk load moment during the pelvic rotation and a deformation of the disk itself (Chaffin et al., 1999). On the other hand, adding a lumbar support and inclining the backrest backward decreases disk pressures (Andersson et al., 1974a). This effect is proportional to the thickness of the lumbar support (approximately an 8% decrease for each 1 cm of pad thickness, see Figure 10.4) and to the inclination of the backrest (approximately a 1.3% decrease for 1° backward movement). The first serves to maintain lumbar lordosis and transfers some of the load to the support, thus reducing the load on the disk, as was also verified indirectly by the reduction of pressures on the seat pan (Shields and Cook, 1988). The second, similarly, transfers some of the load to the backrest and reduces the load on the disks as measured by spinal shrinkage (Corlett and Eklund, 1984a,b). The use of armrests to reduce the loading on the spine decreases the disk pressures by up to 16% (Andersson and Örtengren, 1974b).

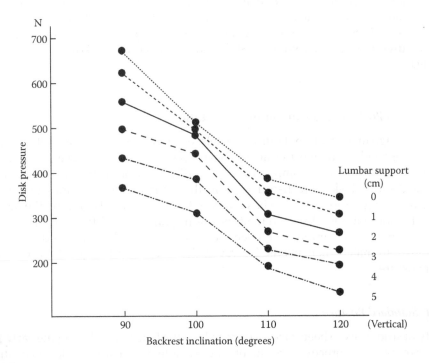

FIGURE 10.4
Disk pressures measured with different backrest inclinations and different size lumbar supports. (Reproduced from Chaffin, D.B. et al., *Occupational Biomechanics*, John Wiley & Sons, New York, 1999. With permission.)

10.2.1.3 Electromyography

Electromyography (EMG) of the back erector spinae muscles has also been used to measure the stresses or loading during a sitting posture. Generally, the EMG levels are low and comparable to a standing posture (Floyd and Silver, 1955; Andersson and Örtengren, 1974a). More forward-leaning postures increase the EMG. However, once forward movement reaches full flexion, i.e., slumping, the EMG levels decrease almost to zero, indicating a relaxation of the erector spinae muscles, with the load being supported by ligaments (Floyd and Silver, 1955). EMG levels also decrease when the arms are supported, reducing some of the load on the muscle (Andersson and Örtengren, 1974b). Similar to disk pressure, EMG levels decrease as the angle between the seat pan and backrest is increased and more of the load is supported by the backrest. However, the effect levels off at angles greater than 110° (Andersson et al., 1974b). Coincidentally, at such angles, it would become increasingly difficult to maintain good visibility of the visual task on the working surface.

One consequence of prolonged sitting is the potential for increased risk of low-back pain (Magora, 1972; Grieco, 1986), although the results are not conclusive (Svensson and Andersson, 1983). The problem appears to be mainly one of postural rigidity, i.e., of remaining too long in one posture, whether standing or sitting (Grieco, 1986). In a large-scale study of 3300 workers, Magora (1972) found that both excessive and minimal time spent in a seated postures are associated with a high frequency of low-back pain, while subjects who varied their working postures, had negligible frequencies. Unfortunately, with higher use of computer workstations, there is a greater tendency toward postural rigidity as found by Grieco (1986) in the telecommunications industry. Specifically, reorganizing a job to include postural flexibility either through a variety of work activities or the use of chairs that promote movements of the body (Festervoll, 1994) such as a sit–stand chair (discussed in Section 10.2.5) is recommended. For further details and guidelines on sitting postures, refer to Åkerblom (1948), Grandjean (1969), Zacharkow (1988), and Chaffin et al. (1999).

10.2.2 Seated Posture at a Computer Workstation

Twenty years ago in a traditional office workplace, the wide variety of activities performed by workers precluded any worries about constrained postures. However, with the almost ubiquitous use of personal computers in the office environment, the risk of incurring work-related musculoskeletal disorders from the static loading of limbs in constrained postures over long periods of time has increased dramatically. Therefore, the availability of adjustable computer workstation to fit the anthropometry of differently sized individuals to an optimal is very important. Even more important is that these individuals adjust the furniture to match their needs. However, there remains the question of what is an optimal posture.

10.2.2.1 Standard Posture

A variety of studies were been carried primarily in the laboratory during the early 1980s as computers entered the office environment. These resulted in postures selected by the tested individuals as their preferred postures and are summarized in Table 10.1. Simultaneously, seating design guidelines were being developed independently based on anthropometric

TABLE 10.1

Preferred Settings and Design Recommendations for a Computer Workstation (Mean Values or Ranges without Wrist of Support)

Workstation Feature	Brown and Schaum (1980)	Miller and Suther (1983)	Grandjean et al. (1982)	Rubin and Marshall (1982)	Grandjean et al. (1983, 1984)	Weber et al. (1984)	AIHA Guide (Kroemer, 1983)	Human Factors and Ergonomics Society (2002)	Traditional Rule of Thumb
Keyboard height (cm)[a]	74	71	77	71	80	78	47–73	56–72	Elbow rest height
Screen height (cm)	99[b]	93[b]	109[b]	87[b]	103[b]	97[b]	91–130[c]	67–84 est.[c]	Seated eye height
Screen angle (°)[d]	10	3	0	—	5	11	±10	±20	Small to avoid glare
Screen distance (cm)	59[e]	—	66[e]	—	76[e]	71[f]	—	>40[f]	Resting focus
Seat height (cm)	50	44	47	42	48	47	36–53	38–56 est.	Popliteal height
Type of study	Lab	Lab	Lab	—	Field	Lab	Design guidelines: 1st per. female to 99th per. male	Design guidelines: 5th per. female to 95th per. male	Basis for design guidelines
Number of subjects	40 females 60 males	15 females 22 males	30 females	—	48 females 20 males	20			

a Home row from floor.
b Center of screen from floor.
c Top of screen from floor.
d Upward tilted screen relative to vertical.
e From center of screen to keyboard edge.
f From center of screen to eyes.

measurements taken in a "standard" seating posture with the trunk vertical and with 90° angles at the elbow, hips, knees, and ankles (see Figure 10.5; Branton, 1974; Diffrient et al., 1974; Webb Associates, 1978). These measurements then evolved into various national and international guidelines or standards such as BSR/HFES 100 (United States), BS EN 1135 (2000; United Kingdom), DIN EN 1135 (1996; Germany), ISO 9241-5 (1998; International), and JIS Z 8513 (1994; Japan). Not unexpectedly, there can be considerable variation in these standards with some of the differences due to ethnic anthropometric differences and others due to trade-offs between interacting parameters assigned different weights. Also, some differences may result from practical considerations, such as the comments of Lueder (1983) that German DIN standards are moving away from excessive workstation adjustability because people tend not to use them. Two of the guidelines for various workstation features are listed in Table 10.1. Specific adjustment ranges for various chair features are given in Figure 10.6 and Table 10.2.

FIGURE 10.5
Standard anthropometric sitting position. (From Webb Associates, *Anthropometric Source Book, Vol. I. Anthropometry for Designers,* National Aeronautics and Space Administration, Washington, DC, 1978.)

The preferred settings for seat height are quite consistent and fall within the design guidelines of 5th percentile female to 95th percentile male popliteal heights. Keyboard preferences tend to be consistent in the range of 71–80 cm above the floor, but tend to be on the high side of the design guidelines based on elbow resting height. Other researchers have observed a similar tendency for operators to prefer the home row of the keyboard to be anywhere from 6 to 9 cm above resting elbow height (Grandjean et al., 1983; Life and Pheasant, 1984; Sauter et al., 1991; Liao and Drury, 2000). In such cases, many of the operators actually tended to lean back, acquiring a 104° trunk angle as opposed to the expected 90° vertical trunk position (Grandjean et al., 1983).

FIGURE 10.6
Adjustable chair. Specific seat parameter values found in Table 10.2. (Reproduced from Freivalds, A., *Niebel's Methods, Standards, and Work Design*, The McGraw-Hill Companies, New York, 2009. With permission.)

Side view

TABLE 10.2

Recommended Seat Adjustment Ranges

Seat Parameter	Design Value (cm)	Comments
A = seat height	38–56	Too high, compresses thighs; too low, disk pressure increases
B = seat depth	<43	Too long, cuts popliteal region; use waterfall contour
C = seat width	>46	Wider seats recommended for overweight individuals
D = seat pan angle	−3°–+3°	Downward tilting requires more friction in the fabric
E = seat back to pan angle	90°–120°	<90° leads to fatigue, >120° requires headrest
F = seat back width	>36	Measured in the lumbar region
G = lumbar support	15–25	Vertical height from compressed seat pan to center of lumbar support
H = foot rest height	2.5–23	—
I = foot rest depth	30.5	—
J = foot rest distance	42	—
K = leg clearance	66	—
L = work surface height	~81	Determined by elbow rest height
M = work surface thickness	<5	Maximum value
N = thigh clearance	>20	Minimum value

Sources: Lines A to G adapted from Human Factors and Ergonomics Society, *Human Factors Engineering of Computer Workstations*, Santa Monica, CA, 2002; lines H to M adapted from Eastman Kodak, *Ergonomics Design for People at Work*, Lifetime Learning Publications, Belmont, CA, 1983.

10.2.2.2 Screen Height

Preferred screen height also varied considerably and tended to be higher than the recommendation based on the top of the screen being at seated eye height (discounting the Kroemer, 1983 recommendation, which was hard to interpret). In both cases, preferred values obtained after short periods in a laboratory could be vastly different from those that result after many hours of work a day for many months or years.

10.2.2.3 Screen Distance

The preferred screen distance is relatively consistent and corresponds closely to the mean intermediate resting focus of 59 cm found in young adults. This position is hypothesized by Leibowitz and Owens (1975) to provide the least amount of stress for the accommodative system of the eyes and should be the most comfortable reading distance. Preferred screen angles were generally small (i.e., the screen was almost vertical), which is the desired position so as to reduce reflection from overhead lights and consequent glare.

10.2.2.4 Arms Support

As mentioned previously, if the arms are unsupported, as during typewriting, disk pressure increased to 16% from a normal seated posture with the arms handing comfortably down (Andersson and Örtengren, 1974b). Therefore, the use of a wrist or forearm support during keyboarding would be recommended as long as the support does not impede the activity. Later studies specifically examining keyboards and supports, found that the use of a wrist support decreased trapezius EMG activity by 25% and was preferred by two-thirds of the subjects (Weber et al., 1984), especially by those with existing shoulder pains and elbows bent at 105° (Erdelyi et al., 1988). Similarly, trapezius EMG activity remained below 1% MVC for almost 50% of the working time with use of wrist supports while the same could be achieved for only 10% of the time without the use of wrist supports (Aarås et al., 1997). The use of wrist supports also significantly decreased wrist flexion (Gerr et al., 2000) and significantly increased the number of keystrokes entered on the second day after practice (Smith et al., 1998). On the other hand, other studies found no improvements with wrist supports (Fernström et al., 1994), with some subjects even reporting an increase in musculoskeletal discomfort (Parsons, 1991). Potentially, the greatest problem with wrist rests may be with the increase of pressures in the carpal tunnel from 14 mm Hg in unsupported wrists to 31 mm Hg while using wrist rests (Horie et al., 1993). Prolonged pressures of 30 mm Hg have been associated with altered nerve function in animal studies (Hargens et al., 1979; Lundborg et al., 1983; Powell and Myers, 1986), which could be the first step in the sequence of events leading to carpal tunnel syndrome (CTS) (Dahlin et al., 1987).

10.2.2.5 Alternate Posture

A cautionary note should be given regarding the traditional 90° seating posture. This posture is not necessarily the posture chosen by all people (Barkla, 1964; Mandal, 1981) and as few as 10% of individuals will actually sit with the trunk vertical (Grandjean et al., 1983). Also, this approach is based on a static posture and ignores the fact that sitting should be a dynamic activity, which should be further encouraged through job design or the use of sit–stand stools. Similarly, although physical workstation dimensions are important determinants of operator posture, the correlations between specific workstation and anthropometric dimensions are not always very high. For example, Gerr et al. (2000) found highest correlations of $r = 0.7$ for line of sight and monitor height and $r = 0.6$ between keyboard height and elbow resting height. However, monitor height and seated eye height showed only a correlation of $r = 0.18$. Overall, the most critical feature is adjustability of the workstation and its furniture, especially seat height, keyboard height, work surface and thus monitor height, and wrist/forearm support.

10.2.3 Determination of Seated Comfort

Seated comfort is obviously a very subjective issue, very much dependent on each individual's preferences as well as the task being performed. Thus, there is no one easy approach to determining a unique value for comfort. Shackel et al. (1969), Branton (1969), Drury and Coury (1982), Lueder (1983), Zacharkow (1988), and Zhang et al. (1996) have suggested a variety of approaches, including (1) comparison with anthropometric data and guidelines, (2) fitting trials, (3) observation of postural changes, (4) observation of task performance, (5) subjective assessment techniques, and (6) physical measures of comfort.

10.2.3.1 Fitting Trials

In fitting trials, the subjects are allowed to adjust the dimensions of the chair or work place until subjective comfort is attained (Jones, 1969; Drury and Coury, 1982). These then can be used as a reference point about which the dimensions are varied so as to establish a tolerable range (LeCarpentier, 1969). The method is reasonably accurate and repeatable in that the selected values compared favorably to anthropometric guidelines (Jones, 1969) and day-to-day variations in mean comfort positions were relatively small, varying only by a couple of degrees or centimeters (LeCarpentier, 1969).

10.2.3.2 Postural Changes

A variety of body movements occur while sitting, ranging from small involuntary motor responses such respiration and heart beat to large intentional movements required for the task. Among these are also restless postural changes attempting to compensate for uncomfortable seating conditions. Grandjean et al. (1960) found a good correlation between the number of body movements and subjective ratings of seat discomfort. Branton and Grayson (1967) were able to identify differences in train seat designs based on both long-term filming of subjects and short-term observations with a larger sample. Cantoni et al. (1984) found a significant decrease in postural changes, ranging from 44% to 71%, at ergonomically designed chairs and VDT workstations as compared to the traditional switchboard workstation being replaced for telephone operators. Fenety et al. (2000) found good reliability in using a pressure mat to track a subject's center of pressure as a means of evaluating sitting discomfort. Unfortunately, postural changes are not solely due to uncomfortable chairs. Heat, humidity, general work stress as well as individual variability and circadian rhythms can also affect restlessness (Jürgens, 1980). The furniture itself may constrain movements and, thus, further limit the usefulness of postural measures as tool for evaluating seating comfort (Karvonen et al., 1962).

10.2.3.3 Task Performance

Intuitively, there should be a relationship between comfort and task performance. Various office surveys (cited in Lueder, 1983) have found that the majority of office workers felt that increased comfort would enhance their productivity. Operationally, in an office setting, this may be harder to prove. Although many studies (Smith et al., 1981; Springer, 1982; Ong, 1984) have shown improved task performance at an ergonomically redesigned VDT workstation, the improvements were probably not solely due to a more comfortable chair, but most likely included all of the other improvements as well, the reduced glare, the copy holders, the arm rests, etc.

10.2.3.4 Subjective Assessment

Subjective assessment of seat comfort is probably the most common evaluation technique due to ease of use and apparent face validity. Typically, overall comfort is elicited through a relatively simple unstructured scale, perhaps with two points (e.g., comfortable/uncomfortable—cited in Drury and Coury, 1982) or three points (uncomfortable, medium, comfortable—Grandjean et al., 1973). More levels, seven (Shvartz et al., 1980), eleven (Shackel et al., 1969), or even the use of a continuous visual analogue scale (Drury and Coury, 1982), in principle, may provide greater precision. Five to seven categories is the optimum number for general psychometric testing (Guilford, 1954). Similarly, a five-category scale, but further partitioned into 10 scale points, was found to be the most reliable and valid scale for rating seating pressure discomfort (Shen and Parsons, 1997).

Since ratings of overall comfort may be influenced by specific factors of the chair design or even factors beyond the chair itself, it may be useful to focus the ratings on selected features of the chair as well as various regions of the body. In the first case, a chair features checklist (see Figure 10.7) was developed by Shackel et al. (1969) and used

FIGURE 10.7
Chair features checklist. (Reprinted from Drury, C.G. and Francher, M., *Appl. Ergon.*, 16, 41, 1985. With permission.)

later by Drury and Coury (1982) to recommend specific design changes in a prototype chair. In the second case, a body discomfort chart, similar to Figure 8.6, has been used to rate specific areas of the body separately using one of the above rating scales (Drury and Coury, 1982). Later, factor analysis was used successfully on an expanded list of comfort/discomfort descriptors in quantifying the multidimensional complexity of seating (Zhang et al., 1996; Helander and Zhang, 1997). The combination of all of the above approaches may give the best overall assessment for a particular chair and especially for the evaluation of a group chairs.

In terms of the actual assessment, a smaller number of pretrained testers may be preferable to a larger sample of untrained subjects, because the former will be more sensitive to lower levels of discomfort (Jones, 1969). Subjects having back pain are particularly sensitive discriminators of seating comfort (Hall, 1972). However, then the ratings might be particularly weighted by back and buttock comfort as found even in normal subjects (Wachsler and Lerner, 1960). The duration of assessment has not been specifically established. Although Wachsler and Learner (1960) found no differences in rank ordering at 5 min with ranking at 4 h, most others (Barkla, 1964; Shackel et al., 1969; Drury and Coury, 1982) have advocated and used longer periods with regular, periodic evaluations.

Perhaps the most important aspects of subjective feelings of comfort for seated workers are having the ability to easily adjust the chair, being provided with sufficient training to be able to make these adjustments, and, most of all, feeling that they have the ability to control their own working environment (Groensteijn et al., 2009; Robertson et al., 2009).

10.2.3.5 Physical Measures

The physical measures discussed in Section 10.2.1 can also be used to assess the comfort of a particular chair. They are especially desirable because of the objective and quantitative nature of the measurements. Although the correlation between physiological parameters and the overall state of comfort or discomfort is not well understood, first signs of discomfort, imperceptible to the subject, appear in EMG of the back muscles. Once the discomfort becomes perceptible, arousal increases with concurrent signs in heart rate and EMG in other muscles not directly related to sitting (Lueder, 1983). A novel alternative is to use an activity monitor (see Section 7.2.4) to measure discomfort-related body movements of a sitting individual. Telfer et al. (2009) found a significant correlation with these movements and subjective discomfort ratings. Also, the pressure on the buttocks is a common reason for feeling discomfort (Slechta et al., 1959; Wotzka et al., 1969), discussed in greater detail in Section 10.2.4.

There are also disadvantages to physical measures. The measurements can be equipment intensive, costly, time consuming, and intrusive to the subject, perhaps even changing the person's responses. A low level of EMG activity in one muscle group may not imply comfort, but may show compensation for an increased level in another group, requiring the measurement of a large number of muscle groups, which further increases the cost and complexity of experimentation. Therefore, no one technique yields a good measure of sitting comfort, and, consequently, a variety or combination of approaches may need to be used.

10.2.4 Seat Pressure

During sitting most of the body weight (65%) is transferred to the seat pan. Some of the weight is also transferred to the floor through the feet (18%), the backrest (4%–5% at 15° posterior inclination), and the armrests (12%) (Swearingen et al., 1962). The weight transfer to the backrest would be even greater if the backrest included a lumbar support (Diebschlag and Müller-Limmroth, 1980). In an anterior-leaning posture or with forward-sloping seat pans, up to 38% of the weight can be transferred through the feet (Jürgens, 1969).

10.2.4.1 Seat Pressure Distribution

Since most of the weight, though, is transferred through the buttocks, it is very important to provide proper seat contour, padding, and shape to achieve an optimum pressure distribution. Within the buttocks and the undersides of the thighs, the major weight-bearing areas are the *ischial tuberosities* or sit bones, which can withstand a pressure of 9 kPa (90 g/cm²) for short periods of time (Rebiffé, 1969). The pressure then decreases as one progresses from these bones to the periphery of the buttocks or thighs, where the values decrease to below 1 kPa (see Figure 10.8). Even given such a small area, each ischial tuberorsity supports up to 18% of the body weight, while each thigh, with a much larger area, supports up to 21% of the body weight. The sacral area supports roughly 5% of the weight (Drummond et al., 1982). Maintaining such a skewed weight distribution can be aided by the use of slightly contoured seats. On the other hand, overly contoured seats may increase pressure on the softer tissues of the undersides of the thighs, restrict movement, and restrict postural flexibility. Therefore, there must be a compromise design between the different constraints. Similarly, the density and thickness of the seat-pan cushioning will affect the pressure distribution, with most guidelines limiting the thickness to 4 cm, with an outer covering that breathes. Similarly, individuals with their own internal padding in the form thick gluteal musculature develop discomfort and pain later than individuals with thin

FIGURE 10.8
Seated pressure distribution (g/cm²).
(Reproduced from Rebiffé, R., *Ergonomics*, 12, 246, 1969. With permission.)

gluteal musculature (Hertzberg, 1972). Further details on instrumentation for measuring seat pressure distributions can be found in Section 7.3.

10.2.4.2 Sores and Ulcers

Excessive localized pressure has been linked to pressure sores and *ischemic ulcers*, which is a major problem in long-term health care (Kosiak, 1959). Pressures above 4.7 kPa (35 mm Hg) for extended time periods are undesirable because they exceed capillary blood pressure (30–35 mm Hg), causing ischemia and putting tissues at risk. However, sitting on unpadded flat wooden chairs yields mean pressures of 43 kPa, exceeding by a magnitude of 10 the pressures causing ischemia (Kosiak et al., 1958). Perhaps the continuous variation in pressure patterns observed during restless sitting allows blood to return to the areas that were temporarily ischemic. Such postural flexibility can be purposefully encouraged through task design similar to the approach used in preventing pressure sores for mobility-impaired workers (Swarts et al., 1988). Houle (1969) even suggested using an automatic device to artificially shift pressure concentrations from one area to another. Kosiak (1959) also found a clear inverse relationship between pressure required to start forming ischemic ulcers and time (see Figure 10.9). Assuming a reduction in pressures to more tolerable levels, this could serve as the basis for sitting-time guidelines.

10.2.4.3 Adaptive Seats

The ultimate approach may be the "intelligent seat system" as prototyped by Ng et al. (1995). Since the buttocks have nonuniform pressure support capability and the material properties of most surfaces have relatively uniform hardness (a hard surface would be

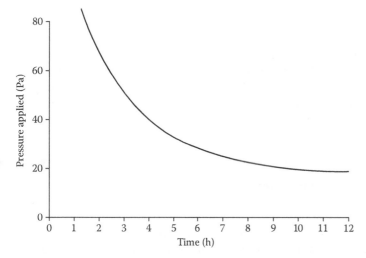

FIGURE 10.9
Pressure–time relationship for the formation of ischemic ulcers. (Adapted from Kosiak, M., *Arch. Phys. Med. Rehabil.*, 40, 62, 1959.)

very uniform, a softer cushion would be less uniform), it would make logical sense to provide an interactive seat that automatically adjusts itself to the individual's pressure distribution by making pressure-sensitive adjustments. In their design, air-filled bladders embedded in the seat were automatically inflated or deflated to optimize seating comfort based on previously collected data on subjective evaluations and pressure distributions. As the seated subject changed posture or position the system would readjust itself accordingly.

10.2.4.4 Cushioning

Overly contoured and cushioned seats or fluid- or gel-filled seats will tend to distribute pressures uniformly across the seat pan and buttocks. Although advocated by some (Sprigle et al., 1990), this approach allows the prominent areas to sink into the support surface, increases pressures on surrounding softer tissues (Lindan et al., 1965), and impedes transport within tissues (Krouskop et al., 1985). Furthermore, regardless of which type of cushioning material is used, including specialized resin-filled foam cushions designed to reduce ulcerations in wheelchair-bound patients, the pressures on the ischial tuberosities always exceeded capillary blood pressures (Mooney et al., 1971).

10.2.4.5 Two-Stage Seats

Given these potential problems with a uniform pressure distribution, Goonetilleke (1998) presents a contrarian view of purposefully promoting localized force concentrations, even beyond those areas that can withstand them (such as the ischial tuberosities) and cites the popular use of beaded seat covers, massage rollers, and knobby health sandals as examples of this approach. Of course, too high pressure concentrations over extended periods of time will lead to localized ischemia, sores, and ulcerations (Kosiak, 1959). Ultimately, the ideal pressure profile for seats may be a two-stage strategy, with an initial distributed-force comfort, followed by a concentrated-force discomfort that encourages postural flexibility. Undoubtedly, seating comfort also depends very much on individual preferences and further research in the area is needed.

10.2.4.6 Foot Pressure

As mentioned previously, the transfer of up to 25% of the body weight to the feet favors the buttocks, but at the cost of the feet. Over the course of a workday, the legs increase in volume by almost 5% and lead to discomfort in the feet, especially in late afternoon (Winkel, 1981; Winkel and Jørgensen, 1986). A higher seat height with a forward-sloping seat pan increased foot swelling as compared to a lower seat with a slightly upward-sloping seat pan (Bendix et al., 1985b). However, modest leg movements every 10–15 min, can reduce the swelling by as much as 50% (Winkel and Jørgensen, 1986).

10.2.5 Sit–Stand, Forward-Sloping, and Saddle Chairs

10.2.5.1 Sit–Stand Chairs

The idea of *sit–stand chairs* or stools (no backrest) has been around for some time, first suggested by Staffel (1884) for maintaining lumbar lordosis and then appearing in the design of school furniture as a chair that could be adjusted for supported standing, sitting, and plain standing (Burgerstein, 1915). Later it was promoted for situations when extreme mobility and reach are required (Laurig, 1969), for assembly work on large vertical frames, high workplaces, areas with inadequate leg room, or certain surgical procedures (Bendix et al., 1985a). Obviously, the change between sitting and standing postures is quick and simple, and the larger angle between the trunk and thighs preserves lumbar lordosis, even without the use of a backrest (Bendix and Biering-Sørensen, 1983). Similarly, spinal loading as measured by spinal compression was found to be lower than with ordinary office chairs (Eklund and Corlett, 1987; Michel and Helander, 1994). More importantly, musculoskeletal complaints are decreased with minimal performance decrements (Husemann et al., 2009). For situations, where users have a choice, even though the users were in general positive to sit–stand workstations, utilization of such workstations may need to be improved with education, motivation, and also the use of electrically controlled adjustments (Wilks et al., 2006).

Two necessary features for a sit–stand chair or stool are height adjustability and a large base of support, so that the stool does not tip over when leaning back and sitting down. If the base is large enough, the feet can even rest on and assist in counterbalancing the backward tipping (see Figure 10.10). The major disadvantage of sit–stand chairs is the decreased used of the backrest and increased pressure on the feet so as to avoid sliding out of the seat. As a note, standing workstations have been modified so as to allow computers users to walk or cycle while performing computer tasks. Straker et al. (2009) found that task performance decreased significantly from a seated workstation, especially for mouse work, probably due to a combined effect of dual-task interference and eye–hand motor control impairment. The reasoning behind this was to counteract some of the effects of a computerized office environment as one of the factors for current sedentary

FIGURE 10.10
Industrial   sit/stand   stool. (Courtesy of Biofit, Waterville, OH.)

FIGURE 10.11
X-ray drawings on the spine in various postures. Normal lying position of balanced muscle relaxation is with a 135° trunk–thigh angle. (Reproduced from Keegan, J.J., *J. Bone Joint Surg.*, 35A, 589, 1953. With permission.)

lifestyles. However, whether this gain is offset by the loss in productivity is something that has to be studied further.

10.2.5.2 Trunk–Thigh Angle

The biomechanical advantages of an increased angle between trunk and thigh was first detailed by Keegan (1953) who took x-rays of individuals lying on their sides (Figure 10.11) and concluded that a posture of about 45° of hip flexion or 135° included trunk–thigh angle to be normal, because that was the posture most typically assumed by individual when lying relaxed on one's side. This is also the posture assumed by individuals under weightless conditions (see Figure 10.12). Similarly, Schoberth (1962) analyzed the sacral base angle with respect to horizontal, which for lordosis of a standing posture is typically around 40°. Upon sitting and the loss of lordosis, the sacral angle was almost parallel with the seat. However, when the seat pan was tilted forward 20°, the base angle increased to 20°, with a noticeable lordosis. Similar results from x-ray studies (Burandt, 1969) led to further recommendations of using forward-sloping seats in office chairs (Burandt and Grandjean, 1969). The forward tilting chair concept was further promoted by Mandal (1976, 1981, 1982) after observing school children tipping their chairs forward and horseback riders having similar large trunk–thigh angles.

10.2.5.3 Forward Sloping Chairs

Objective comparisons of forward-sloping chairs with more conventional chairs confirmed that kyphosis of the lumbar spine tended to decrease with increasing forward-sloping seat pans (Bendix, 1984; Bridger, 1988; Bridger et al., 1989). However, as much as two-thirds

FIGURE 10.12
Typical relaxed posture assumed by individuals in weightless conditions. (From Thornton, W., Anthropometric changes, In: weightlessness, in Webb Associates (ed.), *Anthropometric Source Book*, National Aeronautics and Space Administration, Houston, TX, 1978.)

of the body's adaptation to the forward-sloping seat may have occurred in the hip joints, with only one-third occurring in the lumbar spine (Bendix and Biering-Sørensen, 1983). Still, increasing seat height, along with the forward-sloping seat, tended to increase lordosis. Coincidentally, subjects preferred freely tiltable rather than fixed forward-sloping seats (Bendix, 1984). In either case, seat heights need to be raised approximately 3–5 cm above popliteal height, with a concurrent rise in table heights of 4–6 cm above elbow height (Bendix and Bloch, 1986). Note that the same effect can be obtained by using a pelvic support pad, with angles in the range of 4°–10°, on a conventional chair (Wu et al., 1998).

One of the disadvantages of forward-sloping chairs is the tendency to slide forward in the seat, placing more weight on the feet and increasing foot swelling (Bendix et al., 1985b), with the beneficial effects limited to a forward inclination of 10° unless friction is increased (Rasmussen et al., 2009). To avoid this problem, H.C. Mengshœl of Norway introduced the Balans stool with a 15° forward-sloping seat pan and a knee-support pad to prevent sliding off (Vandraas, 1981). Because of the forward thigh inclination, he did not think a backrest was necessary, thus resulting in a stool. Initial subjective evaluations elicited mixed responses, with complaints of knee and shin pains and problems of entry and egress (Drury and Francher, 1985). Later, in more objective evaluations, the Balans stool approximated standing lumbar lordosis significantly better than conventional chairs (Frey and Tecklin, 1986; Link et al., 1990). When compared to a forward tiltable chair, the Balans stool was again significantly better for lumbar lordosis, but produced no significant difference in spinal shrinkage and heart rate (Bendix et al., 1988). Over extended periods of time, the subjects reported greater fatigue in the Balans stool. Similar results were also reported by Lander et al. (1987) with increased cervical and lumbar EMG readings over time as compared to a conventional chair. Finally, Ericson and Goldie (1989) found significantly greater spinal shrinkage with the Balans stool than with a conventional chair, which they attributed to the lack of a backrest. Thus, the Balans stool may have some benefits for some individuals in some situations, but overall may not be the cure for back pain as claimed by the manufacturers.

Recently, it has become popular to use stability balls as an alternative to traditional office chairs. One common claim is that these balls encourage more trunk movement and muscle activity which would increase core stability and consequently reduce low-back injuries. Gregory et al. (2006) in a controlled study, did find significantly increased muscle activation in the thoracic erector spinae muscles, decreased pelvic tilt in the posterior direction, but increased reported discomfort while on the ball. Similarly, Kingma and van Dieën (2009) found 33% greater trunk motion, 78% greater mean lumbar EMG, but significantly more spinal compression while sitting on the ball as compared to a chair. Therefore, one may wonder whether the advantages of increased trunk and back activity outweigh the disadvantages of increased discomfort and increased spinal loading, and whether these balls should be utilized for prolonged sitting.

10.2.5.4 Saddle Chairs

The main disadvantages of the forward-sloping chairs, slipping forward and out in conventional designs, and increased pressure on the knees in the Balans stool, have been eliminated in another alternative design, the saddle chair. Bendix et al. (1985a) first introduced a saddle like sit–stand chair with the operator straddling the seat and allowing the thighs to slope downward 45° from the conventional horizontal position. This approach was extended by Congleton et al. (1985) by adding a pommel to the forward-sloping seat, forming a more sculpted saddle-like seat (see Figure 10.13). Specifically designed as a sit–stand chair for surgeons, who rated it superior over conventional surgical stools, the chair was later commercially modified for the office environment.

10.2.5.5 Compromise Seat Pan

A final and, perhaps, simplest alternative is a compromise design that maintains the area under the ischial tuberosities horizontal and slopes the front part of the seat pan forward. This design, first suggested by Jürgens (1969) and later studied by Ericson and Goldie (1989) and Graf et al. (1993), allows most of the body weight to be supported by the area best suited for that, preventing forward slippage, but still opens up the trunk–thigh angle to decrease spinal kyphosis. Spinal shrinkage for this design was intermediate between a conventional chair and a Balan's chair (Ericson and Goldie, 1989), erector spinae EMG levels and user discomfort ratings were lower than for a conventional chair (Graf et al., 1993). The only disadvantage of the design appears to a greater percentage of body weight being placed on the feet with concomitant complaints of leg discomfort.

FIGURE 10.13
Saddle chair allowing the operator to straddle the seat. (Courtesy of Neutral Posture Inc., Bryan, TX, http://www.igoergo.com/)

FIGURE 10.14
Electromyographic recordings of shoulder muscle activity: (a) optimal height of home row and (b, c) home row too high, resulting in either elevation of shoulders by trapezius muscle or the abduction of the arms by the deltoid muscle. (Reproduced from Grandjean, E., *Ergonomics in Computerized Offices*, Taylor & Francis, London, U.K. 1987. With permission.)

10.2.6 Work Surface and Line of Sight

10.2.6.1 Work Surface Height

The placement of the work surface is of critical importance in the design of an office environment. If the working height is too high, above the resting elbow height, the shoulders may be elevated with increased activity of the trapezius muscle (see Figure 10.14b) or the upper arms may be abducted with increased activity of the deltoid muscle (see Figure 10.14c). In either case, eventual fatigue and discomfort to the neck, shoulders, and arms will occur. If the working height is too low, below the resting elbow height, the neck or back will be excessively flexed, resulting in neck and back discomfort. In fact, most of the muscles observed in Figure 10.14b,c are in nonoptimum postures and exceed the recommended static muscular loading limit of 5% of maximal voluntary contraction (Jonsson, 1988). At the optimum working height (see Figure 10.15a), the home row of the keyboard or the level of the writing surface is set at the resting elbow height. In this posture, muscle activity is at a relative minimum (Hagberg, 1982; cited in Grandjean, 1987), task performance is at a maximum (Ellis, 1951). These studies support the often cited principle for determining work surface height: upper arms hang down naturally and elbows flexed at 90° so that the forearms are parallel to the ground (see Figure 9.8 and 10.14a).

FIGURE 10.15
Tilting of work surface to bring details closer to line of sight.

There are modifications to the principle with the work surface height being adjusted to the task being performed (Ayoub, 1973). For difficult to see material such as poor-quality typeface or fine assembly, it is advantageous to raise the work surface 10–20 cm above elbow height, to bring details closer to the normal line of sight (see Figure 10.15). Another, perhaps better, alternative is to tilt the work surface approximately 15°. However, rounded parts then have a tendency to roll off the surface. It is also desirable to support the elbow and reduce the previously mentioned static loading. During manual work with heavier parts, the work surface should be lowered up to 10 cm to take advantage of the stronger trunk muscles. However, this distance will be limited by knee height and the thickness of the work surface and one should consider a standing workplace with the work surface height as much as 40 cm below elbow height. In any case, an easily adjustable work surface to accommodate different-sized individuals and various tasks should be the norm. Also, the bottom height of the work surface should allow sufficient leg room for the worker.

10.2.6.2 Line of Sight

The *normal line of sight* for seated workers has often been quoted at approximately 15° (±15°) below horizontal (McCormick, 1970; VanCott and Kinkade, 1972; Eastman Kodak, 1983; Grandjean, 1988), but with little definitive research to substantiate these recommendations and without a clear definition of horizontal. Early researchers (see Table 10.3) simply related the viewing angle to an undefined "horizontal," whereas later researchers used either the *Frankfurt plane* (FP), the *eye–ear line* (EEL), or *Reid's base line* (RBL) as a reference line (see Figure 10.16). The Frankfurt plane is delineated by a line (in the sagittal plane) passing through the *tragion* (notch above the piece cartilage that is just anterior to the auditory passage) and the lower ridge of the eye socket and roughly corresponds to horizontal when the head is held erect (Hill and Kroemer, 1986). The eye–ear line passes through the outer corner of the eyelid and the center of the auditory canal. The two differ by roughly by 13°, 11° as reported by Menozzi et al. (1994) or 15° as reported by Jampel and Shi (1992).

TABLE 10.3

Normal Line of Sight for a 0.5 m Reading Distance

Reference	Type of Study	Preferred Line of Sight (°)		
		Original	Ref.	Converted to FP
Lehmann and Stier (1961)	Lab	−38	Unknown	—
Grandjean et al. (1983)	Field—VDT	−9	Unknown	—
Kroemer and Hill (1986)	Lab—Landolt rings	−33	FP	−33
Heuer et al. (1991)	Lab—non-VDT	−11.3	~10° from FP	−21.3
	Lab—vergence	−13.5		−23.5
Menozzi et al. (1994)	Lab—LEDs	−12.3	FP	−12.3
Villanueva et al. (1996)	Lab—VDT (force positions)	−27.9 to −43.2	EEL	−14.9 to −30.2
Jaschinski et al. (1998)	Field—VDT	−8.6	Unknown	—
Burgess-Limerick et al. (1998)	Lab—VDT	−22 to −27	EEL	−9 to −14
Mon-Williams et al. (1999)	Lab—VDT	−26.8 to −33	EEL	−13.8 to −20
Sommerich et al. (2001)	Lab—VDT	−36.5 (of three choices)	EEL	−23.5
Psihogios et al. (2001)	Field—VDT	−24.3	EEL	−11.3

Note: See Figure 10.17; FP, Frankfurt plane; EEL, eye–ear line; est, estimated.

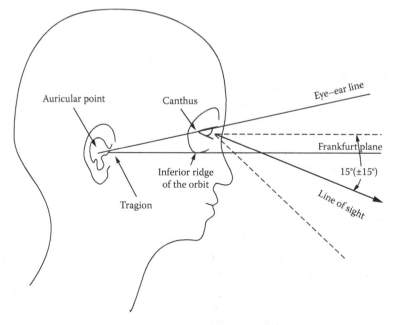

FIGURE 10.16
Normal line of sight with reference to the Frankfurt plane and eye–ear line.

Reid's base line is delineated by a line passing through the center of the auditory canal and the lower ridge of the eye socket, and roughly corresponds to the line created by the Frankfurt plane in the sagittal plane. Unfortunately, in many cases it has been confused with the eye–ear line. There also appears to a difference in the values for normal line of sight obtained from field studies as opposed to laboratory studies. Whereas the latter probably measure the preferred line sight implicitly or explicitly (Heuer et al., 1991) based on resting vergence and resting accommodation, field studies are based on longer time periods and probably take into account musculoskeletal strain due to neck flexion. The true normal line of sight may depend on the task or workplace situation due to the trade-off of various factors including muscular and visual strain.

Most of the reported values for normal line of vision (see Table 10.3) range between −9° and −23.5° (with respect to FP), with a mean of the self-selected positions of approximately −16°. Larger angles of up to −33° were found by Kroemer and Hill (1986) and Villanueva et al. (1996) and may aid vision by improving eye moisture. Sotoyama et al. (1996) reported that larger downward gaze angles decrease the ocular surface area exposed to the atmosphere, potentially reducing the dry-eye problems and the reduced blink rate that arise during VDT use (Yaginuma et al., 1990). However, excessively low-screen positions of −40 (defined by center of screen) significantly increased muscle activity in 6 of 10 neck, shoulder, and back muscles studied (Turville et al., 1998) and cannot be recommended for extended periods of time. Thus, overall, the original recommendation of 15° below horizontal is still quite reasonable, even with the more current larger monitors (Seghers et al., 2003). Also, given that neck flexion of up to 15° produced no subjective discomfort or EMG changes over a 6 h time period (Chaffin, 1973) and line-of-sight standard deviations having a range of ±13° (Hill and Kroemer, 1986), the recommended range of ±15° is also quite reasonable. In practical terms, this means that the center of the screen should be positioned 15° below horizontal, with the top of the screen roughly at horizontal eye level (OSHA, 1991). Similarly, if a copy holder is used, it should be positioned at the same line of sight, only at one side of the screen (Bauer and Witting, 1998).

10.2.6.3 Tilted Work Surface

Tilting the work surface to reduce neck flexion and tension in the neck muscles has been recommended as early as the nineteenth century, especially for school furniture (Staffel, 1984). This practice seems to have decreased over the years, both in the classroom and architectural design studios, but recent epidemiological (Ferguson, 1976) and biomechanical (Less and Eichelberg, 1976) data have revived interest in tilted work surfaces. A sitting horizontal work surface places strain on the cervical spine due to increased torque from the forward inclination of the head (Less and Eichelberg, 1976), increased kyphosis of the lumbar spine, and lack of elbow support (Andersson et al., 1974a). A 15° sloping table top was found to decrease neck flexion angles by approximately 6° (Bridger, 1988) while a 45° sloping desk decreased neck angles by 14° and decreased trapezius activity (Bendix and Hagberg, 1984). This latter steep slope was found to be very acceptable for reading but quite unacceptable for writing, with pencils and paper tending to slide down. Therefore, a compromise design of 10° inclination has been recommended (de Wall et al., 1991; Freudenthal et al., 1991). This resulted in a mean reduction in neck angle of 9°, a mean reduction in trunk angle of 8° and a decrease in back torque of 29%. A slightly larger desk inclination of 15° (along with a forward-sloping chair) was tested in a primary school setting with very favorable ratings as well as a decrease in neck flexion (4°), an increase in hip angle (12°), and a decrease in muscle activity (Marschall et al., 1995). Whether the ratings were due solely to the inclined desk surface or the combination with the sloping chair was difficult to determine. Coincidentally, university students also preferred a slope of 10°–15° for a lecture hall desk (Hira, 1980). In any case, the traditional sloping desk may be returning to favor in the classroom.

10.2.6.4 Working Area

The work surface should be large enough accommodate the items used for the task but critical or more frequently used items should be placed within the *normal working area* as defined by the area circumscribed by the forearm when it is moved in an arc pivoted at a fixed elbow (Maynard, 1934). This area represents the most convenient zone within which motions may be made by that hand with minimum muscle action and expenditure of effort. The maximum working area is defined the area circumscribed by the extended arm. This area defined by a pivoting elbow was defined quantitatively by Farley (1955) for an average male and female while Squires (1956) further modified this area into a "windshield wiper" pattern, by allowing the elbow to move along the arc CD, with the outer edge being limited by 25° lateral shoulder rotation. Since the elbow was allowed to move, the normal working area was increased substantially. Konz and Goel (1969) used Squires (1956) concept to mathematically generate more detailed normal working areas, which, however, did not conform well with the shape of Squires (1956) curve. Therefore, Das and Grady (1983) examined these differences in greater detail, eventually modifying Squires (1956) approach to define coverage on both sides of the body median for 5th, 50th, and 95th percentile males and females (see Figure 10.17; Das and Behara, 1995).

10.2.6.5 Work Space Envelope

The working area concept can be expanded into a *work space envelope*, or the three-dimensional (3D) space within which an individual can work. This is typically determined for a seated person via functional arm reach, which, as can be expected, will depend on the type of task performed as well as the type of grip or function performed. A fingertip action (e.g., activating a push button) will be roughly 5 cm longer than a thumb tip action (e.g., turning a knob), while a full grip action will be roughly 5 cm shorter than a thumb tip action (Bullock, 1974). In a classic study, Dempster (1955) determined work space envelopes for different hand actions in various postures (supine, prone, inverted, five angles) for 22 "median and

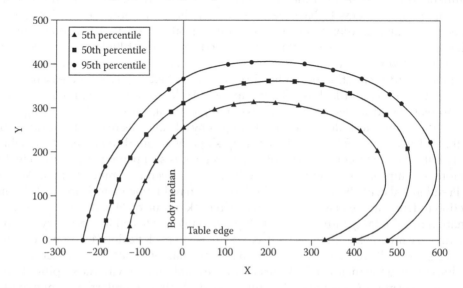

FIGURE 10.17
Normal working area for males. (Reproduced from Das, B. and Behara, D.N., *Ergonomics*, 38, 734, 1995. With permission.)

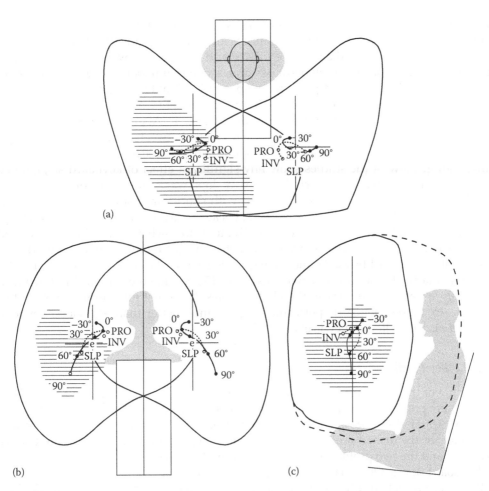

FIGURE 10.18
Optimum (shaded) and maximum (dark lines) workspace envelopes for males in three planes. (From Kennedy, K.W., *Reach Capability of the USAF Population: Phase I. The Outer Boundaries of Grasping-Reach Envelopes for the Shirt-Sleeved, Seated Operator*, TDR 64–59, USAF Aerospace Medical Research Laboratory, Dayton, OH, 1964.)

muscular" males. The heavy line is the enveloping outline of many photographic traces of contours of hand movements while the shaded areas depict the region common to all hand motions and postures and, thus, perhaps the optimum region (see Figure 10.18). More detailed data on U.S. Air Force personnel was collected by Kennedy (1964).

10.3 Keyboard

10.3.1 Standard Keyboard Features

10.3.1.1 Keyboard Slope

The standard computer keyboard evolved, more or less, from the manual typewriter. Characteristics that carried over include the shape, slope, and profile of the keyboard, as well as the size and shapes of the individual keys. The standard keyboard slope of 30° for manual typewriters as reported by Moneta (1960; cited in Alden et al., 1972) appeared to be based on convention rather any data since Scales and Chapanis (1954) found most individuals preferred slopes in the range of 15°–25° and Dreyfuss (1959) in his anthropometric tables indicated an optimum slope of 11° and a maximum slope of 20°. Later research on computer keyboards found preferred slopes of 21° (Galitz, 1965; cited in Alden et al., 1972), 18° with higher rates of keystrokes (Emmons and Hirsch, 1982), 10°–15° (Suther and McTyre, 1982), 18° (Miller and Suther, 1983), and 14.4°–16.1° (Abernethy, 1984). These results have lead to the recommendation of a keyboard slope between 0° and 15°, with an upper maximum at 25° (Human Factors and Ergonomics Society, 2002).

Interestingly, few of the studies show any significant effect of keyboard slope on typing performance. However, preferred keyboard slope was to found to correlate inversely and significantly with seat height ($r = -0.71$) with shorter individuals preferring steeper slopes. Miller and Suther (1983) reasoned that because stature correlates with hand length, a steeper slope makes it easier for shorter individuals to reach all keys. On the other hand, flatter keyboards satisfy more easily work surface height requirements and work better in adjustable keyboard trays. As such, low-profile keyboards, defined as having less than 3 cm height at the home row and slope less than 15°, became the standard in Europe and eventually, a defacto standard in the United States. Note that for standing workstations, flat and −15° slope keyboards performed significantly better than +15° slope keyboards (Najjar et al., 1988; cited in Lewis et al., 1997).

10.3.1.2 Key Profile

The profile of the keyboard can be stepped, sloped, or dished (see Figure 10.19). Although no data were presented, the dished profile was reported to improve keying speed for skilled operators (Çakir et al., 1980). Similarly, Paci and Gabbrielli (1984) claimed that performance was better for the dished profile as compared to a stepped profile. However, no data were presented and the two profiles were confounded with different keyboard slopes. Only Magyar (1985; cited in Lewis et al., 1997) indicated statistically significant lower performance on a sloped keyboard as compared to a stepped or a dished profile. However, these results were not sufficient to clearly identify as one profile superior to another. It is, perhaps, more important that the key itself be indented to provide an accurate location of the user's finger, minimize reflections (45% or less), provide a surface for the labels and prevent accumulation of dirt and dust, either on the key or falling between keys into the mechanism (Çakir et al., 1980). A matt surface will reduce reflections, but an excessively rough surface will tend to accumulate dirt.

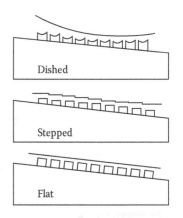

FIGURE 10.19

Keyboard profiles. (Reprinted from Lewis, J.R., Potosnak, K.M., and Magyar, R.L., Keys and keyboards, In: M. Helander, T.K. Landauer and P. Prabhu (eds), *Handbook of Human-Computer Interaction*, Elsevier, North Holland, Amsterdam, the Netherlands, 1997. With permission.)

10.3.1.3 Key Size, Displacement, and Resistance

In terms of key design characteristics, it appears that as computer input devices came into being during the late 1950s and 1960s, a wide variety of key configurations existed. Key resistances ranged from 0.6 to 2.3 N, key displacements ranged from 0.71 to 1.59 cm and key sizes were generally around 1.27 cm (0.5 in.) in width and separated

1.81 cm (0.75 in.) from center to center, similar to those found on typewriters (Pollock and Gildner, 1963; cited in Alden et al., 1972; Harkins, 1965). Biomechanical and anthropometrical considerations first appeared with Dreyfuss (1959) recommendations of key resistances in the range of 1.15–3.06 N, a 0.47 cm displacement, and key sizes of 1.27 cm in width by 1.11 cm in length. The first reliable experimental data came from the Deininger (1960a,b) study on 10 button key sets for push-button telephones. Overall, there were rather small differences in operator responses, but smaller key resistances (around 1 N) were preferable to larger resistances (around 4 N) and intermediate displacements (0.3 cm) were preferable to very small (0.1 cm) or very large (0.5 cm) displacements. Keying times decreased 8% and keying errors decreased from 7.1% to 1.3% as the key size was increased from 1 to 1.27 cm^2.

Kinkead and Gonzalez (1969; cited in Lewis et al., 1997) found optimum keying performance at low levels of resistance (0.25–1.5 N) and travel (0.13–0.64 cm). These results were further confirmed by Clare (1976) who recommended 1.27 cm square keys with a 1.9 cm separation distance, by Loricchio and Lewis (1991) who found that keying rates increased 8.8% (p < .05) in going from 1 to 1.4 cm keys, and by Loricchio (1992) who found 8.2% increase in keying rate in going from 0.75 to 0.5 N (p = .08) key resistance. However, going to even lower key resistances may be counterproductive in that Akagi (1992) found more errors for 0.35 N resistance than a 0.7 N resistance. Furthermore, 0.5 N seems to be lower limit for preventing accidental key activation (Rose, 1991). Thus, the 0.5 N value might be optimal and, as such, have led to recommendations of key resistances between 0.5 and 0.6 N with a maximum range of 0.25–1.5 N. Key width should be a minimum of 1.2 cm with a horizontal separation of 1.8–1.9 cm and a vertical separation of 1.8–2.1 cm. Key displacement should be in the range of 0.15–0.6 cm but with a preferred range of 0.2–0.4 cm (Human Factors and Ergonomics Society, 2002). Later on, more detailed testing and analysis based on Fitts' (1954) Law confirmed the 1.9 cm spacing as optimum but found that a smaller key size of 0.8 cm may be more appropriate based on the size of the average finger pad (Drury and Hoffman, 1992).

10.3.1.4 Key Feedback

It would be expected from basic human factors principles that feedback would be necessary for optimum keying performance. However, Deininger's (1960a,b) classic study on push-button telephones did not indicate a need for auditory feedback. He reasoned that the force–displacement characteristics of the keys provided sufficient feedback for efficient operator performance. Diehl and Seibel (1962) also found no differences in typing performance under four feedback conditions (none, auditory, visual, and both auditory and visual) and Deininger's (1960a,b) conclusions were supported. On the other hand, Monty and Snyder (1983) found a small but significant improvement with a keyboard having an audible click.

Kinkead and Gonzalez (1969; cited in Lewis et al., 1997) found that keys with a snap-action response caused significantly more errors than without while Brunner and Richardson (1984) found the linear-spring response to be least preferred and the with largest number of errors, followed by the snap-action response. The fewest errors and up to a 6% faster typing speed was obtained with an elastomer-type of response (see Figure 10.20). In this type of a response, there are two force or resistance peaks, the first being the *make point*, which activates the key switch. The second occurs after a reduction in resistance, the *break point*, which breaks the circuit and deactivates the switch and signals the user that the keystroke has been completed. Due to the inertia of the hand, the key is continues to depress

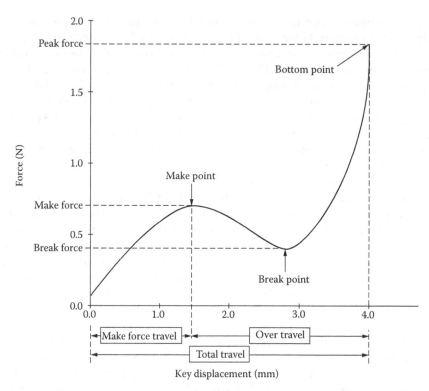

FIGURE 10.20
Optimum force–displacement characteristic in key switches.

until it bottoms out at the *bottom point*. As a consequence, BSR/HFES 100 recommends, at the minimum, tactile feedback with the elastomer-type of response (Human Factors and Ergonomics Society, 2002). If possible, auditory feedback should also be provided. Later research showed the even the type of elastomer response can have an effect on performance. Increasing the make force for keys from 0.47 to 1.02 N increased fingertip forces by 40% and EMG activity by 20% (Rempel et al., 1997b). In a later study, Tomatis et al. (2009) found that key factor was not so much the flexor force increase, but instead an increase in the co-activation of forearm extensor and flexor muscle activity. They recommend that make forces be maintained below 0.59 N. Another factor could be the time to reach the make force. Rempel et al. (1999) found that longer times to reach the make point decreased hand pain over 12 weeks of use. The authors hypothesized that this longer lag created a feeling of looseness, less tension, and less fear of accidental activation of the keys in the operators as compared to a short make force travel distance.

10.3.1.5 Keying Forces

Clare (1976) recommended that the force–displacement characteristics for keys should vary depending on finger distance from the base row. However, actual keying forces were not measured until Rempel et al. (1994) instrumented a keyboard with piezoelectric load cells. They identified three distinct phases and forces exerted by the finger in a keystroke corresponding roughly to the pattern of key resistance shown in Figure 10.20: (1) key switch compression to reach *make force* which preceded the break point in an elastomer key,

(2) finger impact on bottoming out, typically registering the peak force, and (3) finger pulp compression as the key is being released. Mean keying forces ranged from 1.4 to 2.2 N, but anywhere from 2.5 to 3.9 times greater than the make force or key resistance (Armstrong et al., 1994). Although keying forces were greater for higher key resistances, individuals typed much harder than necessary, 4.1–7.0 times more force than needed, on lower resistance (0.28 N) keyboards as compared to higher resistance (0.83 N), in which case they exerted 2.2–3.5 times more force (Gerard et al., 1996). This effect could either result of from a hypothesized motor program of a sequence of fast ballistic movements (Martin et al., 1996) or simply from the inertial properties of the hand (Gerard et al., 1999). In the first case, the authors reasoned that if the two factors, force and speed, could be programmed separately, then, through appropriate training, typing stress levels could be reduced.

In terms of muscle exertion measured by EMG, typists exerted anywhere from 6% to 20% of maximum voluntary contraction (MVC), which is fairly high for a very repetitive task (Martin et al., 1996). Given that Byström and Fransson-Hall (1994) found that fatigue in intermittent hand grip tasks appeared at EMG levels as low 17% MVC. There is the possibility of muscular fatigue arising from keyboarding, especially if key forces are high or the operators are overexerting. Interestingly, Sommerich et al. (1996) found a significant positive correlation between forced typing speed and keying forces, implying that the problem of muscular fatigue is exacerbated in situations where operators may be attempting to meet deadlines. Preferred typing speed, in less stressful conditions, did not correlate with keying force. This is further supported by two later studies which found a significant increase in discomfort and shoulder and neck muscle activation in "faster" and "harder" conditions as compared to baseline conditions (Szeto et al., 2005a,b). A possible confounding factor in many of these studies is the proficiency of the operators, i.e., practiced and proficient typists, who are also faster, may use different muscle recruitment patterns that allow them to be more efficient than less proficient and slower typists. This hypothesis is supported by the observations of Gerard et al. (2002) in that faster typists did not experience more discomfort than slower typists and that relative pace may be more important that absolute typing speed.

Another possible approach to decreasing keying forces is to increase over travel, which would allow for more time for the finger to decelerate, decreasing the resulting forces. Radwin and Jeng (1997) found a 24% decrease (p < .01) in peak force as over travel was increased from 0 to 3 mm. Interestingly, there was a corresponding, although a much smaller (2%) but still significant (p < .01) increase in keying rates. Reducing make force also reduced peak forces, but is limited to the threshold value of 0.5 N in preventing accidental key activation (Rose, 1991). A good summary of the most recent research on key forces can be found Fagarasanu and Kumar (2003).

10.3.2 Split and Sloped Keyboards

10.3.2.1 Standard Keyboard Problems

The standard keyboard creates several biomechanical problems for the operator. First, the hands tend to be ulnarly deviated up to 40° (mean values of 25°; Smutz et al., 1994) placing additional loading on the carpal tunnel and increasing the pressure within the tunnel up to 13% (Werner et al., 1997). Second, to obtain a flat palm, the forearm tends to be pronated close to the anatomical limit (mean values of 76°), which requires the activation of the forearm muscles (mainly pronator teres and pronator quadratus). Such tension over extended time periods can also lead to muscular fatigue. Third, to compensate for this

FIGURE 10.21
Split keyboard with improved hand/
wrist postures.

tension, there is a tendency for the operator to lift the upper arms laterally and forward, which requires the activation of the shoulder muscles (primarily the deltoid and teres minor). Again, static tension may lead to fatigue. Fourth, depending on the height and slope of the keyboard, there is a tendency for the wrists to be extended up to 50° (mean values of 23°; Serina et al., 1999). Of all the possible wrist deviations, this wrist extension may be the most critical with carpal tunnel pressures increasing to 63 mm Hg (for finger tip forces of 6 N), considerably above 30 mm Hg, the threshold level for potential injury (Rempel et al., 1997a).

Such problems at a typewriter keyboard were noticed as early as 1926 by Klockenberg, who proposed that the keyboard be split into two halves, each angled 15° from the center line (see Figure 10.21, included angle is 30°), as well as tilted laterally down (sometimes termed *tented*). Furthermore, Klockenberg (1926) suggested an arching of the key rows for each half of the keyboard so as to better configure with the natural layout of the fingers. The lateral tilting was more specifically examined by Creamer and Trumbo (1960) with a mechanical typewriter cut into two halves and tilted at five different angles. Keying at the middle position of 44° was 5% significantly faster than at the extremes of 0° (flat) or 88° (nearly vertical). Kroemer (1964, 1965, 1972) performed a more detailed analysis by varying also the upper arm position and found that the subjects preferred a similar hand orientation of 40° for the upper arms hanging down naturally. Although the subjects preferred typing a split and tilted keyboard over a standard keyboard, typing speed did not show any differences. Error rates, however, decreased by 39%.

10.3.2.2 Optimum Split Angles

Further experimentation by Zipp et al. (1981, 1983) using EMG measurements of the shoulder, arm, and hand muscle indicated optimal ranges of 0°–60° for pronation and 0°–15° for ulnar deviation, with the standard position for keyboards of 90° pronation and 20°–25° ulnar deviation clearly beyond the optimal range. A 13° angulation from center line (26° included angle) showed lower EMG than a 26° angulation. Also, preferred lateral tilt angles of 10°–20° were smaller than the 44° found by Kroemer (1964, 1965, 1972). Since only three subjects had been utilized in the above experiments, Nakaseko et al. (1985) performed further testing on 20 experienced typists and found similar results with subjective preferences, which led to the first commercial split model standardized at a 25° split (internal angle), a 10° lateral tilt and also a 10° horizontal tilt (far edge higher) (Buesen, 1984). Since then, several other split or tilted models have been introduced and evaluated scientifically to provide better hand and wrist postures (Gerard et al., 1994; Tittiranonda et al., 1999; Zecevic et al., 2000; Rempel et al., 2007b). The latter study provided perhaps the best comparison and found that and opening angle of 12° (along with a 14° lateral tilt) provided the most neutral posture.

10.3.2.3 Performance Effects

Although most research studies confirmed decreased muscular tension with split keyboards, no one examined performance effects until Price and Dowell (1997) found 9.2% slower typing speeds with split keyboards as compared to standard keyboards and Swanson et al. (1997) found a 5.5% decrease in performance with no improvement in discomfort ratings after 2 days' exposure. Similar performance decrements of 4% were found by Smith et al. (1998) and of 6% by Marklin et al. (1999). The performance decrement in novice users (new to split keyboards) may be due to poor visual feedback from the lateral tilt and in skilled typists, even after prolonged familiarization (seven or more hours), may be due to a difficulty in changing motor patterns (Çakir, 1995). In that case, an adjustable split angle may be preferable over a fixed splint angle to allow the user to become accustomed to gradual changes over time (Marklin et al., 1999).

Most of the above studies exposed their subjects, typically healthy typists, to the split keyboards for several hours or, at most, several days. Therefore, although the preferences tended toward the split keyboards, there is the possibility that subjects responded to the novelty effect of the keyboards. Similarly, although postures approached more neutral positions, full adaptation to the new configuration with corresponding changes in motor patterns may not have fully occurred either, as exhibited by the above-mentioned performance decrements. Only Tittiranonda et al. (1999) specifically examined computer users with musculoskeletal disorders in a 6 month prospective, observer-blinded, epidemiological study with three different split keyboards and a standard keyboard as a control. At the end of the study, the group with the keyboard with a 24° split angle, 10° lateral inclination, and −2° downward tilt exhibited a significant decrease in pain severity and hand function, but not in clinical signs. Satisfaction with keyboards correlated directly with improvement in pain severity. Interestingly, there was a placebo effect for the first week, in which all keyboards, even the standard but cosmetically altered one, were rated better than standard keyboard. This may indicate that some of the earlier studies may have been influenced by a placebo effect. In general, split keyboards seems to provide the best posture (Rempel et al., 2007b), with decreased angular velocities and accelerations for most joints (Baker et al., 2007) with no decrements in performance. Therefore, split keyboards could be considered a successful ergonomics intervention in the office environment (Rempel, 2008).

10.3.2.4 Negative Slope Keyboards

While the split angle and vertical tilt had substantial effects on decreasing ulnar deviation and pronation, respectively, these are not the most critical factors in decreasing carpal tunnel pressures. Wrist extension was found to increase carpal tunnel pressures more dramatically (Rempel et al., 1997a) perhaps due to the 25% MVC or greater exertions found in wrist extensors once the wrist is extended to 30°. Interestingly, wrist extension is not affected by the split or tilted keyboard designs (Marklin et al., 1999).

Wrist extension has been reduced by the use of negative-slope (i.e., tilted forward) keyboards (Hedge and Powers, 1995). Whereas users on a standard keyboard exhibited 13° of wrist extension, those on a 12° negative-slope keyboard (self-selected by the users) showed a slight 1° wrist flexion. A later field study of 38 typists confirmed decreased wrist extension with and increased satisfaction of the negative-slope keyboard as compared to a standard flat keyboard (Hedge et al., 1999).

10.3.3 Layout of Keys

10.3.3.1 Standard QWERTY Layout

The standard layout of keys, termed *QWERTY* because of the sequence of the first six leftmost keys in the third row, was patented by C.L. Sholes in 1878 as the eighth of a series of patents on typing machines (see Figure 10.22). Although no specific technical claims were made regarding the layout of the keys, it can be hypothesized that Sholes, being a printer by trade, used an arrangement similar to that in the printer's type case. Another possible explanation is that the most commonly used keys (or letters) are separated from each other such they would not jam upon rapid sequential activation (Kroemer and Kroemer, 2001), although a statistical analysis of close type bars (keys typed in succession or less than four intervening keystrokes) shows that the QWERTY keyboard has more close type bars (26%) than a random keyboard (22%) (Noyes, 1998). Also, there are some alphabetic patterns found on QWERTY keyboard. In following years, many other variations of and potential improvements to the layout of the keys were patented, including one by F. Heidner in 1915 that included a split and tiltable keyboard.

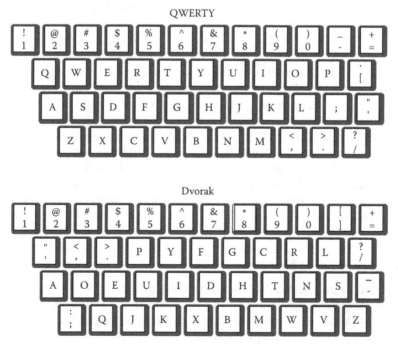

FIGURE 10.22
Standard QWERTY and alternative Dvorak keyboards.

10.3.3.2 Dvorak Layout

The most notable and scientifically based alternative layout was patented by A. Dvorak in 1936 (see Figure 10.22). He allocated the most commonly used keys to the strongest (middle) fingers, more work to the right hand, and the most frequently used letters to the home row such that movement from row to row was minimized (Dvorak, 1943). Extensive investigations into *Dvorak* layout were carried out by the U.S. Navy in 1944, the Australian Post Office in 1953, and the U.S. National Bureau of Standards (cited in Noyes, 1983a). Unfortunately, although all claimed the superiority of the Dvorak arrangement, especially in the speed of training new typists, none of these studies provided much experimental evidence. The only controlled study by Strong (1956) found no performance difference on a 1 min, typing test and superiority of the QWERTY arrangement both in speed and accuracy on a 5 min, test. However, only experienced QWERTY typists were used, who were then retrained on the Dvorak arrangement, which gave them an unfair bias against Dvorak. Also, interestingly, Fox and Stansfield (1964) found that fastest digram keying times occur when successive taps are done with alternate hands, which is precisely what the QWERTY keyboard does.

10.3.3.3 Other Layouts

There have been a variety of other post-Dvorak layouts, either balanced (Griffith, 1949; Maxwell, 1953) or alphabetical (Michaels, 1971) in layout, none of which have received the notoriety of the Dvorak layout, failed to show improved performance (Hirsch, 1970), and suffer the same fate as the Dvorak layout (Noyes, 1983a). Perhaps the best conclusions are given by Norman and Fisher (1982). Performance of alphabetical keyboards is quite slow, at best reaching within 2% of the QWERTY keyboard, because of additional mental processing and visual search requirements. Performance on the Dvorak keyboard shows at best a 5% improvement over the QWERTY keyboard, which is, probably, not great enough to justify switching and retraining of millions of people.

10.3.4 Chord Keyboards

Data entry on a typical keyboard is in a sequential manner, i.e., individual characters are keyed in a specific sequence. On the other hand, in a *chord* keyboard entering one character requires the simultaneous activation of two or more keys. The basic trade-off is that with such activation, fewer keys are required and considerably more information can be entered. Research on chord keyboards was conducted primarily in the 1960s for use in post office mail sorting. Using 46 postal employees unskilled in using either a standard typewriter or a chord keyboard and randomly assigned to two groups, Conrad and Longman (1965) found that functional proficiency was achieved roughly 2 weeks more quickly on the chord keyboard. However, the performance in keystrokes per minute was lower because of the shorter practice time. When each group was allowed to continue the keyboarding task for a total of 33 days of effective practice, the chord keyboard group had caught up and surpassed standard typewriter group by approximately 10 strokes per minute (approximately 10% better). However, the learning curve had not yet leveled off and so peak performance had not yet been achieved. The overall error rate, though, for the chord keyboard was double the standard keyboard. Similarly, Bowen and Guinness (1965) found that when memory encoding was required (i.e., specific patterns of keys had to be remembered), subjects could encode up to 55 items per minute on the chord keyboards versus 40 items per minute on the standard keyboard. Seibel (1964), based on his previous research of response times for all possible finger pattern (chord) combinations and comparisons of stenotypists (using chord keyboards but confounded in that a shorthand technique is also used) versus regular typists, estimated that chord keyboards allowed anywhere from 50% to 100% greater data input per time.

A more recent study compared Dvorak, chord, split, and contoured split keyboards with the standard QWERTY keyboard by calculating learning curves (Anderson et al., 2009). The simple split keyboard at a learning curve of 90.4% was significantly different from the other three, Dvorak at 79.1%, chord at 77.3%, and contoured split at 76.9%. The authors concluded that productivity decrements could be quickly regained for the split and contoured split keyboards, but would be much more difficult for the chord and Dvorak keyboards because of the very large (four to five times larger) task completion times. Perhaps Noyes (1983b) provides the best conclusion regarding chord keyboards. They have distinct advantages of small size and portability and one-handed operation (for a small set of keys), allowing the other hand to perform other tasks. For special tasks, such as stenotyping or mail-sorting, where special patterns are remembered, they are especially useful. However, for general usage, sequential keyboards fulfill the majority of everyday requirements without the need for additional specialized training.

10.3.5 Numeric Keypads

Of the wide variety of digit arrangements possible on a ten-key numeric keypad, the general characteristic preferred by users is that numerals increase from left to right and then from top to bottom as shown in Figure 10.23a (Lutz and Chapanis, 1955). In selecting an appropriate arrangement for push-button telephones, Deininger (1960a,b) found an average keying time of 4.92 s for the above arrangement as opposed to a slightly longer time of 5.08 s for an alternate arrangement used on calculators in which the numbers increased from the bottom to the top (see Figure 10.23b). Interestingly, the push buttons arranged in an identical pattern to a rotary dial yielded even faster times. However, because of "engineering advantages" the first layout was selected for push-button telephones. In a direct comparison of the two layouts using postal office clerks, Conrad (1967; cited in Seibel, 1972) found faster keying rates (0.67 s per stroke versus 0.73 s per stroke) and fewer errors (0.55% versus 1.16%) for the telephone arrangement. Similar advantages for the telephone arrangement were found by Paul et al. (1965; cited in Seibel, 1972) for air traffic controllers.

A study by Conrad and Hull (1968) divided 90 inexperienced housewives into three groups, one to each of the two layouts and a third that alternated layouts while eight-digit codes into the keypads. Not surprisingly, the alternating group had lowest performance at 6.77 codes per minute, while the telephone layout was best at 7.75 codes per minute as compared to 7.41 codes per minute for the calculator layout. However, this latter difference was not statistically significant, although the difference between telephone and alternating layouts was significant. More importantly, on all measures of accuracy (% wrong codes, % wrong digits, % codes and digits uncorrected), the telephone layout was significantly

1	2	3
4	5	6
7	8	9
	0	

7	8	9
4	5	6
1	2	3
	0	

(a)   (b)

FIGURE 10.23
Numeric keypad arrangements: (a) telephone and (b) calculator.

better than the calculator layout, contrary to what would have been expected from a speed–accuracy trade-off. A survey of 100 college students in a variety of simulated scenarios found preferences for the telephone layout ranging from 50% to 82% (Straub and Granaas, 1993). In a further study of layouts with respect to type of task performed found no significant differences between the two layouts, other than the zero digit should be placed at the bottom of the keypad (Marteniuk et al., 1997). Probably, because of the relatively small advantage of the telephone layout, BSR/HFES 100 (Human Factors and Ergonomics Society, 2002) has not come out in favor of either layout, but recommends the use of both. This, however, would produce the worst situation in terms of performance, especially if an office environment included both layouts as could typically be expected, e.g., a telephone next to a PC keyboard having a numeric keypad.

10.3.6 Forearm and Wrist Supports

One important change that occurred as office workers switched from paper and pencil tasks to computer work and keyboard entry was that the forearm support from the writing surface was lost, placing more stress on the upper limb musculature. Consequently, the use of wrist and forearm supports during computer work has been recommended. In one of the first studies, five different wrist pads were tested using EMG, electrogoniometers, and contact pressure sensors. Key findings were keyboard wrist pads should be at least 48 cm long and 5–6 cm wide (smaller ones exerted higher pressures potentially impairing blood circulation and impinging on nerves); thicker pads maintained a more neutral wrist posture; flat surfaces were better as contoured surfaces induced wrist deviation; and firm cushions with moderate softness were most comfortable (Paul and Menon, 1994). Hedge and Powers (1995) used video-motion analysis to examine wrist postures for three conditions: normal keyboard without arm support, the same with support, and a negative slope keyboard support system. Ulnar deviation was comparable in all conditions, but wrist extension was significantly reduced with the negative slope keyboard. In effect, the arm supports didn't have much effect. A similar result was found by Cook et al. (2004). There were no significant differences in muscle activity, ulnar deviations for either hand, and right wrist flexion/extension for use or no use of wrist rest. Only left-wrist extension was significantly higher with a wrist rest during keyboard use. Finally, Nag et al. (2009) measured EMG for various muscles in comparing no forearm support, forearm support, and two types of wrist rests. Forearm support significantly reduced forearm extensor activity and upper trapezius activity over no support. Wrist rests, however, increased activity in the upper trapezius (similar to what Bendix and Jessen [1986] found with typewriters). Gel-filled wrist rests were better in reducing forearm muscle activity as compared to bead-packed wrist rests. One can conclude from these studies that forearm supports are better than wrist rests, which are probably better than no support at all.

10.4 Mouse and Other Cursor-Positioning Devices

10.4.1 Cursor Positioning

The primary data entry device for the computer has been the keyboard. However, with the growing ubiquitousness of graphical user interfaces and depending on the task performed, the operator may actually spend less than half the time using the keyboard. Especially for windows- and menu-based systems, some type of cursor-positioning device, better than the cursor keys on a keyboard, was needed. For this, a wide variety of devices have been developed and tested. The *touch screen* uses either a touch-sensitive overlay on the screen or senses the interruption of an infrared beam across the screen as the finger approaches the screen. This approach is quite natural with the user simply touching the target directly on the screen. However, the finger can obscure the target and, in spite of the fairly large targets required, accuracy can be poor (Beringer and Petersen, 1985). The *light pen* is a special stylus linked to the computer by an electrical cable that senses the electron scanning beam at the particular location on the screen. The user has a similar natural pointing response as with a touch screen, but usually with more accuracy.

A *digitizing tablet* is a flat pad placed on the desktop, again linked to the computer. Movement of a stylus is sensed at the appropriate position on the tablet, which can either be absolute (i.e., the tablet is a representation of the screen) or relative (i.e., only direct movement across the tablet is shown). This then gets into tablet size versus accuracy trade-offs and optimum control–response ratios (Arnaut and Greenstein, 1986). Also, the user needs to look back at the screen to receive feedback. Both displacement and force *joysticks* (currently termed *track sticks* or *track points*) can be used to control the cursor and have a considerable background of research on types of control systems, types of displays, control–response ratios, and tracking performance (Poulton, 1974). The keyboard cursor (arrow) keys can also be utilized, but are slow and poor for drawing. The *mouse* is a handheld device with a roller ball in the base to control position and one or more buttons for other inputs. It is a relative positioning device and requires a clear space next to the keyboard for operation. The *trackball* is an upside-down mouse without the mouse pad, is a good alternative for work surfaces with limited space. For a more detailed review of cursor-positioning devices, refer to Greenstein and Arnaut (1988) or Sanders and McCormick (1993).

When computers first became popular, several studies examined the above-mentioned cursor-positioning devices for performance, typically speed or time to complete various tasks, accuracy, and user preferences. Typically, a limited number of inexperienced subjects were tested. Although the lack of experience would allow for an unbiased evaluation of the device, learning effects were confounded with performance, and, in one case, perhaps due to inexperience, a subject had to be discarded do very poor performance (Card et al., 1978). Also, the small number of subjects would limit generalizability. The results of four such studies are summarized in Table 10.4. A final recommendation for the optimum device is difficult to make because different studies examined different devices and direct comparisons cannot be made. However, overall, there are clear speed–accuracy trade-offs, with the fastest devices (touch screens and light pens) being quite inaccurate. Therefore, consideration may need to be given to the type of task being performed. Keyboard cursor keys were slow and probably are not acceptable. Touch pads were a bit faster than joysticks, but were less preferred by users. Mice tended to rank high in all studies, both in speed and accuracy, which, probably, indicates why mice are so ubiquitous.

10.4.2 Mouse

Along with the increased use of the mouse, there has been an increase in WRMSDs associated with the mouse. Fogleman and Brogmus (1995) reviewed workers' compensation claims, showing that, although a very small percentage of all claims (0.04%) are related to the mouse, a larger portion of WRMSDs (1%) and computer-related claims (6.1%) are related to the mouse. Furthermore, the problem grew rapidly from 1990 to 1993 and needed further attention.

TABLE 10.4

Comparison of Cursor-Positioning Devices

Device	Card et al. (1978)		Albert (1982)			Epps (1987)		MacKenzie et al. (1991)		Average Ranking (Two or More Entries)		
	Sp	Acc	Sp	Acc	Pref	Sp	Pref	Sp	Acc	Sp	Acc	Pref
Touch screen			1	6.5	2							
Light pen			2	6.5	2							
Digitizing tablet			3	2	2			1	2	2	2	
Joystick, force	2	3	5	3	6.5	6	4			4.3	3	5.3
Joystick, displacement			6	4	6.5	5	3			5.5		4.8
Cursor keys, step	4	4	7	5	5		1			4.5	4.5	
Cursor keys, text	3	2										
Track ball			4	1	4	2	1	3	3	3	2	2.5
Mouse	1	1				1	2	2	1	1.3	1	
Touch pad, linear gain						3	6					
Touch pad, increasing gain						4	5					
Number of subjects	4		8			6		—		—		

Abbreviations: Sp, speed; Acc, accuracy; Pref, preference; rankings, 1 = fastest, most accurate, or most preferred.

There are several problems associated with mouse usage. Depending on the placement of the mouse, there are large ulnar deviations (up to 60°) and large lateral shoulder rotations (up to 45°) (Karlqvist et al., 1994) with consequential increased activity in the mouse-side shoulder muscles, primarily the trapezius and the deltoid (Jensen et al., 1998). Depending on the task, pinch and finger tip pressure forces can be quite high. The two main mousing tasks are pointing, i.e., moving and positioning the mouse, sometimes termed *point and click*, and dragging, i.e., manipulating the icons or windows with mouse, sometimes termed *drag and drop*. Mice have been specifically instrumented with strain gages to measure the forces during these tasks (Johnson et al., 1997). Mean pinching forces ranged from 0.55 to 1.40 N during pointing tasks and two to three times greater for dragging tasks. The finger-tip forces during button operation did not differ significantly (1.51–1.99 N) between the tasks (Johnson et al., 1994). Similar finger-tip forces were found by Kotani and Horii (2001) in a more complex Fitts' Law mouse targeting task, with lowest forces for the highest index of difficulty. However, the forces were up to twice as large as the minimum force necessary to activate the control. Park (1999) also found fingertip forces to exceed the minimum by 2.3–2.8 times, which again confirms that individuals tend to overgrip objects or tools by as much as to five times the minimum necessary force (Lowe and Freivalds, 1999).

One suggestion to reduce at least the pinch forces in the dragging task is for computer manufacturers to include a drag-lock on the mouse similar to what is found on trackballs (Johnson et al., 1994). Another approach may be to redesign the mouse with an upright handle gripped with a power grip so as to provide a more neutral forearm posture and decreased EMG levels in hand, forearm, and shoulder muscles (Aarås and Ro, 1997). An added feature of this particular mouse design (although not specifically discussed by the authors) is that the control button is activated by the thumb, which is 23% stronger than the index finger (Hertzberg, 1973). Furthermore, the button could just as well be placed on the side of the handle, allowing it to be activated directly from the power grip. Later field testing over a 6 month period found a significant reduction in pain intensity and frequency for the wrist/hand, forearm, shoulder, and neck (Aarås et al., 1999).

Keir et al. (1998, 1999) measured carpal tunnel pressure during mouse usage and found mean pressures of 33.1 mm Hg during dragging and 28.0 mm Hg during pointing as compared to 5.3 mm Hg during a neutral resting state. The higher pressures during dragging were attributed to the button being depressed for a greater percentage of time and greater pinch forces. Also, mouse usage, in general, promoted wrist extension and forearm rotation, both of which also increased carpal tunnel pressure (Werner et al., 1997; Rempel et al., 1998). Prolonged pressures of 30 mm Hg have been associated with altered nerve function in animal studies (Hargens et al., 1979; Lundborg et al., 1983; Powell and Myers, 1986), which could be the first step in the sequence of events leading to CTS (Dahlin et al., 1987). Interestingly, Keir et al. (1999) also tested three different mouse designs, each of which promoted slightly different radioulnar deviations. However, there were no significant differences in the carpal tunnel pressures attributed to the relatively small changes in angle.

Researchers have examined various workstation parameters to reduce the stress of mousing. Using forearm supports significantly decreased trapezius muscle activity (Aarås et al., 1997). Considering that the mouse is typically placed to the right of the numeric keypad, the large lateral shoulder rotations and ulnar deviations (Karlqvist et al., 1994) are not unexpected. Removing the numeric keypad and moving the mouse closer to the body median significantly decreased deltoid muscle activity and improved RULA scores (Cook and Kothiyal, 1998). Alternatively, they suggested using the mouse with left hand. Unfortunately, this results in a 30% slower response times for right-handed individuals

(Hoffman et al., 1997). Left-handed individuals showed no such decrement, presumably because of previous experiences using the nondominant hand. Even after a 3–4 weeks of using the mouse with the left hand with continued improvements, the task performance time may still be slightly longer than when using the mouse with the right hand, 14% longer in one study (Delisle et al., 2004) and 6.7% longer in another study (Ackland and Hendrie, 2005).

Another potential problem with mouse work is *hovering behavior*, gripping the mouse without using it, with the negative effects of prolonged extended wrists with potential muscle exertion. If mouse users could relax the hand, the static loading could be reduced. De Kraker et al. (2008) instrumented a mouse to provide tactile vibrating feedback signal if the mouse was not clicked or scrolled for more than 10 s. Subjects did decrease their hovering behavior by 14% (compared to 5% for the control group) without any negative effect on productivity. An interesting alternative for reducing the stress on the upper limbs from mouse work is to use foot pedals. Kim and Kaber (2009) examined four different combinations of foot pedals for a text editing task and found that none came close to mousing performance (best was 18.5% slower), although the subjects considered them to be useful in reducing workload. Overall, foot pedals may have some use for special populations, including those with upper limb WRMSDs as well for some complex, dynamic test editing tasks.

Karlqvist et al. (1998) examined several alternative mouse positions, found similar results to Cook and Kothiyal (1998) and recommended an optimum position of a neutral shoulder rotation with a relaxed and supported arm. Park (1999) measured fingertip forces, wrist angles, shoulder abduction angles, and deltoid EMG for a total of 18 different mouse positions, three lateral positions, three heights, and two posterior/anterior positions. The optimum position based on lowest stress for most variables was the lowest height, 90% of the subject's elbow resting height, the most posterior position, at the edge of the keyboard, and the most medial position, 31.5 cm from the body median, centered with the GH keys on the keyboard. Not surprisingly, only wrist extension showed an opposite trend with the highest level yielding the smallest extension angle. Ultimately, as in most ergonomic designs, there will need to be trade-offs, as all variables cannot be optimized.

10.4.3 Mouse Alternatives

The trackball as a similar but alternate device for the mouse has been reexamined. Harvey and Peper (1997) found lower trapezius and deltoid EMGs with a centrally located trackball, below the center of the keyboard, as compared to a mouse positioned to the right of the keyboard. However, type of input device was confounded with placement. For the same operating position, to the right of the numeric keypad, Burgess-Limerick et al. (1999) found that a trackball decreased ulnar deviation but increased wrist extension. Using 3D motion analysis and EMG measurements, Karlqvist et al. (1999) found very similar results. However, female operators had elevated and rotated shoulders as compared to male operators and increased muscle activity, which they attributed to anthropometric differences and varying working styles. Given the trade-offs and the large individual variations, they suggested that the use of trackball for interventions be linked to follow-up evaluations of postures. Also there may be concern, not yet examined, with the large amounts of thumb motion.

An early precursor to the *touch pad*, in the form of tiltable push button, was first compared to the mouse and cursor keys by Loricchio (1992). Experienced mouse users did significantly better with the mouse, while non-experienced users had mixed results. However, both experienced and non-experienced mouse users found the pushbutton difficult to use.

Çakir et al. (1995) found an improved version of the touch pad to yield performance levels comparable to a mouse within 5 h of usage. Wrist deviations with the touch pad were less than for the mouse with implications (although not tested) of decreased long-term postural discomfort. Latest research by Akamatsu and MacKenzie (2002) indicates that applied forces with a touch pad are significantly lower than for a mouse (1.24 versus 1.6 N). Interestingly, the applied forces on a touch pad decrease as the operator approaches the target, while the forces on a mouse increase. The authors attributed this effect as a compensatory effect to increase friction with the mouse and consequently improve the precision of the movement. Since the hand and forearm movements used for controlling the mouse are less precise than finger movements used with a touch pad (Langolf et al., 1976), one would suspect that the touch pad should yield more precise movements than a mouse. However, the exact opposite was found. Also, the touch pad yielded 19% significantly slower movements and 16% lower throughput. The authors alluded to the increased jitter with increased forces in the touch pad, suggesting that the dynamics of the touch pad be altered to be comparable to a mouse for increased precision.

Batra et al. (1998) compared the touch pad to a track ball, and a *track point*, an isometric joystick in middle of laptop keyboards. The touch pad and track ball had similar performance on various pointing, box-sizing, and text selection tasks. However, the track point performed consistently worse and was judged not well suited as an input device. Fernström and Ericson (1997) also examined the track point as an alternative to the mouse, but in terms of muscular loading. Shoulder loading decreased significantly, but at the expense of added forearm loading because the forearm was not supported. Subjects were free to use armrest but none except one did so. This again indicates the need for proper training in the adjustment of computer workstation furniture. Also, subjects preferred to use the track point so as to keep their hands on the keyboard, i.e., they resisted the postural variation in reaching for the mouse. Interestingly, highest muscle loading was found for manual handwriting. Thus, overall, the touch pad may prove to be a practical alternative to the mouse, especially for use on notebook PCs.

10.5 Notebooks and Handheld PCs

Portable PCs, or laptop or notebook computers (earlier distinction based on size, but which is continually changing), are becoming very popular, rising from 34% of the U.S. PC market in 2000 (Sommerich, 2000) to 60.7% in 2009 (http://news.cnet.com/crave/?keyword=IDC). Its main advantage over a desktop is reduced size (and weight) and portability. However, with the smaller size, there are distinct disadvantages; smaller keys and keyboard, keyboard attached to screen, and the lack of a peripheral cursor-positioning devices. Yoshitake (1995) found that touch typists with wide fingers performed worse on small keyboards (16.7 mm width versus 19–21 on standard keyboards) than typists with narrow fingers. Similar results had been found previously (Loricchio and Lewis, 1991) on numeric keypads with narrower inter-key spacing and narrow keys.

The lack of adjustability in placing the screen has been found to give rise to excessive neck flexion (44°–50°, beyond the recommended 15°), increased shoulder flexion (22°–34°, rather than arms hanging naturally), and elbow angles greater than 90° (101°–110°) (Harbison and Forrester, 1995). Straker et al. (1997) found similar neck flexions (mean of 57°) with greater discomfort after 20 min of work as compared to a desktop PC. This discomfort is most likely due to the increased neck extensor muscle activity as observed by Villanueva et al. (1998) for four different types of notebook computers. Part of the problem is the trade-off between best line of sight, at a screen tilt angle of approximately 100°, and the increased likelihood of glare with such tilt angle, which causes users to push the notebook farther away from the user (Jonai et al., 2002).

Price and Dowell (1998) found that raising the notebook to a higher surface to reduce neck flexion only worsened shoulder flexion. Adding an external keyboard and raising the notebook computer or adding any external monitor improved the body angles comparable to a desktop PC. Jacobs et al. (2009) found similar results in university students using notebooks in that adding a notebook riser and external keyboard and mouse along with receiving proper training resulting in significant reductions in self-reported discomfort ratings from pre- to post-surveys. Interestingly, although termed laptops, the placement of the portable PC on the laptop produced significantly worse discomfort scores as compared to the already poor placement on a desktop (Asundi et al., 2010).

Given that the notebook user does attach an external mouse but relies on the integrated cursor-positioning device, generates the question of the best placement of this device, typically a touch pad. Kelaher et al. (2001) used a Fitts' tapping task to examine five different locations of a touch pad, top/bottom in combination with center/right side and one attached to the middle of the right side. The top and bottom locations exhibited a trade-off between wrist extension and ulnar deviation. The bottom positions were better than top for elbow and shoulder angles as well as discomfort ratings and performance. However, the right-side location proved best, although not significantly, and it would require some sort of clip attachment provided by the manufacturer.

Even smaller handheld computers, termed *personal digital assistants* (PDAs), were introduced in the 1990s but have had few detailed scientific evaluations performed, and currently are being replaced by smart phones. Being pocket sized, they offer much greater portability and flexibility, but at an even greater disadvantage for data entry. Wright et al. (2000) found significant decrements in speed and accuracy when entering text via the touch screen. Most subjects preferred using an external but small keyboard. Older individuals were significantly slower compared to younger individuals, but similar in error rates. The authors recommended alternate input methods such as handwriting or voice input to remedy such an unacceptable form of data entry. Many of the new smart phones, such as the Apple I-Phone utilize a touch screen. Park and Han (2010) studied 4, 7 and 10 mm keys for one-handed thumb pressing and found that the large ones gave significantly fewer errors, faster task completion times and more convenient pressing locations. However, smaller phones have limited number of virtual key locations and they detailed optimal thumb pressing areas (key locations) based on key size. One approach to reducing the number of errors due to the small key sizes and the absence of tactile feedback is to use regional error correction methods. These were found to significantly reduce both the time and the number of touches required to complete the task, especially for small keys, but less so for larger keys (Kwon et al., 2009).

Interestingly, PDAs are still highly utilized in distribution and order centers or even large stores in the form of graphic order terminals. Since they are used for extensive time periods, considerable fatigue is generated both from the weight and gripping force. A reasonable expectation would be that an over-the-shoulder strap support would reduce muscular EMG activity and subjective ratings of perceived fatigue as was found for the first 30–45 min of the 2 h session. However, by the end of the session, the straps did not always decrease the sensation of fatigue (Mamaghani et al., 2009). Perhaps, the later sensation of fatigue was so overwhelming that they obscured the benefits of the strap.

10.6 Interventions for Office Work

10.6.1 Rest Pauses

The general principle for the allocation of rest in heavy work, derived from the intermittent work studies of Karrasch and Müller (1951) and Åstrand et al. (1960a,b), is frequent, short rest pauses, as opposed to less frequent but long pauses. This principle was extended to office work by Çakir et al. (1980) based on its cognitive demands and data from Graf (1960; cited in Çakir et al., 1980). Graf found that providing rest pauses of 2, 4, and 6 min after 45, 90, and 125 min in a 3 h task involving arithmetic calculations increased productivity 5.6% over nonstop work, even though the rest pauses decreased working time by 6.7%. Providing the same amount of rest but in shorter, more frequent pauses of 0.5, 1, and 2 min every 15 min increased productivity even more, 9.8% over baseline conditions. Graf's data showing that increasing the length of a rest pause beyond 5 min produced marginal benefits led Grandjean (1987) to generalize the principle for office work as 3–5 min rest every hour.

Cognitive work is not the sole factor leading to fatigue in office work. Several studies found degradations in color adaptation and accommodation occurring with prolonged viewing of computer screens, then termed visual display terminals (VDTs), in the ever increasing computerization of office work (Çakir et al., 1980; Haider et al., 1980; Krueger, 1980). Such degradations were found to be reversed with 15 min breaks (Haider et al., 1980), leading NIOSH (1981) to recommend a 15 min break every 2 h of continuous but moderate VDT work or a 15 min break every hour for very high visual VDT demands or workload. However, these recommendations were made with few detailed studies to support them. In a more recent study, using electroencephalograms, electrooculograms, EMG and subjective ratings, Hayashi et al. (2004) found that a 20 min nap was significantly more effective than a 20 min simple break between two 1 h VDT work intervals in increasing motivation and task performance and decreasing sleepiness.

Other research also supported the hourly recommendation, with Floru et al. (1985) and Gao et al. (1990) finding that performance on VDT tasks steadily decreased over a 45–60 min period, which was then followed by a rebound in performance. This was attributed to Bills (1931) *blocks* or cycling patterns in mental arousal and, along with associated changes in electroencephalograms and heart rate, indicated a natural point at which a rest pause should be provided. There is some data indicating that these rest pauses should be of an active (walking or stretching) nature rather than a passive nature. Sundelin and Hagberg (1989) found that subjects preferred such pauses and experienced less perceived discomfort, although not a statistically significant level. NIOSH researchers (Galinsky et al., 2000) further confirmed the need for breaks every hour finding significant decreases in perceived discomfort in various body parts in those workers receiving pauses every hour as compared to those receiving pauses every 2 h. Interestingly, although the productivity rate increased slightly, total productivity did not increase, because of the time lost due to the added pauses.

In addition to regular pauses, *micropauses* at irregular, spontaneous intervals may also provide benefit in relieving discomfort and perhaps, some increase in productivity Henning et al., 1997; McLean et al., 2001). Previously, Henning et al. (1989) found that self-selected micropauses of 27 s did not completely reduce the steady in decline in performance over 40 min work periods and recommended that slightly longer pauses were needed. Also, Henning et al. (1994) found that spontaneous pauses provided just as much benefit as regimented pauses and had the added advantage of eliminating unnecessary task inter-ruptions. In a later study, Balci and Aghazadeh (2003) compared thee different work/rest schedules: 60 min work/10 min rest, 30 min work/5 min rest, and 15 min work with micro-breaks. The schedule with microbreaks produced significantly lowest neck, back, and chest discomfort; highest speed, accuracy, and task performance; and second lowest eyestrain and blurred vision. Although no specific recommendations for the length of micropauses were ever fully determined, the need for such pauses was clearly supported.

The original recommendation of 15 min rest for every hour for computer data-entry work does not correspond well with the principle of frequent, short pauses and may not be sufficient, based on empirical data. A more flexible schedule of 5–15 min rest for every hour, 5 min for good working conditions, 15 min for very poor conditions, with fre-quent spontaneous micropauses (at least every 10 min) may be a better recommendation (Pheasant, 1991).

10.6.2 Exercises

Although the primary emphasis for control measures has been on proper workstation design, Winkel (1987) and Sundelin and Hagberg (1989) have recommended dynamic rest pauses to relieve the stresses of sedentary work. Although more than 14 exercise pro-grams, specifically designed for VDT users, have been cited in literature (summarized in Lee et al., 1992), few have been tested for effectiveness in and well-controlled laboratory experiments or even well-designed field studies.

Muscle groups typically fatigue during extended periods at a computer workstation include the shoulder elevators (levelator scapulae, trapezius, latissimus dorsi, rhomboid), back muscles (erector spinae), chest muscles (pectoralis, infrspinatus, serratus), and fore-arm flexors (flexor carpi, flexor digitorum). As a consequence, a majority of the exercises (54%) are designated for the shoulders and upper limbs. However, exercises are also sug-gested for the neck, trunk, back, and legs. At the least the exercises should be (1) practical, i.e., requiring minimum time, causing minimal disruption of work activities and embar-rassment to the operator, and corresponding to the ability and motivation levels of the operators and (2) safe, i.e., should be based on accepted biomechanical and physiotherapy principles and not pose added risks to the operator. However, some of the exercises were found to require excessive amounts of time and, with considerable flexing, rotation, and extension of joints, may pose risks for those individuals with preexisting WRMSDs of the upper limbs (Lee et al., 1992).

More recent research shows some positive effect from exercises. Although not tested statistically, Sucher (1994) found some improvement in the range of motion for the wrist and an increase in nerve conduction velocities of symptomatic patients. This was attrib-uted to exercises specifically stretching the carpal ligament which opened the carpal canal. Rozmanryn et al. (1998) divided 197 patients symptomatic with CTS into two groups. Both were treated conservatively, but one group also performed nerve and ten-don gliding exercises. Of the control patients, 71% still underwent surgery, while only 43% of the exercising patients underwent surgery, of which 70% remained relatively symptomatic 2 years later. This was a significant ($p < .001$) difference which the authors attributed to the exercise. Other more recent studies have also found that tendon and *nerve gliding* exercises in combination with other conservative treatments provide signifi-cant improvements (Akalin et al., 2002; Pinar et al., 2005; Baysal et al., 2006). However, tendon and nerve gliding exercises alone are not sufficient to produce improvements (Bardark et al., 2009) and most typically these exercises work best for mild to moderate cases, with all severe cases still requiring surgery (Seradge et al., 2002). More information on specific tendon and nerve gliding exercises can be found in Wehbé (1987) and Webhé and Schlegel (2004).

While the above studies examined specific exercises as a means of reducing the symptoms for those individuals already diagnosed with CTS, a more critical question is whether exercise programs can prevent or reduce the development of CTS in typical workers subject to occupational stressors. Seradge et al. (2000) introduced an exercise program in a meat packing plant with 286 production workers. With no other ergonomic controls being implemented and the CTS incidence rate decreasing by 45% in 1 year, one could consider the exercise program a success. However, with no control group, the results could also be due to overall heightened ergonomics awareness or some other extraneous or confounded factor not directly measured.

Disregarding the direct effectiveness of these programs on the individual, there is also the major problem of overall effectiveness. Most such worksite programs attract only a small proportion of the company's workforce (unless they are made mandatory), exhibit high drop-out rates (Song et al., 1982), and provide smaller benefits than predicted from a controlled laboratory setting (Blair et al., 1986). There are many theories of psychosocial factors that either motivate a person or cause perceived barriers to exercise (Godin and Gionet, 1991). However, these factors are no different in the workplace than in a personal setting. Therefore, the same principles that foster exercise in a general population should also guide the promotion of exercise in the workplace (Godin and Gionet, 1991).

Note that, although not specifically tested as an intervention, increased general aerobic exercise and its resultant decrease in percent body fat and increase in peak aerobic capacity have been found to correlate significantly with decreased median nerve sensory latency (Nathan et al., 2001). Consequently, the authors recommended aerobic exercise programs as a means of reducing hand CTS symptoms. Also, one should not excessively overdue any strengthening exercise programs, lest the exercise become equivalent to the stressful work of high forces and excessive joint deviations ergonomists are attempting to redesign. Mauer et al. (1991) found the same CTS symptoms appear in a group of 30 body builders, especially for those training more than 6 years.

10.6.3 Splints

As mentioned in Section 6.3, for most patients with mild CTS, initial treatment is usually simple and conservative: anti-inflammatory medications, applying heat/cold, exercise, and restriction of motion through wrist splints or *orthoses*. Typically, it is recommended that a wrist splint be worn at night while sleeping to avoid placing the wrist in a position in which the median nerve could become pinched. Unfortunately, the splints are often worn continually throughout the day, the thought process being that if the splint provides benefit for 8 h, 24 h would even be better. In such cases, the splint could possibly interfere with task performance and place additional stress on the affected upper limb. It might be useful to first examine the efficacy of splints.

Most surgical, controlled studies with randomized trials have concluded that for severe cases of CTS, surgical treatment relieved symptoms significantly better than splinting (Gerritsen et al., 2002; Verdugo et al., 2008) and can even be less expensive (Korthals-deBos et al., 2006). The same conclusion also applies to lateral epicondylitis (Derebery et al., 2005). However, for mild cases of CTS splinting (especially if with a cock-up or volar part) will improve median nerve latencies and nerve conduction velocity (Mishra et al., 2006; Brininger et al., 2007; De Angelis et al., 2009). However, if after 5 months no improvements are seen, then surgery may be required (Nobuta et al., 2008). In addition, the combination of splinting with some other treatment, ultrasound, steroid injections, laser, or ultrasound therapy is typically more efficacious than splinting alone (Sevim et al., 2004; Baysal et al., 2006; Yagci et al., 2009). Splints work best if positioned so as to maintain a neutral wrist posture (Walker et al., 2000; Kuo et al., 2001) because this minimizes the carpal tunnel pressure (Weiss et al., 1995). One could conclude that, in the short term, splinting with steroid injections or other conservative treatments may improve symptoms, but, in the long term, surgery will give significantly better results (Ucan et al., 2006).

As to whether the wearing of splints has a negative effect during work is less conclusive because so few studies have examined this aspect. Perez-Balke and Buchholz (1994) found that splinting decreases maximum grip force by 18% for females and 10% for males, most likely due to the 30° extension required by the manufacturer to fit the splint. With regards to the hypothesis that splinting reduces wrist extensor muscle load, Johansson et al. (2004) found no reduction in EMG activity in either the wrist extensor or wrist flexor muscles. Therefore, one could conclude that wearing wrist splints while actively working could increase additional stress on the affected limb.

Questions

1. What are some of the factors that may cause musculoskeletal problems in an office environment?
2. How does the spine change in going from a standing to a seated posture?
3. What factors may help reduce the increased disk pressure found in a seated posture?
4. Why may the standard seated posture with 90 angles not be the best posture?
5. How is optimum chair height determined?
6. What are important chair parameters that need to be adjusted for optimum comfort?
7. How can seating comfort be measured? Compare and contrast the approaches.
8. What is the theory behind seat pressure distribution and seat design?
9. What are the advantages of sit–stand chairs?
10. How is work surface height determined and how does it relate to chair height?
11. How is the normal line of sight and how is it determined?
12. How is normal working area determined?
13. What are the trade-offs with a tilted work surface?
14. What are important characteristics of key design for keyboards?
15. Why is feedback important in key stroking? How it is best incorporated?
16. What biomechanical advantages do split and adjustable keyboards provide?
17. What are the trade-offs of a Dvorak layout as compared to the standard QWERTY layout? That is, why haven't they become popular in spite of the scientific design?
18. What is a chord keyboard?

19. Compare and contrast different approaches to cursor positioning. Which seems to have the most optimum characteristics?

20. Why are wrist rests not especially recommended in reducing arm fatigue?

21. What are some the problems encountered with laptop or notebook computers?

References

Aarås, A. and Ro, O. (1997). Workload when using a mouse as an input device. *International Journal of Human-Computer Interaction* 9:105–116.

Aarås, A., Fostervold, K.I., Ro, O., Thoresen, M., and Larsen, S. (1997). Postural load during VDU work: A comparison between various work postures. *Ergonomics* 40:1255–1268.

Aarås, A., Ro, O., and Thoresen, M. (1999). Can a more neutral position of the forearm when operation a computer mouse reduce the pain level for a visual display unit operators? A prospective epidemiological intervention study. *International Journal of Human-Computer Interaction* 11:79–94.

Abernethy, C.N. (1984). Behavioural data in the design of ergonomic computer terminals and workstations—A case study. *Behavioural and Information Technology* 3:399–403.

Ackland, T. and Hendrie, G. (2005). Training the non-preferred hand for fine motor control using a computer mouse. *International Journal of Industrial Engineering* 35:149–155.

ACTU-VTHC. (1982). Guidelines for the prevention of repetition strain injury (RSI), Australian Council of Trades Unions and Victorian Trades Hall Council Health and Safety Bulletin 18, Melbourne, Victoria.

Akagi, K. (1992). A computer keyboard key feel study in performance and preference. *Proceedings of the Human Factors Society* 36:523–527.

Akalin, E., El, O., Peker, O., Senocak, O., Tamci, S., Gülbahar, S., Cakmur, R., and Oncel, S. (2002). Treatment of carpal tunnel syndrome with nerve and tendon gliding exercises. *American Journal of Physical Medicine* 81:108–113.

Akamatsu, M. and MacKenzie, I.S. (2002). Changes in applied force to a touchpad during pointing tasks. *International Journal of Industrial Ergonomics* 29:171–182.

Åkerblom, B. (1948). *Standing and Sitting Posture*. Stockholm, Sweden: A.B. Nordiska Bokhandeln.

Albert, A.E. (1982). The effect of graphic input devices on performance in a cursor positioning task. *Proceedings of the Human Factors Society* 26:54–58.

Alden, D.G., Daniels, R.W., and Kanarick, A.F. (1972). Keyboard design and operation: A review of the major issues. *Human Factors* 14:275–293.

Andersson, G.B.J. and Örtengren, R. (1974a). Lumbar disc pressure and myoelectric back muscle activity during sitting: II. Studies on an office chair. *Scandinavian Journal of Rehabilitation Medicine* 6:115–121.

Andersson, G.B.J. and Örtengren, R. (1974b). Lumbar disc pressure and myoelectric back muscle activity during sitting: III. Studies on a wheel chair. *Scandinavian Journal of Rehabilitation Medicine* 6:122–127.

Andersson, G.B.J., Örtengren, R., Nachemson, A., and Elfström, G. (1974a). Lumbar disc pressure and myoelectric back muscle activity during sitting: I. Studies on an experimental chair. *Scandinavian Journal of Rehabilitation Medicine* 6:104–114.

Andersson, G.B.J., Örtengren, R., Nachemson, A., and Elfström, G. (1974b). Lumbar disc pressure and myoelectric back muscle activity during sitting: IV. Studies on a car driver's seat. *Scandinavian Journal of Rehabilitation Medicine* 6:128–133.

Andersson, G.B.J., Murphy, R.W., Örtengren, R., and Nachemson, A.L. (1979). The influence of backrest inclination and lumbar support on the lumbar lordosis in sitting. *Spine* 4:52–58.

Anderson, A., Mirka, G.M., Joines, S.M.B., and Kaber, D.B. (2009). Analysis of alternative keyboards using learning curves. *Human Factors* 51:35–45.

Armstrong, T.J., Foulke, J.A., Martin, B.J., Gerson, J., and Rempel, D.M. (1994). Investigation of applied forces in alphanumeric keyboard work. *American Industrial Hygiene Association Journal* 55:30–35.

Arnaut, L.Y. and Greenstein, J. (1986). Minimizing the touch table: The effects of control-display gain and method of cursor control. *Human Factors* 28:717–726.

Åstrand, I., Åstrand, P.O., Christensen, E.H., and Hedman, R. (1960a). Intermittent muscular work. *Acta Physiologica Scandinavica* 48:443–453.

Åstrand, I., Åstrand, P.O., Christensen, E.H., and Hedman, R. (1960b). Myohemoglobin as an oxygen-store in man. *Acta Physiologica Scandinavica* 48:454–460.

Asundi, K., Odell, D., Luce, A., and Dennerlein, J.T. (2010). Notebook computer use on a desk, lap and lap support: Effects on posture, performance and comfort. *Ergonomics* 53:74–82.

Ayoub, M.M. (1973). Work place design and posture. *Human Factors* 15:265–268.

Baker, N.A., Cham, R., Hale, E., Cook, J., and Redfern, M.S. (2007). Digit kinematics during typing with standard and ergonomic keyboard configurations. *International Journal of Industrial Ergonomics* 37:345–355.

Balci, R. and Aghazadeh, F. (2003). The effect of work-rest schedules and type of task on the discomfort and performance of VDT users. *Ergonomics* 46:455–465.

Bardark, A.N., Alp, M., Erhan, B., Paker, N., Kaya, B., and Onal, A.E. (2009). Evaluation of the clinical efficacy of conservative treatment in the management of carpal tunnel syndrome. *Advances in Therapy* 26:107–116.

Barkla, D.M. (1964). Chair angles, duration of sitting, and comfort ratings. *Ergonomics* 7:297–304.

Batra, S., Dykstra, D., Hus, P., Raddle, K.A., and Wiedenbeck, S. (1998). Pointing device performance for laptop computers. *Proceedings of the Human Factors and Ergonomics Society* 42:536–540.

Bauer, W. and Witting, T. (1998). Influence of screen and copy holder positions on head posture, muscle activity and user judgment. *Applied Ergonomics* 29:185–192.

Baysal, O., Altay, Z., Ozcan, C., Ertem, K., Yologlu, S., and Kayhan, A. (2006). Comparison of three conservative treatment protocols in carpal tunnel syndrome. *International Journal of Clinical Practice* 60:820–828.

Bendix, A., Jensen, C.V., and Bendix, T. (1988). Posture, acceptability and energy consumption on a tiltable and a knee-supported chair. *Clinical Biomechanics* 3:66–73.

Bendix, T. (1984). Seated trunk posture at various seat inclinations, seat heights, and table heights. *Human Factors* 26:695–703.

Bendix, T. and Biering-Sørenson, F. (1983). Posture of trunk when sitting on forward inclining seats. *Scandinavian Journal of Rehabilitation Medicine* 15:197–203.

Bendix, T. and Bloch, I. (1986). How should a seated workplace with a tiltable chair be adjusted? *Applied Ergonomics* 17:127–135.

Bendix, T. and Hagberg, M. (1984). Trunk posture and load on the trapezius muscle whilst sitting at sloping desks. *Ergonomics* 27:873–882.

Bendix, T. and Jessen, F. (1986). Wrist support during typing—A controlled, electromyographic study. *Applied Ergonomics* 17:162–168.

Bendix, T., Krohn, L., Jessen, L., and Aarås, A. (1985a). Trunk posture and trapezius muscle load whilst work in standing, supported standing, and sitting postures. *Spine* 54:378–385.

Bendix, T., Winkel, J., and Jessen, F. (1985b). Comparison of office chairs with fixed forwards or backwards inclining, or tiltable seats. *European Journal of Applied Physiology* 54:378–385.

Beringer, D. and Petersen, J. (1985). Underlying behavioral parameters of the operation of touch-input devices: Biases, models, and feedback. *Human Factors* 27:445–458.

Bills, A.G. (1931). Blocking: A new principle in mental fatigue. *American Journal of Psychology* 42:230–245.

Blair, S.N., Piserchia, P.V., Wilbur, C.S., and Crowder, J.H. (1986). A public health intervention model for work-site health promotion. *Journal of the American Medical Association* 255:921–926.

Bowen, H.M. and Guinness, G.V. (1965). Preliminary experiments on keyboard design for semiautomatic mail sorting. *Journal of Applied Psychology* 49:194–198.

Branton, P. (1969). Behaviour, body mechanics and discomfort. *Ergonomics* 12:316–327.

Branton, P. (1974). Seating in industry. *Applied Ergonomics* 1:159–165.

Branton, P. and Grayson, G. (1967). An evaluation of train seats by observation of sitting behaviour. *Ergonomics* 10:35–51.

Bridger, R.S. (1988). Postural adaptations to a sloping chair and work surface. *Human Factors* 30:237–247.

Bridger, R.S., von Eisenhart-Rothe, C., and Henneberg, M. (1989). Effects of seat slope and hip flexion on spinal angles in sitting. *Human Factors* 31:679–688.

Brininger, T.L., Rogers, J.C., Holm, M.B., Baker, N.A., Li, Z.M., and Goitz, R.J. (2007). Efficacy of a fabricated customized splint and tendon and nerve gliding exercises for the treatment of carpal tunnel syndrome: A randomized controlled trial. *Archives of Physical Medicine and Rehabilitation* 88:1429–1435.

Brown, C.R. and Schaum, D.L. (1980). User-adjusted VDU parameters. In: E. Grandjean and E. Vigliani (eds), *Ergonomic Aspects of Visual Display Terminals*. London, U.K.: Taylor & Francis, pp. 195–200.

Brunner, H. and Richardson, R.M. (1984). Effects of keyboard design and typing skill on user keyboard preferences and throughput performance. *Proceedings of the Human Factors Society* 28:267–271.

BS EN 1135. (2000). *Office Furniture, Office Work Chair, Dimensions, Determination of Dimensions*. London, U.K.: British Standards Institution (http://www.bsi-global.com/ index.html).

Buesen, J. (1984). Product development of an ergonomic keyboard. *Behaviour and Information Technology* 3:387–390.

Bullock, M.I. (1974). The determination of functional arm reach boundaries for operation of manual controls. *Ergonomics* 17:375–388.

Burandt, U. (1969). Röntgenuntersuchung über die Stellung von Becken und Wirbelsäule beim Sitzen auf vorgeneigten Flächen (X-ray study of the position of the pelvis and spin while sitting in forward-sloping surfaces). *Ergonomics* 12:356–364.

Burandt, U. and Grandjean, E. (1969). Untersuchungen über das Sitzverhalten von Büroangestellten und über die Auswirkungen verschiedenartiger Sitzprofile (Research on seated office workers and on the consequences of various postures). *Ergonomics* 12:338–347.

Burgerstein, L. (1915). *School Hygiene*. New York: Stokes.

Burgess-Limerick, R., Plooy, A., and Ankrum, D.R. (1998). The effect of imposed and self-selected computer monitor height on posture and gaze angle. *Clinical Biomechanics* 13:584–592.

Burgess-Limerick, R., Shemmell, J., Scadden, R., and Plooy, A. (1999). Wrist posture during computer pointing device use. *Clinical Biomechanics* 14:280–286.

Byström, S. and Fransson-Hall, C. (1994). Acceptability of intermittent handgrip contractions based on physiological response. *Human Factors* 36:158–171.

Çakir, A. (1995). Acceptance of the adjustable keyboard. *Ergonomics* 38:1728–1744.

Çakir, A. Reuter, H.J., Schmude, L., and Armbruster, A. (1978). *Untersuchungen zur Anpassung von Bildschirmarbeitsplatzen an Die Physische und Psychische Funktionsweise des Menschen (Research on the Adjustment of VDT Workplaces and the Physical and Psychological Functioning of Workers)*. Bonn, Germany: Der Bündesminister für Arbeit und Sozialsordnung.

Çakir, A., Hart, D.J., and Stewart, T.F.M. (1980). *Visual Display Terminals*. New York: John Wiley & Sons.

Çakir, A.E., Çakir, G., Müller, T., and Unema, P. (1995). The TrackpadTM—A study on user comfort and performance. In: *CHI '95 Conference on Human Factors in Computing Systems*, Vol. 2, pp. 97–98.

Cantoni, S., Colombini, D., Occhipinti, E., Grieco, A., Frigo, C., and Pedotti, A. (1984). Posture analysis and evaluation at the old and new work place of a telephone company. In: E. Grandjean (ed.), *Ergonomics and Health in Modern Offices*. London, U.K.: Taylor & Francis, pp. 456–464.

Card, S.K., English, W.K., and Burr, B.J. (1978). Evaluation of mouse, rate-controlled isometric joystick, step keys and text keys for text selection on a CRT. *Ergonomics* 21:601–613.

Chaffin, D.B. (1973). Localized muscle fatigue—Definition and measurement. *Journal of Occupational Medicine* 15:346–354.

Chaffin, D.B., Andersson, G.B.J., and Martin, B.J. (1999). *Occupational Biomechanics*, 3rd edn, New York: John Wiley & Sons.

Clare, R.C. (1976). Human factors: A most important ingredient in keyboard designs. *Electronic Design News* 21(April): 99–102.

Congleton, J.J., Ayoub, M.M., and Smith, J.L. (1985). The design and evaluation of the neutral posture chair for surgeons. *Human Factors* 27:589–600.

Conrad, R. (1967). Performance with different push-button arrangements. *Hett PTT Bendriff* 15:110–113.

Conrad, R. and Hull, A.J. (1968). The preferred layout for numeral data-entry keysets. *Ergonomics* 11:165–173.

Conrad, R. and Longman, D.J.A. (1965). Standard typewriter versus chord keyboard—An experimental comparison. *Ergonomics* 8:77–92.

Cook, C.J. and Kothiyal, K. (1998). Influence of mouse position on muscular activity in the neck, shoulder and arm in computer users. *Applied Ergonomics* 29:439–443.

Cook, C., Burgess-Limerick, R., and Papalia, S. (2004). The effect of wrist rests and forearm support during keyboard and mouse use. *International Journal of Industrial Ergonomics* 33:463–472.

Corlett, E.N. and Eklund, J.A.E. (1984a). How does a backrest work? *Applied Ergonomics* 15:111–114.

Corlett, E.N. and Eklund, J.A.E. (1984b). Shrinkage as a measure of the effect of load on the spine. *Spine* 9:189–194.

Creamer, L.R. and Trumbo, D.A. (1960). Multifinger tapping performance as a function of the direction of tapping movements. *Journal of Applied Psychology* 44:376–380.

Dahlin, L.B., Nordborg, C., and Lundborg, G. (1987). Morphologic changes in nerve cell bodies induced by experimental graded compression. *Experimental Neurology* 95:611–621.

Das, B. and Behara, D.N. (1995). Determination of the normal horizontal working area: A new model and method. *Ergonomics* 38:734–748.

Das, B. and Grady, R.M. (1983). The normal working area in the horizontal plane—A comparative analysis between Farley's and Squires' concepts. *Ergonomics* 26:449–459.

De Angelis, M.V., Pierfelice, F., Di Giovanni, P., Staniscia, T., and Uncini, A. (2009). Efficacy of a soft hand brace and a wrist splint for carpal tunnel syndrome: A randomized controlled study. *Acta Neurologica Scandinavica* 119:68–74.

De Kraker, H., De Korte, E.M., Van Mil, F.L.K., Rijs, B.P., and Bongers, P.M. (2008). The effect of a feedback signal in a computer mouse on hovering behaviour, productivity, comfort and usability in a field study. *Ergonomics* 51:140–155.

de Wall, M., van Riel, M.P.J.M., and Snijders, C.J. (1991). The effect of sitting posture of a desk with a 10°inclination for reading and writing. *Ergonomics* 34:575–584.

Deininger, R.L. (1960a). Human factors engineering studies of the design an use of pushbutton telephone sets. *The Bell System Technical Journal* 39:995–1012.

Deininger, R.L. (1960b). Desirable push-button characteristics. *IRE Transactions on Human Factors in Electronics* 1:24–30.

Delisle, A., Imbeau, D., Santos, B., Plamondon, A., and Montpetit, Y. (2004). Left-handed versus right-handed computer mouse use: Effect on upper-extremity posture. *Applied Ergonomics* 35:21–28.

Dempster, W.T. (1955). *Space Requirements of the Seated Operator*, WADC TR 55-159. Dayton, OH: Wright-Patterson AFB.

Derebery, V., Devenport, J., Giang, G., and Fogarty, W. (2005). The effects of splinting on outcomes for epicondylitis. *Archives of Physical Medicine and Rehabilitation* 86:1081–1088.

Diebschlag, W. and Müller-Limmroth, W. (1980). Physiological requirements on car seat: Some results of experimental studies. In: D.J. Oborne and J.A. Levis (eds), *Human Factors in Transport Research*, Vol. 2. London, U.K.: Academic Press, pp. 223–230.

Diehl, M.J. and Seibel, R. (1962). The relative importance of visual and auditory feedback in speed of typewriting. *Journal of Applied Psychology* 46:365–369.

Diffrient, N., Tilley, A.R., and Bardagjy, J.C. (1974). *Humanscale 1/2/3*. Cambridge, MA: MIT Press.

DIN. (1996). DIN EN 1135 Office furniture—Office Work Chair. Berlin D-10772: Deutsches Institut für Normung (http://www.din.de/or http://www2.beuth.de/)

Dreyfuss, H. (1959). *Anthropometric Data*. New York: Whitney Publications.

Drummond, D.S., Narechania, R.G., Rosenthal, A.N., Breed, A.L., Lange, T.A., and Drummond, D.K. (1982). A study of pressure distributions measured during balanced and unbalanced sitting. *The Journal of Bone and Joint Surgery* 64A:1034–1039.

Drury, C.G. and Coury, B.G. (1982). A methodology for chair evaluation. *Applied Ergonomics* 13:195–202.

Drury, C.G. and Francher, M. (1985). Evaluation of a forward-sloping chair. *Applied Ergonomics* 16:41–47.

Drury, C. and Hoffman, E. (1992). A model for movement time on data-entry keyboards. *Ergonomics* 35:129–147.

Dvorak, A. (1943). There is a better typewriter keyboard. *National Business Education Quarterly* 12:51–58.

Eastman Kodak. (1983). *Ergonomics Design for People at Work*, Vol. 1. Belmont, CA: Lifetime Learning Publications.

Eklund, J.A.E. and Corlett, E.N. (1987). Evaluation of spinal loads and chair design in seated work tasks. *Clinical Biomechanics* 2:27–33.

Ellis, D.S. (1951). Speed of manipulative performance as a function of work surface height. *Journal of Applied Psychology* 35:289–296.

Emmons, W.H. and Hirsch, R.S. (1982). Thirty millimeter keyboards: How good are they? *Proceedings of the Human Factors Society* 26:425–429.

Epps, B.W. (1987). A comparison of cursor control devices on a graphics editing task. *Proceedings of the Human Factors Society* 31:442–446.

Erdelyi, A., Sihvonen, T., Helin, P., and Hänninen, O. (1988). Shoulder strain in keyboard workers and its alleviation by arm supports. *International Archives for Occupational and Environmental Health* 60:119–124.

Ericson, M.O. and Goldie, I. (1989). Spinal shrinkage with three different types of chair whilst performing video display unit work. *International Journal of Industrial Ergonomics* 3:177–183.

Fagarasanu, M. and Kumar, S. (2003). Carpal tunnel syndrome due to keyboarding and mouse tasks: A review. *International Journal of Industrial Ergonomics* 31:119–136.

Farley, R.R. (1955). Some principles of methods and motion study as used in development work. *General Motors Engineering Journal* 2:20–25.

Fenety, P.A., Putnam, C., and Walker, J.M. (2000). In-chair movement: Validity, reliability and implications for measuring sitting discomfort. *Applied Ergonomics* 31:383–393.

Ferguson, D. (1976). Posture aching and body build in telephonists. *Journal of Human Ergology* 5:183–186.

Ferguson, D. (1984). The "new" industrial epidemic. *The Medical Journal of Australia* 140:318–319.

Fernström, E. and Ericson, M.O. (1997). Computer mouse or trackpoint—Effects on muscular load and operator experience. *Applied Ergonomics* 28:347–354.

Fernström, E., Ericson, M.O., and Malker, H. (1994). Electromyographic activity during typewriter and keyboard use. *Ergonomics* 37:477–484.

Festervoll, I. (1994). Office seating and movement. In: R. Lueder and K. Noro (eds), *Hard Facts about Soft Machines: The Ergonomics of Seating*. London, U.K.: Taylor & Francis, pp. 413–421.

Fitts, P. (1954). The information capacity of the human motor system in controlling the amplitude of movement. *Journal of Experimental Psychology* 47:381–391.

Floyd, W.F. and Silver, P.H.S. (1955). The function of the erectores spinae muscles in certain movements and postures in man. *Journal of Physiology* 129:184–203.

Floru, R., Cail, F., and Elias, R. (1985). Psychophysiological changes during a VDU repetitive task. *Ergonomics* 28:1455–1468.

Fogleman, M. and Brogmus, G. (1995). Computer mouse use and cumulative trauma disorders of the upper extremities. *Ergonomics* 38:2465–2475.

Fox, J.G. and Stansfield, R.G. (1964). Digram keying times for typists. *Ergonomics* 7:317–320.

Freivalds, A. (2009). *Niebel's Methods, Standards & Work Design*, 11th edn, New York: McGraw-Hill.

Freudenthal, A., van Riel, M.P.J.M., Molenbroek, J.F.M., and Snijders, C.J. (1991). The effect on sitting posture of a desk with a ten-degree inclination using an adjustable chair and table. *Applied Ergonomics* 22:329–336.

Frey, J.K. and Tecklin, J.S. (1986). Comparison of lumbar curves when sitting on the Westnofa Balans® multi-chair, sitting on a conventional chair, and standing. *Physical Therapy* 66:1365–1369.

Galinsky, T.L., Swanson, N.G., Sauter, S.L., Hurrell, J.J., and Schleifer, L.M. (2000). A field study of supplementary rest breaks for data-entry operators. *Ergonomics* 43:622–638.

Galitz, W.O. (1965). *CRT Keyboard Human Factors Evaluation*. Rosemont, IL: UNIVAC.

Gao, C., Lu, D., She, Q., Cai, R., Yang, L., and Zhang, G. (1990). The effects of VDT data entry work on operators. *Ergonomics* 33:917–924.

Gerard, M.H., Armstrong, T.J., Foulke, J.A., and Martin, B.J. (1996). Effects of key stiffness on force and the development of fatigue while typing. *American Industrial Hygiene Association Journal* 57:849–854.

Gerard, M.J., Jones, S.K., Smith, L.A., Thomas, R.E., and Wang, T. (1994). An ergonomic evaluation of the Kinesis Ergonomic Computer keyboard. *Ergonomics* 37:1661–1668.

Gerard, M.J., Armstrong, T.J., Franzblau, A., Martin, B.J., and Rempel, D.M. (1999). The effects of key-switch stiffness on typing force, finger, electromyography, and subjective discomfort. *American Industrial Hygiene Association Journal* 60:762–769.

Gerard, M.J., Armstrong, T.J., Martin, B.J., and Rempel, D.M. (2002). The effects of work pace on within-participant and between participant key forces, electromyography and fatigue. *Human Factors* 44:51–61.

Gerr, F., Marcus, M., Ortiz, D., White, B., Jones, W., Cohen, S., Gentry, E., Edwards, A., and Bauer, E. (2000). Computer users' postures and associations with workstation characteristics. *American Industrial Hygiene Association Journal* 61:223–230.

Gerritsen, A.A., de Vet, H.C., Scholten, R.J., Bertelsmann, F.W., de Krom, M.C., and Bouter, L.M. (2002). Splinting vs surgery in the treatment of carpal tunnel syndrome: A randomized controlled trial. *Journal of the American Medical Association* 266(10):1245–1251.

Godin, G. and Gionet, N.J. (1991). Determinants of an intention to exercise of an electric power commission's employees. *Ergonomics* 34:1221–1230.

Goonetilleke, R.S. (1998). Designing to minimize comfort. *Ergonomics in Design*, July:12–19.

Graf, M., Guggenbühl, U., and Krueger, H. (1993). Investigations on the effects of seat shape and slope on posture and back muscle activity. *International Journal of Industrial Ergonomics* 12:91–103.

Graf, O. (1960). Arbeitsphysiologie, Wiesbaden.

Grandjean, E., ed. (1969). *The Sitting Posture*. London, U.K.: Taylor & Francis.

Grandjean, E. (1987). *Ergonomics in Computerized Offices*. London, U.K.: Taylor & Francis.

Grandjean, E. (1988). *Fitting the Task to Man*, 4th edn, London, U.K.: Taylor & Francis.

Grandjean, E., Jenni, M., and Rhiner, A. (1960). Eine indirekte Methode zur Erfassung des Komfortgefühls beim Sitzen (An indirect method for understanding seating comfort). *Internationale Zeitschrift für Angewandte Physiologie einschliesslich Arbeitsphysiologie* 18:101–106.

Grandjean, E., Hünting, W., Wotzka, G., and Schärer, R. (1973). An ergonomic investigation of multi-purpose chairs. *Human Factors* 15:247–255.

Grandjean, E., Nishiyama, K., Hünting, W., and Pidermann, M. (1982). A laboratory study on preferred and imposed settings of a VDT workstation. *Behaviour and Information Technology* 1:289–304.

Grandjean, E., Hünting, W., and Pidermann, M. (1983). VDT workstation preferred design: preferred settings and their effects. *Human Factors* 25:161–175.

Grandjean, E., Hünting, W., and Nishiyama, K. (1984). Preferred VDT workstation settings, body posture and physical impairments. *Applied Ergonomics* 15:99–104.

Greenstein, J.S. and Arnaut, L.Y. (1988). Input devices. In: M. Helander (ed.), *Handbook of Human-Computer Interaction*. Amsterdam, the Netherlands: Elsevier/North-Holland, pp. 495–519.

Gregory, D.E., Dunk, N.M., and Callaghan, J.P. (2006). Stability ball versus office chair: Comparison of muscle activation and lumbar spine posture during prolonged sitting. *Human Factors* 48:142–153.

Grieco, A. (1986). Sitting posture: An old problem and a new one. *Ergonomics* 29:345–362.

Griffith, R.T. (1949). The minimotion typewriter keyboard. *Journal of the Franklin Institute* 248:399–436.

Groensteijn, L., Vink, P., de Looze, M., and Krause, F. (2009). Effects of differences in office chair controls, seat and backrest angle design in relation to tasks. *Applied Ergonomics* 40:362–370.

Guilford, J.P. (1954). *Psychometric Methods*. New York: McGraw-Hill.

Hagberg, M. (1982). *Arbetsrelaterade Besvär I Halsrygg och Skuldra (Working Report on Neck, Back and Shoulder Disorders)*. Stockholm, Sweden: Arbetsmiljöinstitutet.

Haider, M., Kundi, M., and Weißenböck, M. (1980). Worker strain related to VDUs with differently coloured characters. In: E. Grandjean, and E. Vigliani (eds), *Ergonomics Aspects of Visual Display Terminals*. London, U.K.: Taylor & Francis, pp. 53–64.

Hall, M.A.W. (1972). Back pain and car seat comfort. *Applied Ergonomics* 15:82–91.

Harbison, S. and Forrester, C. (1995). The ergonomics of notebook computers: Problems or just progress. *Journal of Occupational Health and Safety, Australia New Zealand* 11:481–487.

Hargens, A.R., Romine, J.S., Sipe, J.C., Evans, K.L., Mubarak, S.J., and Akeson, W.H. (1979). Peripheral nerve-conduction block by high compartment pressure. *Journal of Bone and Joint Surgery* 61A:192–200.

Harkins, W.H. (1965). Switch system for consoles. *Industrial Design* 12(6):39–43.

Harvey, R. and Peper, E. (1997). Surface electromyography and mouse use position. *Ergonomics* 40:781–789.

Hayashi, M., Chikazawa, Y., and Hori, T. (2004). Short nap versus short rest: recuperative effects during VDT work. *Ergonomics* 47:1549–1560.

Hedge, A. and Powers, J.R. (1995). Wrist postures while keyboarding: Effects of a negative slope keyboard system and full motion forearm supports. *Ergonomics* 38:508–517.

Hedge, A., Morimoto, S., and McCrobie, D. (1999). Effects of keyboard tray geometry on upper body posture and comfort. *Ergonomics* 42:1333–1349.

Helander, M.G. and Zhang, L. (1997). Field studies of comfort and discomfort in sitting. *Human Factors* 40:895–915.

Henning, R.A., Sauter, S.L., Salvendy, G., and Krieg, E.F. (1989). Microbreak length, performance, and stress in a data entry task. *Ergonomics* 32:855–864.

Henning, R.A., Kissel, G.V., and Maynard, D.C. (1994). Compensatory rest breaks for VDT operators. *International Journal of Industrial Ergonomics* 14:243–249.

Henning, R.A., Jacques, P., Kissel, G.V., Sullivan, A.B., and Alteras-Webb, S.M. (1997). Frequent short rest breaks from computer work: Effects on productivity and well-being at two-field sites. *Ergonomics* 40:78–91.

Hertzberg, H.T.E. (1972). *The Human Buttocks in Sitting: Pressures, Patterns, and Palliatives*. SAE Technical Paper No. 720005. Warrendale, PA: Society of Automotive Engineers.

Hertzberg, H. (1973). Engineering anthropometry. In: H. VanCott and R. Kincaid (ed.), *Human Engineering Guide to Equipment Design*. Washington, DC: U.S. Government Printing Office, pp. 467–584.

Heuer, H., Brüwer, M., Römer, T., Kröger, H., and Knapp, H. (1991). Preferred vertical gaze direction and observation distance. *Ergonomics* 34:379–392.

Hill, S.G. and Kroemer, K.H.E. (1986). Preferred declination of the line of sight. *Human Factors* 28:127–134.

Hira, D.S. (1980). An ergonomic appraisal of educational desks. *Ergonomics* 23:213–221.

Hirsch, R.S. (1970). Effects of standard versus alphabetical keyboard formats on typing performance. *Journal of Applied Psychology* 54:484–490.

Hocking, B. (1987). Epidemiology aspects of repetitive strain injury in Telecom Australia. *Medical Journal of Australia* 147:218–222.

Hoffman, E.R., Chang, W.Y., and Yim, K.Y. (1997). Computer mouse operation: Is the left-handed user disadvantaged? *Applied Ergonomics* 28:245–248.

Horie, S., Hargens, A., and Rempel, D. (1993). Effect of keyboard wrist rest in preventing carpal tunnel syndrome. *Proceedings of the APHA Annual Meeting*. Washington, DC: American Public Health Association, p. 319.

Houle, R.J. (1969). Evaluation of seat devices designed to prevent ischemic ulcers in paraplegic patients. *Archives of Physical Medicine and Rehabilitation* 50:587–594.

Human Factors and Ergonomics Society. (2002). *Human Factors Engineering of Computer Workstations*, Santa Monica, CA: HFES.

Hünting, W., Läubli, T., and Grandjean, E. (1981). Postural and visual loads at VDT workplaces. *Ergonomics* 24:917–944.

Husemann, B., Von Mach, C.Y., Borsotto, D., Zepf, K.I., and Scharnbacher, J. (2009). Comparisons of musculoskeletal complains and data entry between a sitting and a sit-stand workstation paradigm. *Human Factors* 51:310–320.

ISO 9241-5. (1998). *Ergonomics Requirements for Office Work with Visual Display Terminals (VDTs)—Part 5: Workstation Layout and Postural Requirements*. Geneva, Switzerland: International Organization for Standardization (http://www.iso.ch/iso/en/ISOOnline.frontpage).

Jacobs, K., Johnson, P., Dennerlein, J., Peterson, D., Kaufman, J., Gold, J., Williams, S., Richmond, N., Karban, S., Firn, E., Ansong, E., Hudak, S., Tung, K., Hall, V., Pencina, K., and Pencina, M. (2009). University students' notebook computer use. *Applied Ergonomics* 40:404–409.

Jampel, R.S. and Shi, D.X. (1992). The primary position of the eyes, the resetting saccade, and the transverse visual head plane. *Investigative Ophthalmology and Visual Science* 33:2501–2510.

Jaschinski, W., Heuer, H., and Kylian, H. (1998). Preferred position of visual displays relative to the eyes: A field study of visual strain and individual differences. *Ergonomics* 41:1034–1049.

Jensen, C., Borg, V., Finsen, L., Hansen, K., Juul-Kristensen, B., and Christensen, H. (1998). Job demands, muscle activity and musculoskeletal symptoms in relation to work with the computer mouse. *Scandinavian Journal of Work and Environmental Health* 24:418–424.

JIS Z 8513. (1994). *Ergonomics, Office Work with Visual Display Terminals (VDTs)*. Tokyo 100-8921, Japan: Japanese Industrial Standards Committee (http://www.jisc.org/).

Johansson, L., Björing, G., and Hägg, G. (2004). The effect of wrist orthoses on forearm muscle activity. *Applied Ergonomics* 35:129–136.

Johnson, P.W., Tal, R., Smutz, W.P., and Rempel, D.M. (1994). Fingertip forces measured during computer mouse operation: a comparison of pointing and dragging. *Proceedings of the 12th Triennial Congress of the International Ergonomics Association*, Vol. 2, pp. 208–210.

Johnson, P., Rempel, D., and Hagberg, M. (1997). Developing and evaluating force sensing mice for use in epidemiological studies. *Proceedings of the 13th Triennial Congress of the International Ergonomics Association*, Vol. 5, pp. 47–49.

Jonai, H., Villanueva, M.B.G., Takata, A., Sotoyama, M., and Saito, S. (2002). Effects of the liquid crystal display tilt angle of a notebook computer on posture, muscle activities and somatic complaints. *International Journal of Industrial Ergonomics* 29:219–239.

Jones, J.C. (1969). Methods and results of seating research. *Ergonomics* 12:171–181.

Jonsson, B. (1988). The static load component in muscle work. *European Journal of Applied Physiology* 57:305–310.

Jürgens, H.W. (1969). Die Verteilung des Körperdrucks auf Sitzfläche und Rückenlehne als Problem der Industrieanthropologie (Distribution of body weight on the seat pan and seat back as an ergonomics problem). *Ergonomics* 12:198–205.

Jürgens, H.W. (1980). Body movements of the driver in relation to sitting conditions in the car: A methodological study. In: D.J. Oborne and J.A. Lewis (eds). *Human Factors in Transport Research*, Vol. 2. London, U.K.: Academic Press, pp. 249–256.

Kaji, R. (2000). Facts and fancies on writer's cramp. *Muscle Nerve* 23:1313–1315.

Karlqvist, L., Hagberg, M., and Selin, K. (1994). Variation in upper limb posture and movement during word processing with and without mouse use. *Ergonomics* 37:1261–1267.

Karlqvist, L.K., Bernmark, E., Ekenvall, L., Hagberg, M., Isaksson, A., and Rostö, T. (1998). Computer mouse position as a determinant of posture, muscular load and perceived exertion. *Scandinavian Journal of Work and Environmental Health* 24:62–73.

Karrasch, K. and Müller, E.A. (1951). Das Verhalten der Pulsfrequenz in der Erholungsperiode nach körperlicher Arbeit (Heart rate recovery during rest after heavy work). *Arbeitsphysiologie* 14:369–382.

Karvonen, M.J., Koskela, A., and Noro, L. (1962). Preliminary report on the sitting postures of school children. *Ergonomics* 5:471–477.

Keegan, J.J. (1953). Alteration of the lumbar curve related to posture and seating. *Journal of Bone and Joint Surgery* 35A:589–603.

Keir, P.J., Bach, J.M., and Rempel, D.M. (1998). Fingertip loading and carpal tunnel pressure: Differences between a pinching and a pressing task. *Journal of Orthopaedic Research* 16:112–115.

Keir, P.J., Bach, J.M., and Rempel, D.M. (1999). Effects of computer mouse design and task on carpal tunnel pressure. *Ergonomics* 42:1350–1360.

Kelaher, D., Nay, T., Lawrence, B., Lamar, S., and Sommerich, C.M. (2001). An investigation of the effects of touchpad location within a notebook computer. *Applied Ergonomics* 32:101–110.

Kennedy, K.W. (1964). *Reach Capability of the USAF Population: Phase I. The Outer Boundaries of Grasping-Reach Envelopes for the Shirt-Sleeved, Seated Operator*, TDR 64-59. Dayton, OH: USAF Aerospace Medical Research Laboratory.

Kim, S.H. and Kaber, D.B. (2009). Design and evaluation of dynamic text-editing methods using foot pedals. *International Journal of Industrial Ergonomics* 39:358–365.

Kingma, I. and van Dieën, J.H. (2009). Static and dynamic postural loadings during computer work in females: Sitting on an office chair versus sitting on an exercise ball. *Applied Ergonomics* 40:199–205.

Kinkead, R.D. and Gonzalez, B.K. (1969). *Human Factors Design Recommendations for Touch Operated Keyboards*. Doc. 12091-FR. Minneapolis, MN: Honeywell, Inc.

Klockenberg, E.A. (1926). *Rationalisierung der Schreibmaschine und Ihrer Bedienung (Rationalization of Typewriters and Their Operation)*. Berlin, Germany: Springer-Verlag.

Komoike, Y. and Horiguchi, S. (1971). Fatigue assessment on key punch operators, typists and others. *Ergonomics* 14:101–109.

Konz, S. and Goel, S.C. (1969). The shape of the normal work area in the horizontal plane. *American Institute of Industrial Engineers* 1:70–74.

Korthals-deBos, I.B., Gerritsen, A.A., van Tulder, M.W., Rutten-vanMölken, M.P., Ader, H.J., de Vet, H.C., and Bouter, L.M. (2006). Surgery is more cost-effective than splinting for carpal tunnel syndrome in the Netherlands: Results of an economic evaluation alongside a randomized controlled trial. *BMC Musculoskeletal Disorders* 7:86.

Kosiak, M. (1959). Etiology and pathology of ischemic ulcers. *Archives of Physical Medicine and Rehabilitation* 40:62–69.

Kosiak, M. Kubicek, W.G., Olsen, M., Danz, J.N., and Kottke, F.J. (1958). Evaluation of pressure as a factor in the production of ischial ulcers. *Archives of Physical Medicine and Rehabilitation* 39:623–629.

Kotani, K. and Horii, K. (2001). A fundamental study on pointing force applied to the mouse in relation to approaching angles and the index of difficulty. *International Journal of Industrial Ergonomics* 28:189–195.

Kroemer, K.H.E. (1964). Über den Einfluss der räumlichen Lage von Tastenfeldern auf die Leistung an Schreibmaschinen (Influence of keyboard spatial positioning on the efficiency of typewriters). *Internationale Zeitschrift für Angewandte Physiologie einschliesslich Arbeitsphysiologie* 20:240–251.

Kroemer, K.H.E. (1965). Vergleich einer normalen Schreibmaschinen-Tastatur mit einer "K-tastatur" (Comparison of a standard typewriter keyboard with a K-keyboard). *Internationale Zeitschrift für Angewandte Physiologie einschliesslich Arbeitsphysiologie* 20:453–464.

Kroemer, K.H.E. (1972). Human engineering the keyboard. *Human Factors* 14:51–63.

Kroemer, K.H.E. (1983). *Ergonomics Guides, Ergonomics of VDT Workplaces*. Fairfax, VA: American Industrial Hygiene Association.

Kroemer, K.H.E. and Hill, S.G. (1986). Preferred line of sight angle. *Ergonomics* 29:1129–1134.

Kroemer, K.H.E. and Kroemer, A.D. (2001). *Office Ergonomics*. London, U.K.: Taylor & Francis.

Krouskop, T.A., Williams, R., Krebs, M., Herszkowicz, I., and Garber, S. (1985). Effectiveness of mattress overlay in reducing interface pressures during recumbency. *Journal of Rehabilitation Research and Development* 22:7–10.

Krueger, H. (1980). Ophthalmological aspects of work with display workstations. In: E. Grandjean and E. Vigliani (eds), *Ergonomics Aspects of Visual Display Terminals*. London, U.K.: Taylor & Francis, pp. 31–40.

Kuo, M.H., Leong, C.P., Cheng, Y.F., and Chang, H.W. (2001). Static wrist position associated with least median nerve compression: Sonographic evaluation. *American Journal of Physical Medicine and Rehabilitation* 80:256–260.

Kwon, S., Lee, D., and Chung, M.K. (2009). Effect of key size and activation area on the performance of a regional error correction methods in a touch-screen QWERTY keyboard. *International Journal of Industrial Ergonomics* 39:888–893.

Lander, C., Korbon, G.A., DeGood, D.E., and Rowlingson, J.C. (1987). The Balans chair and its semi-kneeling position: An ergonomic comparison with the conventional sitting position. *Spine* 12:269–272.

Langolf, G.D., Chaffin, D.B., and Foulke, J.A. (1976). An investigation of Fitts' law using a wide range of movement amplitudes. *Journal of Motor Behavior* 8:113–128.

Laurig, W. (1969). Der stehsitz als physiologisch günstige Alternative zum reine Steharbeitsplatz (Sitstanding as a physiologically favorable alternative for a tidy standing workstation). *Arbeitsmedizin, Sozialmedizin, und Arbeitshygiene* 4:219.

LeCarpentier, E.F. (1969). Easy chair dimensions for comfort—A subjective approach. *Ergonomics* 12:328–337.

Lee, K., Swanson, N., Sauter, S., Wickstrom, R., Waikar, A., and Mangums, M. (1992). A review of physical exercises recommended for VDT operators. *Applied Ergonomics* 23:387–408.

Lehmann, G. and Stier, F. (1961). Mensch und Gerät (Humans and tools). In: *Handbuch der Gesamten Arbeitsmedizin*, Vol. 1. Berlin, Germany: Urban und Schwarzenberg, pp. 718–788.

Leibowitz, H.W. and Owens, D.A. (1975). Anomalous myopias and the intermediate dark focus of accommodation. *Science* 189:646–648.

Less, M. and Eichelberg, W. (1976). Force changes in neck vertebrae and muscles. In: P. Komi (ed.), *Biomechanics*, Vol. V-A. Baltimore, MD: University Park Press, pp. 530–536.

Lewis, J.R., Potosnak, K.M., and Magyar, R.L. (1997). Keys and keyboards. In: M. Helander, T.K. Landauer and P. Prabhu (eds), *Handbook of Human-Computer Interaction*, 2nd edn, North Holland, the Netherlands: Elsevier, pp. 1285–1315.

Liao, M.H. and Drury, C.G. (2000). Posture, discomfort and performance in a VDT task. *Ergonomics* 43:345–359.

Life, M.A. and Pheasant, S.T. (1984). An integrated approach to the study of posture in keyboard operation. *Applied Ergonomics* 15:83–90.

Lindan, O., Greenway, R.M., and Piazza, J.M. (1965). Pressure distribution on the surface of the human body: I. Evaluation in lying and sitting positions using a "bed of springs and nails." *Archives of Physical Medicine* 46:378–385.

Link, C.S., Nicholson, G.G., Shaddeau, S.A., Birch, R., and Gossman, M.R. (1990). Lumbar curvature in standing and sitting in two types of chairs: Relationship of hamstring and hip flexor muscle length. *Physical Therapy* 70:611–618.

Loricchio, D.F. (1992). A comparison of three pointing devices: Mouse, cursor keys, and a key-board integration pushbutton. *Proceedings of the Human Factors Society* 36:303–305.

Loricchio, D.F. and Lewis, J.R. (1991). User assessment of standard and reduced-size numeric key-pads. *Proceedings of the Human Factors Society* 35:251–252.

Lowe, B.D. and Freivalds, A. (1999). Effect of carpal tunnel syndrome on grip force coordination on hand tools. *Ergonomics* 42:550–564.

Lueder, R.K. (1983). Seat comfort: A review of the construct in the office environment. *Human Factors* 25:701–711.

Lundborg, G., Myers, R., and Powell, H. (1983). Nerve compression injury and increased endoneurial fluid pressure: A "miniature compartment syndrome." *Journal of Neurology, Neurosurgery, and Psychiatry* 46:1119–1124.

Lutz, M.C. and Chapanis, A. (1955). Expected locations of digits and letters on ten-button keysets. *Journal of Applied Psychology* 39:314–317.

MacKenzie, I.S., Sellen, A., and Buxton, W. (1991). A comparison of input devices in elemental pointing and dragging tasks. *Proceedings of the CHI '91 Conference on Human Factors in Computing Systems*. New York: ACM, pp. 161–166.

Maeda, K. (1977). Occupational cervicobrachial disorder and its causative factors. *Journal of Human Ergology* 6:193–202.

Maeda, K., Horiguchi, S., and Hosokawa, M. (1982), History of the studies on occupational cerviobrachial disorder in Japan and remaining problems. *Journal of Human Ergology* 11:17–29.

Magora, A. (1972). Investigation of the relation between low back pain and occupation, 3. Physical requirements: Sitting standing and weight lifting. *Industrial Medicine and Surgery* 41:5–9.

Magyar, R.L. (1985). *Effects of Curved, Flat, and Stepped Keybutton Configurations of Keyboard Preference and Throughput Performance*. Boca Raton, FL: International Business Machine Corp.

Mamaghani, N.K., Shimomura, Y., Iwanaga, K., and Katsuura, T. (2009). Effects of strap support in a hand-held device on the muscular activity in female workers assessed by electromyography an subjective rating. *Ergonomics* 52:848–859.

Mandal, Å.C. (1976). Work-chair with tilting seat. *Ergonomics* 19:157–164.

Mandal, Å.C. (1981). The seated man (Homo Sedens). *Applied Ergonomics* 12:19–26.

Mandal, Å.C. (1982). The correct height of school furniture. *Human Factors* 24:257–269.

Marklin, R.W., Simoneau, G.G., and Monroe, J.F. (1999). Wrist and forearm posture from typing of split and vertically inclined computer keyboards. *Human Factors* 41:559–569.

Marschall, M., Harrington, A.C., and Steele, J.R. (1995). Effect of work station design on sitting posture in young children. *Ergonomics* 38:1932–1940.

Marteniuk, R.G., Ivens, C.J., and Brown, B.E. (1997). Are there task specific performance effects for differently configured numeric keypads? *Applied Ergonomics* 27:321–325.

Martin, B.J., Armstrong, T.J., Foulke, J.A., Natarajan, S., Klinenberg, E., Serina, E., and Rempel, D. (1996). Keyboard reaction force and finger flexor electromyograms during computer keyboard work. *Human Factors* 38:654–664.

Mauer, U.M., Lotspeich, E., Klein, H.J., and Rath, S.A. (1991). Body building–effect on neural conduction velocity of the median nerve in the carpal tunnel (in German). *Zeitschrift für Orthopaedie und ihre Grenzgebiete* 129:319–321.

Maxwell, W.C. (1953). The rhythmic keyboard. *Journal of Business Education* 27:327–330.

Maynard, H.B. (1934). Workplace layouts that save, time effort, and money. *Iron Age* 134(Dec. 6): 28–30, 92.

McCormick, E.J. (1970). *Human Factors Engineering*, 3rd edn, New York: McGraw-Hill, p. 427.

McLean, L., Tingley, M., Scott, R.N., and Rickards, J. (2001). Computer terminal work and the benefit of microbreaks. *Applied Ergonomics* 32:225–237.

Menozzi, M., von Buol, A., Krueger, H., and Miège, C. (1994). Direction of gaze and comfort: Discovering the relation for the ergonomic optimization of visual tasks. *Ophthalmology and Physiological Optics* 14:393–399.

Michaels, S.E. (1971). QWERTY versus alphabetic keyboards as a function of typing skill. *Human Factors* 13:419–426.

Michel, D.P. and Helander, M.G. (1994). Effects of two types of chairs on stature change and comfort for individuals with healthy and herniated discs. *Ergonomics* 37:1231–1244.

Miller, I. and Suther, T.W. (1983). Display station anthropometrics: Preferred height and angle settings of CRT and keyboard. *Human Factors* 25:401–408.

Mishra, S., Prabhakar, S., Lal, V., Modi, M., Das, C.P., and Khurana, D. (2006). Efficacy of splinting and oral steroids in the treatment of carpal tunnel syndrome: A prospective randomized clinical and electrophysiology study. *Neurology India* 54:286–290.

Mon-Williams, M., Burgess-Limerick, R., Plooy, A., and Wann, J. (1999). Vertical gaze direction and postural adjustment: An extension of the Heuer model. *Journal of Experimental Psychology: Applied* 5:35–53.

Moneta, K.B. (1960). Optimum physical design of an alphabetical keyboard, post office. Research Report No. 20412.

Monty, R.W. and Snyder, H.L. (1983). Keyboard design: An investigation of user preference and performance. *Proceedings of the Human Factors Society* 27:201–105.

Mooney, V., Einbund, M.J., Rogers, J.E., and Stauffer, E.S. (1971). Comparison of pressure distribution qualities in seat cushions. *Bulletin of Prosthetic Research* 10–15:129–143.

Nachemson, A. and Morris, J.M. (1964). In vivo measurements of intradiscal pressure. *The Journal of Bone and Joint Surgery* 46A:1077–1092.

Nag, P.K., Pal, A., Nag, A., and Vyas, H. (2009). Influence of arm and wrist support on forearm and back muscle activity in computer keyboard operation. *Applied Ergonomics* 40:286–291.

Najjar, L.J., Stanton, B.C., and Bowen, C.D. (1988). *Keyboard Heights and Slopes for Standing Typists.* Technical Report 85–0081. Rockville, MD: International Business Machine Corp.

Nakaseko, M., Grandjean, E., Hünting, W., and Gierer, R. (1985). Studies on ergonomically designed alphanumeric keyboards. *Human Factors* 27:175–187.

Nathan, P.A., Wilcox, A., Emerick, P.S., Meadows, K.D., and McCormack, A.L. (2001). Effects of an aerobic exercise program on median nerve conduction and symptoms associated with carpal tunnel syndrome. *Journal of Occupational and Environmental Medicine* 43:840–843.

National Research Council. (1984). *Video Displays, Work and Vision.* Washington, DC: National Academy of Press.

National Research Council. (2001). *Musculoskeletal Disorders and the Workplace.* Washington, DC: National Academy of Press.

Ng, D., Cassar, T., and Gross, C.M. (1995). Evaluation of an intelligent seat system. *Applied Ergonomics* 26:109–116.

NIOSH. (1981). *Potential Health Hazards of Video Display Terminals.* Report No. 81–129. Cincinnati, OH: National Institute for Occupational Safety and Health.

NIOSH. (1989). *Carpal Tunnel Syndrome: Selected References.* Cincinnati, OH: National Institute for Occupational Safety and Health.

NIOSH. (1995). *Cumulative Trauma Disorders in the Workplace: Bibliography.* Report No. 95–119. Cincinnati, OH: National Institute for Occupational Safety and Health.

NIOSH. (1997). *Musculoskeletal Disorders and Workplace Factors.* Report No. 97-141. Cincinnati, OH: National Institute for Occupational Safety and Health.

Nobuta, S., Sato, K., Nakagawa, T., Hatori, M., and Itoi, E. (2008). Effects of wrist splinting for carpal tunnel syndrome and motor nerve conduction measurements. *Upsala Journal of Medical Sciences* 113:181–192.

Norman, D. and Fisher, D. (1982). Why alphabetic keyboards are not easy to use: Keyboard layout doesn't much matter. *Human Factors* 24:509–519.

Noyes, J. (1983a). The QWERTY keyboard: A review. *International Journal of Man-Machine Studies* 18:265–281.

Noyes, J. (1983b). Chord keyboards. *Applied Ergonomics* 14:55–59.

Noyes, J. (1998). QWERTY—The immortal keyboard. *Control & Computing Engineering Journal* 9(3):117–122.

Ong, C.N. (1984). VDT work place design and physical fatigue: A case study in Singapore. In: E. Grandjean (ed.), *Ergonomics and Health in Modern Offices.* London, U.K.: Taylor & Francis, pp. 484–494.

OSHA. (1991). *Working Safely with Video Display Terminals.* Washington, DC: U.S. Department of Labor, Occupational Safety and Health Administration.

Paci, A.M. and Gabbrielli, L. (1984). Some experiences in the field of design of VDU work stations. In: E. Grandjean (ed.), *Ergonomics and Health in Modern Offices.* London, U.K.: Taylor & Francis, pp. 391–399.

Park, S.K. (1999). The development of an exposure measurement system for assessing risk of work-related musculoskeletal disorders (WMSDs). Unpublished PhD thesis. University Park, PA: Penn State University.

Park, S.Y. and Han, S.H. (2010). Touch key design for one-handed thumb interaction with a mobile phone: Effects of touch key size and touch key location. *International Journal of Industrial Ergonomics* 40:68–76.

Parsons, C.A. (1991). Use of wrist rest by data input VDU operators. In: E.J. Lovesey (ed.), *Contemporary Ergonomics 1991: Proceedings of the Ergonomics Society's Annual Conference.* London, U.K.: Taylor & Francis, pp. 319–321.

Paul, L.E., Sarlanis, K., and Buckley, E.P. (1965). A human factors comparison of two data entry keyboards. Presented at the *Sixth Annual Symposium of the Professional Group on Human Factors in Electronics,* IEEE.

Paul, R. and Menon, K.K. (1994). Ergonomic evaluation of keyboard wrist pads. *Proceedings of the International Ergonomics Association* 2:204–207.

Perez-Balke, G. and Buchholz, B.O. (1994). A study of the effect of a resting splint on peak grip strength. *Proceedings of the Human Factors and Ergonomics Society* 38:544–548.

Pheasant, S. (1991). *Ergonomics, Work and Health.* London, U.K.: MacMillan Press.

Pinar, L., Enhos, A., Ada, S., and Gübgör, N. (2005). Can we use nerve gliding exercises in women with carpal tunnel syndrome? *Advances in Therapy* 22:467–475.

Pollock, W.T. and Gildner, G.G. (1963). *Study of Computer Manual Input Devices,* ESD-TDR-63-545. Bedford, MA: USAF, Hanscom Field.

Pooni, J.S., Hukins, D.W.L., Harris, P.F., Hilton, R.C., and Davies, K.E. (1986). Comparison of the structure of human intervertebral discs in the cervical, thoracic, and lumbar regions of the spine. *Surgical and Radiologic Anatomy* 8:175–182.

Poulton, E.C. (1974). *Tracking Skill and Manual Control.* New York: Academic Press.

Powell, H.C. and Myers, R.R. (1986). Pathology of experimental nerve compression. *Laboratory Investigation* 55:91–100.

Price, J.M. and Dowell, W.R. (1997). A field evaluation of two split keyboards. *Proceedings of the Human Factors and Ergonomics Society* 41:410–414.

Psihogios, J.P., Sommerich, C.M., Mirka, G.A., and Moon, S.D. (2001). A field evaluation of monitor placement effects in VDT users. *Applied Ergonomics* 32:313–325.

Radwin, R.G. and Jeng, O.J. (1997). Activation force and travel effects on overexertion in repetitive key tapping. *Human Factors* 39:130–140.

Rasmussen, J., Tørholm, S., and de Zee, M. (2009). Computational analysis of the influence of seat pan inclination and friction on muscle activity and spinal joint forces. *International Journal of Industrial Ergonomics* 39:52–57.

Rebiffé, R. (1969). Le siège to conducteur: Son adaptation aux exigences fonctionelles et anthropometriques (Driver seating: Derived from functional and anthropometric requirements). *Ergonomics* 12:246–261.

Rempel, D. (2008). The split keyboard: An ergonomics success story. *Human Factors* 50:385–392.

Rempel, D., Dennerlein, J., Mote, C.D., and Armstrong, T. (1994). A method of measuring fingertip loading during keyboard use. *Journal of Biomechanics* 27:1101–1104.

Rempel, D., Keir, P.J., Smutz, W.P., and Hargens, A. (1997a). Effects of static fingertip loading on carpal tunnel pressure. *Journal of Orthopaedic Research* 15:422–426.

Rempel, D., Serina, E., Klinenberg, E., Martin, B.J., Armstrong, T.J., Foulke, J.A., and Natarajan, S. (1997b). The effect of keyboard keyswitch make force on applied force and finger flexor muscle activity. *Ergonomics* 40:800–808.

Rempel, D., Bach, J.M., Gordon, L., and Tal, R. (1998). Effects of forearm pronation/supination and metacarpophalangeal flexion on carpal tunnel pressure. *Journal of Hand Surgery* 23A:38–42.

Rempel, D., Tittiranonda, P., Burastero, S., Hudes, M., and So, Y. (1999). Effect of keyboard keyswitch design on hand pain. *Journal of Occupational and Environmental Medicine* 41:111–119.

Rempel, D., Barr, A., Brafmann, D., and Young, E. (2007). The effect of six keyboard designs on wrist and forearm postures. *Applied Ergonomics* 38:293–298.

Rose, M.J. (1991). Keyboard operating posture and actuation force: Implications for muscle over-use. *Applied Ergonomics* 22:198–203.

Robertson, M., Amick III, B.C., DeRango, K., Rooney, T., Bazzani, L., Harrist, R., and Moore, A. (2009). The effects of an office ergonomics training and chair intervention on worker knowledge, behavior and musculoskeletal risk. *Applied Ergonomics* 40:124–135.

Rozmanryn, L.M., Dovelle, S., Rothman, E.R., Gorman, K., Olvey, K.M., and Bartko, J.J. (1998). Nerve and tendon gliding exercises and the conservative management of carpal tunnel syndrome. *Journal of Hand Therapy* 11:171–179.

Rubin, T. and Marshall, C.J. (1982). Adjustable VDT workstations: Can naive users achieve a human factors solution? *International Conference on Man-Machine Systems*, Conference Publication No. 121. Manchester, U.K.: Institution of Electrical Engineers.

Sanders, M.S. and McCormick, E.J. (1993). *Human Factors in Engineering and Design*, 7th edn, New York: McGraw-Hill, p. 361.

Sauter, S.L., Schleifer, L.M., and Knutson, S.J. (1991). Work posture, workstation design, and musculoskeletal discomfort in a VDT data entry task. *Human Factors* 33:151–167.

Scales, E.M. and Chapanis, A. (1954). The effect of performance of tilting the toll-operators' keyset. *Journal of Applied Psychology* 38:452–456.

Schoberth, H. (1962). *Sitzhalten, Sitzschaden, Sitzmöbel (Sitting Postures, Sitting Disorders, Chairs)*. Berlin, Germany: Spring Verlag.

Seghers, J., Jochem, A., and Spaepen, A. (2003). Posture, muscle activity and muscle fatigue in prolonged VDT work at different screen height settings. *Ergonomics* 46:714–730.

Seibel, R. (1964). Data entry through chord, parallel entry devices. *Human Factors* 6:189–192.

Seibel, R. (1972). Data entry devices and procedures. In: H.P. VanCott and R.G. Kinkade (eds), *Human Engineering Guide to Equipment Design*. Washington, DC: American Institutes for Research, pp. 311–344.

Seradge, H., Bear, C., and Bithell, D. (2000). Preventing carpal tunnel syndrome and cumulative trauma disorder: Effect of carpal tunnel decompression exercises: An Oklahoma experience. *Journal of the Oklahoma State Medical Association* 93:150–153.

Seradge, H., Parker, W., Baer, C., Mayfield, K., and Schall, L. (2002). Conservative treatment of carpal tunnel syndrome: An outcome study of adjunct exercises. *Journal of the Oklahoma State Medical Association* 95:7–14.

Serina, E.R., Tal, R., and Rempel, D. (1999). Wrist and forearm postures and motions during typing. *Ergonomics* 42:938–951.

Sevim, S., Dogu, O., Camdeviren, H., Kaleagasi, H., Aral, J., Arslan, E., and Milcan, A. (2004). Long-term effectiveness of steroid injections and splinting in mild and moderate carpal tunnel syndrome. *Neurological Sciences* 25:48–52.

Shackel, B., Chidsey, K.D., and Shipley, P. (1969). The assessment of chair comfort. *Ergonomics* 12:269–306.

Sheehy, M.P. and Marsden, C.D. (1982). Writer's cramp—A focal dystonia. *Brain* 105:461–480.

Shen, W. and Parsons, K.C. (1997). Validity and reliability of rating scales for seated pressure discomfort. *International Journal of Industrial Ergonomics* 20:441–461.

Shields, R.K. and Cook, T.M. (1988). Effect of seat angle and lumbar support on seat buttock pressure. *Physical Therapy* 68:1682–1686.

Shvartz, E., Guame, J.G., White, R.T., Riebold, R.C., and Glassford, E.J. (1980). Effect of the circutone seat on hemodynamic, subjective and thermal responses during prolonged sitting. *Proceedings of the Human Factors Society* 24:639–642.

Silverstein, B.A., Fine, J.L., and Armstrong, T.J. (1986). Hand wrist cumulative trauma disorders in industry. *British Journal of Industrial Medicine* 43:779–784.

Slechta, R.F., Forrest, J., Carter, W.K., and Forrest, J. (1959). *Comfort Evaluation of the C-124 Crew Seat (Weber)*. WADC Technical Report 58-136. Dayton, OH: Wright Air Development Center, Wright-Patterson Air Force Base.

Smith, M.J., Cohen, B.G.F., and Stammerjohn, L.W. (1981). An investigation of health complaints and job stress in video display operations. *Human Factors* 23:387–400.

Smith, M.J., Karsh, B.T., Conway, F.T., Cohen, W.J., James, C.A., Morgan, J.J., Sanders, K., and Zehel, D.J. (1998). Effects of a split keyboard design and wrist rest on performance, posture, and comfort. *Human Factors* 40:324–336.

Smutz, P., Serina, E., and Rempel, D. (1994). A system for evaluating the effect of keyboard design on force, posture, comfort, and productivity. *Ergonomics* 37:1649–1660.

Sommerich, C.M. (2000). Inputting to a notebook computer. *Proceedings of the IEA/HFES 2000 Congress*, pp. 671–674.

Sommerich, C.M., Marras, W.S., and Parnianpour, M. (1996). Observations on the relationship between key strike force and typing speed. *American Industrial Hygiene Association Journal* 57:1109–1114.

Sommerich, C.M., Joines, S.M.B., and Psihogios, J.P. (2001). Effects of computer monitor viewing angle and related factors on strain, performance, and preference outcomes. *Human Factors* 43:39–55.

Song, T.K., Shepard, R.J., and Cox, M.H. (1982). Absenteeism, employee turnover, and sustained exercise participation. *Journal of Sports Medicine and Physical Fitness* 22:392–399.

Sotoyama, M., Jonai, H., Saito, S., and Villanueva, M.B.G. (1996). Analysis of ocular surface area for comfortable VDT workstation layout. *Ergonomics* 39:877–884.

Springer, T.J. (1982). VDT workstations: A comparative evaluation of alternatives. *Applied Ergonomics* 13:211–212.

Sprigle, S., Chung, K.C., and Brubacker, C.E. (1990). Reduction of sitting pressures with custom contoured cushions. *Journal of Rehabilitation Research and Development* 27:135–140.

Squires, P.C. (1956). *The Shape of the Normal Working Area*. Report No. 275. New London, CT: U.S. Navy Department, Bureau of Medicine and Surgery.

Staffel, F. (1884). Zur Hygiene des Sitzens (Seating health). *Zentralblatt für algemeine Gesundheitspflege* 3:404–421.

Straker, L., Jones, K.J., and Miller, J. (1997). A comparison of the postures assumed when using laptop computers and desktop computers. *Applied Ergonomics* 28:263–268.

Straker, L., Levine, J., and Campbell, A. (2009). The effects of walking and cycling computer workstations on keyboard and mouse performance. *Human Factors* 51:831–844.

Straub, H.R. and Granaas, M.M. (1993). Task-specific preference for numeric keypads. *Applied Ergonomics* 24:289–290.

Strong, E.P. (1956). *A Comparative Experiment in Simplified Keyboard Re-Training and Standard Keyboard Supplementary Training*. Washington, DC: General Services Administration.

Sucher, B.M. (1994). Palpatory diagnosis and manipulative management of carpal tunnel syndrome. *Journal of the American Osteopathic Association* 94:647–663.

Sundelin, G. and Hagberg, M. (1989). The effects of different pause types on neck and shoulder EMG activity during VDU work. *Ergonomics* 32:527–537.

Suther, T.W. and McTyre, J.H. (1982). Effect on operator performance at thin profile keyboard slopes of 5°, 10°, 15°, and 25°. *Proceedings of the Human Factors Society* 26:430–434.

Svensson, H.O. and Andersson, G.B.J. (1983). Low back pain in 40–47 year old men: Work history and work environment factors. *Spine* 8:272–276.

Swanson, N.G., Galinsky, T.L., Cole, L.L., Pan, C.S., and Sauter, S.L. (1997). The impact of keyboard design on comfort and productivity in a text-entry task. *Applied Ergonomics* 28:9–16.

Swarts, A.E., Krouskop, T.A., and Smith, D.R. (1988). Tissue pressure management in the vocational setting. *Archives of Physical Medicine and Rehabilitation* 69:97–100.

Swearingen, J.J., Wheelwright, C.D., and Garner, J.D. (1962). *An Analysis of Sitting Areas and Pressures of Man*. Rep. No. 62-1. Oklahoma City, OK: U.S. Civil Aero-Medical Research Institute.

Szeto, G.P.Y., Straker, L.M., and O'Sullivan, P.B. (2005a). The effects of speed and force of keyboard operations on neck-shoulder muscle activities in symptomatic and asymptomatic office workers. *International Journal of Industrial Ergonomics* 35:429–444.

Szeto, G.P.Y., Straker, L.M., and O'Sullivan, P.B. (2005b). The effects of speed and force on motor control in symptomatic and asymptomatic office workers. *International Journal of Industrial Ergonomics* 35:779–795.

Telfer, S., Spence, W.D., and Solomonidis, S.E. (2009). The potential for actigraphy to be used as an indicator of sitting discomfort. *Human Factors* 51:694–704.

Thornton, W. (1978). Anthropometric changes in weightlessness. In: Webb Associates (ed.), *Anthropometric Source Book*, Vol. 1, NASA RP1024. Houston, TX: National Aeronautics and Space Administration.

Tittiranonda, P., Rempel, D., Armstrong, T., and Burastero, S. (1999). Effect of four computer keyboards in computer users with upper extremity musculoskeletal disorders. *American Journal of Industrial Medicine* 35:647–661.

Tomatis, L., Nakaseko, M., and Läubli, T. (2009). Co-activation and maximal EMG activity of forearm muscles during key tapping. *International Journal of Industrial Ergonomics* 39:749–755.

Turville, K.L., Psihogios, J.P., Ulmer, T.R., and Mirka, G.A. (1998). The effects of video display terminal height on the operator: A comparison of the 15° and 40° recommendations. *Applied Ergonomics* 29:239–246.

Ucan, H., Yagci, I., Yilmaz, L., Yagmurlu, F., Keskin, D., and Bodur, H. (2006). Comparison of splinting, splinting plus local steroid injection and open carpal tunnel release outcomes in idiopathic carpal tunnel syndrome. *Rheumatology International* 27:45–51.

Udo, H., Otani, T., Udo, A., and Yoshinaga, F. (2000). A electromyographic study of two different types of ball point pens. *Industrial Health* 38:47–50.

VanCott, H.P. and Kinkade, R.G. (1972). *Human Engineering Guide to Equipment Design*. Washington, DC: U.S. Government Printing Office, p. 400.

Vandraas, K. (1981). Necessary for some, unusable for others, an alternative for many. *Fysioterapueuten* 48:546–550 (in Norwegian).

Verdugo, R.J., Salinas, R.A., Castillo, J.L., and Cea, J.G. (2008). Surgical versus non-surgical treatment for carpal tunnel syndrome. *Cochrane Database System Review* 3:CD001552.

Villanueva, M.B.G., Sotoyama, M., Jonai, H., Takeuchi, Y., and Saito, S. (1996). Adjustments of posture and viewing parameters of the eye to changes in the screen height of the visual display terminal. *Ergonomics* 39:933–945.

Villanueva, M.B.G., Jonai, H., and Saito, S. (1998). Ergonomics aspects of portable personal computers with flat panel displays: Evaluation of posture, muscle activities, discomfort and performance. *Industrial Health* 36:282–289.

Wachsler, R.A. and Lerner, D.B. (1960). An analysis of some factors influencing seat comfort. *Ergonomics* 3:315–320.

Walker, W.C., Metzler, M., Cifu, D.X., and Swartz, Z. (2000). Neutral wrist splinting in carpal tunnel syndrome: A comparison of night-only versus full-time wear instructions. *Archives of Physical Medicine and Rehabilitation* 81:424–429.

Waters, T.R., Putz-Anderson, V., Garg, A., and Fine, L.J. (1993). Revised NIOSH equation for the design an evaluation of manual lifting tasks. *Ergonomics* 36:749–776.

Webb Associates. (1978). *Anthropometric Source Book, Vol. I. Anthropometry for Designers*. NASA Ref. Pub. 1024, Washington, DC: National Aeronautics and Space Administration.

Weber, A., Sancin, E., and Grandjean, E. (1984). The effects of various keyboard heights on EMG and physical discomfort. In: E. Grandjean (ed.), *Ergonomics and Health in Modern Offices*. London, U.K.: Taylor & Francis, pp. 477–483.

Wehbé, M.A. (1987). Tendon gliding exercises. *Journal of Occupational Therapy* 41:164–167.

Webhé, M.A. and Schlegel, J.M. (2004). Nerve gliding exercises for thoracic outlet syndrome. *Hand Clinics* 20:51–55.

Weiss, N.D., Gordon, L., Bloom, T., So, Y., and Rempel, D.M. (1995). Position of the wrist associated with the lowest carpal-tunnel pressure: Implications for splint design. *Journal of Bone and Joint Surgery American* 77:1695–1696.

Werner, R., Armstrong, T.J., Bir, C., and Aylard, M.K. (1997). Intracarpal canal pressures: the role of the finger, hand wrist and forearm position. *Clinical Biomechanics* 12:44–51.

Wilks, S. (1878). *Lectures on Diseases of the Nervous System*. London, U.K.: Churchill, pp. 452–460.

Wilks, S., Mortimer, M., and Nylén, P. (2006). The introduction of sit-stand worktables; aspects of attitudes, compliance and satisfaction. *Applied Ergonomics* 37:3559–365.

Winkel, J. (1981). Swelling of lower leg in sedentary work—A pilot study. *Journal of Human Ergology* 10:139–149.

Winkel, J. (1987). On the significance of physical activity in sedentary work. In: G. Knave and P.G. Wideback (eds), *Work with Display Units 86*. Amsterdam, the Netherlands: Elsevier Science, pp. 229–236.

Winkel, J. and Jørgensen, K. (1986). Evaluation of foot swelling and lower-limb temperatures in relation to leg activity during long-term seated office work. *Ergonomics* 29:313–328.

Wotzka, G., Grandjean, E., Burandt, U., Kretzschmar, H., and Leonhard, T. (1969). Investigation for the development of an auditorium seat. *Ergonomics* 12:182–197.

Wright, P., Bartram, C., Rogers, N., Emslie, H., Evans, J., Wilson, B., and Belt, S. (2000). Text entry on handheld computers by older users. *Ergonomics* 43:703–716.

Wu, C.S., Miyamoto, H., and Noro, H. (1998). Research on pelvic angle variation when using a pelvic support. *Ergonomics* 41:317–327.

Yagci, I., Elmas, O., Akcan, E., Ustun, I., Gunduz, O.H., and Guven, Z. (2009). Comparison of splinting and splinting plus low-level laser therapy in idiopathic carpal tunnel syndrome. *Clinical Rheumatology* 26:1059–1065.

Yaginuma, Y., Yamada, H., and Nagai, H. (1990). Study of the relationship between lacrimation and blink in VDT work. *Ergonomics* 33:799–809.

Yoshitake, R. (1995). Relationship between key space and user performance on reduced keyboards. *Journal of Physiological Anthropology and Applied Human Science* 14:287–292.

Zacharkow, D. (1988). *Posture: Sitting, Standing, Chair Design and Exercise.* Springfield, IL: Charles C. Thomas.

Zecevic, A., Miller, D.I., and Harburn, K. (2000). An evaluation of the ergonomics of three computer keyboards. *Ergonomics* 43:55–72.

Zhang, L., Helander, M.G., and Drury, C.G. (1996). Identifying factors of comfort and discomfort in sitting. *Human Factors* 38:377–389.

Zipp, P., Haider, E., Halpern, N., Mainzer, J., and Rohmert, W. (1981). Untersuchung zur ergonomischen Gestaltung von Tastaturen (Research on the ergonomic shape of keyboards). *Zentralblatt für Arbeitsmedizin* 31:326–330.

Zipp, P., Haider, E., Halpern, N., and Rohmert, W. (1983). Keyboard design through physiological strain measurements. *Applied Ergonomics* 14:117–122.

Glossary

Abduction: Raising the arm or thigh away from the body, in the coronal plane; *opp.* adduction.

Abscissa: The vertical axis of a coordinate system, also termed the y-axis.

Accommodation: Adjustment in sensory threshold to a constant level stimuli, resulting in a decreased the rate of firing in the accompanying neuron.

Accuracy: The extent to which a measurement is close to the "true value" or has small deviations from the value being assessed.

Actin: The globular proteins comprising thin filaments within muscles.

Action potential: The active disturbance of nerve and muscle membrane potentials, which creates the means for transmission of information.

Activation heat: Heat in muscle tissue coinciding with the active state.

Active state: Condition in which there are still some calcium ions left in the myofibrils after a previous muscle contraction, causing a potentiating effect for the following contraction.

Adduction: Lowering the arm or bringing the thigh closer to the midline of the body, in the coronal plane; *opp.* abduction.

Adenosine triphosphate: The most basic energy molecule in the body, with energy being stored and released with the forming and breaking of its phosphate bonds.

Adson's test: Test for thoracic outlet syndrome in which the patient is seated with the head extended and turned to the affected side, a positive sign is the weakening of the pulse at the wrist while raising the affected arm and taking a deep breath.

Aerobic: Requiring oxygen, typically referring to metabolism; *opp.* anaerobic.

Afferent: Direction of information flow, typically sensory, from the periphery to the central nervous system; *opp.* efferent.

Agonists: Muscles that act as the prime activators of motion; *opp.* antagonists.

Algebraic approach: Method for finding the inverse Laplace transform by algebraically manipulating the fractional form of a transfer function.

All-or-nothing response: Once an initial depolarization reaches the threshold level, the production of an action potential cannot be stopped. Also, refers to the fact that once a motor neuron is stimulated all its collaterals will transmit the same action potential to the associated muscle fibers.

Anaerobic: Not needing oxygen, typically referring to metabolism; *opp.* aerobic.

Anisotropic: Material whose properties vary depending on the direction of applied forces; *opp.* isotropic.

Annulospiral: Type of receptor found in the equatorial region of the muscle, sensitive both to changes in length and velocity, also termed primary ending.

Annulus fibrosus: The outer onion like fiber casings of an intervertebral disk.

Anode: The positive pole or terminal to which electrons are attracted or current flows.

Antagonists: Muscles that counteract the agonists and oppose the original motion.

Antenna effect: Tendency of long leads to pick up stray electromagnetic radiation and create noise on top of the desired signal.

Anterior interosseous syndrome: Compression of the anterior interosseous branch of the median nerve by the deep anterior forearm muscles, resulting in motor difficulties producing a thumb–index finger tip pinch.

Anthropometers: Specialized calipers for measuring body dimensions.

Antidromic: Nerve conduction along an axon in the direction reverse of normal. *opp.* orthodromic.

Arthritis: Inflammation or degeneration of joint structures; in the form *rheumatoid arthritis* or *osteoarthritis*.

Atari thumb: See *DeQuervain's disease*.

Attributable risk: Estimate of the proportion by which the rate of the disease status among exposed individuals would be reduced if the exposure were eliminated.

Axial bones: Bones found in the skull, vertebrae, pelvis, etc.

Axial rotation: Rotation of a limb or the trunk along the long axis.

Axon: The long part of the neuron, which carries the action potential.

Bandwidth: The amount of information that can be transferred over a channel, defined by the inverse of the Fitts' Law slope; also the range of continuous frequencies that can be processed by a system.

Basal ganglia: Part of the brain above the brain stem associated with motor processing.

Bicipital tendinitis: Inflammation of the long head of the biceps tendon as it passes over the head of the humerus through the bicipital groove caused by hyperabducting the elbow or forceful contractions of the biceps.

Biomechanics: The science that deals with forces and their effects, applied to biological systems.

Bipennate muscles: Muscles whose fibers are arranged obliquely on both sides of the long axis, as in a complete bird feather.

Bipolar: Type of electromyographical recording in which two active electrodes are placed over different areas of the muscle in order to obtain a differential reading.

Bit: Acronym for binary digit, the amount of information obtained from two equally likely alternatives.

Block diagram: System representation using block elements.

Blocks: Cycling patterns in mental arousal.

Bode plot: Linearized frequency analysis plots on a log–log scale.

Body discomfort map: A type of symptom survey in which the worker marks each body part where pain or discomfort is experienced and then rates the level of pain.

Bottom point: Point on keystroke travel at which the key mechanically bottoms out.

Bowler's thumb: See *digital neuritis*.

Brain stem: Part of brain connecting with the spinal cord associated with a variety of motor and sensory processing.

Break force: The minimum force needed to break the circuit and deactivate a key switch; it also signals the user that the keystroke has been completed.

Break frequency: A critical value of frequency at which point the plotted values change suddenly.

Break point: Point on keystroke travel at which the circuit is broken and the key switch is deactivated; it also signals the user that the keystroke has been completed.

Bursae: Closed sacs filled with synovial fluid to reduce friction and with facilitate the motion of tendons and muscles over bony protuberances around joints.

Bursitis: Inflammation of bursae.

Cancellous bone: Spongy and less dense bone material found in the center of bone; also termed spongy bone.

Capitate: The central wrist bone in the distal row.

Carbohydrate loading: Eating increased amounts of carbohydrates two or three days prior to an intense physical activity.

Carpal: Refers to the wrist area; typically the eight carpal bones of the wrist.

Carpal tunnel: Area of the wrist formed by the eight carpal bones on the dorsal side and the flexor retinaculum on the palmar side of the wrist.

Carpal tunnel syndrome: Entrapment of the median nerve in the carpal tunnel, leading to sensory and motor impairment of the middle three fingers.

Carpometacarpal joint: The wrist joint.

Cartesian coordinate system: A two- or three-dimensional coordinate system with perpendicular axes, same as rectangular coordinate system.

Cartilage: Connective tissue covering articular bony surfaces or found in the ear and nose.

Case–control study: Type of epidemiological study in which individuals are selected based on the presence (cases) or absence (controls) of a disease, then information is collected about earlier exposure to a risk factor of interest.

Cases: Individuals having the disease or disorder of interest.

Category ratio scale: A scale with verbal anchors for rating muscular exertion, pain, or discomfort.

Cathode: The negative pole or terminal from which electrons or current flows.

Causality: The extent to which the occurrence of risk factors is responsible for the subsequent occurrence of the disease.

Cell membrane: The outer edge of a cell that acts as a selective barrier for the passage of nutrients, wastes, and hormones.

Center of gravity: The exact center of an object's mass or equilibrium point of that object, also termed center of mass.

Center of mass: The exact center of an object's mass or equilibrium point of that object, also termed center of gravity.

Central nervous system: The portion of the nervous system that includes the brain and the spinal cord; *opp.* peripheral nervous system.

Centrifugal force: Force acting on the body acting along the radius of the rotation.

Cerebellum: Posterior part of the brain that process feedback control for muscles.

Cerebral cortex: Part of the brain which receives sensory information from the neuromusculature and which controls muscle action; also termed sensorimotor cortex.

Cervical radiculopathy: Compression of the spinal nerve roots that form the brachial plexus (C5, C6, C7, C8) in between the intervertebral openings.

Cervical spine: The portion of the spinal column consisting of the seven vertebrae in the neck.

Characteristic function: The denominator of a transfer function, the roots of which characterize the system response.

Cherry pitter's thumb: See *digital neuritis.*

Choice-reaction time: Average time interval for an operator to respond to one or more stimuli with one or more appropriate responses.

Chondrocytes: Cartilage cells arranged in a layered zones.

Chord: Type of keyboard in which entering one character requires the simultaneous activation of two or more keys.

Clasp knife reflex: A reflex involving Golgi tendon organs, in which the limbs collapse due to an overload of force.

Clinical trials: Formal intervention study in which individuals are randomly assigned to one of two study groups, an intervention group and a control group, typically to study the effectiveness of a new drug or treatment.

Closed-loop system: Type of system in which there is some form of comparison between the system output and the command input, also feedback system; *opp.* open-loop system.

Closed-loop transfer function: Complete transfer function representation of a system.

Coefficient of friction: A characteristic of the interaction of the material properties of two surfaces, such as the roughness; for a grip, the ratio of peak shear force as a function of the normal (perpendicular to shear) gripping force.

Coefficient of variability: Simple measure of reliability expressed as the standard deviation of a series repeat measurements divided by the mean.

Cohort study: A type of epidemiological study in which subjects are selected based on the presence or absence of a risk factor, they are then followed over time for the development of the disease of interest.

Collagen: Type of fiber providing strength and stiffness to soft connective tissue.

Common-mode signal-to-noise rejection ratio: The ability of a device to reject a signal that is common to or applied to both input terminals (typically undesired noise) expressed as the ratio of the differential signal gain to the common-mode signal gain.

Compact bone: Denser bone material with higher mineral content, found in the outer edge of the diaphysis, also known as cortical bone.

Compression: Loading mode in which the load is applied axially toward the surface, compressing the material.

Concentric: A dynamic muscle contraction in which the muscle is shortening; *opp.* eccentric.

Congruity: The state of agreement between exposure and disease status.

Construct validity: Type of validity that refers to the physiological or psychological construct or characteristic being measured by the test.

Content validity: See *face validity*.

Contralateral: See *crossed*.

Control: Individual without the disease or disorder of interest.

Correlation coefficient: A formal calculation of the agreement between two or more sets of measurements; typically the Pearson product moment correlation coefficient.

Cortical bone: Denser bone material with higher mineral content, found in the outer edge of the diaphysis, also known as compact bone.

Creep: See *strain retardation*.

Criterion validity: Type of validity that refers to the relationship of scores obtained using the test and the actual cases incurred.

Critically damped: System response for a damping ratio of one.

Cronbach's alpha: An estimate of a test's reliability based on a ratio of the variance of item scores and the variance of test scores.

Crossed: Pertaining to the other side of the body.

Cross product: Manipulation of vectors using the right-hand rule to calculate the moment of the force, resulting in a vector.

Cross-sectional study: Type of epidemiological study in which individuals are sampled at a point in time and then subdivided into distributions of exposures and disease status; *syn.* prevalence study.

Crosstalk: A measurement problem in which a signal is communicated from one channel to another channel, where it is not desired.

Cubital tunnel syndrome: Entrapment of the ulnar nerve at the ulnar groove or cubital tunnel formed by the two heads of the flexor carpi ulnaris near the elbow, often from direct pressure on that area.

Cytoplasm: Cell material other than the nucleus, roughly 80% water.

Damping element: A dashpot-like element in Hill's muscle model representing the viscous nature of the internal water.

Damping ratio: A factor defining the reduction of oscillations in a dynamic system.

Delta function: See *unit impulse.*

Dendrites: The long branches off the cell body that serve to collect nerve impulses from other neurons.

Depolarization: A positive change in the membrane potential.

DeQuervain's disease: Tendinitis of the abductor pollicis longus and extensor pollicis brevis of the thumb; some times termed Atari thumb or Nintendo thumb due to chronic overuse of the thumb with video games.

Diaphysis: The tubular shaft of a long bone.

Digital neuritis: Numbness due to direct pressure on the digital nerves while grasping tools or other items with sharp edges; depending on the aggravating task, may be termed also as bowler's thumb or cherry pitter's thumb.

Digitizing tablet: A flat pad with a stylus, connected to a computer, the movement of which is sensed at the appropriate position on the tablet and produces input to the computer.

Digram: Two-letter keying sequences.

Direction: The line of action of a force.

Disk compression forces: Compressive forces found in the lumbar disks due to external loads.

Disk herniation: The bulging of the intervertebral disks or the even more catastrophic extrusion of the nucleus pulposus gel material.

Distal: Referring to the portion of the body that is furthest from the central longitudinal axis of the trunk.

Distributed model: Type of modeling approach in which all elements are modeled individually; *opp.* lumped model.

Dorsiflexion: Movement of the foot or toes upward; *opp.* plantar flexion.

Dose–response relationship: The direct association between the intensity and duration of exposure and the risk or degree of disease status.

Dot product: Manipulation of vectors in the same direction resulting in a purely scalar value.

Double crush syndrome: Multiple nerve entrapment, which may lead to multiple and/or conflicting symptoms.

Drag and drop: A mouse operation in which an icon the screen is moved and positioned in a new location.

Dupuytren's contracture: Formation of nodules in the palmar fascia, an extension of the tendon of the palmaris longus muscle, leading to permanent contracture of the ring and little fingers.

Dvorak: Type of keyboard layout in which the most commonly used keys are assigned to the strongest (middle) fingers; the home row has the sequence AOEIUDHTNS.

Dynamics: Biomechanical principles applied to a system of bodies in motion.

Eccentric: A dynamic muscle contraction in which the muscle is lengthening; *opp.* concentric.

Efferent: Direction of information flow, typically motor control, from the central nervous system to the periphery; *opp.* afferent.

Efficiency of electrical activity: A type of analysis for the slope of the EMG amplitude–force curve.

Elastic cartilage: Type of cartilage found in the ear and epiglottis of the throat.

Elastic region: Initial region of a stress–strain curve that is linear and repeatable.

Elasticity: A spring-like property of a material which enables it to recover from a deformation produced by an external force.

Elastin: Type of fiber providing elasticity to soft connective tissue.

Electrical impedance: The total resistance to electric current flow.

Electromyography: The recording and analysis of the electrical activity of muscles.

Endomysium: The inner layer of fascia that covers individual muscle fibers.

Energy: The capacity of a system to do work.

Enslaving: Involuntary force production by fingers not explicitly recruited in the grasp.

Enthesopathy: Specific form of tendinitis occurring at the tendon–bone interface.

Epidemiology: Branch of medicine that studies the distribution and control of epidemic diseases.

Epimysium: The outer layer of fascia covering muscle.

Epiphysis: The two enlarged rounded ends of a long bone.

Etiologic fraction: See *attribulable risk*.

Etiology: The study of the cause or development of a disease.

Eversion: Moving the sole of the foot outward; *opp.* inversion.

Excitatory post synaptic potentials: Excitatory inputs that depolarize a section of a motoneuron cell body making it easier to create an action potential.

Extension: Joint movement such that the included angle between the two limbs increases, for trunk or neck, bending backward; *opp.* flexion.

External force: Forces acting outside the body, e.g., weight held in hand.

Exteroreceptors: Receptors on the body surface that respond to an external sensation.

Extrafusal: With reference to the outside of the muscle spindle, typically regular muscle fibers; *opp.* intrafusal.

Extra-pyramidal tract: Indirect motor control pathway from the sensory cortex, passing through the basal ganglia, cerebellum, and brain stem, with slower processing than the pyramidal tract.

Extrinsic: Refers to a mechanism which originates outside the structure on which it acts; typically the finger muscles that are located in the forearm; *opp.* intrinsic.

Eye–ear line: Imaginary line passing through the outer corner of the eye-lid and the center of the auditory canal.

Face validity: Type of validity that refers to the content or format of a tool or test, which, on its face level, should measure what it is intended to measure.

Failure point: Point at which material loses its structural integrity.

Fascia: Soft connective tissue covering organs and muscles.

Fasciculi: A bundle of muscle fibers.

Feed-forward system: See *open-loop system*.

Feedback system: See *closed-loop system*.

Fenn-effect: See *heat of shortening*.

Fibrocartilage: Type of cartilage found in the intervertebral disks.

Fibromyalgia: Chronically painful and spastic muscles, with tingling sensations, may result in nervousness and sleeplessness; also termed fibrositis, also termed fibrositis.

Fibrositis: See *fibromyalgia*.

Final value theorem: Method for finding the final value of an output response.

Finkelstein's test: Test for DeQuervain's disease in which the patient wraps the fingers around the thumb and deviates the wrist in the ulnar direction, pain at the base of the thumb is a positive sign.

First-class lever: The fulcrum is located between the opposing forces, e.g., a playground teeter-totter.

First-order system: System whose transfer function has only one pole.

Fitts' law: Rule describing the movement time as a function of the difficulty of the movement.

Flexion: Joint movement such that the included angle between the two limbs decreases, for trunk or neck, bending forward; *opp.* extension.

Flexor digitorum profundus: One of the two major finger flexor muscles, the other being the flexor digitorum superficialis.

Flexor digitorum superficialis: One of the two major finger flexor muscles, the other being the flexor digitorum profundus.

Flexor retinaculum: The ligament which forms one surface of the carpal tunnel and acts to prevent bowstringing of the flexor tendons; also termed transverse carpal ligament.

Flower spray: Type of receptor found in the polar regions of the muscle spindle, sensitive only to change in length.

Focal dystonia: See *writer's cramp*.

Force: An action that cause bodies to be pushed or pulled in different directions.

Force ratio: The ratio of grip force to the tool-application force.

Frankfurt plane: Imaginary plane delineated by a line (in the sagittal plane) passing through the tragion and the lower ridge of the eye socket and roughly corresponds to horizontal when the head is held erect.

Free-body diagram: The isolation of a body or a part of the body such that it is in static equilibrium.

Frequency analysis: A type of signal analysis in which the phase relationship and the ratio of magnitudes of the output to the input are plotted against the frequency characteristics of the input signal.

Friction: The interaction between two surfaces when coming into contact as one slides over the other.

Frontal plane: Reference plane dividing the body into front and back halves, as observed face to face, *ant.* coronal plane.

Fulcrum: The pivot point in a lever system.

Fusiform: Spindle shaped, tapering at both ends, usually in reference to muscle spindles.

Fusiform muscles: Muscles whose fibers lie parallel to the long axis.

Gain: The ratio of the output signal to the input signal in a system.

Ganglionic cysts: Nodules of synovial fluid that form under the skin of the hand as a by-product of tenosynovitis.

Gleno-humeral joint: Strictly the shoulder joint, as opposed to the complete shoulder girdle.

Gold standard: The best measurement system that is currently available.

Golgi tendon organs: Receptors at the tendon–muscle junction that respond to tension.

Gray matter: The central H-shaped darker region of the spinal cord containing moto-neuron cell bodies.

Guyon canal syndrome: Entrapment of the ulnar nerve at Guyon's canal on the medial side of the hand, leading to tingling and numbness of the little and ring fingers.

Hamate: The hook shaped wrist bone in the distal row.

Hand–arm vibration syndrome: Tingling, numbness, and loss of fine control due to ischemia of the blood supply to nerves and muscles of the hand; from power tool vibrations, cold temperatures, or direct pressure; *syn.* white-finger syndrome.

Haversian canal system: Internal structure of bone formation with repeated layers of collagen fibers and hydroxy apatite crystals.

Hawthorne effect: A phenomenon in which employee-perceived interest by the employer may result in increased productivity; however, more generally, it applies to the difficulty in teasing apart confounded variables in an uncontrolled study, as happened in the original study at the Western Electric Hawthorne Works plant.

Heat of shortening: Heat in muscle tissue due to the act of shortening as opposed to a simple isometric contraction; also termed the Fenn effect.

Heavy meromyosin: The head subunit of the myosin molecule which acts the rotational bridge between the thick and thin filaments.

Hick–Hyman law: Rule that choice-reaction time is linearly related to the amount of information presented.

Hovering behavior: Gripping the mouse without using it.

Hyaline cartilage: Type of cartilage covering articular bony surfaces.

Hydrodynamic lubrication: Type of joint lubrication in which translational joint motion creates a wedge effect, forcing synovial fluid between the articular surfaces.

Hydrolysis: The splitting of a molecules into two with the use of water.

Hydrophilic: Water loving or allowing water molecules to adhere to the surface.

Hydrostatic lubrication: Type of joint lubrication in which loading of the joint forces synovial fluid out of the pores of the cartilage, into the space between the articular surfaces.

Hydroxy apatite: A crystalline structure of calcium forming the ground substance within bone.

Hypothenar: Muscle group located at the base and acting on the little finger.

Hypothenar hammer syndrome: Compression of the ulnar artery against the hypothenar eminence during hand hammering.

Hysteresis: A measurement error in which the current value depends both on the present condition as well as past conditions.

Iatrogenesis: An argument, that some disorders may result from the course of the professional activities of a physician, such as autosuggestion from discussions, examinations, or treatments.

Impulse response: The output obtained by using a unit impulse function for the input, useful in characterizing a transfer function.

In vitro: Muscle preparation maintained in a glass container; *opp.* in vivo.

In vivo: Muscle preparation maintained within a living body; *opp.* in vitro.

Incidence rate: The degree of new cases of disease with respect to exposure time.

Index of difficulty: The amount of information found in a movement, defined as a function of the distance of movement and target size.

Information theory: Theory in which the coding and content of messages can be quantified, typically in bits.

Inhibitory post synaptic potentials: Inhibitory inputs that hyperpolarize a section of a motoneuron cell body, making it more difficult to create an action potential.

Initial heat: The combined effect of activation heat and heat of shortening.

Initial value theorem: Method for finding the initial value of an output response.

Innervation ratio: The ratio of muscle fibers to motor neurons, a measure of motor control.

Insertion: Muscle attachment to a bone that is furthest from the midline of the trunk.

Integrated: An outdated type of EMG processing in which the raw signal is charged through a capacitor; now typically used in reference to a smoothed signal.

Internal forces: Forces acting inside the body, e.g., muscular forces.

Interphalangeal: Refers to the joints between the phalanges.

Intervention studies: Type of epidemiological study in which the factor of interest is directly manipulated.

Intraclass correlation: An estimate of a test's reliability for more than two analysts, based on analysis of variance of the analysts' scores.

Intrafusal: With reference to the inside of a muscle spindle, typically intrafusal muscle fibers; *opp.* extrafusal.

Intrinsic: Refers to a mechanism which is located in the structure on which it acts; typically, the finger muscles that are located in the hand; *opp.* extrinsic.

Invasive: Procedure which breaks the skin; for electromyography, using needle electrodes within the muscle.

Inversion: Bringing the sole of the foot inward; *opp.* eversion.

Ischemia: Lack of blood flow.

Ischemic ulcers: Inflammation and lesions on the surface of the buttocks due loss of blood flow from direct pressure of seating for extended periods of time; more typically found in patients with limited mobility.

Ischial tuberosities: The major weight-bearing areas of the buttocks; *syn.* sit bones.

Isoinertial: A dynamic muscle contraction in which the muscle contracts at a constant acceleration.

Isokinetic: A dynamic muscle contraction in which the muscle contracts at a constant velocity.

Isometric: Type of muscle contraction in which force production is achieved without changes in muscle length; also static contraction.

Isometric experiment: Experiment in which a muscle is contracted isometrically, i.e., with both ends rigidly fixed so that it cannot shorten.

Isotonic: A dynamic muscle contraction in which the muscle force remains constant.

Isotropic: Material whose properties are independent of the direction of applied forces; *opp.* anisotropic.

Joysticks: A lever type computer input control device with two degrees of freedom, either proportional to displacement or proportional to force.

Kappa statistic: An estimate of a test's reliability based on the proportion of agreement observed between analysts but corrected for the proportion of agreement expected by chance.

Kinematics: Type of dynamics in which only pure motion, displacement, velocities, and acceleration are studied.

Kinetic energy: Capacity of a body to do work associated with linear displacement of the body.

Kinetics: Type of dynamics in which the forces that produce a motion are studied in addition to the motion itself.

Kyphosis: Distinctive posterior convex curvature of the spinal column in thoracic area; *opp.* lordosis.

Lactic acid: Breakdown product of anaerobic metabolism, typically associated with fatigue.

Lamellar bone: Bone layers formed through repeated deposits of collagen fibers and hydroxy apatite crystals.

Laptop computers: Small, portable computers that can be operated when placed in the lap.

Latency period: Delay in the rise of muscle tension due to conduction delays.

Lateral: Reference direction, further away from the midline of the body; *opp.* medial.

Lateral epicondylitis: Inflammation at the tendon insertion on the lateral epicondyle of the humerus, resulting from forceful, twisting motions, also referred to as *tennis elbow*.

Law of acceleration: Newton's second law: the acceleration of a body is proportional to the unbalanced force acting upon it and inversely proportional to the mass of the body.

Law of conservation of mechanical energy: Law of physics stating that energy cannot be created or destroyed, but can only be transformed, i.e., the sum of the various forms will always be constant for any condition of the system.

Law of inertia: Newton's first law: a body remains at rest or in constant-velocity motion until acted upon by an external unbalanced force.

Law of reaction: Newton's third law: for every action there is an equal and opposite reaction.

Lever system: A system of opposing forces acting around a pivot point such that they are in static equilibrium.

Liability: The obligation to provide compensation for damages or injury.

Ligament: Connective tissue attaching bone to bone.

Light meromyosin: The tail subunit of the myosin molecule which serves to bind the long molecules together into a tight filament.

Light pen: Special stylus linked to the computer that senses the electron scanning beam at a particular location on the screen allowing for direct manipulation of the screen.

Logistic function: Function used for fitting dependent variable with binary values, also termed logit function.

Logit function: See *logistic function*.

Long bones: Bones found in the extremities, i.e., the femur, the humerus.

Longitudinal study: See *prospective study*.

Lordosis: Distinctive anterior convex curvature of the spinal column in the cervical and lumbar areas; *opp.* kyphosis.

Lumbar spine: The portion of the spinal column consisting of the five vertebrae of the lower back, below belt level.

Lumped model: Type of modeling approach in which the elements are treated holistically rather than individually; *opp.* distributed model.

Lunate: The half-moon shaped wrist bone in the proximal row.

Magnitude: A scalar quantity that indicates the size of the push or pull action of a force.

Make force: The peak force needed to break the circuit and deactivate a key switch.

Make point: Point on keystroke travel at which a key switch is activated.

Matching: The selection of controls such that key characteristics are the same as for the exposed group of individuals.

Mechanical advantage: The ratio of the opposing forces in a lever system.

Medial: Reference direction, closer to the midline of the body; *opp.* lateral.

Metacarpal: Refers to the palm area; typically the bones that connect the fingers to the wrist.

Metacarpals: The bones forming the palm.

Metacarpophalangeal: Refers to the joint between the proximal phalange and the metacarpal bone.

Micropauses: Small rest pauses at irregular, spontaneous intervals.

Miniature end-plate potential: The depolarization occurring at the motor end plate, as an action potential travels from a neuron to the muscle fiber.

Minimum yield strength: The relative material strength at the yield point.

Mitochondria: Energy production unit in the cell.

Modulation index: The percentage of maximum pinch force utilized as the tool application force modulates between minimum and maximum values.

Moment: The tendency of a force to cause rotation about a point when the force is at a distance from the point of rotation, same as torque.

Moment of inertia: Quantity resisting rotation in a body.

Morbidity: The proportion of individuals within a population having some disease.

Motoneuron: An efferent neuron, with the cell body in the spinal cord, carrying information toward a muscle fiber; also motor neuron.

Motor redundancy: More degrees of freedom than constraints in motor control.

Motor unit: Functional unit of muscle, defined as one motor neuron and all of the muscle fibers innervated by collaterals of that motor neuron.

Mouse: A handheld computer input device with a roller ball in the base-to-control position and one or more buttons for other inputs.

Multipennate muscles: Muscles whose fibers are relatively short and lie in several different oblique directions.

Muscle spindles: Modified muscle fiber receptors that respond to changes in muscle length and velocity.

Myalgia: Simple muscle soreness or pain.

Myelin: Specialized fatty sheath covering an axons, forces an action potential to jump between gaps in the myelin, resulting in very high nerve conduction speeds.

Myofascial pain syndrome: Chronic muscle strain and myalgia.

Myofibrils: Subdivision of a muscle fiber that contains the ultimate contractile mechanism.

Myofilaments: The thick and thin protein filaments in a myofibril.

Myoglobin: Muscle protein that stores oxygen.

Myosin: The long protein molecules with heads comprising thick filaments within muscle.

Myositis: Inflammation of muscle tissue.

Myotendinitis: Inflammation of the muscle–tendon interface.

Natural frequency: The characteristic frequency at which a system tends to oscillate with minimal external input.

Negligence: The failure to exercise a reasonable amount of care in preventing injury.

Nerve gliding: Type of exercise which aims to slide the nerve through the carpal tunnel (or other narrow area) while minimizing strain.

Neuromuscular junction: The interconnection between a neuron and muscle cell.

Neuron: Nerve cell consisting of cell body and its dendrites, axon, and collaterals.

Nintendo thumb: See *DeQuervain's disease.*

Noninvasive: Procedures which do not break the skin; for electromyography, using surface electrodes on the surface of the skin over the belly of the muscle.

Normal line of sight: Line of sight assumed by a seated individual in a relaxed posture, roughly 15° (±15°) below horizontal.

Normal working area: Region of work surface defined by the area circumscribed by the forearm when it is moved in an arc pivoted at a fixed elbow.

Notebook computers: Small notebook-sized computers.

Nuclear bag: Intrafusal muscle fibers with swollen equatorial regions.

Nuclear chain: Intrafusal muscle fibers with no central swelling.

Nucleus: Cell unit containing genetic material.

Nucleus pulposus: The gel-like center of an intervertebral disk.

Odds ratio: The ratio of the odds of a particular exposure among with individuals with a specific disease to the corresponding odds of exposure among individuals without the disease of interest.

Onset latency: The time between nerve stimulation and the initial response detected at the active recording electrode; measures the fastest fibers.

Open-loop system: Type of system in which the command input is independent of the system output; *opp.* closed-loop system.

Open-loop transfer function: Simple representation of a system using only the plant, controller, and feedback element.

Opposition: Movement of the thumb to oppose the other digits, pulpy surface to pulpy surface.

Ordinate: The horizontal axis of a coordinate system, also termed the x-axis.

Origin: The point of intersection of the two axes of a coordinate system from which all points are defined; also the muscle attachment to a bone that is nearest the midline of the trunk.

Orthodromic: Nerve conduction along an axon in the normal direction. *Opp.* antidromic.

Orthosis: Device for correcting maladjustments, also simply termed a splint.

Ossification: Bone formation through repeated deposits of collagen fibers and hydroxy apatite crystals.

Osteoarthritis: Type of arthritis involving a degenerative process of joint cartilage.

Osteoblasts: Bone-forming cells.

Osteoclasts: Cells within bone that reabsorb bone structure.

Osteocytes: Bone cells which have become mineralized.

Overdamped: System response in which oscillations will die quickly out with time.

Pacinian corpuscles: Pressure-sensitive receptors found in loose connective tissues near joints.

Parallel elastic element: Spring-like element in Hill's muscle model representing the different types of fascia and membranes that are parallel to the muscle fibers.

Pareto analysis: An exploratory tool in which items of interest are identified and measured on a common scale and ordered in ascending order, creating a cumulative probability distribution; typically a minority (about 20%) of ranked items will account for a majority (about 80%) of total activity. *Syn.* 80–20 rule.

Partial fraction expansion: Method for finding the inverse Laplace by manipulating the fractional form of a transfer function.

Patellar reflex: A typical stretch reflex created by tapping just below the knee of a free-hanging leg, resulting in it jerking up.

Peak latency: Time between nerve stimulation and peak response detected at the active recording electrode.

Pearson product moment correlation coefficient: Type of correlation coefficient based on least square regression between two variables; the resulting correlation coefficient will range from 0 to ±1, with zero indicating no relationship, a +1 indicating a perfect relationship, and –1 indicating an inverse relationship.

Pennate muscles: Muscles whose fibers are arranged obliquely to the long axis, similar to the fibers in a birds feather; also termed unipennate.

Perimysium: The inner layer of fascia that subdivides bundles of muscle fibers into fasciculi.

Peritendinitis: Type of tendinitis with inflammation of only the tendon proper.

Personal digital assistants: Small handheld computers, typically operated with a stylus and touch screen.

Phalanges: The bones of the fingers.

Phalen's test: Test for carpal tunnel syndrome in which the patient holds the wrist in hyperflexion for 1 min., pain, tingling or numbness in the hand is a positive sign.

Pisiform: The pea-shaped wrist bone in the proximal row.

Plant: A simple transfer function or element that exerts control over the input in a system.

Plantar flexion: Movement of the foot downward; *opp.* dorsiflexion.

Plastic deformation region: Region of a stress–strain curve in which the material will not return to its original shape when unloaded.

Plausibility: The likelihood that an association between exposure and disease status is compatible with a physiological mechanism.

Point and click: A mouse operation in which the cursor is moved to a certain location and a command is executed with the activation of a mouse button.

Polar coordinate system: A two-dimensional coordinates system using an angle θ and a distance r, defined from the origin, to identify points.

Pole-zero diagram: A type of plot showing the poles and zeros of a system.

Poles: The roots of the denominator of a transfer function.

Posterior interosseous syndrome: Entrapment of the interosseous branch of the radial nerve within the supinator muscles of the forearm, resulting in a weakness in the extensor muscles for the wrist and little finger.

Posture targeting: Procedure for recording joint angle on a body diagram with target-like concentric circle arrangements.

Posturegram: System for evaluating posture by plotting the position and angle of each joint with respect to a reference level and independent of other joint positions.

Potential energy: Capacity of a body to do work associated with its position in the gravitational field.

Power grip: Type of grip in which partly flexed fingers and the palm, with an opposing thumb, forming a clamp around the object; intended for power rather than control.

Power spectrum: A plot of the ratio of the magnitudes of the output to the input signals for a given narrow frequency band, typically expressed in decibels.

Precision: The extent to which a measurement shows a small scatter or variance around the "true value"; *syn.* resolution.

Precision grip: Type of grip in which the object is pinched between the flexor aspects of the fingers and the opposing thumb; intended for optimal control rather than power.

Predictive validity: See *criterion validity*.

Predictive value: The ability of a test to predict future occurrences of the undesired state.

Pressure: A force distributed over an area rather than a single point of application.

Prevalence: The proportion of individuals in a given population that have the disease of interest.

Prevalence study: See *cross-sectional study*.

Primary endings: See *annulospiral*.

Principle of moments: Mechanics principle: the moments of the components must be equal to the moment of the whole body.

Pronation: Rotation of the forearm to the palm down position; *opp.* supination.

Pronator teres syndrome: Entrapment of the median nerve at the elbow due to the pronator teres muscle.

Proprioreceptors: Mechanoreceptors in the neuromuscular system needed for motor control, e.g., muscle spindles, Golgi tendon organs.

Prospective study: A cohort study in which the status of the disease state is followed after the start of the study; *syn.* longitudinal study.

Proteoglycan: A polysaccharide composed of hyaluronic acid, proteins, lipids, and water, forming the ground substance of soft connective tissue.

Protraction: Drawing the shoulder forward; *opp.* protraction.

Proximal: Referring to the portion of the body that is closest to the central longitudinal axis of the trunk.

Proximate causation: The direct, legal relationship between two events, the first of which results in an accident and/or injury.

Pyramidal tract: Direct motor control pathway from the sensory cortex to the spinal cord; *opp.* extra pyramidal tract.

Quick release: Type of muscle experiment in which the quick release of a stop mechanism exposes the muscle to a constant load.

QWERTY: The standard keyboard in which the sequence of the first six left-most keys in the third row up is QWERTY.

Radial deviation: Movement of the hand closer to radius bone in the forearm (toward the little finger); *opp.* ulnar deviation.

Radial tunnel syndrome: Compression of the radial nerve at the lateral epicondyle of the radius, resulting in tingling and numbness in the thumb.

Radius: One of the forearm bones, the other being the ulna.

Radius of gyration: The effective distance from the axis of rotation for which a point mass yields an equivalent moment of inertia to the complete body segment.

Ramp function: A function whole value increases linearly with time.

Rate coding: Theory for EMG signal increase, attributed the increase in frequency of neuronal firing.

Raynaud's syndrome: Constriction of the blood supply to the hand from cold temperatures.

Reaction torque: The torque that is transferred from the action of a power tool to the operator's arm due to the time lag in the operator releasing the trigger or due to the delay in the tool's shut-off mechanism.

Receiver operating characteristic: The plot of sensitivity as a function of (1-specificity), showing the power of test in discriminating cases from controls.

Reciprocal inhibition: Reflex in which antagonistic muscles are inhibited while the agonists are contracting.

Rectangular coordinate system: A coordinate system with perpendicular axes, same as Cartesian coordinate system.

Refractory period: The period of time during which the cell membrane potential returns to normal steady state and cannot be easily stimulated.

Reid's base line: Imaginary line passing through the center of the auditory canal and the lower ridge of the eye socket, corresponding roughly to the line created by the Frankfurt Plane in the sagittal plane.

Relative risk: See *risk ratio.*

Relaxation heat: Heat in muscle tissue observed after muscle contraction; also termed recovery heat.

Reliability: Refers to the consistency or stability of a measure, i.e., are multiple measurements in agreement.

Reliability coefficient: See *correlation coefficient.*

Residue approach: Method for finding the inverse Laplace by differentiating the fractional form of a transfer function.

Resolution: See *precision*.

Resting heat: Steady-state heat of muscle tissue due to simply being alive.

Resting length: Muscle length in a relaxed state, typically yielding maximum tension when contracted isometrically.

Reticulin: Bulk filler in soft connective tissue.

Retraction: Drawing the shoulders backward; *opp.* protraction.

Retrospective study: A cohort study in which the development of the disease state occurred before the start of the study.

Rheumatoid arthritis: Type of arthritis involving a generalized inflammatory process.

Right-hand rule: Procedure to identify the direction of a vector cross product, the fingers of the right hand. pointing in the direction of the first vector. are curled toward the second vector so as to cover the included angle between the two vectors, the extended thumb points in the resultant cross-product vector direction, which is perpendicular to both of the original vectors.

Risk ratio: The ratio of the risk of a particular disease occurring among exposed individuals divided by the corresponding risk among unexposed individuals; also termed relative risk, *syn.* relative risk.

Root locus: Analytical procedure for graphing the poles and zeros of the open-loop transfer function for determining system stability.

Root-mean-square (RMS) signal: An effective "average" value of a time varying signal, calculated as the square root of the of the average value of the signal squared over one cycle.

Roots: Solutions of a polynomial function such that the function equals to zero.

Rotational equilibrium: Condition in which the net moments about any point in the body due to the external forces are zero.

Rotator cuff tendinitis: Inflammation of tendons of various muscles around the shoulder caused from chronically raised or abducted arms.

RULA (rapid upper limb assessment): A posture-targeting procedure yielding a rudimentary musculoskeletal injury risk level.

Sacrum: The portion of the spinal column consisting of five fused vertebrae primarily within the pelvis.

Safety margin: The amount of grip force exceeding the minimum grip force required to avoid the object from slipping out of the hand.

Sagittal plane: Anatomical reference plane dividing the body into right and left halves, as observed from either the side of the body.

Sarcomere: Repeating unit within the myofibril, delineated by the z-disks.

Sarcoplasmic reticulum: Series of tubules and sacs surrounding the myofibrils from which calcium ions are released into the filaments.

Scaphoid: The boat-shaped wrist bone in the proximal row.

Second-class lever: A lever system in which the resistance force is located between the effort force and the fulcrum, resulting in a mechanical advantage greater than one.

Second-order system: System whose transfer function has two poles, typically used to represent the mass-spring-dashpot systems.

Secondary endings: See *flower spray*.

Sensitivity: The probability that an individual who actually has the disease will have a positive test result; or a test's ability to identify injurious jobs.

Series elastic element: Spring-like element in Hill's muscle model representing the tendon in series with muscle fibers.

Shear: Loading mode in which the load is applied perpendicular to the surface.

Shunt muscles: Muscle with the origin close to the joint and the insertion point far from the joint, creating a large moment arm and a relative stabilizing effect on the joint; *opp.* spurt muscles.

Signal-detection theory: A model for explaining the decision making process for an individual detecting a signal against background noise based on specific criteria provided; similarly applied to a test in diagnosing a disease.

Simple-reaction time: Time interval for an operator to respond to a single predetermined stimuli with a single predetermined response.

Sit–stand chairs: A fairly high chair or stool that allows the user to easily switch from a semi-sitting posture to a standing posture, allowing for postural mobility.

Size principle: Specific pattern of motor unit recruitment by the size of the neuron, starting with the smallest slow twitch units and ending with the largest fast twitch units.

Sliding-filament theory: Theory of muscle contraction in which the myofilaments slide over one another.

Slip reflex: The reflexive increase in pinch force which occurs approximately 75 ms after the onset of slip between the fingertips and the object being held.

Smoothed-rectified signal: Type of EMG processing in which the raw signal is first rectified to all positive values, and then smoothed with a resistor-capacitor circuit to eliminate large spikes.

Spearman–Brown prophecy formula: Method for computing the reliability coefficient for a full test using the split-half procedure.

Specificity: The probability that an individual who does not have the disease will have a negative test result; or a test's ability to correctly identify safe jobs.

Spherical coordinate system: A coordinates system using distance r and two angles θ and φ to identify points from the origin.

Split-half procedure: A procedure for establishing the reliability of a test; two halves of the test are scored separately for each person and correlation coefficient is calculated for the two sets of scores; the reliability coefficient for the full test is computed using the Spearman–Brown prophecy formula.

Spurt muscles: Muscles that originate far from the joint of rotation but insert close to the joint, causing the limb to move very rapidly; *opp.* shunt muscles.

Squeeze-film lubrication: Type of joint lubrication in which fluid is squeezed out from the areas of high pressure to areas of lower pressure.

Stadiometry: Measurement of spinal shrinkage as an indirect assessment of extended spinal loading.

Standard anatomical position: Standard reference position of the upright human body with palms facing forward.

Static equilibrium: Result of Newton's first law such that bodies are at rest or in constant-velocity motion.

Statics: Biomechanical principles applied to a system of bodies at rest.

Stenosing tenosynovitis: Acute form of tenosynovitis with localized swelling, a narrowing of the sheath, and the formation of a nodule on the tendon, causing the tendon to be become temporarily entrapped as it attempts to slide through the sheath.

Stenosing tenosynovitis crepitans: Extreme form of tenosynovitis, in which the trapped tendon will crackle or crepitate as it is pulled from the entrapment.

Strain: Deformation of a material normalized to its initial length.

Strain index: An upper limb musculoskeletal injury risk assessment tool that rates six different occupational factors.

Strain retardation: The resulting strain response for a unit step input of stress, also termed creep.

Stratified sampling: An approach in which the population is divided into mutually exclusive strata with random sampling performed within each stratum.

Stress: Load applied per unit area.

Stress relaxation: The resulting stress response for a unit step input of strain.

Stress–strain curve: A plot of stress as a function of strain during compressive or tensile loading of a material.

Stretch receptors: Collectively the annulospiral and flower spray endings of a muscle spindle.

Stretch reflex: The contraction of a muscle following a sudden stretch.

Striated muscle: Another term for skeletal muscle because of the striated appearance from the various bands.

Strict liability: Higher level of liability, in which the plaintiff need not prove negligence or fault.

Supination: Rotation of the forearm to the palm up position; *opp.* pronation.

Surveillance: Ongoing observation of a population in order to detect changes in the occurrence of a disease.

Survivor bias: The tendency for workers who are resistant to injury to stay on high-exposure jobs, leading to skewed sampling results.

Symptom survey: Questionnaire to assess the extent of medical problems.

Synapse: The specific gap between a neuron and muscle cell.

Synovia: Membranes lining joints and tendons which secrete the low-friction synovial fluid for lubrication.

Tangential force: Force acting at the center of mass of the body, perpendicular to the radius of rotation.

Tarsal: Referring to the instep of the foot.

Temporal contiguity: The timeliness of the precedence of an exposure with respect to the disease.

Temporality: The fact that the exposure precedes the disease in time.

Tendinitis: Inflammation of the tendon, typically due to chronic overuse.

Tendon: Connective tissue attaching muscle to bone.

Tennis elbow: See *lateral epicondylitis*.

Tenosynovitis: Inflammation of the tendon and its sheath and the tendon, typically due to chronic overuse.

Tension: Loading mode in which the load is applied axially away from the surface, stretching the material.

Tension-neck syndrome: A type of myofascial syndrome characterized by pain and tenderness in the shoulder and neck region, characteristic of clerical workers and small-parts assemblers, who have contracted the upper back and neck muscles in hunched forward postures for better visibility.

Tented: Term used for a keyboard split in the middle and laterally tilted down.

Test–retest reliability: Measurement of the consistency or agreement of measurements with intervening time intervals.

Tetanic frequency: The minimum frequency at which the state of tetanus can be achieved.

Tetanus: Series of muscle contractions, in which the summation of individual contractions attains a steady level of force higher than the individual contractions.

Thenar: Muscle group located at the base and acting on the thumb.

Thermocouple: A very sensitive temperature gage using two dissimilar metals, which, when connected, create an electrical potential proportional to the surrounding temperature.

Thermoelastic heat: Heat gained or lost when a material is forcibly stretched or contracted.

Third-class lever: A lever system in which the effort force is located between the fulcrum and the resistance force, resulting in a mechanical advantage less than one.

Thoracic outlet syndrome: Entrapment of the brachial plexus in one or more shoulder sites: the scalenus muscles in the neck, between the clavicle and first rib and between the chest wall and the pectoralis minor muscle, resulting in numbness or tingling in the arm and hand.

Thoracic spine: The portion of the spinal column consisting of the 12 vertebrae of the upper back.

Tide mark: Boundary between calcified cartilage and bone.

Time constant: The time required for a function to fall to 36.8% ($= e^{-1}$) of its initial value or rise to 63.2% ($= 1 - e^{-1}$) of its final value.

Tinel's test: Test for carpal tunnel syndrome in which the median nerve at the wrist is tapped, pain, tingling, or numbness in the hand is a positive sign.

Torque: The tendency of a force to cause rotation about a point when the force is at a distance from the point of rotation, same as moment.

Touch pad: A computer input device located on keyboard that performs similarly to a digitizing tablet but without the special stylus, i.e., direct touch with a finger tip manipulates the cursor.

Touch screen: Type of display using a touch-sensitive overlay for direct manipulation of the screen.

Trabeculae: The three-dimensional lattice-like structure of fibers in bone, serves to better distribute stress.

Track point: A force joystick.

Track stick: A displacement joystick.

Trackball: A computer input device similar to an upside-down mouse, the rotary displacement of the ball being converted to cursor position.

Tragion: The notch above the piece cartilage that is just anterior to the auditory passage.

Transfer function: An operator that acts on an input function and transforms it into an output function.

Translational equilibrium: Condition in which the net forces on a body are zero.

Transverse carpal ligament: See *flexor retinaculum*.

Transverse plane: Anatomical reference plane parallel to the ground, as observed directly above the head.

Trapezium: A four-sided wrist bone in the distal row.

Trapezoid: A four-sided wrist bone (with two sides parallel) in the distal row.

Tremor: Involuntary physiological oscillations of a limb, that are smaller than volitional motions.

Trigger finger: Stenosing tenosynovitis of the index finger, typically from repeated, forceful activations of a power tool.

Trigger points: Small areas of spastic muscle that are tender to touch.

Triquetrum: The triangle-shaped wrist bone in the proximal row.

Tropomyosin: Thin-filament protein which serves to link globular actin molecules together in chain.

Troponin: Thin-filament protein which acts as an inhibitor of the cross bridging.

Two-point discrimination test: Test for nerve impairment in which individuals are pricked with either one pin or two pins simultaneously, a positive sign is when they cannot distinguish two pricks separated by at least 5 mm.

Ulna: One of the forearm bones, the other being the radius.

Ulnar deviation: Movement of the hand closer to the ulna in the forearm (toward the thumb); *opp.* radial deviation.

Ultimate tensile strength: Material strength at the failure point.

Undamped: System response for a damping ratio of zero in which the system will oscillate at steady state.

Underdamped: System response in which oscillations will die out with time.

Unipennate: See *pennate*.

Unipolar: Type of electromyographical recording in which one active electrode is attached over the belly of the muscle to obtain the largest signal possible from the greatest number of motor units.

Unit impulse: A function in the form of a pulse whose magnitude approaches infinite height as the width of the pulse approaches zero with an area remaining constant and equal to one.

Unit-membrane theory: Theory in which the cell membrane is modeled as a protein and phospholipid bilayer structure covered with mucopolysaccharide surface.

Unit-step function: A function of value zero for time less than zero and value one for time greater than or equal to zero.

Validity: The appropriateness, meaningfulness, and usefulness of a tool or survey to measure what it is supposed to measure.

Vector: The combination of a magnitude and direction into one quantity.

Viscoelastic theory: An approach in which a material and its properties can be modeled using of springs and dashpots.

Viscosity: A dashpot-like property of a material of a material or fluid that resists the force tending to make it flow.

Visual analogue scale: Method for indicating the degree of perceived pain by putting a mark on a line, such that the distance indicated is comparable to the pain experienced.

Wald statistic: Ratio of regression coefficient to its standard error, used in evaluating the significance of the coefficient.

White-finger syndrome: The blanching of skin due to ischemia of the blood supply from hand–arm vibration syndrome or Raynaud's syndrome.

White matter: The lighter outer region of the spinal cord containing the myelin sheaths and axons of descending neuronal tracts.

Wolff's law: "Form follows function" with reference to the trabeculae structure bone adapting to external stress.

Work-space envelope: The three-dimensional space within which an individual can work, typically defined by the spherical surface circumscribed by a function arm reach while pivoting about the shoulder.

Woven bone: The first layers of bone formation.

Writer's cramp: Excessive and repeated muscle contraction while holding a pen or pencil, also termed focal dystonia.

Yield point: Point on a stress–strain curve at which the material leaves the elastic region and enters the plastic deformation region.

Z-disks: Myofilament element holding the thin filaments together.

Zero drift: A measurement error in which the baseline tends to shift over time.

Zeroes: The roots of the numerator of a transfer function.

Author Index

Subject Index